# 4TH EDITION
# Pregnancy
# Childbirth
## and the
# Newborn
## THE COMPLETE GUIDE

Penny Simkin, PT
Janet Whalley, RN, IBCLC
Ann Keppler, RN, MN
Janelle Durham, MSW, ICCE, LCCE
April Bolding, PT, DPT, CD, CCE
of Parent Trust for Washington Children

 Meadowbrook Press
Distributed by Simon & Schuster
New York

Library of Congress Cataloging-in-Publication Data

Pregnancy, childbirth, and the newborn : the complete guide / by Penny
Simkin ... [et al.].
    p. cm.
  Includes index.
  ISBN 978-0-88166-531-4 (Meadowbrook) — ISBN 978-1-4391-7511-8 (Simon & Schuster)
  1. Pregnancy. 2. Childbirth. 3. Newborn infants—Care. I. Simkin,
Penny, 1938-
  RG525.S583 2010
  618.2—dc22
                        2010011641

Executive Editor: Megan McGinnis
Editor: Alicia Ester
Creative Director: Tamara JM Peterson
Production Manager: Paul Woods
Index: Beverlee Day

Although the authors and publisher have made every effort to ensure that the information in this book is
accurate and current, only your caregiver knows you and your health history well enough to make specific
recommendations. The authors, editors, reviewers, and publisher disclaim any liability from the use of this book.

Published by
Meadowbrook Press
6110 Blue Circle Drive, Suite 237
Minnetonka, MN 55343

www.meadowbrookpress.com

BOOK TRADE DISTRIBUTION by
Simon and Schuster, a division of Simon and Schuster, Inc.
1230 Avenue of the Americas
New York, NY 10020

15  14  13  12         15  14  13  12  11  10  9  8  7  6  5

Printed in the United States of America

# Praise for
## *Pregnancy, Childbirth, and the Newborn*

Women who use this book to prepare themselves for labor
will be leagues ahead of women who don't, and ahead of most
of the professionals who take care of women during labor.

—Judith Rooks, CNM; author of *Midwifery in America*

"The single best book for understanding pregnancy and birth."

—Carol Jones, CNM; Director of Midwifery, Virginia Mason Clinic, Seattle, WA

"This book is authoritative without feeling overwhelming. It keeps
the woman and her family in focus and provides a range of options.
If expectant parents could have one book, this would be the one."

—Trish Booth, MA, LCCE, FACCE; childbirth education consultant, Manlius, NY

"A truly wonderful book for expectant families. It's informative, thorough,
and helpful. We give it to all our patients, and they think it's great, too!"

—Carolyn Kline, MD, MPH; perinatologist, Eastside Maternal Fetal Medicine, Kirkland and Bellevue, WA

"The material is beautifully organized and the presentation is crystal clear."

—Sheila Kitzinger, author of *The Complete Book of Pregnancy and Childbirth*

"For the most part, pregnancy books are written for and read by women,
but if you're a caring father (or father-to-be), this is an outstanding book.
It gives the fairest and most complete descriptions of the myriad medical
options available during childbirth. It is the best of the many books available."

—Tom Seager, father of three, Potsdam, NY

# Dedication

To our husbands:

Peter Simkin, Doug Whalley,
Jerry Keppler, Peter Durham, and Tim Hunt.


To our children and their families:

Andy, Bess, Freddy, Charlie, and Eva Rose Simkin;
Linny Simkin and Jeff, Peter, and Callie Jobson;
Mary Simkin-Maass and Greg, Sara Jane, and Amelia Maass;
Elizabeth Simkin, Nick Boyar, and Cole Simkin-Boyar.

Scott, Heidi, Kate, and Adelyn Whalley; Mike Whalley;
Kristin, Max, and Tyler Rose; Brian Platt.

Eric, Courtney, Lucas, and Noah Keppler; Heidi Keppler.

Amelia and Izzi Durham.

Lily and Maya Rose Bolding Hunt.


To the thousands of expectant and new parents whom
we have taught and who have taught us so much.

And to the Great Starts Program of Parent Trust for Washington
Children, which since 1950 has educated, supported, and
encouraged families in their transitions to parenthood.

# Contents

# Acknowledgments

This book, originally conceived as a class manual called *Becoming Parents*, was first published by the Childbirth Education Association of Seattle (CEAS) in 1976. Gillian Mitchell, Penny Simkin, Janet Whalley, and Ann Keppler wrote and edited it. In 1984, Meadowbrook Press published the first edition of *Pregnancy, Childbirth, and the Newborn* (an extensive revision of the original book) with the help of editor Tom Grady. The second edition was published in 1991 with the help of editor Kerstin Gorham. The third edition was published in 2001, with the help of editors Joseph Gredler, Nancy Campbell, and Christine Zuchora-Walske. Editors Megan McGinnis and Alicia Ester helped with the publication of the fourth edition.

Many other people have helped with the creation of this latest edition. We are grateful to:

- The fabulous Great Starts instructors, who provided suggestions for revisions, input on content, recommended resources, and more. And especially to Kim James, for always providing intriguing food for thought.
- The staff of Parent Trust for Washington Children, especially Jack Edgerton for his leadership, Linda McDaniels for cheerleading the project, and Michele Sonntag for running the Great Starts program so effectively that Janelle Durham could focus her attention on the book revision process.
- The Penny Simkin, Inc. staff of Candace Halverson, Tanya Baer, and Molly Kirkpatrick for their assistance and support.
- Professional consultants: Diana Koala, MD, and Michelle M. Grandy, RN, CNM.

We also wish to thank the following for their contributions to the artwork of this edition:

Illustrations: Ruth Ancheta and Shanna Alvarez; special thanks to Susan Spellman, for being so easy to work with on so many details of the illustrations.

Photographs: Carlos A. Arguelles; Charlotte R. Brown, Ineffable Images; Bob Cerelli; Sandra Coan; Jan Dowers; Sofia Zadra Goff; Sindea Horste; Samantha Kroop, Park Avenue Art; Willa Kveta; Spike Mafford; Katie McCollough; Medela; Marilyn Nolt; Elisha Rain; Stevens Hospital, Edmonds, WA; and Well-Rounded Maternity Center, Menomonee Falls, WI.

Models: Lisa Black Avolio; April Bolding; Heidi and Kate Whalley; Dina Apostlou with Kosta and Melina; Courtney, Eric, Noah, and Lucas Keppler; Michele Sonntag, Kathleen Porch, and the attendees of First Weeks in April 2010.

# Introduction

Although society, culture, and family life are in constant flux, our basic needs haven't changed. For survival, we'll always require food, drink, shelter, physical safety, emotional satisfaction, spiritual fulfillment, and love and support.

Similarly, while maternity care practices are continually changing the way women are helped to give birth, childbirth itself hasn't changed. How a woman's body functions during pregnancy, labor, birth, and the postpartum period—and what she needs during these times—hasn't changed since the beginning of humankind.

This fourth edition of *Pregnancy, Childbirth, and the Newborn: The Complete Guide* reflects maternity care in today's society, but it also promotes the fundamental truth that many aspects of pregnancy, childbirth, and the postpartum period remain unchanged. Our approach is to first describe those normal, healthy processes along with their typical variations and accompanying emotions; at the same time, we discuss the usual maternity care practices for monitoring them. We next describe comfort measures and self-help techniques for coping with labor, which you and your partner can master during pregnancy. We then cover possible complications and the care practices and procedures that may be needed to resolve them.

This edition presents revised and expanded discussions on:

- Maternity care and self-care, including the Three Rs (relaxation, rhythm, and ritual), a self-help approach to finding comfort in labor
- Your relationships with your baby, partner, parents and other relatives, friends and coworkers, and caregivers (physicians, midwives, nurses, doulas, and breastfeeding counselors)
- Informed decision-making (Maternity care is full of options, and you have the legal and moral right to choose the best ones for you.)
- Transitions from woman to mother, man to father, partner to parent, fetus to newborn, only child to big sister or brother

This book also includes revised discussions on nutrition and fitness during pregnancy, new information on complementary medicine methods such as acupuncture, new summaries of warning signs of complications, up-to-date research-based information on interventions during childbirth, revised statistics on cesarean birth and vaginal birth after cesarean (VBAC), plus much more.

If you're familiar with our previous editions of *Pregnancy, Childbirth, and the Newborn,* you'll notice that this edition has a completely new look, with more photos, illustrations, and boxed features that allow us to highlight important information.

Also included in this new design are fun and informative sidebars, such as "Common Q&A" about pregnancy, childbirth, and newborn care; "Two Views" (two first-person accounts) on these topics; "In Their Own Words," in which parents describe their pregnancy, childbirth, and parenting experiences from their points of view; "Fact or Fiction?" in which we present common misinformation and the facts; and helpful, timely "Advice from the Authors."

An exciting new feature for this edition is our web site, **http://www.PCNGuide.com**. Throughout the book, we refer to our web site whenever we have more to say about a topic or want to provide the most current information on changing health care practices and recommendations. By visiting our web site, you can learn up-to-date facts on medical interventions, medications, care procedures, and much more. You can also download a number of charts, work sheets, and forms to help you record important information during pregnancy, birth, and beyond.

With abundant information on pregnancy and maternity care available on the Internet and TV and in bookstores, you may wonder if there's a need for a book like *Pregnancy, Childbirth, and the Newborn*. Our resounding response is, "Yes, more than ever!" As expectant parents, you should have a portable, comprehensive, and unbiased source of factual information and sound advice. We hope the following chapters will give you the insight and wisdom you need to sift through all the other information you'll encounter and make the choices that are best for you and your family.

From the moment you learned of your pregnancy, you've undoubtedly had several questions and concerns. You also have strengths and weaknesses, hopes and dreams, and ideas about how to raise and care for your child. Although we don't know you personally, we have a pretty good idea of what you want and need to know. At the same time, we understand that you're an individual; "one size fits all" doesn't apply to maternity care or child care. Our intent is to supply you with accurate information and let you decide how best to use it.

It's our privilege to offer you guidance during this life-changing journey. Our cumulative years of experience working with women and their families total more than 130 years. We're constantly asking expectant and new parents what's helpful and what's not. Based on their answers, we're continuously adapting the way we teach, guide, and advise women, couples, and families. It's our wish that with the knowledge you gain from our collective wisdom gathered in these chapters, you'll have a safe, satisfying pregnancy and birth and a joyful introduction to parenting.

Penny Simkin, PT

Janet Whalley, RN, IBCLC

Ann Keppler, RN, MN

Janelle Durham, MSW, ICCE, LCCE

April Bolding, PT, DPT, CD, CCE

P.S. In recognition of the fact that babies do indeed come in two sexes, throughout the book we've alternated the use of masculine and feminine pronouns when referring to the baby. We've also used inclusive language to reflect various family configurations, including traditional mother-father-children families, single-parent families, blended families formed by second marriages, families with gay and lesbian parents, and families formed by open adoption or surrogate mothers.

# CHAPTER 1

# You're Having a Baby!

Having a baby presents some of life's greatest challenges and rewards. During pregnancy, childbirth, and your newborn's first weeks, you'll experience everything from wonder and joy to bewilderment and stress—often at the same time. You can be glad that pregnancy lasts around nine months so you have time to learn, plan, adjust, and prepare.

Day by day, your developing baby is becoming capable of thriving outside the protective environment of your body. You're becoming physically and emotionally ready to give birth, and your partner is learning how to support you during labor. Together, you'll prepare to meet your baby's needs.

This book provides reliable information and guidance for staying healthy, finding good prenatal care and support, learning about your options for maternity care, and making decisions that reflect your preferences and priorities. Your baby is getting ready to join your family, so let's turn the page and start preparing for his birth!

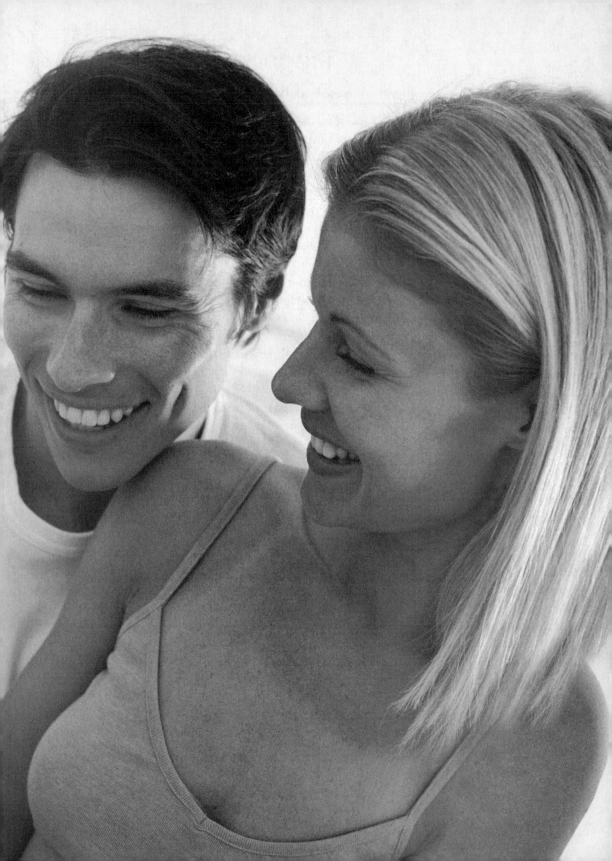

# Pregnancy: A Time for Change and Preparation

Like most expectant parents, you want a healthy pregnancy so you can provide a safe environment for your developing baby. Pregnancy is the time to assess your diet, fitness level, lifestyle, finances, and relationships—and make any necessary changes for optimal health. It's also the time to arrange for prenatal care and seek help to resolve or manage any medical problems or mental health challenges. Chapters 4 through 6 discuss ways to have the healthiest pregnancy possible for you and your baby.

Because pregnancy puts extra demands on your body, you may have questions about the health of your pregnancy. Chapter 3 describes common changes and concerns that can arise in pregnancy and what you can do to address them, and Chapter 19 discusses what changes you can expect if this pregnancy isn't your first. During pregnancy, you'll also discover that you want to talk with other pregnant women, expectant partners, and new parents so you can learn from their experiences and benefit from their support. Use this time to draw upon or develop a support system that can help you long after your baby is born.

Looking ahead to the birth, you may wonder how you'll manage labor. Will you want to use medications to reduce or eliminate pain? Will you want a natural, drug-free birth? What kind of support will you want your partner to provide? Pregnancy is the time to prepare for how you'll cope with childbirth; reading this book is a good place to start, and taking childbirth preparation classes will enhance your knowledge of your options. Chapters 9 and 12 describe when and how labor begins and what childbirth is really like, while Chapters 10 and 11 provide information on the various medications and non-medicated options for managing labor pain.

Just as most pregnancies are normal, so are most labors and births. However, just as problems can arise in pregnancy, complications can develop during childbirth, and medical interventions may become necessary for the health of the mother and baby. If your pregnancy, labor, or birth becomes complicated, it's helpful to be aware of the possible problems and potential solutions. Chapters 7, 13, and 14 describe pregnancy and childbirth complications and the options for treatment, including cesarean birth.

As you anticipate parenthood, questions and deep feelings may come up about your childhood, and about your parents' relationships with each other and with you. Your partner may have the same experience. Pregnancy is a good time to strengthen bonds, mend fences, or clarify boundaries with your parents so you can enter parenthood on your own terms.

You and your partner may also spend a lot of time thinking about the amazing responsibility of physically, emotionally, and spiritually nurturing a child. Pregnancy is a good time for you and your partner to explore your expectations of parenthood and develop the qualities essential for parenting, perhaps by taking parenting classes, reading parenting books, or speaking to friends and relatives about their parenting experiences.

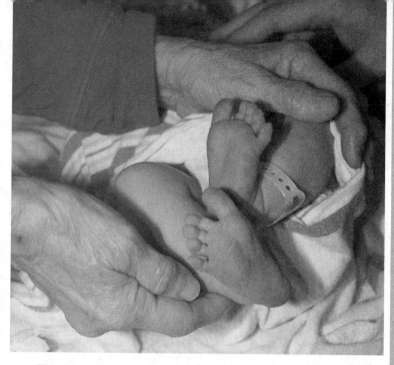

# Birth as a Long-term Memory

## Your Mother's Memories of Giving Birth

Ask your mother to tell you her story of giving birth to you, and have your partner do the same with his or her mother. What does your mother remember about going into labor? What did your father do? What did her caregivers do and say? What did she feel when she first saw you and held you? How does your mother feel now about your birth? Unless she was heavily drugged during labor, she'll probably have clear and detailed memories, and the intensity of her emotions as she recalls them may surprise you.

Research shows that women vividly recall their birth experiences for many years.[1] After you give birth to your baby, you'll remember the major facts of the experience, such as how long you were in labor, the time of her birth, and her birth weight. But you'll also remember other details such as how you knew you were in labor, how you felt during contractions, what you did to relieve the pain, and how others comforted you and helped you cope. This information will make up your unique, unforgettable story of giving birth to your child.

Some women have positive, fulfilling, and empowering memories of giving birth. These women feel that they were treated with kindness and their priorities and preferences for care were respected—even if labor was long and complicated. Other women remember their birth experiences with shame, anger, remorse, or resignation. These women feel that they were disrespected, abandoned, or powerless during childbirth, and this negative treatment tarnished their memories of the experience.

No one has complete control over pregnancy and childbirth, but the decisions you make during pregnancy will affect your memory of your birth experience. By making decisions that will help you have a satisfying birth, you increase your chances of having good memories of the experience. (See page 30 for steps to improve your chances of having a satisfying birth experience.) Conversely, if you make decisions that will hinder your ability to have a satisfying birth—or if the decisions you make aren't respected—you increase your risk of having unhappy memories of the experience.

## Different Views on Childbirth

When asked to describe their childbirth experiences to their children, women gave a variety of responses. Here are a few examples:

*It was the best day of my life!*

*I have always felt I shortchanged you. I didn't welcome you the way you deserved.*

*After giving birth, I knew I could do anything!*

*Labor with you seemed to go on forever. But it didn't matter how tired I was or how hard it was: You were worth every minute!*

# Making Decisions for a Satisfying Pregnancy and Birth

Because pregnancy and birth are normally healthy processes and highly personal, emotionally significant experiences, you typically have more choices for care than you would for a medical condition that involves disease or injury. These choices include: where you have your baby, who your caregivers are, how educated you become about pregnancy and childbirth, who provides you companionship and support in labor, how you want to manage labor pain, and to what extent you want your caregivers to manage your care.

If you're surprised by the number of decisions you'll have to make during pregnancy, you may be overwhelmed by the staggering amount of information available to you on maternity care. Some resources provide sound, reliable advice (such as this book); others don't. Chapters 2 and 8 discuss how you can find and evaluate maternity care information so you can make decisions that are right for you and your family.

This book is based on the importance of your active participation in every aspect of your care. When you're well informed of your choices and can communicate your questions, needs, and preferences, you help ensure maximum safety for you and your baby, and enhance your satisfaction with the birth experience.

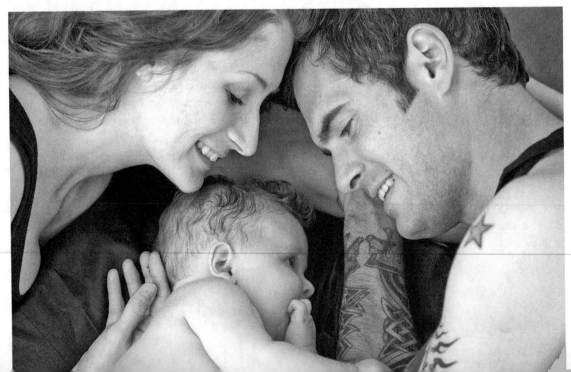

# More than the Birth of a Baby

Cultures around the world celebrate birth as a significant, joyous event marked by rituals of hope, promise, and new life. At the moment of birth, many lives are transformed. For you and your partner, your baby's birth marks your birth as parents. For your family, the birth creates their new roles as siblings, grandparents, aunts, uncles, and cousins.

When you meet your baby, you may feel that you've always known him—or you may be totally surprised by him. As you gaze at him and stroke, sniff, and snuggle him, you'll begin to fall in love as only parents and babies can. During the first few hours and days of your baby's life, you'll begin to fully appreciate the fact that this tiny person is the same mystery being you knew in the womb.

After the initial awe of new parenthood fades, you'll realize that your life has permanently changed and is more uncertain and less simple than it was before you became a parent. You may wonder how our species has ever survived when birth, breastfeeding, and baby care seem so challenging. A newborn's needs are almost constant and sometimes hard to understand. When your baby cries, you may ask yourself: "Is he hungry, wet, cold, sleepy, lonely, in pain? How do I soothe him, hold him, change him, bathe him, feed him? How do I know I'm doing a good job?" Chapters 17 and 18 describe the basics of baby care and feeding; your confidence will grow as you become more experienced with nurturing and nourishing your baby.

In the first few weeks of your newborn's life, you may have other worries, such as: "How can I get enough sleep? Can we afford a longer maternity leave? Will I ever have time to be romantic with my partner again? Will I ever *want* to be romantic again?" Chapters 15 and 16 describe what life is like for a new mother, and discuss concerns, doubts, and problems that can arise in the postpartum period and what you can do to address them.

After these early challenges, the rewards will start to come. Your baby will settle down when you cuddle him. He'll gain weight. He'll smile and coo. He'll stop crying when you sing to him. His sleeping pattern will become more predictable. He won't be able to take his eyes off you, and you won't be able to take your eyes off him. At that point, you'll realize that you wouldn't return to your prebaby life, even if you could.

The time spanning pregnancy, childbirth, and your newborn's first weeks will be an unforgettable experience, one that will have a lasting impact on your life. This book will help you discover that you already know how to grow your baby, give birth to him, and nourish and nurture him. Besides good health and good care, all you really need are confidence, support, and the practical skills and knowledge provided in the following chapters.

## *Key Points to Remember*

- Pregnancy is marked by physical and emotional changes, and it's a time to prepare for childbirth and parenthood.
- Birth is an unforgettable experience. You'll remember giving birth to your baby for years to come.
- The decisions you make for your care will have a great impact on you, your family, and your baby.
- The birth of your baby will have profound emotional significance, and your journey as a new parent will be one of wonder, doubt, and self-discovery.

# So Many Choices

After you discover that you're pregnant, you begin to make choices that will affect your entire childbearing experience. You choose how you'll gather information on pregnancy and birth. You select the kind of maternity care you'll want. You decide how you'll communicate your choices to your caregivers. Because these choices most affect you, your baby, and your family, it's important that you play a key role in the decision-making process. Your active participation now will give you satisfaction and fulfillment for years to come, because you'll feel that your wishes were honored with kindness and respect.

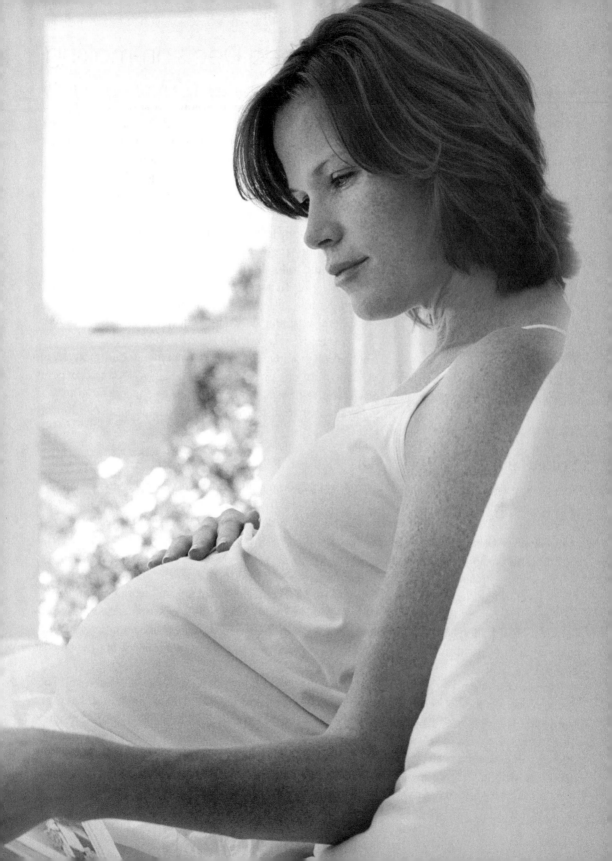

# Informed Decision-making

In the United States and Canada, it's your legal right to play a central role when making decisions that affect you and your baby. To help you make an *informed decision* (or *informed choice*) about a health care option or medical treatment (a procedure, test, intervention, or medication), you can consult with your caregiver and other knowledgeable medical professionals, as well as with supportive friends and family.

If you agree to an option or treatment after becoming informed about it, you've given your *informed consent*. By law, your caregivers can't give you medical treatment in either of the following cases:

- You're insufficiently informed about the treatment (and therefore can't give your informed consent).
- After becoming sufficiently informed about the treatment, you refuse it (*informed refusal*).

A more collaborative approach to making an informed decision is *shared decision-making*, in which you and your caregiver discuss the medical risks and benefits of treatment and any possible alternatives. You also discuss any questions or concerns you may have, as well as your priorities and preferences. Shared decision-making enhances trust and understanding between you and your caregiver.[1]

## YOUR CAREGIVER'S ROLE IN DECISION-MAKING

Your caregiver's approach to maternity care depends on training, experience, and general perception of pregnancy and birth. If your caregiver believes that the childbearing process is normal unless proven otherwise, he or she won't recommend medical interventions unless problems develop. If your caregiver believes the process is abnormal, he or she may recommend medical procedures and drugs to ensure a good outcome.

Sometimes, treatment is *routine*, which means it's offered to all pregnant women or newborns. Other times, it's designed for individuals and their current situations. Before recommending any treatment, your caregiver considers many factors, including your health; care standards set by professional organizations or government agencies; his or her personal experience and preferences for interventions, hospital routines, and policies; the usual care practices among his or her peers; cost; and staffing issues.

In addition, your caregiver considers whether treatment will achieve the desired results or create problems, then weighs the treatment's benefits against its risks. This *benefit-risk analysis* sometimes shows that a relatively risk-free option is the best treatment to achieve desired results. Other times, the analysis reveals that the best treatment is the one with the greatest risk of side effects. Some caregivers always choose the treatment that best achieves results, despite any risks that come with it. Others choose a less risky option first, even if its chances of success are low, then consider trying a more risky option if the first option is unsuccessful.

## Online Resources to Help You Make Informed Decisions

- Learn more about your maternity care choices at http://www.childbirthconnection.org.
- Learn more about mother-friendly hospitals at http://www.motherfriendly.org.
- Find a birth center at http://www.birthcenters.org/find-a-birth-center/.
- Find an obstetrician at http://www.acog.org/member-lookup/.
- Learn more about family physicians at http://familydoctor.org.
- Learn more about midwifery at http://cfmidwifery.org.
- Find a nurse-midwife at http://www.acnm.org/find.cfm.
- Find a licensed midwife or certified professional midwife at http://www.mana.org/memberlist.html and http://cfmidwifery.org/find/.
- Learn more about the midwifery and medical models of care at http://www.childbirthconnection.org.
- Find a childbirth educator at http://www.icea.org, http://www.lamaze.org, http://www.bradleybirth.com, or http://www.birthingfromwithin.com.
- Find a birth or postpartum doula at http://www.dona.org or http://www.doulamatch.net.

You may also visit the web sites of specific hospitals, birth centers, caregivers, doulas, and childbirth educators in your area.

### *What to Do If You and Your Caregiver Disagree about Treatment*

Almost all treatment carries some risks or disadvantages, but you and your caregiver may disagree on just how risky or disadvantageous a treatment is. For example, your caregiver may believe a medical procedure is safe and low-risk, but you may have a medical history that has made you uncomfortable with any procedure. Or you may have religious or cultural beliefs that guide you to seek alternatives to procedures.

If disagreement about treatment arises, you and your caregiver can usually settle it with respectful discussion and good communication—the foundation of shared decision-making.

But what if a disagreement can't be settled? Although rare, relationships between caregivers and pregnant women may fall apart because of a troubling mismatch in attitudes or opinions. When this happens, one person may feel bullied to change his or her wishes to match those of the other person. Or one person may believe that following the other person's wishes will cause harm.

When settling a disagreement is unlikely, in the United States and Canada a pregnant woman has the legal right (in most circumstances) to change to a different caregiver, and a caregiver has the right to discontinue care if there are other care options available to the pregnant woman. Given the limited time frame of pregnancy and labor, it's best to avoid this situation by carefully choosing your caregiver and birthplace (see pages 11–21). See page 20 for further information on changing caregivers.

## MAKING AN INFORMED DECISION

This chapter covers many of the important decisions you'll make during pregnancy, birth, and after the birth. You should make some decisions early in pregnancy (such as finding your caregiver); you can delay making other decisions until mid- to late-pregnancy (such as choosing your baby's caregiver). The following sections discuss topics that require you to make decisions, and they're presented roughly in the order that you should address them.

## Key Questions for Making an Informed Decision

When you're offered a test or treatment, first ask how urgent the situation is and whether you have time to ask questions, discuss options, and consider the information you've learned. Then, ask these key questions.

**Benefits:** What's the problem we're trying to identify, prevent, or fix? How's the test or procedure done? How likely is it to work?

**Risks:** What are the possible risks or side effects for my baby or me, and how are they handled? Are there other tradeoffs or disadvantages, such as additional procedures or precautions that will be necessary to maintain safety? What's the cost (if paying out of pocket)?

**Alternatives:** What other options are available? Are there other procedures that may work? Can I delay the treatment or choose not to do it? What are the risks and benefits of the alternatives and how effective are they? (Keep in mind that low-risk options are sometimes less effective, so ask for guidance when analyzing benefits against risks.)

**Next steps:** If the procedure identifies or solves the problem, what can we expect to happen afterward? If the procedure doesn't identify or solve the problem, what will we need to do next?

There's no universal agreement among either medical professionals or the general public on the safest, most satisfying ways to manage pregnancy and give birth, especially for a healthy woman having a normal pregnancy. Many types of maternity care are available, but not everyone has access to them. Use this chapter to help you investigate your choices and decide what kind of care best suits your needs, beliefs, and priorities.

Whenever you're asked to make a choice about your or your baby's health care, ask the key questions above to learn more about your options. Always remember that your caregiver can provide information about treatment and recommend options, but only you can decide what's best for you and your baby.

# Health Care Coverage

Having a baby can be expensive, and different kinds of maternity care have different costs. In the United States, a licensed midwife may charge as little as $2,500 for prenatal care and attendance at an uncomplicated home birth. Using a midwife for prenatal care and a birth center for the birth may cost $4,000 to $4,500. Using an obstetrician for prenatal care and having an uncomplicated vaginal birth in a hospital can cost more than $7,500. A complicated cesarean birth can increase that cost to more than $20,000.[2]

If you have private health insurance, find out which caregivers and birthplaces it fully or partially covers. Also find out the coverage for a hospital stay after a vaginal birth and after a cesarean birth. Learn whether the coverage includes complications (and to what extent) and whether it includes a follow-up visit for you and your baby within the first few days after the birth.

If you don't understand the extent of your coverage, contact an insurance company representative for clarification so you know what services you may have to pay for (partially or fully). Visit our web site, http://www.PCNGuide.com, to download a work sheet to track this information. That way, if you decide to have an uncovered or partially covered service, you'll know how much you'll pay out of pocket.

Some insurance plans cover—but don't directly pay for—such services as midwifery care, childbirth preparation classes, birth or postpartum doulas (see pages 23 and 26), home birth, and breastfeeding assistance. Instead, you pay for these services and your insurance company reimburses you. If you have such an insurance plan and use these services, ask the service providers how to submit your request for reimbursement.

You may also use a flexible spending account (FSA) to pay for uncovered or partially covered services. Health care FSAs are employer-established benefit plans that let employees set aside a portion of their salaries to pay for specified medical expenses. An added benefit of FSAs is that employees avoid paying income and Social Security taxes on contributions to the account.

Roughly 25 percent of people in the United States can't afford health insurance or don't work for employers who offer health insurance as a benefit. If you're in this situation, check with your local public health department about Medicaid coverage for maternity care to help cover your costs. If you qualify for assistance, be prepared to choose among only a limited number of caregivers and birthplaces. Because Medicaid doesn't reimburse caregivers and hospitals as fully as private insurance companies do, many caregivers accept only a limited number of Medicaid clients; others refuse to accept any.

If you live in Canada, tax revenues pay for all citizens' health care, including maternity care (except for out-of-hospital birth or midwifery care in some provinces—check your province's regulations).

## Consumer Reviews of Caregivers and Health Care Facilities

In 2008, the Coalition for Improving Maternity Services launched an online consumer survey that allows new mothers in the United States to share information about their experiences with their caregivers and health care facilities. The aim is to help improve transparency in maternity care practices. To see the continuously updated results of this feedback and view public health data about intervention rates at local hospitals, visit http://www.thebirthsurvey.com.

# Choosing a Birthplace

Ideally, the best place to give birth is somewhere you feel safe and comfortable. It should be somewhere you can get the help and expertise you want—not only for the birth, but also during pregnancy and after the birth. That birthplace may be a hospital, a birth center, or your home.

If you can, choose your birthplace before selecting your caregiver. That way, you can select a caregiver who attends births at the place you've chosen.

## BIRTHING IN A HOSPITAL

Most women in North America give birth in hospitals, and these institutions vary widely in the services they offer, their staff's attitudes toward patients, and their philosophies of care. Knowing the philosophy, policies, and services of each hospital you're considering helps you choose wisely. Depending on your health care coverage and where you live, you might or might not have a choice of hospitals. If you do, try to learn about several hospitals, take their tours, then choose the one that best suits your needs. If you don't have a choice of hospitals, you can at least learn what to expect when you give birth at the only available hospital.

Some hospitals provide only primary maternity care for women having normal, low-risk pregnancies. Other hospitals also have tertiary care, which offers intensive care, complete obstetrical and anesthetic services, a blood bank, 24-hour laboratory services, and a neonatal intensive care unit (NICU). If you have a difficult pregnancy or expect complications in labor or birth, you may need a hospital that provides tertiary care.

## In Their Own Words

Perhaps because my first birth was at a teaching and research hospital, I felt my care was "by the book." My partner liked that the providers performed every test and asked every question for the health and safety of my baby and me.

I gave birth to my second baby at a different hospital, and from start to finish, my caregivers were experienced women, most of them mothers. I felt empowered by the calm, efficient way they took care of business. The time after the birth was more peaceful than it was for my first birth, with many fewer interruptions by staff.

—*Anita*

When choosing a hospital, consider asking about its staffing policies for laboring women having low-risk pregnancies and for those having high-risk pregnancies. Hospital administrators know the value of having one nurse continuously attend to just one patient, but most don't guarantee pregnant women one-to-one nursing care throughout labor. Because of nursing-staff shortages, many hospitals must rely on nurses who work in several departments ("floating" nurses) and who might not have experience in maternity nursing. Some hospitals hire temporary "traveling" nurses, who may be unfamiliar with the hospital's policies. Others use licensed practical nurses or nursing assistants, either of whom might have limited training and might not be legally allowed to perform some tasks.

Hospitals don't allow pregnant women to choose who administers anesthesia. If you want or need epidural anesthesia when laboring at the hospital, the anesthesia staff member who's on call administers it. This person may be a nurse anesthetist, an anesthesiologist, or a resident (physician-in-training). When considering a hospital, you can find out the credentials and experience of its anesthesia staff. You can also meet with a staff member to discuss anesthesia services, especially if you have fears or a physical condition that may make anesthesia problematic.

Many hospitals provide birthing rooms, where women labor, give birth, and stay with their families until they're discharged. Other hospitals have separate postpartum rooms, where mothers and babies stay after the birth until they go home. Rooms usually have a TV, a chair-bed for the father or partner, and bathtubs to use during labor and afterward. Some hospitals' maternity rooms are designed to look like hotel rooms, with emergency equipment hidden in cupboards or a closet.

Some hospitals try to honor pregnant women's wishes by offering flexible, individualized, and culturally sensitive care. To determine how "mother-friendly" a hospital is, visit http://www.mother friendly.org to view questions you can ask. These questions are based on the Coalition for Improving Maternity Services' "Ten Steps of Mother-Friendly Care."

Many hospitals have received the World Health Organization's Baby-Friendly award, designating that the institution adheres to practices that best support and promote breastfeeding. Visit http://www.babyfriendlyusa.org for the locations of "baby-friendly" hospitals.

To learn about a hospital's routines and policies, ask the questions on page 13 when touring the hospital and when seeing your caregiver. If you dislike a particular routine, your caregiver may be able to write orders that override it. (See also Chapter 8 for additional questions that may arise as you create your birth plan.)

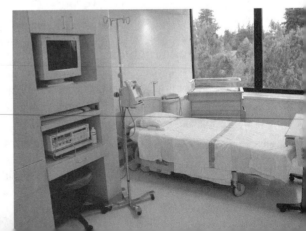

# Questions to Ask When Choosing a Hospital

Here are questions to ask your caregiver at a prenatal visit, a hospital representative, or the guide during the hospital tour. The answers will give you a good idea of what to expect when birthing at that hospital. Visit our web site, http://www.PCNGuide.com, to download a work sheet to record the answers. If the person can't answer your questions, find someone who can.

- What's the ratio of patients to nurses during early labor? Active labor? Birth? After the birth? Are these registered nurses or paraprofessionals (aides, practical nurses, or technical assistants)? Do you use floating or traveling nurses who aren't familiar with the hospital's policies?
- Do you encourage birth plans? (See Chapter 8.)
- What equipment do you use to monitor the baby's heart rate? Can I move around while being monitored? (See pages 252–253.)
- Do most laboring women have intravenous (IV) fluids? Do you allow women to eat and drink during labor?
- Is anesthesia available at all times? (See Chapter 10.)
- What non-drug methods of pain relief do you encourage?
- How many bathtubs do you have? How often do women use them to relieve labor pain? Do women give birth in the tubs? (See page 211 for more information on water births.)
- Who can be with me during labor? Do you welcome doulas?
- If I have a cesarean, how many people do you allow to attend?
- How long is the usual hospital stay after a vaginal birth? Cesarean birth?
- What usually happens to a baby immediately after birth? Will my baby go to the nursery or stay with me? May I hold my baby for the initial assessments? Who will examine my baby after birth? When?
- Do you have breastfeeding specialists on staff? May I call them after I go home?
- Do you offer any postpartum and newborn follow-up after I go home?

## *The Hospital Tour*

For many expectant parents, seeing where they'll give birth helps boost confidence and reduce uneasiness. For this reason, most hospitals offer tours of their maternity departments. To learn details about a tour, visit the hospital's web site or call the prenatal education department or labor-and-delivery unit. Tours typically involve a visit to the triage area (see page 249), a birthing room, a postpartum room (if separate from the birthing room), the nursery, and the family waiting area. Tours usually don't include the operating room where cesarean deliveries are performed. The tour guide discusses some usual routines and policies, gives practical advice (for example, which entrance to use in the middle of the night), and answers questions you may have.

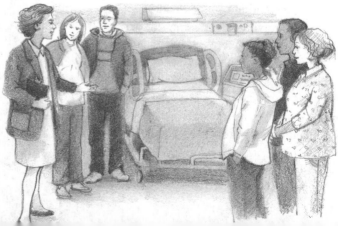

# BIRTHING OUTSIDE A HOSPITAL

In some areas of the United States and Canada, women with low-risk pregnancies have the option of giving birth with highly qualified midwives in a *freestanding birth center* (unaffiliated with a hospital) or at home. A woman who chooses this option prefers to give birth in a relaxed, low-tech, and cozy environment. She desires the continuous personal care of her caregiver during pregnancy, birth, and the postpartum period. During labor, she wants the freedom to move and act as she wishes, surrounding herself only with people of her choosing and permitting only essential interventions.

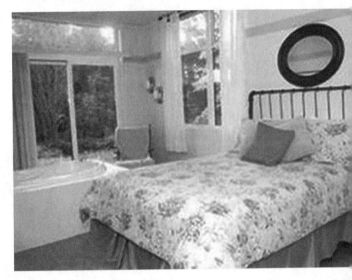

For women with low-risk pregnancies, good prenatal care, skilled caregivers, and hospital backup, planned out-of-hospital births are as safe for mothers and babies as planned hospital births—sometimes even safer.[3] Because planned out-of-hospital births are usually uncomplicated and normal, they require fewer routine interventions and less medical equipment. As a result, the cost of a birth-center birth or home birth is less than the cost of a hospital birth. Medicaid and many health insurance plans often cover the cost of out-of-hospital births. If a woman is transferred from a birth center or home to a hospital, however, insurance plans might not cover some costs resulting from the transfer.

You're a good candidate for out-of-hospital birth if you're physically and mentally healthy when you become pregnant and remain so throughout pregnancy. You also should have a well-trained, highly qualified midwife assess your and your baby's condition throughout pregnancy, screening for problems that make out-of-hospital birth unsafe.

Even after carefully screening women who intend to have an out-of-hospital birth, 15 to 25 percent of first-time mothers and 5 to 10 percent of second-time mothers are transferred to the hospital during labor or after the birth for problems judged to require medical intervention.[4] Almost all transfers

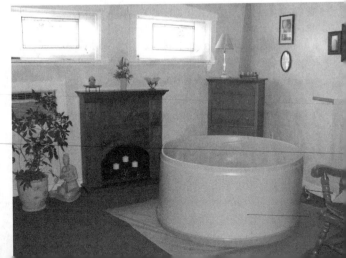

during labor (96 percent) are for non-emergencies such as prolonged labor, meconium in the amniotic fluid, prolonged ruptured membranes, or desire for pain medication.[5] In these situations, procedures or medications aren't immediately necessary for the welfare of the baby or mother.

For 3 to 4 percent of home births, urgent transfers to the hospital are necessary during labor.[6] In these cases, the women were screened and had uncomplicated, normal pregnancies, but a condition arises during labor that requires immediate medical action, such as cord prolapse, hemorrhage, or concerns about the baby's heart rate and oxygen supply. After a home birth, just over 1 percent of mothers and just under 1 percent of babies require a transfer to the hospital for reasons such as bleeding in the mother, retained placenta, and respiratory problems in the baby.[7]

Qualified midwives are trained for emergencies such as these. Their immediate response is similar to the first response of medical personnel in hospitals. To handle emergencies, midwives carry oxygen tanks, IV fluids, and suctioning devices, as well as medications to stop contractions temporarily, to stop bleeding, and to lower blood pressure. When further medical care is needed, they arrange for quick transfer to the hospital.

Although emergency transfers to the hospital are rare, they can be frightening and stressful. If you're considering an out-of-hospital birth, take this possibility into account and consider how far away your home or birth center is from the hospital. (See Chapters 13 and 16 for further discussion on problems that can arise during labor and after the birth and how they're treated in hospital and out-of-hospital settings.) Visit our web site, http://www.PCNGuide.com, to download a list of questions to ask your midwife and yourself about out-of-hospital birth.

# Choosing Your Caregiver

When you begin your search for a maternity caregiver, first ask yourself the following questions:

1. *What options do I have?*

    Learn what kinds of caregivers are available in your area, which ones your insurance covers, and which ones attend births at your chosen birthplace. Then, consult a trusted medical professional, local childbirth preparation group, or knowledgeable friend to further narrow your list.

2. *How does group care work? Who's in the group?*

    Most often when you choose a caregiver, you select a group of caregivers, not just one person. Your prenatal appointments may rotate among the group members, or you may see one or two caregivers throughout your pregnancy. The caregiver who attends your labor is the one on call at the time—and may be a stranger to you.

3. *What type of caregiver do I want? Does the sex of the caregiver matter to me? What approach to maternity care do I prefer?*

The following sections provide further information to help you answer these questions.

## TYPES OF MATERNITY CAREGIVERS

Different types of providers care for women during pregnancy, birth, and after the birth. Some have extensive medical training, while others acquire much of their knowledge through hands-on training.

When choosing a caregiver, it's important to consider the state of your health. A healthy pregnant woman can safely choose among any of the following types of caregivers. If your pregnancy is complicated or if your caregiver anticipates problems in labor, your safest option is most likely an obstetrician or perinatologist, either as the sole caregiver or as a consultant with a family physician or midwife.

For any caregiver, find out his or her educational background, credentials, training, and experience, especially if you're considering a caregiver whose practice is unregulated. Also learn about the caregiver's backup and referral arrangements, in case you need to transfer to a specialist during pregnancy or labor.

## Physicians

*Obstetricians/gynecologists (OB-GYNs)* have graduated from medical school or a school of osteopathic medicine. They've had three or more years of additional training in obstetrics (a surgical subspecialty focused on pregnancy, birth, and the postpartum period) and gynecology (medical and surgical treatment of diseases of women). Much of their education focuses on detection and treatment of problems. To qualify for board certification (which demonstrates an OB-GYN's exceptional expertise), they must pass an exam administered by the American College of Obstetricians and Gynecologists. In the United States, obstetricians provide most maternity care (85 percent), and pregnant women in Canada commonly use their services (although many choose to use those of family physicians).

*Perinatologists* are OB-GYNs who have received further training and certification in managing very high-risk pregnancies and births. They often consult with other physicians and midwives or accept referrals from them. These specialists practice only in major medical centers in urban areas.

*Family physicians* have graduated from medical school or a school of osteopathic medicine and have completed two or more years of additional training in family medicine, including maternity and pediatric care. Their education focuses on the health care needs of the entire family, which many expectant parents find appealing. They refer to specialists if their patients develop complications. To qualify for board certification, they must pass an exam administered by the American Academy of Family Physicians.

## Midwives

Midwives are the typical maternity caregivers in most countries and are becoming increasingly popular in the United States and parts of Canada.

*Certified nurse-midwives (CNMs)* have graduated from nursing school, passed an exam to become registered nurses, and completed one or more years of additional training in midwifery. Their education and practice are based on the Midwifery Model of Care (see page 18), which focuses on the needs of healthy women during the childbearing year. When compared to obstetricians, CNMs tend to spend more time in prenatal visits with their clients, individualizing their care; however, they refer clients to obstetricians if serious medical problems arise. To become certified, CNMs must pass an exam administered by the American College of Nurse-Midwives. They deliver babies in homes, hospitals, and birth centers.

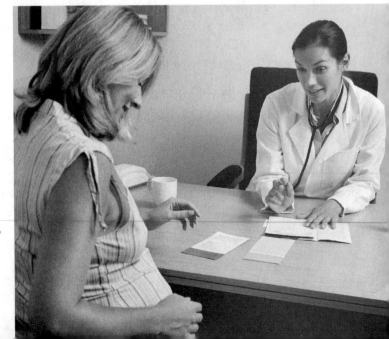

## Do Women Make Better Caregivers?

Some pregnant women believe they'll feel more comfortable with a female caregiver than with a male caregiver, because she can better understand and empathize about what happens to a woman during pregnancy and birth.

It's true that many female caregivers are sensitive, caring, understanding, and competent—but so are many male caregivers. Some caregivers, regardless of their sex, can be impersonal, rushed, and uninterested in you as an individual. Try not to choose a caregiver based on gender. Instead, focus on a caregiver's personal qualities, philosophy of care, and professional qualifications.

If you prefer a female caregiver for cultural, religious, or personal reasons, remember that many caregivers work in groups, and anyone from that group may attend your birth. Most physicians' groups include both men and women. Most midwives' groups are all women.

*Licensed midwives (LMs)* have completed up to three years of formal training according to their state's requirements. The focus of their education and style of care is based on the midwifery model, and is similar to that of CNMs, although a nursing background isn't required. They refer to obstetricians when medical problems arise. To become licensed, LMs must complete the educational requirements, attend a minimum number of births, and pass an exam administered by their state licensing board. Twenty-one states recognize LMs and offer these exams. Most LMs provide care only for women planning births in homes or birth centers.

*Certified professional midwives (CPMs)* have received training from a variety of sources, including apprenticeship, school, and self-study, and have been the primary attendant at twenty or more births. They practice outside hospitals and their care is similar to that of LMs. CPMs must pass an exam administered by the North American Registry of Midwives. Many LMs are also CPMs.

## Other Caregivers

*Advanced practice nurse practitioners* provide prenatal and postpartum care, although they don't attend women during labor. They often work with a group of physicians or midwives.

*Naturopathic doctors (NDs)* have completed three or four years of postgraduate training in natural medicine; some take an additional year of midwifery training to be able to provide prenatal care and attend births.

*Lay or empirical midwives* also provide care for pregnant women. Their qualifications and standards of care vary—some are well-trained and highly skilled; others aren't. Some are legally registered in their state or province, while others practice in states in which no laws regulate their practice. Some object to certification or licensure and have chosen to practice outside the law.

# Models of Care

## Midwifery Model of Care

This model of care is designed to maintain and enhance a woman's physiological and psychological resources for giving birth. It's based on these premises:

- Birth is a normal physiological process and an emotionally transformative experience.
- A woman's state of mind influences the labor process, so individualized care is necessary.
- Because a woman's participation contributes to a healthy pregnancy, labor, and birth, childbirth preparation is necessary.
- Low intervention and cesarean rates are desirable.
- Caregivers monitor the mother's and baby's well-being and provide education and support. If problems arise, they start with tools that cause the least intervention to regain a healthy physiological process.

## Medical Model of Care

This model of care is designed to replace or alter the body's own resources with medical and technological interventions. It's based on these premises:

- The natural childbirth process is unpredictable, unreliable, and potentially unsafe. Routine care protocols for all women give the caregiver a sense of control over the birth process.
- Medical interventions improve labor and birth.
- Cesareans are no less safe for the mother or baby than natural labor and vaginal birth; in fact, they may be safer.
- Caregivers use routine interventions before problems arise. If problems arise, they intervene quickly with the tool most likely to have the quickest effect.

## A Caregiver's Approach to Maternity Care

Education, training, peers' attitudes, and personal experiences influence a caregiver's approach to pregnancy and birth. A caregiver's philosophy of care typically follows either the midwifery model or the medical model (see above). Despite the names of these models, some physicians' practices resemble the midwifery model, and some midwives' practices lean more toward the medical model. Caregivers who follow the midwifery model treat pregnancy and birth as a normal family-centered event; they use medical interventions only when problems arise.

Caregivers who adhere to the medical model rely heavily on technology, interventions, or surgery, even when caring for a woman having a normal, healthy pregnancy. They frequently induce labor; prescribe medications and IV fluids; use continuous electronic fetal monitoring, vacuum extraction, or forceps; or perform an episiotomy or cesarean delivery. Some expectant couples may feel reassured with a caregiver who's prepared to intervene should a problem arise. But research shows that the routine use of technology and intervention isn't always safer for mothers and babies. In fact, this approach to maternity care sometimes causes side effects that lead to more medical problems. (See Chapter 13 for more information.)

Some caregivers (often those following the midwifery model) practice holistic care, focusing not only on the medical parts of pregnancy but also on a woman's emotional, spiritual, and physical well-being. If a caregiver doesn't provide holistic care, a woman can discuss non-medical problems with friends or relatives, other pregnant women, a childbirth educator, a doula, a birth counselor, or a psychotherapist.

When choosing a caregiver, find one who's qualified to provide the care that meets your health needs and whose approach to care appeals to you. You may learn about a caregiver's (or group's) approach to pregnancy and birth on his or her web site. Some midwife or physician groups have open "meet and greet" sessions in which you can talk with the caregivers in person. Others are glad to schedule a private consultation.

## Interviewing a Potential Caregiver

The initial interview can help you decide whether a potential caregiver inspires your confidence and trust. During an interview, you can learn whether a caregiver is open and comfortable with you, responds thoughtfully to your questions, and is happy to provide additional explanation upon request. If a caregiver seems impatient and defensive during the interview, it's likely you'll see that behavior in his or her care.

If you have a choice of caregivers, feel free to interview more than one, but schedule the appointments early. Appointments for many caregivers have long waiting periods, and it's easier to cancel appointments than to make them quickly. When scheduling an appointment, make it clear that it's only to learn more about the caregiver and his or her practice.

Because an interview typically lasts only ten to thirty minutes—and because most caregivers charge for office visits—you may want to first visit a caregiver's web site to learn about his or her qualifications and experience, fees, backup care when off duty, and birthplaces. (You may also learn this background information by calling the caregiver's office.) That way, during the interview you can focus on three or four essential questions to help you decide whether the caregiver is a good fit for you.

## Questions to Ask a Potential Caregiver

- Will I see you or another caregiver at each prenatal appointment? Does a nurse sometimes handle prenatal visits?
- Do the caregivers in your group share a similar philosophy of care? What are the chances you'll attend my birth? Do you think it's a good idea to induce labor so I'll give birth when you're on call? Will your colleagues respect the birth plan I've made with you? Will the hospital staff?
- Do you recommend childbirth preparation classes? Doulas? Birth plans?
- What do you think of trying for natural childbirth and how do you support this approach? Do you use non-drug ways to relieve labor pain and avoid routine interventions if possible? How many of your clients attempt natural childbirth? How many succeed?
- How often do you use interventions such as labor induction, IV fluids, artificial rupture of membranes, continuous electronic fetal monitoring, episiotomy, forceps, and vacuum extraction?
- How often do you find it necessary to perform an unplanned cesarean birth with a first-time mother having a low-risk pregnancy? How many of your clients—low- and high-risk—have a cesarean? What can I do to help reduce the likelihood of needing a cesarean?
- If I develop complications during pregnancy or labor, will you manage my care or will you refer me to another caregiver? Who is that person?
- When and how often will I see you for checkups after the birth?

If you're taking medications or have a medical or mental health problem, disclose that information to the caregiver during the interview. It may affect the care he or she can provide you.

To prepare for the interview, read the questions on page 19 and become as knowledgeable about them as possible so you can better judge the caregiver's answers. Visit our web site, http://www.PCNGuide.com, to download a work sheet to record the caregiver's responses at the interview.

If you're concerned about whether the caregiver will respect your legal right to informed consent and refusal (see page 8), visit http://www.solaceformothers.org/tools/Informed_with_notes.pdf for a list of questions that you may want to ask.

## CHANGING CAREGIVERS IF YOU'RE DISSATISFIED WITH YOUR CARE

To have a satisfying birth experience, it's essential that you feel comfortable with your caregiver. You need to feel you can trust your caregiver's recommendations and believe that he or she listens to you and cares about your well-being.

But what if you *don't* feel comfortable with your caregiver? Here are three ways to handle the situation:

1.  Express your discomfort and explain what will make you feel more at ease, but do so calmly and without using accusatory language.

    For example, you may say something such as: "Dr. Jones, this is hard for me to say, but I get the impression that my questions are an inconvenience to you. When I need to know more about something, I feel that you brush me off and I shouldn't ask you anything."

    By using the pronoun *I* often, you communicate that *you* are the one experiencing a problem with the relationship. You're not directly criticizing your caregiver's behavior by saying something such as: "Dr. Jones, you're always in a rush and you don't let me ask any questions. You don't even care about your patients." Such language will likely make your caregiver defensive and less willing to improve your relationship.

    Expressing yourself with direct but respectful language may evoke an effort to work together as equals and may improve communication, perhaps convincing one of you to agree to the other's way of thinking on some matter or to agree to a compromise. Your birth plan should contain these joint decisions. (See Chapter 8.)

    Especially if you anticipate this conversation to be challenging, practice what you want to say ahead of time with your partner or a friend.

2.  If the above approach doesn't work, consider changing caregivers. Although it's always uncomfortable to change caregivers, doing so may be better than staying with someone who makes you feel uneasy.

    Don't drop your caregiver until you've found someone who better suits you and who has agreed to become your caregiver. If your original caregiver is in a group practice, try to select a new caregiver who's not in that group. (By choosing another caregiver in the same group, you risk having your original caregiver attend you in labor.)

3.  If you can't change caregivers (or don't want to) and you can't discuss your feelings with your caregiver, consider talking with the office nurse, a childbirth educator, doula (see page 23), or others to help you cope with the relationship. Try to work with your caregiver as best you can by asserting your position reasonably and calmly. For example, you may say something such as: "I realize you don't agree with some of my choices, but I've learned that they're not unreasonable, and many caregivers allow them. Please work with me." If your caregiver continues to push for options that go against your wishes, remember that you have the right to refuse unacceptable care practices. It's unlikely you'll need to take this step, but in case you do, having the support of family, friends, and other advocates will be essential.

# Choosing Childbirth Preparation Classes

Many hospitals, colleges and universities, nonprofit community organizations, groups of caregivers, and independent childbirth educators offer childbirth preparation classes. The programs vary in size, philosophy, cost, topics covered, and number of classes in the series. The background and training of the instructors vary (they may be registered nurses, physical therapists, teachers, psychologists, social workers, college graduates, or others), as does the quality of the classes.

Colleges and universities, community groups, and independent educators usually sponsor *consumer-oriented classes*, which prepare parents to take responsibility in decision-making and self-care. Hospitals or caregivers usually sponsor *provider-oriented classes*, which inform parents about the type of care provided by a hospital or caregiver group, but avoid discussion of reasonable alternatives or controversial topics in maternity care.

Visit the web sites of organizations and institutions offering childbirth classes in your area. If possible, compare your options to determine which class best suits your needs.

## CHILDBIRTH PREPARATION ON DVD OR ONLINE

Childbirth preparation classes on DVD or online cost less than traditional childbirth classes, and you can watch them whenever you have time and whenever you need to review topics.

But in key ways, these classes can't compare to in-person classes. They can't address local practices and incorporate up-to-date research data. They can't provide opportunities for asking the instructor questions or getting feedback and advice on comfort measures if they're not working for you. Lastly, they can't provide an opportunity for developing new friendships with other expectant parents.

## Different Views on Childbirth Classes

After the birth, new parents were asked to comment on how well childbirth classes prepared them for birth. Although there were many different views, the responses shared the following sentiments:

*Childbirth classes prepared us for what to expect and do at each stage of labor and delivery. They took a lot of the "shock value" out of the process.*

*The classes gave us a better understanding of the big picture of birth. Although the class was well taught and formatted, we discovered that some things can be learned only from experience.*

*The class gave me confidence and a sense of security. I didn't feel scared or unsure. It gave me the chance to clarify my preferences before I went into labor.*

## Questions to Ask When Choosing Childbirth Preparation Classes

- Who sponsors the classes?
- What's the instructor's background and training?
- What's the instructor's experience with birth and childbirth education? Does the instructor participate in continuing education in the field? Is she certified by a reputable organization?
- Does the instructor cover normal childbirth as well as complications? Does she cover all choices and include their pros and cons? Does she teach self-help comfort measures and natural childbirth techniques? Does she describe disadvantages and risks as well as advantages of various procedures and medications?
- Does the series cover postpartum adjustment, newborn care, development, and feeding?
- How are the classes scheduled? As a series of four to eight weekly meetings? A one- or two-day course? (Classes that last only one or two days may be convenient, but they can be exhausting and overwhelming. Classes that meet regularly over a longer period let you better absorb the information, practice the techniques, and think of questions to ask at the next class.)
- What is the cost of the series? (A few health insurance plans and government assistance programs cover the cost of childbirth classes.)
- What is the ratio of students to instructor?
- Is the instructor available to students by phone, e-mail, or in person for questions outside of class and after the series?

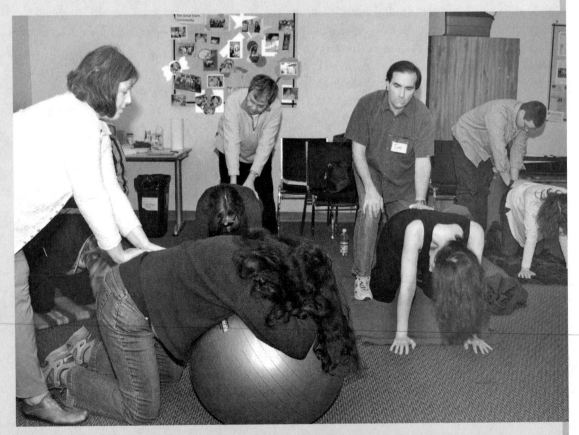

# All about Birth Doulas

In 2007, the Cochrane Library (a prestigious collection of databases that contain high-quality, independent evidence to inform people when making decisions about health care) issued a report about the "dehumanization" of women's birth experiences, caused by a lack of continuous support for laboring women. Concerned by this development, maternity experts and professionals have called for a "rehumanization" of childbirth by reestablishing continuous support of laboring women. The review found that support was most effective when provided by women who weren't hospital staff.[8]

Many studies show that continuous support benefits laboring women, especially when the support begins in early labor and is given by someone whose only role is to provide it. Benefits include the following:

- Shorter labors, with less need for medication to speed up labor
- More spontaneous vaginal births (that is, births that don't require forceps, vacuum extraction, or cesarean delivery.)
- Fewer requests for pain medications
- Less dissatisfaction with birth experiences

The desire to provide laboring women with continuous support has led to the emergence of the *birth doula*, a person (almost always a woman) who's trained and experienced in supporting women and their partners during labor and birth. Unlike a caregiver or a nurse, a birth doula doesn't concentrate on the clinical parts of labor or give medical advice, and she doesn't work in shifts (and leave a laboring woman when the shift is done). Instead, she stays with a laboring woman continuously throughout labor and birth, giving encouragement, reassurance, advice, and help. Her presence can help ease the stress, unpredictability, and pain of labor.

Consider hiring a birth doula if you want someone you trust to be with you throughout your labor and birth. She can give you and your partner confidence and a sense of well-being. If necessary, she can guide your partner through the comfort measures to help make you more comfortable. See page 190 for more information about doulas.

## FINDING A BIRTH DOULA

To find birth doulas in your area, ask your friends, childbirth educator, or caregiver for recommendations. You can also search online. Try to consult with several doulas by phone or e-mail to help you decide which ones you want to interview in person.

During the interview, ask the questions on page 24. Pay attention not only to *what* the doula says, but also *how* she says it. Her behavior and body language will help you decide whether she's a good fit for you.

Most doulas charge a fee for their services, although some doulas-in-training charge a small fee (if any) and some experienced doulas may waive or reduce their fees for clients with tight finances. A few hospitals provide doula services at low cost or no cost to the patient, and some charitable agencies or public health departments cover doulas' fees for women who can't afford the services. Given doulas' contributions to improved outcomes in maternity care, their services make financial sense; however, health insurance plans rarely cover doula services.

## Questions to Ask a Potential Birth Doula

DONA International is the world's oldest, largest, and most respected doula association. The following questions are based on those found on its web site (http://www.dona.org/mothers /how_to_hire_a_doula.php).

- What training, education, and experience do you have?
- What's your philosophy of childbirth and supporting women and their partners through labor?
- When do you try to join a woman in labor—in early labor, later in labor, or whenever she feels she needs you? Do you go to her home or the birthplace?
- Will you meet with me before the birth to discuss my birth plans and the role that you'll play in supporting me through labor? Will you visit me after my baby is born?
- May I contact you with questions or concerns before or after the birth?
- Do you work with one or more backup doulas for times when you're unavailable? May I meet them?
- What's your fee? What services does it include? What are your refund policies? (If her fee is more than you can pay, ask if she provides a sliding scale or can refer you to someone who does.)
- Will you provide references?

# Your Baby's Health Care

After your baby is born, adjusting to new parenthood will be easier if you make some decisions about his health care well before the birth. (See Chapter 8 for more information on developing a postpartum plan.)

While you're pregnant, you can research early health care choices you'll make for your baby after the birth, including circumcision (see page 372) and vaccinations (see page 386). Learning about these options before the birth prepares you to make an informed decision when the time comes.

You can also learn about the types of health care available for your newborn. Considering these options before the birth gives you time to arrange for the best available health care for your baby.

## CHOOSING A CAREGIVER FOR YOUR BABY

By choosing your baby's caregiver before the birth, you'll have someone to call whenever you're concerned about your newborn's health, from the moment she's born. You can also find out the schedule of well-baby checkups ahead of time.

Several types of caregivers provide care for children. *Pediatricians* specialize in children's health care. They've graduated from medical school and completed a pediatric residency. Their offices and waiting rooms are geared for children.

*Family physicians* provide care for the entire family. They've spent several months in pediatrics during medical school and as part of their residency training. They diagnose and treat most illnesses, but refer seriously ill children to pediatricians. If a family physician provides your care before, during, and after pregnancy, it may be a comfortable decision to have him or her care for your baby.

*Pediatric and family nurse practitioners* are registered nurses who have additional training in pediatrics or family health. They provide well-child care and treat common illnesses. They usually work with a group of physicians, and refer serious problems to a physician. Nurse practitioners are knowledgeable about children's emotional, social, and physical development.

*Naturopathic doctors (NDs)* and other alternative practitioners provide well-child care and emphasize non-medical complementary treatment of illness. Their education varies but may consist of four years' training after college. Most care for the entire family, although some don't provide care for babies or children. They don't have hospital privileges, and refer seriously ill children to physicians.

## HEALTH CARE COVERAGE FOR YOUR BABY

The cost of your baby's health care depends on your health insurance coverage and on where your baby visits a caregiver. In most cases, your baby will see a caregiver for well-child visits, during which the caregiver checks your baby's growth, development, and overall health, and gives immunizations. If you have a choice of health insurance plans, compare coverage of well-child visits. Some plans don't pay for well-child visits but cover nearly all expenses to care for an ill child.

Some caregivers practice out of private offices; others practice in clinics. Private-practice care is more expensive than clinic care, but it may be more personalized and convenient. Many health insurance plans cover most (or part) of the costs of private care and provide a list of approved caregivers.

Children's health clinics usually cost less than private practices, but they may have longer waiting times. If the clinic is associated with a medical school, its staff may change frequently. Its caregivers are physicians or nurse practitioners who are rotating through their advanced training under the supervision of fully trained professionals. Other community-based children's clinics offer low-cost care and a consistent staff (which means you see the same caregiver at each visit). Such clinics usually also provide social services and other services to low-income families.

Community health clinics or well-child clinics associated with a public health department offer free or low-cost checkups and vaccinations, but they usually don't provide care for sick children.

## Questions to Ask a Potential Caregiver for Your Baby

- Do you support breastfeeding? Formula feeding? Do you have expertise in breastfeeding? Do you work with lactation consultants or other breastfeeding resources? Do you refer to them?
- What are your thoughts on circumcision?
- What are your thoughts on vaccinations? Do you support delayed schedules? How about the refusal of vaccinations?
- How comfortable are you with the use of home remedies or alternative therapies for minor ailments and common illnesses? Are you concerned about the overuse of antibiotics?
- How available are you (or your office) for phone consultation? Who takes calls when you're unavailable?
- Do you have hospital privileges? Where? If my child must be hospitalized, how involved will you be in his or her care?
- Will you be available to examine my baby soon after the birth (at the hospital or in my home)?
Visit our web site, http://www.PCNGuide.com, to download a work sheet to record the answers to these questions.

## FINDING A CAREGIVER FOR YOUR BABY

After choosing a type of caregiver for your baby and the setting for the visits (private office, clinic, or other), you can focus on choosing a caregiver that suits your needs. A helpful way to start your search is to ask your caregiver, childbirth educator, local hospital, and family and friends to recommend pediatric caregivers. Visit these caregivers' web sites to learn information about their practices (such as the convenience of their locations and office hours). Or call the caregivers' offices to learn the information from the receptionist.

If possible before the birth, schedule an interview with one or more caregivers. Check your health insurance plan to determine whether it covers such appointments. If it doesn't, find out whether the caregiver will charge a fee for the appointment, and if so, the amount.

During the interview, time may be limited, so make sure you ask the questions you most want answered. (See page 25.) Pay attention to *how* a caregiver answers your questions. Does the caregiver seem competent, caring, and considerate? Does his or her style and philosophy match yours? It's important that the person who will care for your baby's health has your confidence and trust.

# Finding Help after Your Baby's Birth

For the first several weeks after the birth, you and your partner may be surprised by how time-consuming baby care is, leaving you few free moments for meal preparation, basic housework, sleep, and socializing. (See Chapter 15.) During this period, it's important to arrange for someone (or more than one person) to help you as you adjust to life with a newborn.

## WHO CAN HELP YOU?

For many new parents, family members (typically, a mother, mother-in-law, or sister) and friends provide help by cooking meals, running errands, doing laundry, housecleaning, and watching the baby so the parents can sleep or relax by themselves.

If family and friends don't live near you or have little time to help, or relationships are strained, others can provide much-needed help. Baby nurses or nannies can take care of your baby, allowing you to do other activities. Mother's helpers cook and clean, but they don't help with baby care or give advice.

An especially knowledgeable source of help is a *postpartum doula*, a person (almost always a woman) who's trained and experienced to help a woman and her family adjust to postpartum life by teaching them about newborns' needs and abilities, and about infant feeding, sleep, and cues. A postpartum doula focuses on enhancing a new mother's confidence and competence and fostering her bond with her baby.

Postpartum doulas and other helpers typically charge by the hour, and the potential costs may seem daunting to expectant parents. But many parents find that the help and care are well worth the price, especially years later when recalling those first few days and weeks with their newborns.

Heath insurance plans rarely cover the services of a postpartum doula or other helper. To pay for these services, put money aside during pregnancy. Or if friends and relatives ask how they can help you after the birth, suggest they contribute money for this purpose, or request the money as a shower gift.

## Questions to Ask a Potential Postpartum Doula

DONA International is the world's oldest, largest, and most respected doula association. The following questions are based on those found on its web site (http://www.dona.org/mothers/how_to_hire_a_doula.php).

- What training and education do you have? Tell me about your experience.
- Have you had a criminal background check?
- Have you had a recent TB test (for tuberculosis) and DTaP vaccination (for pertussis and other illnesses)? Is your CPR certification current?
- What's your philosophy of parenting and of supporting women and their families after the birth?
- May we meet before the birth to discuss our needs and the role you'll play in supporting us after the birth?
- What additional services do you offer?
- May we call you with questions or concerns before the birth?
- When do your services begin after the birth?
- What's your experience with breastfeeding support?
- What's your fee? What's your refund policy?

## FINDING A POSTPARTUM DOULA

If you decide you want a postpartum doula, try to hire one before the birth. You may have trouble finding a doula who suits your needs if you wait until after the birth to start your search.

To find postpartum doulas in your area, ask your friends, childbirth educator, or caregiver for recommendations. You can also search online. Try to consult with several doulas by phone or e-mail to help you decide which ones you want to interview in person.

During the interview, ask the questions above. Pay attention not only to *what* the doula says, but also *how* she says it. Her behavior and body language will help you decide whether she's a good fit for you.

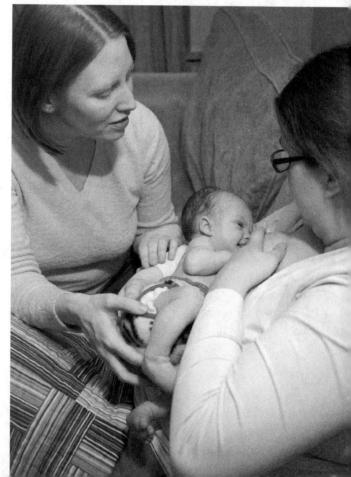

# RETURNING TO WORK

In the United States, the length of maternity and family leave policies is generally short, and parents must return to work earlier than do parents in Canada and other industrialized countries whose leave policies are generous.

Typically before the birth, families decide who will return to work after the baby is born. For some new families, only one parent is able or available to work (such as a single parent). For many other families, both parents return to work for the family's financial well-being, for career development, or because they love their jobs.

Some families can explore the option of having only one parent return to work, letting the other parent stay at home full-time to care for the baby. If this option interests you, discover whether it's possible for your family by answering the following questions. Visit our web site, http://www.PCN Guide.com, for a list of additional questions to consider.

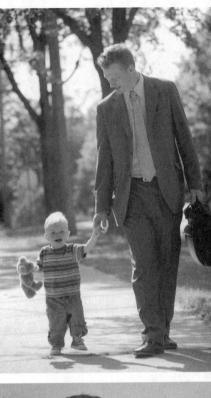

- Can you or your partner delay returning to work until your baby is older?
- Can you or your partner work part-time or job-share? Can either of you work from home?
- What are the costs of returning to work? These may include clothing, transportation, child care, convenience foods, and more visits to your baby's caregiver. (Your baby may become sick more often from exposure to ill children in child care.)
- Will your income exceed the total costs of working outside the home and make working worthwhile?
- Can you simplify your lifestyle and lower your cost of living to offset the loss of income?
- How will the person who works feel about the other's staying at home?

After you've made the best choice for you and your family, make sure you and your partner support each other to accommodate the change. Whether you stay home with your baby or work outside the home, life is more challenging with a baby—it's helpful to have an ally!

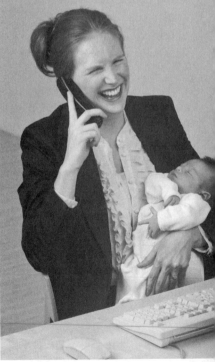

# Finding Child Care for Your Baby

If you and your partner decide to return to work (or you're a single parent who must), your first priority is finding affordable, safe, dependable child care. The best time to arrange for child care is well before the birth, but that might not be possible for some families. If you can't make arrangements before the birth, try to wait three to four months after the birth before returning to work. This will give you time to recover and focus on your baby. When you start your search, allow at least a month to find child care that best suits your needs.

Start your search by asking coworkers or other working parents about their child-care arrangements. Contact local agencies that can help you find licensed child-care facilities, homes, or other providers such as nannies. If you're considering using a nanny or babysitter, see whether you can share his or her services (and the costs) with another family.

If you don't want a stranger caring for your baby, consider asking family members or friends to care for him. Or think about staggering your and your partner's work schedules or working part-time so you and your partner can provide at least some child care. In some work settings, it may be possible for you to bring your baby to work and care for him during the workday. (Some companies even offer on-site child care for their employees.)

If you decide to have someone care for your child outside your home, first visit http://www.saferchild.org/caregiver.htm and http://www.childcareaware.org for advice on evaluating child-care providers. Then visit potential child-care facilities and homes with your baby. How do the providers behave with babies in their care? With gentleness and kindness or with impatience and detachment? How do they deal with crying babies? What do they do when a baby becomes ill? How do they support breastfeeding mothers? How will they feel about your visiting when you can? Find out the facility's or home's hours of operation and holiday and vacation schedules, and ask to see their licenses to ensure they're current. Pay attention to how the providers respond to you and your baby, and trust your instincts about the home or facility.

If you decide to hire a nanny or other in-home provider, interview candidates in your home. Ask the same questions you'd ask providers at a child-care facility or home (see above). Also ask candidates how they plan to cover their child-care duties should they become ill or go on vacation. Pay attention to how candidates interact with your baby and you, and trust your instincts on what you observe. Request references and contact them.

After you've chosen suitable child care, remember that you're establishing a partnership with the child-care workers. Always treat them with respect. Offer compliments and acknowledge their valuable service by giving appropriate holiday gifts.

If at any point you decide a child-care arrangement is no longer right for your baby, be willing to find another provider so you can be assured your baby is receiving the best care.

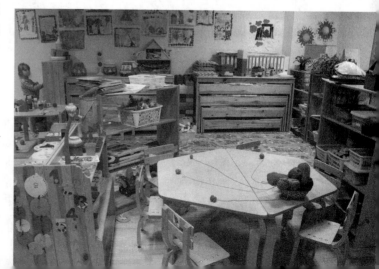

# Ten Steps to Improve Your Chances of Having a Safe and Satisfying Birth

Here's a summary of things to do and choices to make to increase the likelihood of having a safe, satisfying birth and avoiding a cesarean birth and other unwanted interventions.

1. Take care of yourself during pregnancy so you begin labor in the best possible health. Exercise in moderation and eat well. (See Chapters 5 and 6.) If you're overweight when you become pregnant, aim to gain a small or moderate amount of weight. Seek prenatal care to help you detect and manage any health problems that may arise.

2. Choose a birthplace that has a low rate of cesarean birth and minimal routine interventions. (Ask the questions on page 13.) If your pregnancy is low-risk and you prefer minimal interventions, consider birthing at a birth center or at home. Several studies show that women having low-risk pregnancies undergo fewer interventions in an out-of-hospital setting and their birth outcomes are just as good as those of women birthing in hospitals.[9]

3. Find a caregiver who has low intervention rates and encourages the use of self-help techniques in labor. (See Chapters 10 and 11.) If your pregnancy is low-risk, consider using a midwife (if available). Midwives typically use fewer medical interventions than physicians do. If intensive medical care becomes necessary during pregnancy, a midwife will refer you to an obstetrician.

4. Educate yourself and prepare a birth plan. (See Chapter 8.) Take childbirth preparation classes that emphasize informed decision-making and self-help methods to relieve pain and aid progress. Visit http://www.childbirthconnection.org to read and download a copy of "The Rights of Childbearing Women," which outlines a set of basic maternity rights for all childbearing women. Keep these rights in mind as you create and review your birth plan with your caregiver.[10]

5. Hire a birth doula. The continuous labor support a doula provides often leads to a shorter labor, reduced need for pain medication, increased chance of normal vaginal birth, and increased satisfaction with the birth experience.[11]

6. Avoid labor induction for non-medical reasons. If your caregiver suggests induction for a debatable medical reason (such as a suspected big baby), ask about other alternatives. (See page 276.)

7. Use medical interventions only when clearly necessary, not because they're routine. For example, avoid routine IV fluids, continuous electronic monitoring, and augmentation with Pitocin or artificial rupture of membranes. (See Chapter 13.) In some situations, interventions may be the best option for you or your baby. Ask questions to ensure that you make informed decisions. That way, when you remember the birth in the years to come, you'll know you made the right choices. (See page 10.)

8. Learn to differentiate between early labor and active labor so you can delay hospital admission until active labor. (See page 170.) Use labor-coping skills at home to manage pain and aid progress. (See Chapter 11.) Eat, drink, and rest as needed to keep up your energy.

9. Use a variety of positions and activities during active labor, such as walking, dancing, rocking in a rocking chair or on a birth ball, or taking a shower or bath. (See page 208.)

10. Push in positions that aid descent, unless the birth is happening fast; then use positions that slow descent. (See page 220.) Use spontaneous pushing if you have an urge to push. Delay pushing if you don't have an urge to push (and you and baby are doing fine).

# *Key Points to Remember*

- As an expectant parent, it's your responsibility and legal right to become informed about the available options in maternity care and to communicate your preferences to your caregivers.
- To help you make informed decisions, ask key questions and consult with your caregiver and other knowledgeable medical professionals. After considering the information you've learned and weighing it against your values and concerns, you can make the best decisions.
- During your pregnancy, you can make many choices that will help make positive experiences of your labor, birth, and postpartum period. You can decide where you want to give birth, who will provide your care, what childbirth preparation classes to take, whether you want a birth doula and postpartum doula, who will provide medical care for your baby, and what child-care arrangement will best suit your needs if you return to work after the birth.

# CHAPTER 3

# Common Changes and Concerns in Pregnancy

Pregnancy brings about profound physical changes in you, dynamic growth and development in your baby, and emotional adjustments for you and your partner. It's an amazing and exciting time, yet you may find yourself wondering and worrying how your pregnancy is affecting you and your baby. You may try to imagine what your baby looks like in your womb. You may be unsure how you'll react to the many changes ahead. Learning what to expect during a normal and healthy pregnancy may help put your feelings and worries into perspective and let you enjoy your pregnancy.

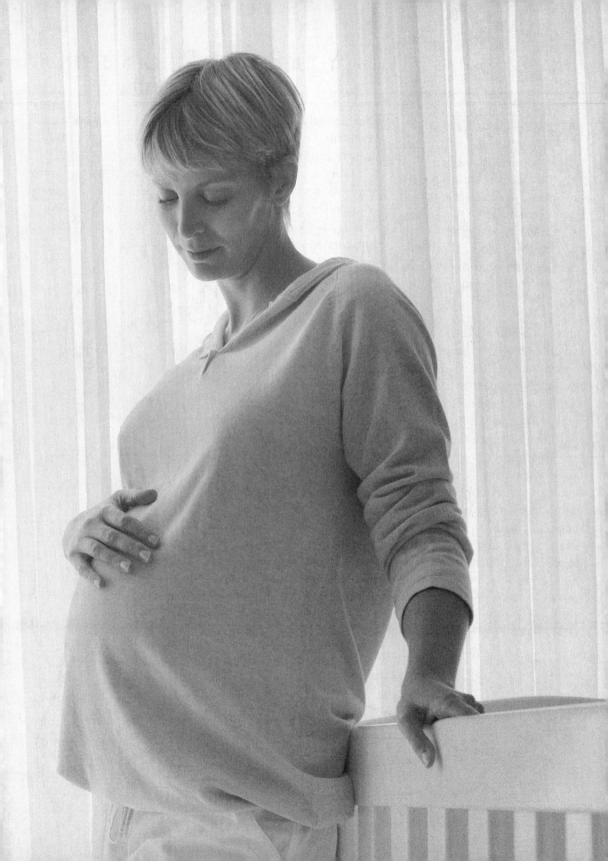

# Your Body's Preparation for Pregnancy

Since roughly the time you reached puberty, your body has naturally been preparing for pregnancy. The design of your body's reproductive system makes pregnancy possible.

Your reproductive anatomy includes both internal and external structures. The labia, urethra, clitoris, and vaginal opening are your external genitals, shown below. These body parts plus your anus are your *perineum*. Many pairs of muscles attached to your pelvis support the perineum and form a strong sling with openings for your urethra, vagina, and anus. These are your *pelvic floor muscles.*

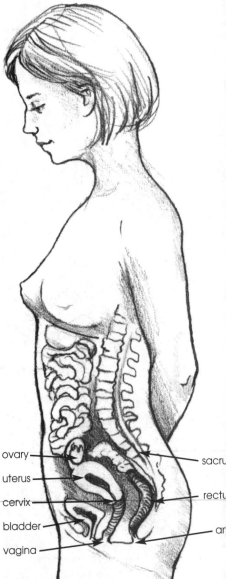

The drawing on page 35 shows your internal reproductive organs. Your *uterus* (or womb) is a hollow, muscular organ the size and shape of a pear, and your *vagina* is a stretchy tube-shaped canal. The lower part of your uterus, which protrudes into your vagina, is your *cervix.* Your *fallopian tubes* provide the paths for an egg (*ovum*) to travel from your *ovaries* (sex glands) to your uterus.

Your ovaries produce the female sex hormones estrogen and progesterone (see page 37). After puberty, your ovaries undergo a cycle of changes every month (give or take a few days), unless you're pregnant. During a cycle, an egg matures in one ovary and causes increased secretion of estrogen, which along with progesterone stimulates growth of the uterine lining (endometrium). Usually only one egg ripens each cycle and is released into one of your fallopian tubes. This process is called *ovulation,* and it usually occurs about halfway through your cycle, but it can occur earlier or later. As the fine hairs in your fallopian tube propel the egg slowly toward your uterus, your ovary

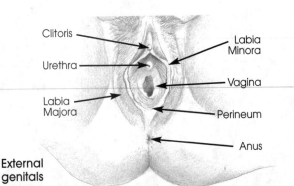

Clitoris

Urethra

Labia Majora

Labia Minora

Vagina

Perineum

Anus

**External genitals**

ovary

uterus

cervix

bladder

vagina

sacru

rect

ar

produces more progesterone, which stimulates the uterine lining to become a rich, nourishing home for a fertilized egg. If fertilization doesn't occur (which means you're not pregnant), your estrogen and progesterone levels diminish and your uterus sheds its unneeded lining. This shedding process is called menstruation.

# Conceiving Your Baby

*Conception* occurs (and you become pregnant) when a sperm from your partner fertilizes (penetrates) your egg.

When your partner has an orgasm, he ejaculates about 1 teaspoon of semen, which contains 150 million to 400 million sperm. If ejaculation occurs during sexual intercourse, these sperm travel from your vagina into your uterus and out to your fallopian tubes. Sperm can live inside you for up to three days, while your egg is viable for only twelve to twenty-four hours after ovulation. Conception usually happens in the part of the fallopian tube farthest from the uterus when a single sperm fertilizes the awaiting egg.

Occasionally, a woman ovulates more than one egg, and a separate sperm fertilizes each one, resulting in fraternal (non-identical) twins, triplets, quadruplets, or higher-order multiples. Sometimes, a single fertilized egg divides into two and produces identical twins. For information on pregnancy with multiples, see page 53.

## Common Q & A

**Q:** If my partner and I have trouble conceiving, what can we do?

**A:** Difficulty conceiving a child can be frustrating. Visit our web site, http://www .PCNGuide.com, for ways you can improve your health before conceiving and ways to enhance fertility. If you've been trying for more than a year, you may want to consult an infertility expert who can look for possible complications with ovulation or a low sperm count. If a problem is discovered, you may choose to use assisted reproductive technology (ART). To learn more about ART, visit http://www.cdc.gov/ART or http://www.marchofdimes .com/pnhec/173_14308.asp.

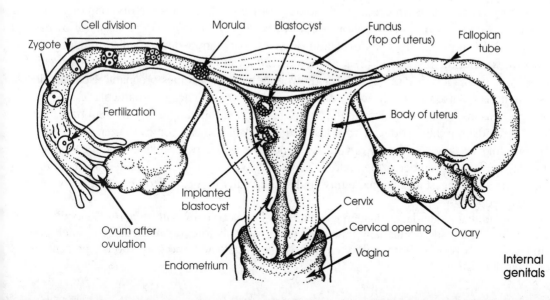

Zygote · Cell division · Morula · Blastocyst · Fundus (top of uterus) · Fallopian tube · Fertilization · Body of uterus · Implanted blastocyst · Ovum after ovulation · Endometrium · Cervix · Cervical opening · Vagina · Ovary

**Internal genitals**

# Now That You're Pregnant

When you suspect that you're pregnant, you may experience some or all of the early signs of pregnancy, which are caused by hormonal changes that begin almost immediately after conception. Here are symptoms that you may notice:

- Breast changes: fullness, tenderness, tingling in the nipple area, and a darkened *areola* (the area around each nipple)
- Missed menstrual period
- Fullness, bloating, or ache in your lower abdomen
- Fatigue and drowsiness
- Feeling lightheaded or faint
- Nausea or vomiting at any time of the day ("morning sickness")
- Frequent urination
- Increased vaginal secretions

## CONFIRMING YOUR PREGNANCY

If you don't experience the above physical symptoms, you might not suspect you're pregnant until you've missed a menstrual period, at which time you may take a home pregnancy test. These do-it-yourself kits check your urine for human chorionic gonadotropin (hCG), a hormone that's produced only during pregnancy. Available in most drugstores and discount stores, they usually provide supplies for two tests. Taking one test after missing a period and another a few days later is more accurate than taking only one test.

To confirm your pregnancy, you can make an appointment for a blood test with a medical professional. If you're pregnant, he or she may give you basic information to help ensure a healthy pregnancy, such as taking folic acid supplements, until you have your first prenatal appointment and can learn more about prenatal health. Even before starting your prenatal visits, it's wise to begin adopting a healthy lifestyle and eating a well-balanced diet. (See Chapters 4, 5, and 6.)

## CALCULATING YOUR DUE DATE

Pregnancy (or *gestation*) lasts an average of 280 days or forty weeks after the first day of your last menstrual period. Although conception occurs within twelve to twenty-four hours of ovulation, it's difficult to know exactly when ovulation occurred. For many women, ovulation happens about two weeks after the first day of their last period, but it can occur earlier or later in the cycle. This uncertainty makes it difficult to know exactly when a woman becomes pregnant, especially if she has sexual intercourse frequently and conception can't be traced back to a particular day.

For these reasons, caregivers calculate the *due date* by using this simple formula: Subtract three months from the date of the first day of your last period (a date you can confirm), then add seven days. For example, let's say the first day of your last period was February 1. Subtracting three months from that day leads to November 1, then adding seven days gives you a due date of November 8. Most caregivers also suggest an optional ultrasound scan in early pregnancy to help estimate your due date. (See page 69.)

Keep in mind that a due date is just an estimate of when your baby will be born. Generally, babies are born healthy and normal any time from three weeks before to two weeks after their due dates. In fact, most babies are born within ten days of their due dates, and only about 5 percent are born on their due dates.

If a due date is just a guess, why is it important? A due date is based on many assessments and decisions that help your caregiver do the following:

- Determine when best to do genetic testing
- Recognize whether results of specific lab tests are within the normal range
- Diagnose a preterm or post-date pregnancy
- Identify a baby who's growing more slowly or rapidly than normal

Because normal pregnancies vary in length, your caregiver will look at a range of normal test results when making these assessments.

# Hormonal Changes during Pregnancy

Changes in hormone production cause many of the physical and emotional changes in pregnancy, helping ensure a healthy pregnancy and the optimal development of your baby. The placenta is the major source of these hormones. (See page 39.) Here's how the various hormones affect you and your pregnancy:

- *Human chorionic gonadotropin (hCG)* is a hormone produced only during pregnancy. (Pregnancy tests check for hCG in your blood or urine.) This hormone ensures that your ovaries produce estrogen and progesterone for the first two to three months of your pregnancy, until your placenta matures and produces the appropriate amount.
- *Estrogen* promotes the growth of your uterine muscles and their blood supply, encourages production of vaginal mucus, and stimulates the development of the ductal system and blood supply in your breasts. Changes in water retention, body fat buildup, and skin pigmentation are related to estrogen levels. In late pregnancy, rising estrogen levels increase the uterus's sensitivity to oxytocin and help start labor.
- *Progesterone* relaxes your uterus during pregnancy, keeping it from contracting too much. It also relaxes the walls of blood vessels (helping you maintain a healthy blood pressure) and the walls of your stomach and bowels (allowing for greater absorption of nutrients and sometimes causing constipation). In late pregnancy, progesterone has less effect on your uterus, letting contractions increase and start labor.
- *Relaxin* from your ovaries relaxes and softens your ligaments, cartilage, and cervix, making these tissues more stretchable during pregnancy and letting your pelvic joints spread during birth.
- *Prostaglandins*, produced in your amniotic membrane, increase in level during late pregnancy. Prostaglandins soften and ripen your cervix in preparation for labor, and stimulate muscles in your uterus and bowels.
- *Corticotropin-releasing hormone (CRH)* comes from your baby, placenta, and tissues within your uterus. Increased levels of CRH in late pregnancy change the ratio of estrogen to progesterone.
- *Oxytocin*, produced in your pituitary gland, stimulates uterine contractions to help trigger the onset of labor and promote labor progress. Often referred to as the "love hormone," oxytocin is present during an orgasm. It's also responsible for the urge to push at the end of labor and for the let-down reflex during breastfeeding. Oxytocin improves mood and produces feelings of calmness and well-being.[1]

Pregnancy also produces greater quantities of many hormones that are present when you're not pregnant. These increased hormone levels cause other physical changes and influence your metabolism, mineral balance, tissue and organ growth, levels of still other hormones, and the onset of labor.

# First Trimester Changes for You and Your Baby

Pregnancy is divided into three *trimesters*, each one lasting about three months. The first trimester is the "formation" period, because by the end of it all of your baby's organ systems are formed and functioning. For you, the first trimester is a time of physical and emotional adjustment to being pregnant.

## THE FIRST FOUR WEEKS OF PREGNANCY

This time marks conception through the first two weeks of your baby's life (four weeks *gestational age*).

### Changes in Your Baby

At conception, your baby gets inherited characteristics from you and her father. Every normal human cell contains forty-six chromosomes of genetic material; an egg and sperm each contains half that number. When a sperm fertilizes an egg, the resulting twenty-three pairs of chromosomes combine to form a unique genetic blueprint for development. This blueprint decides at conception your baby's sex, blood type, eye and hair color, nose and ear shape, and some personality traits and mental capabilities. To a great extent, this blueprint also guides your baby's growth and development throughout her life.

Throughout pregnancy, the terms used to describe a baby change to reflect age and development. After conception, the fertilized egg quickly divides from one cell into two, then four, eight, sixteen, and so on until it becomes a multicellular structure called a *blastocyst*. Within five to nine days, the blastocyst has made its way along the fallopian tube and implants in the uterine lining, usually in the upper part of the uterus. By two weeks, the baby is called an *embryo* and another part of the fertilized egg is developing into the placenta. This primitive placenta has tiny rootlike projections that penetrate the uterine lining and acquire nutrients for the developing embryo.

### Changes in You

While these changes are taking place in your baby, you may have noticed only some breast tenderness or a slight ache in your belly. But you're about to miss your menstrual period, and the remarkable changes that you'll experience have just begun!

## THE 5TH THROUGH 14TH WEEKS OF PREGNANCY

This time marks the third through twelfth weeks of your baby's life (five to fourteen weeks gestational age).

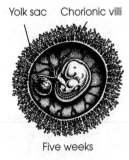

Yolk sac    Chorionic villi

Five weeks

### Changes in Your Baby

During the first few weeks of this trimester, your baby is an embryo that's developing rapidly. His nervous system and circulatory system are forming, and his heart is beating by the twenty-fifth day after conception. Your baby has simple kidneys, a liver, a digestive tract, and a developing umbilical cord. When he's only half the size of a pea, arm and leg buds appear and his face begins to form.

Although your baby's sex is determined at conception, male and female babies appear the same until the embryo is about nine weeks old. Then, if the embryo is male, he begins producing *androgens*, male hormones that signal the development of the scrotum and penis. If female, her external genitals and internal reproductive organs form.

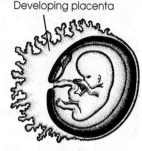

Developing placenta

Eight weeks

By eight weeks after conception (ten weeks gestational age), your baby is structurally complete. His mouth has lips, a tongue, and teeth buds in his gums. His arms have hands with fingers and fingerprints. His legs have knees, ankles, and toes. His arms and legs move at this time, but coordinated movements don't begin until about fourteen weeks. His developing brain begins to send out impulses. His heart is beating strongly and can be seen easily during an ultrasound scan. Your baby grows about 1 millimeter a day. When he's nine weeks old (eleven weeks gestational age), he's called a fetus.

During the first three months, your baby becomes quite active, although you're probably unaware of any movements. Legs kick and arms move. Your baby can suck his thumb, swallow amniotic fluid, and urinate drops of sterile urine into the amniotic fluid, which is completely exchanged about every three hours. Your baby makes breathing movements (that is, his chest rises and falls); "breathing" amniotic fluid into his lungs appears to help with lung development. By ten to twelve weeks (twelve to fourteen weeks gestational age), your baby's eyelids cover his eyes, but his eyes remain closed until the sixth month.

## Development of the Placenta and Changes in the Uterus

During the early weeks of pregnancy, your uterine lining becomes thicker and provides a rich source of nourishment for your growing baby. At the end of the first month of development, projections (chorionic villi) extend into your uterine lining, becoming a primitive placenta. Your baby's blood circulates through the chorionic villi, while your blood circulates into the spaces surrounding them (intervillous spaces). A thin membrane separates the two bloodstreams, which normally don't mix.

The *membranes* (amnion and chorion) create the *amniotic sac* that surrounds your baby. The *amniotic fluid* protects your baby by absorbing bumps from the outside, maintaining an even temperature, and providing a medium for easy movement.

By twelve weeks of pregnancy, the *placenta* is completely formed and serves as an organ for producing hormones and exchanging nutrients and waste products. Most identical twins share the same placenta. Fraternal twins have separate placentas, though the placentas sometimes fuse into one large organ.

The *umbilical cord* links the placenta to your baby's navel, and together the umbilical cord and placenta pass oxygen and nutrients from you to your baby. While the placenta provides a barrier against most (but not all) bacteria in your bloodstream, most viruses and drugs cross to your baby. The placenta also exchanges waste products from your baby, which your blood then carries to your kidneys and lungs for excretion.

By fourteen weeks of pregnancy, your uterus has grown to just above your pubic bone. The cervix is about 4 centimeters long and, though softer than before pregnancy, still fairly firm. The *mucous plug* that fills the cervical opening provides a barrier to help protect your baby.

## Different Views on the First Trimester

Expectant mothers were asked: "What emotional changes did you notice in the first trimester?" Although there were many different views, the responses shared the following sentiments:

*I found myself crying at silly things.*

*I felt like a worrywart over my baby's health.*

*Besides being more emotional, I felt pretty good overall. It feels good to be pregnant.*

## Changes in You

By five weeks (possibly earlier) from the first day of your last menstrual period, a pregnancy test should show a positive result. During the first trimester, you may feel unusually tired and need more sleep because of your changing metabolic rate and your increased energy needs while growing a baby. You may urinate more often as your enlarging uterus presses on your bladder. Many women experience nausea and vomiting during the early months of pregnancy. (See page 119.) Although usually called *morning sickness*, this symptom of pregnancy may occur at any time of the day. While the cause of morning sickness is unknown, it's thought that hormones produced by the developing placenta play a role.

Although your breasts develop in puberty, your milk glands don't fully develop until pregnancy. As hormone levels increase, your breasts change in preparation of providing milk for your baby. Your breasts enlarge, your veins appear bigger, and your nipples may be tender or have a tingling sensation. Your nipples and areolae also enlarge and become darker. Little bumps on your areolae (called *Montgomery glands*) enlarge to produce more lubricant in preparation for breastfeeding.

Although these early pregnancy changes *feel* dramatic to you, you might not *look* much different to others or to yourself.

## Your Emotions

Finding out that you're pregnant may bring about many emotions for both you and your partner. You may be proud that you conceived a child, worried about miscarriage, hesitant to focus on the baby if awaiting genetic testing results, afraid of losing your independence, fretful about changes in your relationship, doubtful of your ability to parent, and happy about becoming parents. You may cry easily or react strongly to minor inconveniences. Your mood swings seem more pronounced, which may be difficult for you and your partner to understand. Talking with your partner and sharing your thoughts and feelings can help you work through this transition together.

# Calendar of Pregnancy: First Trimester

| Gestational Age | Six Weeks | Ten Weeks | Fourteen Weeks |
|---|---|---|---|
| Changes in baby | • About 0.1 inch long<br>• Brain and spinal column begin to form.<br>• Beginning development of gastrointestinal system, heart, and lungs.<br>• Amniotic sac envelops the preliminary tissues of entire body.<br>• Is called a blastocyst from five days to two weeks, then called an embryo. | • About 1 inch long<br>• Face is forming with simple eyes, ears, nose, mouth, and teeth buds.<br>• Arms and legs begin to move.<br>• Fingerprints are present.<br>• Brain is forming.<br>• Fetal heartbeats can be seen on ultrasound scan.<br>• External genitals begin to appear.<br>• Is called an embryo. | • About 3 inches long<br>• Weighs about 1 ounce.<br>• Can move arms, legs, fingers, and toes.<br>• Can smile, frown, suck, and swallow.<br>• Sex is distinguishable.<br>• Bone cells begin to appear.<br>• Can urinate.<br>• Heartbeat can be heard with ultrasound stethoscope.<br>• Vocal cords complete<br>• Is called a fetus. |
| Changes in placenta and uterus | • Uterus is enlarging.<br>• Uterine lining is thick, with increased blood supply.<br>• Placenta and umbilical cord are forming.<br>• Human chorionic gonadotropin (hCG) is present in mother's blood and urine. | • Uterus is size of tennis ball.<br>• Umbilical cord has definite shape.<br>• Amniotic fluid cushions fetus, maintains even temperature, and allows easy movement. | • Uterus is size of grapefruit and reaches just above pubic bone.<br>• Amniotic fluid fills uterine cavity and is continually replaced.<br>• Placenta is small but complete, with full exchange of nutrients and waste products.<br>• Placenta is major source of estrogen and progesterone. |

**First Trimester Changes** (You may experience some or all of these.)

| Common physical changes in mother | • No menstrual periods<br>• Fullness, bloating, or ache in pelvis or lower abdomen<br>• Constipation<br>• Nausea and vomiting (morning sickness)<br>• Fatigue and sleepiness<br>• Feeling faint or lightheaded. | • Frequent urination<br>• Breast changes: fullness, tenderness, tingling of nipples, darkened areolae<br>• Aversions to some foods and odors<br>• Metallic taste<br>• Increased salivation<br>• Increased vaginal secretions<br>• Weight loss or gain up to 5 pounds |
|---|---|---|
| Common emotional changes in mother | • Mood swings<br>• Greater interest in meaning of motherhood | • Increased worries about everything |
| Common emotions of father or partner | • Difficulty acknowledging pregnancy<br>• Difficulty seeing baby as real until proof by ultrasound scan or audible heartbeat | • May gain weight and experience nausea as an empathetic response to her pregnancy. |
| Common changes for both parents | • Mixed feelings about pregnancy: happy, excited, relieved, surprised, proud, anxious, scared, and/or nervous<br>• Concern about mood swings and fatigue<br>• Changes in sexual relationship<br>• Fear that sexual intercourse harms baby | • Examination of feelings toward own parents and their parenting techniques<br>• Determining parenting roles and family values<br>• Concerns about finances<br>• Concern for baby's well-being |

# Second Trimester Changes for You and Your Baby

The second trimester is the "development" period, because your baby's organs and structures begin to enlarge and mature. For you, this trimester is a time of feeling well, energetic, creative, and emotionally sensitive—often at the same time.

## THE 15TH THROUGH 27TH WEEKS OF PREGNANCY

This time marks the thirteenth through the twenty-fifth weeks of your baby's life (fifteen through twenty-seven weeks gestational age).

### Changes in Your Baby

In this trimester, your baby starts to grow hair, eyelashes, and eyebrows. Fine, downy hair (called *lanugo*) develops on her arms, legs, and back. Fingernails and toenails appear. At eighteen weeks of pregnancy, your baby can do all the movements you'll see her do as a newborn.

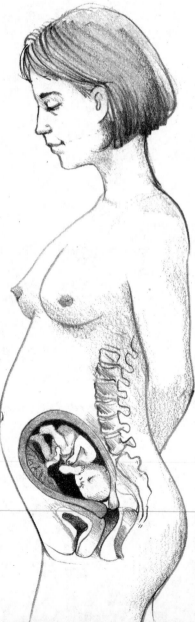

Forming in your baby's intestines is *meconium*, a collection of digestive enzymes and residue from swallowed amniotic fluid. Your baby won't expel the meconium until after birth. (When she does, it'll look like a thick, sticky, greenish-black substance.) Her skin is wrinkled and covered with a creamy protective coating called *vernix caseosa*. During this trimester, you'll probably feel your baby move for the first time (an experience called *quickening*). You may feel a light tapping or fluttering sensation that reminds you of gas bubbles. Or you might not notice your baby's gentle movements. Although still very immature, some babies born near the end of this trimester (twenty-five weeks gestational age) survive.

### Changes in the Placenta and Uterus

Your uterus expands into your abdominal cavity to accommodate your growing baby, placenta, and level of amniotic fluid. During prenatal appointments, your caregiver measures the height of your uterus to check that your baby is growing adequately. Although a baby's size and the amount of amniotic fluid differ among pregnancies, the length of your pregnancy in weeks approximates the distance in centimeters between your pubic bone and the top of your uterus (called the *fundus*). For example, at twenty-five weeks, fundal height is about 25 centimeters.

During this trimester, your uterus normally contracts periodically, although you might not notice it. Called *Braxton-Hicks contractions*, they make your uterus hard for about a minute but aren't painful. Different from labor contractions, Braxton-Hicks contractions don't cause changes in your cervix. If these contractions do cause your cervix to change and it begins to open, you're in preterm (or premature) labor and require medical attention. (See page 136.)

## Changes in You

During these middle months of pregnancy, you probably feel physically well, and your nausea and fatigue likely have disappeared or diminished. The milk glands in your breasts begin making small amounts of *colostrum* (a highly nutritious yellowish fluid produced before breast milk) by mid-pregnancy.

Just as hormonal changes make your nipples and areolae darker, they also make other skin areas more pigmented. A dark line (called linea nigra) may appear between your pubic bone and navel. The skin around your eyes may darken, especially after sun exposure. This "mask of pregnancy" (called chloasma) usually disappears within a few weeks after your baby's birth.

## Your Emotions

Along with these physical changes, you may experience a wide range of emotions. You may enjoy how your pregnant body looks and feels, or your growing body may make you feel unattractive, inconvenienced, and restricted. Heightened emotions may bolster your creativity and make you respond strongly and with more sensitivity to a kind word, a beautiful sunset, or a touching photo. Pregnancy may affect your sleep, and you may recall more of your dreams than you did before becoming pregnant. You also may become introspective and find yourself easily distracted by a need to examine your thoughts and feelings.

During this trimester, your swelling belly usually becomes more obvious, and your pregnancy becomes real and exciting for your partner, family, and friends. Now they can feel the baby wiggle or kick. Being able to see evidence of the growing baby, your partner typically feels more involved in your pregnancy and more interested in your baby. Like you, your partner may have a range of thoughts and feelings about your changing appearance and about becoming a parent. (See pages 53–57.)

Share your feelings and thoughts with your partner often, and make sure to listen when your partner shares his or her feelings with you. You need each other's support, now and in the months and years to come, as you adapt to parenthood. This trimester is a good time to start preparing for parenthood by reading books on parenting and newborn care, visiting web sites about babies, or buying baby clothes and equipment. (See page 160.)

## Different Views on the Second Trimester

Expectant mothers were asked: "What emotional changes did you notice in the second trimester?" Although there were many different views, the responses shared the following sentiments:

*I love feeling the baby move, but it's weird having a separate person inside me.*

*Pregnancy is hard because I have no control over my emotions.*

*I'm looking forward to having the baby, but I like being pregnant. I'll miss it.*

*I haven't exactly "glowed" like my friends, but pregnancy has been a lot easier since I stopped having morning sickness.*

## Calendar of Pregnancy: Second Trimester

| Gestational Age | Nineteen Weeks | Twenty-three Weeks | Twenty-seven Weeks |
|---|---|---|---|
| Changes in baby | • About 5–6 inches long<br>• Weighs about 4 ounces.<br>• Heartbeat is strong.<br>• Skin is thin, transparent.<br>• Downy hair (lanugo) covers body.<br>• Fingernails and toenails are forming.<br>• Has coordinated movements; is able to roll over. | • About 10–12 inches long (6–8 inches crown to rump)<br>• Weighs ½–1 pound.<br>• Heartbeat is audible with ordinary stethoscope.<br>• Hiccups<br>• Hair, eyelashes, eyebrows are present. | • About 11–14 inches long (9–10 inches crown to rump)<br>• Weighs 1–2 pounds.<br>• Skin is wrinkled and covered with protective coating (vernix caseosa).<br>• Eyes are open.<br>• Begins to hear.<br>• Meconium is collecting in bowel.<br>• Has strong grip. |
| Changes in placenta and uterus | • Uterus is 3 inches above pubic bone.<br>• Placenta performs nutritional, respiratory, excretory, and most hormonal functions for fetus.<br>• Amniotic fluid volume increases. | • Uterus is at level of navel.<br>• About 2–3 pints of amniotic fluid<br>• Placenta is fully developed and covers about half the inner surface of uterus. | • Uterus is above level of navel.<br>• Placenta covers less of inner surface of uterus as uterus grows.<br>• Uterus contracts periodically (Braxton-Hicks contractions), which might not be noticeable. |

**Second Trimester Changes** (You may experience some or all of these.)

| | | | |
|---|---|---|---|
| Common physical changes in mother | • Sense of well-being; increased energy<br>• Noticing movement of baby.<br>• Increased appetite<br>• Disappearance of nausea<br>• Constipation<br>• Food cravings or nonfood cravings (pica)<br>• Skin changes: linea nigra, mask of pregnancy (chloasma) | • Less tenderness in breasts<br>• Nasal congestion<br>• Bleeding gums or nosebleeds<br>• Relaxation of pelvic joints<br>• Groin pain from round-ligament contractions<br>• Leg cramps<br>• Weight gain averaging 0.8–1.0 pound per week | |
| Common emotional changes in mother | • Feeling more dependent on others.<br>• Introspective; have trouble concentrating<br>• More daydreaming and dreaming at night | • Developing sense of growth and creativity.<br>• Varying feelings about changing appearance<br>• Increased interest in babies | |
| Common emotions of father or partner | • Feelings of closeness to the baby<br>• Evaluating readiness and ability to be a parent. | • Greater involvement in pregnancy<br>• Varying feelings about partner's changing appearance | |
| Common changes for both parents | • Changes in sexual desire and activity<br>• More enjoyment of pregnancy<br>• Eager to be prepared for baby's arrival | • Increasing interest in and awareness of parenting styles | |

# Third Trimester Changes for You and Your Baby

The third trimester is the "growth" period, because your baby is growing into the size and shape of a newborn. A baby born during this time usually survives, although his chances for an easy transition to life outside the womb improve the closer his birth date is to his due date. (For more information on prematurity, see pages 291–293.)

As your body continues to expand to accommodate your growing baby, you may start looking forward to the end of pregnancy and its physical discomforts and to the long-awaited joy of holding your newborn in your arms.

## THE 28TH THROUGH 38TH WEEKS OF PREGNANCY

This time marks the twenty-sixth through thirty-sixth weeks of your baby's life (twenty-eight through thirty-eight weeks gestational age).

### Changes in Your Baby

In late pregnancy, your baby's lungs mature, and your antibodies pass through the placenta to her, providing some short-term immunity to the diseases to which you're immune.

Your baby's fingernails reach her fingertips and may even need to be cut at birth. The hair on her head grows, the lanugo on her body almost disappears, and fat is deposited under her skin. Buds for her permanent teeth appear behind her primary (baby) teeth buds.

Your baby has periods of sleep and wakefulness. She may move in response to bright light and loud noises. She hears and becomes familiar with your voice and your partner's voice, and with other sounds such as the placental circulation, your gurgling stomach, your heartbeat, and external sounds (for example, music or barking dogs). After birth, your baby will show a clear preference for a familiar voice by turning her head toward the speaker. In addition, sounds that mimic the placental sounds heard in the womb (such as the rhythmic sloshing of water in a dishwasher, the droning of a vacuum cleaner or a fan, or shushing sounds) often soothe a fussy newborn.

As your baby continues to grow and gain weight, she has less room to move around, and you may feel just her arms and legs move rather than her whole body. When your baby has hiccups, you feel a series of rhythmic jolts. At some point during the last trimester, your baby assumes a favorite position—usually head down. During prenatal visits, your caregiver determines the baby's position by feeling your abdomen using a technique called *Leopold's maneuvers*.

## Having Fun with Your Baby before Birth (after Twenty-five Weeks of Pregnancy)

- Every day, sing the same song to your baby or play him your favorite music. He'll recognize it after birth. You also may want to read the same children's book or poem aloud every day.
- Talk to your baby. Have your partner lay his or her head on your lap and "speak" to your belly. Your baby is learning to recognize your voices and may respond when he hears them.
- Press on your belly when you feel your baby's hand or foot push against your uterus. See if he responds to your touch. Try pressing twice (like double-clicking a mouse) and see if your baby mimics your action.
- Shine a flashlight on your belly. See if your baby responds to the light.

## Changes in the Placenta and Uterus

At this point in your pregnancy, changes to the system connecting you to your baby help prepare you to give birth and breastfeed. The changes also help prepare your baby for birth. (See page 165.) Your cervix softens, your uterus becomes more sensitive to oxytocin, and you notice more contractions. The volume of amniotic fluid decreases, from about 1½ quarts at seven months to about 1 quart around your due date.

## Changes in You

In this trimester, your uterus expands, possibly causing shortness of breath or sore lower ribs. High levels of progesterone and pressure from your uterus may cause indigestion, heartburn, varicose veins in your legs, hemorrhoids, or swollen ankles. You may have more backpain as your pelvic ligaments relax for birth, and your heavy uterus and growing baby change your center of gravity. (See Chapter 11 for ways to prevent and treat back pain.)

Small red bumps (called vascular spiders) may appear on the skin of your upper body, along with stretch marks (striae gravidarum) on your abdomen, thighs, or breasts. These marks are reddish during pregnancy and become glistening white lines after birth. Some women attempt to prevent stretch marks by using various lotions or oils, but no evidence shows that these products effectively work.

About two weeks before the birth, your baby "drops" into your pelvic cavity. This descent is called *engagement* or *lightening*. You may feel less pressure on your diaphragm and find breathing and eating easier. The tradeoff is, however, as the baby's head presses on your bladder, you need to urinate more frequently. Some women notice that colostrum leaks from their breasts, but some don't. Either case is normal.

## Your Emotions

In the final trimester, you may think and worry more about labor, birth, and your baby. Talk to your caregiver about your thoughts and fears, and take childbirth preparation classes. Talking to other mothers about birth can be informative and reassuring; however, some of their stories may increase your fears. The same reasoning applies to surfing the Internet for information. Be aware of sources and try to avoid scare stories and alarmist web sites. Aim to balance the points of view so you're accurately informed and not unduly upset.

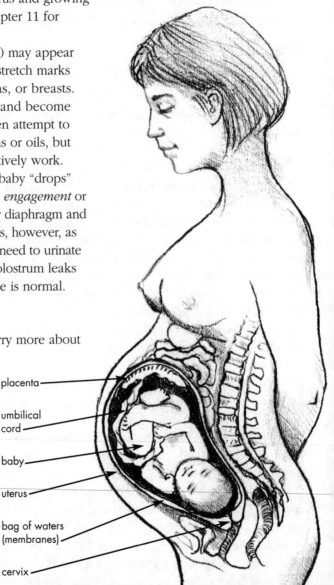

placenta

umbilical cord

baby

uterus

bag of waters (membranes)

cervix

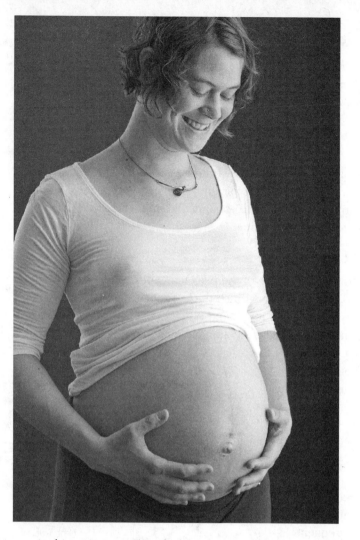

## Different Views on the Third Trimester

Expectant mothers were asked: "What emotional changes did you notice in the third trimester?" Although there were many different views, the responses shared the following sentiments:

*I'm having more loving feelings toward my baby at this time.*

*I'm more sensitive now, a little paranoid and worried—and these feelings are new and strange to me.*

*I just can't get comfortable lying in bed; sometimes I need to sleep in the recliner.*

*I have trouble getting to sleep even though I feel exhausted.*

*I feel special carrying a new life that's a combination of my partner and me.*

At this point, you may feel tired most of the time. You may get more sleep if you lean on a big body pillow or use many pillows. You also may welcome a relaxing warm bath or a soothing massage. As your belly grows and you become less agile, you may depend more on your partner and others. Your sexual relationship also may require some adjustments, due to your physical limitations. (See pages 53–54.)

As you anticipate the responsibilities of parenthood, you may begin thinking more about how your own parents raised you. You may want to follow some of your parents' techniques to raise your child, but you may want to avoid others.

You and your partner may worry about your health or your baby's well-being, especially if you develop a condition that makes your pregnancy high-risk. Know that a healthy lifestyle and early, consistent prenatal care can greatly diminish many of these conditions. If you find yourself worrying excessively, or dreaming about death or harm to you or your baby, share these fears with your partner, your caregiver, a childbirth educator, a relative, or an empathetic friend. Talking about your fears doesn't make them more likely to happen. Instead, sharing your concerns with a supportive person can comfort you and help you put your fears into perspective.

# THE 39TH AND 40TH WEEKS OF PREGNANCY

This time marks the thirty-seventh and thirty-eighth weeks of your baby's life (thirty-nine and forty weeks gestational age).

## Changes in Your Baby

In this last phase of pregnancy, your baby's organs continue to mature in preparation for life outside your uterus. He also adds fat and gains about 1 pound. A newborn averages 20 inches in length, but a range of 18 to 22 inches is normal. At birth, a baby typically weighs 7 to 7½ pounds, although a normal weight for a full-term baby can vary from 5½ to 10 pounds. From the time your baby was just a fertilized egg, his weight has increased six billion times!

## Changes in the Placenta and Uterus

Depending on the size and weight of the baby, the size of the placenta varies. Once you expel the placenta after the birth, it appears round, flat, and about 1 inch thick. The side that was implanted in your uterine wall is divided into lobes and appears rough and bloody. The side that was near your baby is smooth, pale, and shiny, and is covered by the amniotic membrane. The membranes (amniotic and chorionic) extending from the edge of the placenta formed the sac (bag of waters) that contained the amniotic fluid and your baby.

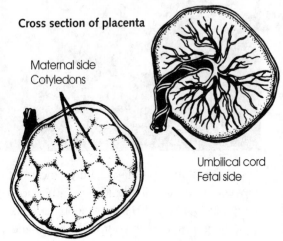

**Cross section of placenta**

Maternal side
Cotyledons

Umbilical cord
Fetal side

The moist, white umbilical cord contains two arteries and one vein. Often twisted like a corkscrew, the umbilical cord measures 12 to 39 inches when pulled straight. At birth, when your baby breathes, her circulation pattern begins to change. Blood flow through her umbilical cord shuts down and more blood flows to her lungs.

Toward the end of pregnancy, prelabor uterine contractions become more obvious and frequent. These contractions enhance circulation in your uterus, press your baby against your cervix, and work with prostaglandins to soften and thin your cervix.

## Changes in You

At this point, you may be looking forward to the end of pregnancy. You may be fed up with the light sleep, fatigue, and other typical discomforts of late pregnancy. At times, you may feel as though you'll be pregnant forever! Visits to your caregiver, childbirth preparation classes, baby showers, nursery preparation, and other common late pregnancy activities should help you realize that your baby is coming soon and a new stage in your life will begin.

# The 41st Week of Pregnancy and Beyond: Post-dates

This time marks the thirty-ninth week (and beyond) of your baby's life in the womb (at least forty-one weeks gestational age).

Although the average length of pregnancy is forty weeks, many pregnancies last longer and are considered *post-date*. Some post-date pregnancies are cases of mistaken due dates; others involve babies who need more time to grow and mature. Occasionally, the baby is ready to be born, but for unexplained reasons, labor doesn't begin.

In a post-date pregnancy, a caregiver determines whether the baby and placenta are healthy by performing specific diagnostic tests. (See Chapter 7.) If all is well, pregnancy can continue until labor begins on its own.

## Changes in Your Baby

Even if your pregnancy lasts beyond your due date, your baby might not be *post-mature*—that is, he doesn't have symptoms such as an absence of lanugo; scant vernix caseosa; long fingernails and toenails; dry, peeling, or cracked skin; and unusual alertness at birth. True post-maturity is rare even in babies born two weeks after their due dates.

If your baby is not post-mature, he's taking the extra time he needs to grow and prepare for life outside your womb.

## Changes in the Placenta

In many post-date pregnancies, the placenta continues to support the growth and well-being of the baby.

In rare cases when the baby is truly post-mature, tests reveal that the placenta isn't functioning as well, that the volume of amniotic fluid is dropping, and that the baby is showing signs of distress. Under these circumstances, the baby's health can't wait for labor to begin on its own, and the caregiver either induces labor or performs a cesarean section.

## Changes in You and Your Emotions

Physically, you may continue feeling much as you did during late pregnancy. Emotionally, however, you may find waiting for labor to begin frustrating, worrisome, or depressing. Consider trying self-induction methods that may encourage labor to begin. (See pages 277–279.)

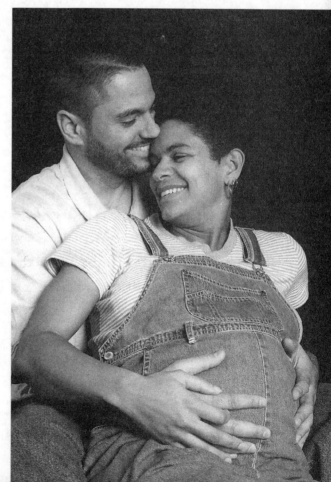

# Calendar of Pregnancy: Third Trimester

| Gestational Age | Thirty-one Weeks | Thirty-five Weeks | Thirty-eight to Forty-two Weeks |
|---|---|---|---|
| Changes in baby | • 14–17 inches long (11–12 inches crown to rump)<br>• Weighs 2½–4 pounds.<br>• Is adding body fat.<br>• Is very active.<br>• Breathing movements are present.<br>• Responds to sound. | • 16½–18 inches long (12–13 inches crown to rump)<br>• Weighs 4–6 pounds.<br>• Has periods of sleep and wakefulness.<br>• May assume birth position.<br>• Bones of head are soft and flexible.<br>• Stores iron in liver. | • 19–21 inches long (13–15 inches crown to rump)<br>• Weighs 6–8 pounds.<br>• More body fat and skin is less wrinkled.<br>• Lanugo is mostly gone.<br>• Vernix caseosa is thick.<br>• Lungs are mature.<br>• Is rapidly gaining antibodies from mother.<br>• In birth position<br>• May descend or "drop" into pelvis (engagement). |
| Changes in placenta and uterus | • Uterus is three finger-breadths above navel. | • Uterus is just below breastbone and ribs.<br>• Uterine contractions (Braxton-Hicks) are more frequent. | • Placenta is 6–8 inches in diameter, 1 inch thick, and about 1 pound.<br>• More frequent uterine contractions<br>• Cervix is softening (ripening) and thinning (effacing).<br>• Amniotic fluid volume is decreasing. |

**Third Trimester Changes** (You may notice some or all of these.)

| | | |
|---|---|---|
| Common physical changes in mother | • Heartburn or indigestion<br>• Shortness of breath<br>• Soreness in lower ribs<br>• Urinary urgency and frequency (not painful urination)<br>• Tingling or numbness in hands<br>• Stretch marks; abdominal itching<br>• Increased perspiration and feeling warmer<br>• Increased colostrum | • Backache<br>• Changes in balance and agility<br>• Light sleep or insomnia<br>• Vascular spiders<br>• Hemorrhoids<br>• Varicose veins<br>• Swollen ankles<br>• Anemia<br>• Total weight gain of 25–35 pounds |
| Common emotional changes in mother | • Excitement and doubts about readiness for baby<br>• Focus on labor and birth, fear of childbirth pain, anxiety about the unknown<br>• Variety of feelings about body changes<br>• Feelings of clumsiness<br>• Difficulty in focusing attention | • Increased dependency on others; desire for protection<br>• Decreased sexual interest<br>• Increased attention from family and friends may be enjoyable at times, tiresome at others<br>• Relief that pregnancy is almost over |
| Common emotions of father or partner | • Protectiveness toward family<br>• Anticipation of parenthood<br>• Fear for health of mother and baby during childbirth<br>• Anxiety over support role in labor | • Longing for relationship to return to normal<br>• Frustration about inability to "fix" partner's discomforts<br>• Worries when something is wrong |
| Common changes for both parents | • Continuing changes in sexual relationship<br>• Fear of harm to baby during sexual activity<br>• Excitement about baby's arrival<br>• Emotional and mental preparation for birth<br>• Eagerness for pregnancy to end | • Choosing names for the baby<br>• Worries about labor pain and responsibilities of parenthood<br>• Simultaneous feelings of anticipation, exhilaration, excitement, and apprehension |

# Common Concerns and Considerations in Pregnancy

The following are typical concerns of pregnant women. Some apply only to women in specific situations. Others are of concern to all.

## AGE OF THE MOTHER

In general, women between the ages of eighteen and thirty-five have few problems in pregnancy. Girls in their early teens and women over age forty may face more pregnancy risks; however, a healthy pregnant woman of any age is likely to have a healthy baby.

### Teenage Pregnancy

If you're a pregnant teenager, you have several strengths and some special needs. A teenager's body is usually fit, and your chances of a healthy pregnancy are good. Because you're young, your uterus is probably strong and your tissues are stretchy. Your labor will likely progress normally and won't need medical interventions.

Because your body is still developing, you must eat well during pregnancy to properly nourish you and your growing baby. Just like every pregnant woman, you need to stay away from drugs, alcohol, and tobacco. Make sure you keep your scheduled prenatal appointments with your caregiver. Taking these steps helps prevent giving birth too early and delivering a baby with low birth weight—the main problems for teen pregnancies.

Some challenges of being a pregnant teenager include:

- Dealing with your parents' reactions to your pregnancy
- Working with your baby's father to address his role and responsibilities
- Attending school with peers who can't relate to your situation
- Deciding whether to keep your baby or consider adoption
- Making decisions about your health care

You can work through these challenges by talking with a school counselor, a city or county health nurse, someone at a pregnancy counseling organization or the YWCA, or understanding friends and family members.

### Pregnancy after Age Thirty-five

More than ever before, women in their thirties and forties are giving birth, many for the first time. Between 1980 and 2004, the birth rate in the United States increased twofold for women in their early thirties, threefold for women older than thirty-four, and fourfold for women forty and older. As an older woman, you may have delayed pregnancy for various reasons such as career or education priorities, financial considerations, infertility, or lack of a partner.

## Advice from the Authors

Pregnant teenagers have unique needs and may require resources geared toward them. Here are some great books on teenage pregnancy:

- *Life Interrupted: The Scoop on Being a Young Mom* by Tricia Goyer (2004). Practical help on juggling school and single parenthood.
- *Your Pregnancy & Newborn Journey: A Guide for Pregnant Teens* by Jeanne Warren Lindsay and Jean Brunelli (2004). Easy-to-read guide on pregnancy.
- *The Unplanned Pregnancy Book for Teens and College Students* by Dorrie Williams-Wheeler (2004). Stories by young women, helpful resources, and useful strategies.

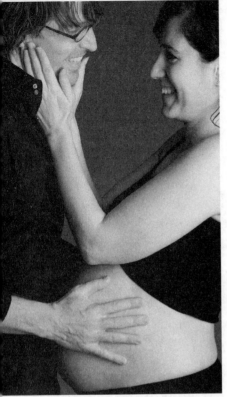

When compared to a younger pregnant woman, your risk of having the following problems is higher: high blood pressure, gestational diabetes, growth problems or inherited disorders in the baby, preterm labor, problems with the placenta, fibroids, labor complications, and cesarean birth.

Why are you at greater risk of having these problems? The answer is simple: The longer a woman lives, the more likely poor health practices, accidents, illnesses, or environmental hazards have affected her body. Also, high blood pressure and diabetes (the two most common risks for older pregnant women) are disorders that increase with one's age.

Despite these possible age-related complications, you're less likely to develop problems in your pregnancy if you've enjoyed good health and taken care of yourself over the years.

As you age, infertility problems increase. If you used fertility drugs or treatments to get pregnant, you may be pregnant with more than one baby. If this is the case, you'll experience many of the same pregnancy risks as women having multiples.

Your risk of problems in pregnancy varies depending on the number of children you've borne. In one study, researchers found that first-time mothers (primiparas) who were older had increased risks of preterm labor, excessive bleeding, or cesarean birth. But pregnant mothers who had birthed before (multiparas) and were older had increased risks of diabetes and chronic or gestational hypertension.[2]

Older women are more likely than younger women to be pregnant with a baby with a genetic disorder such as Down syndrome. Another potential risk factor is the age of the baby's father. The risk of Down syndrome increases for babies whose fathers are older than thirty-five at conception; the risk further increases if both parents are older than thirty-five. In addition, babies whose fathers are older than forty at conception have an increased risk of certain rare congenital disorders such as dwarfism.

Various screening and diagnostic tests offered in early pregnancy can detect these conditions. (See pages 67 and 277.) Because the risk of genetic disorders gradually increases as a woman ages, caregivers typically use thirty-five as the starting age to recommend testing. At this age, the potential benefits from invasive tests, such as amniocentesis and chorionic villus sampling (CVS), begin to outweigh the risks. Now that more noninvasive screening tests are available (such as ultrasound scans and blood tests), younger women are also offered these tests.

As an older pregnant woman, your age and experiences may affect your attitude toward pregnancy. If you have a history of infertility or miscarriage, you may feel vulnerable. You may seek reassurance that your baby is normal and healthy by undergoing numerous tests and procedures designed to detect and treat problems. Be aware that some women find the testing process stressful, especially because the tests don't always give clear results and thus lead to more testing. (See Chapter 7.)

If you're thirty-five or older, what can you do to improve your chances for a healthy pregnancy and baby? Unless you have a preexisting health problem such as high blood pressure or diabetes, you should do what any well-informed pregnant woman does: Take good care of yourself, reduce stress, and have regular prenatal visits with a caring and competent caregiver. Although some problems may arise during your pregnancy, they're almost always treatable or manageable. In fact, most women over age thirty-five give birth to healthy, full-term babies.

## EXPECTING MULTIPLES: TWINS, TRIPLETS, OR MORE

Most often a woman discovers that she's pregnant with *multiples* when an ultrasound scan reveals two or more babies. Your caregiver may suspect a multiple pregnancy if he or she hears two or more heartbeats or if your uterus seems to be growing faster than normal. A comprehensive ultrasound scan confirms a multiple pregnancy.

Twins account for about 3 percent of all births. Although just one-fifth of 1 percent of births results in triplets or more, their incidence has increased in recent years.

A woman pregnant with more than one baby has an increased risk of preterm birth, and thus premature babies. Prematurity causes most problems for multiples. Thankfully, improved medical care for women expecting multiples has helped decrease the risk of preterm birth of extremely small and immature babies.

If you're expecting multiples, you may be both excited and stressed out. Growing more than one baby requires more energy, so you'll probably need to consume more calories and rest more often because of discomfort, fatigue, and the increased risk of preterm labor.

Because birthing multiples is often more complicated than birthing one baby, the chance of cesarean birth rises with the number of babies you're expecting. You may need the care of an obstetrician or a perinatologist. In addition to the increased medical attention, you can also expect more attention from your friends and relatives during your pregnancy. Friends and family usually offer new parents more help in the weeks after the birth of multiples. Be sure to take advantage of any such offer! See Appendix C for a list of resources for parents of multiples.

## SEX DURING PREGNANCY

For most couples, pregnancy changes their sexual relationship, but how it changes isn't the same for every couple. While one pregnant woman may feel clumsy and fat, another may feel ripe, beautiful, and sexual. One woman may feel sick and uncomfortable, while another feels radiant and wonderful. One woman may be alone or in a difficult or abusive relationship, while another may feel secure in a loving relationship. One woman's partner may find the woman's growing belly a turnoff, while another relishes her gorgeous appearance.

## Fact or Fiction?

*The only chance a woman has of conceiving multiples is if multiples run in her family or the baby's father's family.*
**Fiction.** A woman also increases the likelihood of becoming pregnant with multiples if she:

- Is large and tall.
- Is older than thirty-five.
- Is Caucasian or African-American. (Multiples are less common in Asian and Hispanic women.)
- Had at least one other pregnancy.
- Used fertility drugs that increase the number of eggs released during ovulation.
- Had more than one egg implanted during procedures, such as in vitro fertilization.

Most of these factors affect only the rate of fraternal twins, triplets, or higher-order multiples, because the occurrence of identical siblings is an unpredictable and random event.

As your pregnancy progresses, you can expect your sex life to have its ups and downs. For some women in the first trimester, hormonal changes and increased blood flow to pelvic organs (plus, no worries about getting pregnant) increase a desire for sex. For other women, experiencing symptoms such as nausea, vomiting, fatigue, and breast tenderness decrease libido.

During the second trimester, many women notice a stronger libido and experience more sexual pleasure than in the other trimesters. At this stage of pregnancy, many women experience fewer physical discomforts, have more energy, and may be enjoying their new curvy bodies.

In the last trimester many women notice a decreased desire for sexual intercourse, likely because of their bigger bellies and increasing fatigue. If you share this feeling, it's helpful to remember that sex doesn't always mean sexual intercourse. There are other ways you and your partner can stimulate and pleasure each other. Use your imagination and explore new ways to be sensual. *Note:* Avoid having your partner blow air into your vagina. This practice can produce an air embolus (air bubble) in your blood, a potentially fatal condition.

How safe is sex during pregnancy? In general, it's safe; however, your caregiver may suggest that you avoid intercourse for the following high-risk reasons:

- You're at risk for preterm labor (or you're expecting multiples).
- Your partner has a sexually transmitted infection (STI).
- You have placenta previa (low-lying placenta).
- You have an incompetent cervix (one that opens early), which may be the result of previous cervical surgery.
- You have vaginal bleeding during pregnancy (though spotting after intercourse in the first month of pregnancy might not be a complication).
- You have continuing or painful cramps after intercourse.
- Your membranes have ruptured.

If you're not at risk, most caregivers recommend having sex as often as you desire. Uterine contractions are a normal part of having an orgasm and don't harm a healthy pregnancy or baby. Remember that the sealed, fluid-filled amniotic sac cushions and protects your baby from outside forces and elements. If you experience discomfort during sexual intercourse, try positions that don't put your partner's weight on your belly (side-lying, hands-and-knees, or woman on top) or try gentle, shallow penetration.

As your feelings about sex fluctuate throughout pregnancy, your partner might or might not understand or accept them, which can create tension in your relationship. To help prevent long-term problems, keep the lines of communication open. Working through these changes in your sexual relationship can help you prepare for future challenges in your sex life after the birth.

# A Note to Expectant Fathers*

Waiting for fatherhood is a unique emotional experience that's just as meaningful as waiting for motherhood. You may have never felt so important yet so ignored, so committed yet so abandoned, and so deeply in love and sexual yet so afraid of sex. Sharing these feelings with your pregnant partner or close friends may help you through this exciting but challenging time. Consider talking with other expectant fathers (casually or in a discussion group) to help you understand and develop your unique role during the pregnancy and birth, and as a parent.

* Other expectant parents will experience many of the same emotions that expectant fathers feel. See page 57 for further discussion on nontraditional families.

# THE REALITY OF YOUR BABY

During the first trimester, it's difficult to see many physical changes in your pregnant partner, and you might not yet think of your baby as real. When your partner's pregnancy is around sixteen to twenty weeks along, however, changes in her body become obvious and you may begin to feel your baby move inside her. You may even see the bulge of a foot or elbow on her abdomen. Like many expectant fathers, you may fully comprehend your baby's existence when you see her during an ultrasound scan and hear her heartbeat. Plan to be at the appointments when these exams are done.

Although some men emotionally connect with their babies during pregnancy, many men don't begin to attach to their babies until after the birth. Some fall in love upon first seeing their newborns, while others grow to love their babies more gradually over the first months.[3]

# EXCITEMENT, STRESS, AND WORRIES OF BECOMING A FATHER

On one hand, expecting a child may bring you pride and fulfillment because you're creating another generation of your family. On the other hand, you may worry about the health of your partner and baby. It's interesting that many men find life during pregnancy more stressful than life with a newborn. This may be because seeing a healthy mother and baby reduces anxiety and makes parenthood a reality.

If you have worries during the pregnancy, use them as motivation to improve the health of your growing family. You and your partner can eat nutritious foods, avoid potentially risky activities or exposure to illness, and improve your lifestyle.

With a new life soon to come, you may begin to reflect on your own mortality. You may decide to buy more life insurance and write or update your will. One expectant father began riding his motorcycle with a helmet; another quit his job in high-rise construction to take one in a safer trade. These actions show an interest in being present for the baby and providing for him as much as possible.

During pregnancy, some men experience empathy symptoms, which mimic their partners' physical symptoms or discomforts. These include weight gain, food cravings, abdominal cramps or bloating, nausea, vomiting, backaches, toothaches, loss of appetite, and insomnia. If any physical changes or problems concern you, make an appointment with your caregiver for a checkup.

# INCREASED RESPONSIBILITY OF FATHERHOOD

When contemplating fatherhood, many men fear losing their freedom and independence; some feel they've already lost both. To these men, becoming a father means becoming a responsible, mature adult. For example, earning a steady or higher income may become a priority, especially if financial concerns arise. If the duties and responsibilities of impending parenthood overwhelm you, talk to

## Different Views of Expectant Fathers

Expectant fathers were asked: "How did you feel when the pregnancy test was positive?" Some one-word responses included: *excited, relieved, happy, anxious, surprised,* and *proud.* Many men had mixed feelings:

*When we found out we're going to have a baby, I felt terror and excitement.*

*Though I'm excited, I worry about money.*

*I'm happy, but I worry about losing my freedom.*

your partner about your feelings. Together you may be able to create a plan for reducing expenses or increasing your income. You can also begin developing realistic expectations of your role as a parent and provider.

## CHANGES IN YOUR RELATIONSHIP

As your partner focuses on her pregnancy and becomes more preoccupied with your baby's arrival, you may feel left out at times. You may feel displaced if others focus more on her than you, and if she turns to friends and relatives instead of you for emotional support. You may feel that you're expected to care more for her and your relationship, but that she's less available to you emotionally, physically, and sexually. To further complicate matters, you may feel guilty for any resentment or lack of enthusiasm you have about the pregnancy. One way to deal with these emotions is to talk with a friend or relative who has felt the same way. It's also important to share these feelings with your partner; she may be unaware of them and able to help put your mind at ease.

## YOUR ROLE DURING LABOR AND BIRTH

All expectant fathers wonder how they'll perform during labor and birth. They may think, "Will I faint at the sight of blood? Can I handle watching my partner experience pain?" To boost your confidence and prepare for your role during this exciting event, take a childbirth preparation class, watch DVDs or read books on childbirth, and discuss any worries you may have with other fathers and your partner. Also consider having a friend, relative, or doula at the birth to offer additional guidance and help you support your partner. (See page 190.)

## YOUR ROLE AS A FATHER

As the birth of your baby approaches, you may wonder what kind of father you'll be. You may wonder whether you'll act as your own father had when you were a child. You may have already decided that you want to be more emotionally and physically involved with your baby than your father had been with you.

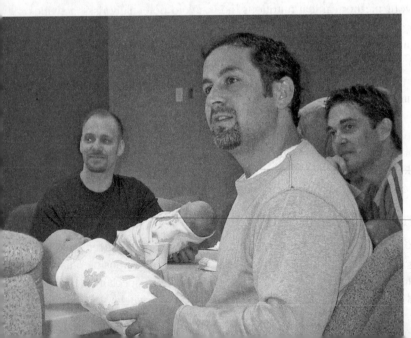

Research shows that certain hormone levels in expectant fathers change during pregnancy. Fathers-to-be have lower levels of testosterone and cortisol and higher levels of estradiol than men who aren't expecting babies. These hormonal changes may explain why many expectant fathers have more caring and nurturing feelings than they had before learning they're to become parents.[4]

The following suggestions may help you adjust to your new role:

- Learn about the normal development and behavior of newborns by reading books on the subject and attending your baby's well-baby checkups.
- Talk with other new fathers about what to realistically expect during the first weeks after the birth.
- After the birth, be prepared for changes in your daily activities. Consider your priorities and those of your family, and create strategies to care for your baby, maintain your relationship with your partner, and find time for yourself.
- Determine how you can get the help that you and your partner will need after the birth.
- Think about how you can care for your new baby (such as holding, rocking, diapering, comforting, or playing with him) and learn more about those skills.
- Plan on having the most amazing adventure in the weeks and months ahead!

# Nontraditional Families

All kinds of relationships make up today's families. The traditional nuclear family (father, mother, and their biological offspring) is no longer the norm. Despite this fact, culture and customs have been slow to acknowledge the changing family structure, and society seems to offer little guidance and support to nontraditional families. While parents in nontraditional families face many of the challenges that all parents face, they also may tackle puzzling or troubling situations.

## IF YOUR PARTNER ISN'T THE BABY'S BIOLOGICAL PARENT

If your partner isn't the baby's biological parent, he or she may feel that the pregnancy is "yours," not "ours." Your partner may question his or her role in making decisions and providing financial support for your growing family. If the baby's biological father is involved in the pregnancy, your partner may feel even less sure about his or her role.

Strangers, acquaintances, friends, relatives—and even you—likely have misplaced or unrealistic expectations and assumptions about your nontraditional family that further challenge your relationship with your partner and with the baby.

## Resources for Expectant Fathers

*Books*

- *The Birth Partner: A Complete Guide to Childbirth for Dads, Doulas, and All Other Labor Companions* by Penny Simkin (2008). Skillfully explains what's involved in the support role during late pregnancy, birth, and afterward.
- *The Expectant Father: Facts, Tips, and Advice for Dads-to-Be* by Armin A. Brott (2001). Information-packed guide to the emotional, financial, and physical changes the father-to-be may experience during the course of his partner's pregnancy.
- *Father's First Steps: 25 Things Every New Dad Should Know* by Robert W. Sears and James M. Sears (2006). Discusses labor support, new fatherhood, bonding with baby, understanding baby talk, and being a good partner and father.
- *The New Dad's Survival Guide: Man-to-Man Advice for First-Time Fathers* by Scott Mactavish (2005). Humorous guide to basic parenting skills, from birth through three months. Its military references might not appeal to some readers.

*Classes*

Classes for dads-to-be focus on learning the basic skills of baby care and fatherhood. Look for Conscious Fathering classes, Boot Camp for New Dads, or another program in your area.

If you're in a lesbian relationship with your partner, the law doesn't sanction your roles as parents to the same extent that it does for married heterosexual couples. Try to seek out the empathy and support of other lesbian parents to help define your roles as two mothers. For example, will one or both of you return to work after a maternity leave? Does your partner want to adopt the baby? What role will the biological father play, if any?

If you're in a heterosexual relationship with someone new since becoming pregnant, the roles and relationships among you, your partner, and the baby's father may be tense or unclear. For example, who will accompany you to prenatal appointments and who will be with you during the labor and birth?

If you conceived your baby with a donor egg or sperm, you or your partner may have difficulty coming to terms with the fact that the baby isn't the biological offspring of one or both of you.

You and your partner can overcome challenges such as these and build a strong and loving family, but it requires creativity, honesty, and respect for each other and the baby. See Appendix C for a list of resources that offer nontraditional families support and advice.

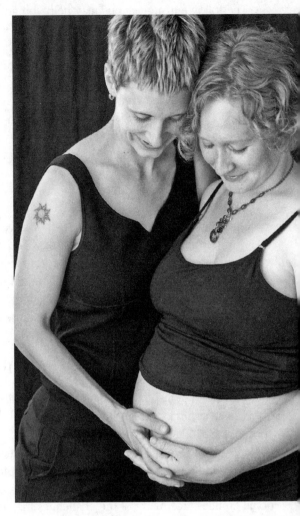

## IF YOU'RE PREGNANT AND SINGLE

If you're pregnant and single, you face a different set of challenges. Although single parenthood is common today, society often offers single parents little support. For example, you may notice that not everyone reacts positively to your pregnancy.

As a single parent, you take on a role usually shared by two people. Parenting is hard work, and at times you may be relieved that you don't have to deal with the added burden of an incompatible partner. But there may be times when you doubt whether you can—or want to—parent alone. You may feel vulnerable or lonely and wish for the companionship and support of a reliable partner. At these times, it's best to reach out to others for help.

If your baby's biological father chooses not to be involved in your baby's life, you have options. You can agree to parent alone, with or without his financial help. Or you can take legal action to confirm his paternity and compel him to provide child support. If you choose this option, you need to create a plan that specifies his involvement in your baby's life.

# Special Challenges in Pregnancy

For some women, past traumatic experiences can present additional challenges in pregnancy. With the proper care and support of trusted caregivers, family, and friends, these women can have positive and healthy pregnancies and childbirth experiences.

## HISTORY OF CHILDHOOD TRAUMA

Early childhood trauma sometimes causes unexpected reactions during pregnancy, birth, or afterward. Women who are physically, sexually, or emotionally abused as adults can also experience these reactions. Some are surprised by their feelings; others know the effects can continue long after the abuse stops. A woman abused as a child learned some long-lasting, damaging lessons about herself and others. For example, many abused women have difficulty trusting others, especially those in authority (such as physicians or midwives).

It's estimated that 25 to 40 percent of women were sexually, physically, or emotionally abused in childhood,[5] so it's not surprising that many survivors (though not all, as it's impossible to generalize the effects of abuse) experience some of the following aftereffects during pregnancy, birth, or afterward.

- A survivor may find vaginal exams, nakedness, or the prospect of a baby coming through her vagina extremely disturbing or even intolerable.
- She may respond to the inevitable loss of control over her body that occurs in labor in the same way she had as a child, when she was helpless to stop her abuser from hurting her.
- She may equate the thought of giving another person total access to her breasts, even for breastfeeding, to her inability to prevent her abuser's violation of her body.

The extent of these problems varies and many factors influence them, including the nature of the abuse, the age at which it occurred, how long it lasted, and the presence or absence of other loving and trustworthy adults in her life. Psychotherapy and emotional support promote healing and help survivors find positive ways to deal with past childhood abuse.

Some caregivers and childbirth educators are more aware than others about the impact of child abuse in adulthood. With empathy and understanding, these professionals can help pregnant survivors have safe, satisfying childbirth experiences and a less stressful postpartum period. If you're an abuse survivor and you trust your caregiver, you may choose to disclose your history of abuse and explain how you think it's affecting your feelings about your body, your baby, the upcoming labor, and your important relationships. If your caregiver has experience working with survivors, he or she may be able to help you address your concerns and communicate them in a birth plan. See Appendix C for a list of resources for survivors of childhood abuse.

## PREGNANCY AFTER A PREVIOUS MISCARRIAGE OR STILLBIRTH

If you've lost a baby during a previous pregnancy or at birth, becoming pregnant again can bring about a wide range of emotions. You may have trouble getting excited about your pregnancy because you fear that you may lose another baby. You may be relieved that you're pregnant again and are hopeful for a healthy pregnancy. You may find that it's easier to remain emotionally detached until you have passed the point in your pregnancy when your last baby died. Or you might not want to become attached to your baby at all until after the birth, when you can see and hear your healthy newborn.

## Common Q & A

**Q:** My previous pregnancy ended in a miscarriage. I worry this pregnancy will end the same way or in a stillbirth. What can I do to help ease my fear?

**A:** After you've suffered the loss of a baby, it's normal to be anxious and worried when you're pregnant again. Consult with your caregiver about the reason for the loss and find out if there's anything you can do this time to ensure a healthy pregnancy. To help put your fears into perspective and focus on the positive, talk with other couples who have lost babies to miscarriage or stillbirth, or with supportive friends and family.

For further information, read these books on pregnancy after a previous loss:

- *Pregnancy after a Loss: A Guide to Pregnancy after a Miscarriage, Stillbirth, or Infant Death* by Carol Cirulli Lanham (1999)
- *Trying Again: A Guide to Pregnancy After Miscarriage, Stillbirth, and Infant Loss* by Ann Douglas, John R. Sussman, and Deborah Davis (2000)

Knowing why a previous pregnancy ended in miscarriage or stillbirth may help you and your caregiver plan for a healthier pregnancy this time. Your caregiver may attempt to diminish your fears by offering more prenatal testing (see page 277), or you may request extra testing yourself to help manage your fears. Another way to help relieve your anxiety is to closely watch your baby's health. For example, you may monitor the baby's activity by counting his movements during a set time. (See page 69.)

Just as each person experiences grief and loss differently, each expectant parent has unique feelings about a pregnancy after a loss. Most people find it helpful to talk with family members, friends, grief counselors, and medical professionals about their feelings and fears. By sharing your concerns with others, you and your partner may learn how to put your grief into perspective and reduce your worries.

## PREGNANCY AND DISABILITY

If you have any physical challenges, you may need extra support with adapting to the changes of pregnancy. What you will need depends on the nature of your disability. You may benefit from a consultation with a physical therapist or occupational therapist, or from connecting with other women with your disability who have managed pregnancy and parenting. (Try searching for online discussion forums to make connections.) Take childbirth preparation classes—although the instructor might not have worked with anyone with your disability before, she can demonstrate ideas that work for many women, and you can figure out how to adapt them to your own needs and abilities.

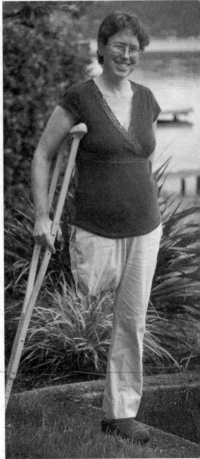

# Key Points to Remember

- Pregnancy lasts about forty weeks from the date of the first day of your last menstrual period. (Ovulation usually takes place about two weeks after your period begins, and for conception to occur, it must happen within twelve to twenty-four hours after ovulation.)
- Normal pregnancies vary in length, so due dates are approximate. Expect your baby to be born any time from two weeks before to two weeks after your due date.
- Pregnancy is divided into three trimesters. The first trimester is your baby's "formation" period, the second is the "development" period, and the third is the "growth" period.
- For better or worse, your previous experiences can affect your feelings about pregnancy and birth. Talking with someone about your circumstances can help you have a more positive and satisfying pregnancy and childbirth experience.

# CHAPTER 4

# Having a Healthy Pregnancy

To have a healthy, safe, and enjoyable pregnancy, it's important to eat well, get enough exercise and rest, and make positive lifestyle choices. It's also essential to have regular prenatal care by a maternity caregiver and to avoid hazards and situations that can harm you or your baby during pregnancy. This chapter discusses the ways you can help prevent pregnancy problems by working with your caregiver, taking care of yourself, and limiting your exposure to potentially harmful substances and circumstances.

Ideally, you began avoiding hazards and consulting with a health care professional *before* you became pregnant. However, getting pregnant might have been a surprise to you. Whether you've planned for this pregnancy or not, you can use the information in this chapter to improve your health and increase your chances of having a healthy pregnancy and baby.

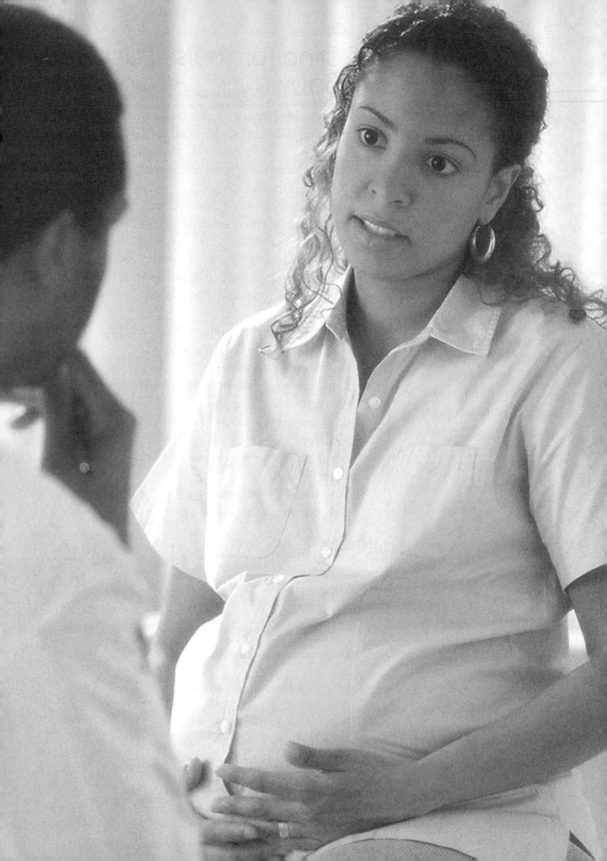

# Caring for Yourself and Your Baby during Pregnancy

Having a healthy lifestyle during pregnancy can benefit not only your physical and mental condition, but also your baby's well-being.

Here's a list of things you can do to stay healthy throughout your pregnancy:

- Attend regular prenatal care appointments with your caregiver to monitor your health and your baby's well-being. (See page 65.)
- Learn the warning signs of pregnancy complications to know when to get medical advice and care. (See page 70.)
- Eat nutritious foods and gain a healthy amount of weight. (See Chapter 6.)
- Maintain your general fitness to stay comfortable as your body changes. (See Chapter 5.)
- Reduce harmful stresses in your life. (See page 71.)
- To relieve symptoms of common ailments and pregnancy discomforts, use safe alternatives to medications. (For home remedies and tips to relieve common discomforts, see pages 73–74.)
- Avoid harmful substances and exposure to hazards. (See pages 76–84.)
- Treat harmful conditions and illnesses before pregnancy and those that develop during pregnancy. (See Chapter 7.)

## A NOTE TO FATHERS AND PARTNERS

Your compassion, care, and encouragement are critical to your partner's well-being during pregnancy. You can help your partner by encouraging her to have a healthy lifestyle. Support her efforts by making healthy changes to your lifestyle as well. For example, if you smoke, you can quit so your partner (and your baby) avoids the harmful effects of secondhand smoke. You can also strive to exercise regularly and avoid consuming unsafe foods and substances.

Get involved in your partner's pregnancy. Attend some or all prenatal appointments, show an interest in prenatal tests and their results, and learn the warnings signs of pregnancy complications (see page 70). Help reduce your partner's pregnancy discomforts by doing the laborious household chores and assisting her with comfort measures (see pages 103–107). If she's upset or distressed, discover what's bothering her and help alleviate anxiety. Review the stress-coping skills discussed on page 72 for ways to decrease your own stress. Because pregnancy can strain a couple's relationship, you may need counseling to help resolve any family problems.

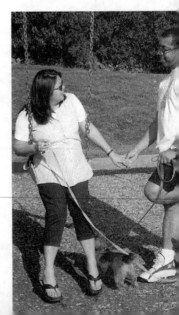

# Prenatal Care

When you know (or strongly suspect) you're pregnant, schedule a visit with your caregiver. (See page 15 for information on the different types of maternity caregivers.) The wait to get an appointment with some caregivers can be several weeks, so call promptly.

Before your first prenatal visit, start making healthy lifestyle changes, such as quitting smoking, avoiding alcohol, eating nutritious foods, and taking folic acid. Consider having your partner accompany you to prenatal appointments so he or she can discuss his or her role at the birth with your caregiver. Visit our web site, http://www.PCNGuide.com, to download a work sheet to bring to appointments.

At your first or second prenatal visit, your caregiver will likely give you a complete physical examination and administer numerous tests. Your caregiver (or an office nurse) will also ask questions about your current life situation and family medical history. At each prenatal appointment, your caregiver will monitor your health and your baby's growth. In midpregnancy, you'll usually have an appointment scheduled for every month. Toward the end of your pregnancy, you'll have an appointment every two weeks, then every week as your due date approaches.

Some caregivers schedule brief appointments; others schedule longer visits so you have time to build a relationship and discuss concerns and questions you may have. If you want a longer appointment than usual, request one in advance.

Toward the end of your pregnancy, schedule a long visit to talk about your birth plan with your caregiver. (See Chapter 8.) Also, if your caregiver is part of a group, try to meet the others in the practice in case one of them is on call when you're in labor. If meeting the others isn't possible, a written birth plan can communicate your specific birth preferences and help introduce you to unfamiliar care providers.

## PRENATAL TESTS

Throughout your pregnancy, your caregiver will offer you routine screening tests and diagnostic tests to detect possible problems with your health or your baby's.

A *screening test* is a quick, easy, and inexpensive way to rule out a particular condition. If the results of your test are negative, you don't have the condition. If the results are positive, you may need further testing to confirm that you have the condition. If additional testing determines you don't have the condition, your screening test gave a "false positive" reading. For inclusion in standard practice, screening tests must have a minimal "false negative" rate; that is, they must be unlikely to miss detecting someone who has the condition. (See pages 67–68 for a list of routine screening tests.)

A *diagnostic test* is more specific and more reliable than a screening test in identifying women with a pregnancy complication or a baby with a problem. Diagnostic tests are often more invasive, more expensive, and usually have more side effects than routine screening tests. As a result, most

## What Information Should I Include in My Medical History?

Your caregiver can provide better prenatal care when he or she is aware of any of the following potentially troubling health or social problems concerning you, your partner, and your families.

- Prior surgeries or illnesses that required medical treatment
- Hereditary conditions or illnesses, including birth defects (such as heart defects), mental retardation, blindness, deafness, stillbirths, and miscarriages
- Prior or current behavioral or mental health conditions, such as depression or eating disorders
- Ethnic or cultural traditions that may affect prenatal care, birth procedures, and postpartum care
- Current prescription medications, drug allergies, and drug reactions
- Prior negative experience with a hospitalization, caregiver, or illness (All may influence your responses to care or medical procedures.)
- Prior sexual abuse, domestic violence, or any other significant mistreatment
- Heavy use of alcohol, tobacco, recreational drugs, or other harmful substances

caregivers use diagnostic tests only if indicated by a positive screening test or other pertinent factors. (See pages 143–145 for more information on diagnostic tests.)

Prenatal tests are reassuring when the results indicate a normal pregnancy or a healthy baby. But if the results are uncertain or if they indicate a problem, you may face difficult choices and considerable anxiety. When your caregiver suggests a prenatal test, ask the following key questions to help you make an informed decision about whether to have the test. These questions are particularly important if the test carries potential risks.

- What are the benefits, risks, and alternatives of the test? (See pages 67–68 and 143–145 for descriptions of prenatal tests.)
- How is the test done?
- Is it a screening test or a diagnostic test?
- How reliable or accurate are its results?
- How will the results influence my prenatal care?
- What happens if the test has a negative result? A positive result?
- How much does the test cost? Will my insurance cover it?
- What are the consequences of not having the test?

Advancing medical technology is improving the ability to detect or diagnose many pregnancy complications or problems with the baby; however, medical technology hasn't advanced the ability to treat or cure many of these problems. For example, amniocentesis can diagnose the presence of Down syndrome in the baby, but the test can't predict how seriously the condition will affect her.

Because Down syndrome is untreatable, families who have a test that can detect it must decide how they'll respond if test results are positive. Some families consider whether to terminate the pregnancy. Other families believe abortion isn't an option for them, even if problems are discovered. These families may choose not to have the test (and avoid the anxiety of waiting for the results), or they may choose to have the test so they can learn what to expect and can prepare for the future.

Some prenatal tests indicate certain conditions that can improve with self-care or medical treatment. For example, glucose screening and a diagnostic glucose tolerance test indicate gestational diabetes (see page 68). To treat the condition, you can make changes to improve your diet and exercise regimen.

With good prenatal care, including screening and diagnostic tests, you'll greatly increase your chances of having a healthy pregnancy and baby. To learn more information about prenatal testing, visit http://www.mymidwife.org/prenatal_guide.cfm and http://www.marchofdimes.com. You can also visit our web site, http://www.PCNGuide.com.

## ROUTINE EXAMS AND SCREENING TESTS

Your caregiver will perform some exams and tests at just one prenatal visit and will perform others periodically throughout your pregnancy. Caregivers typically perform the following assessments at every prenatal visit:

- **Urine test** to detect bacteria, protein, and sugar (At first visit, a urine test may be used to confirm pregnancy.)
- **Blood pressure check** to screen for high blood pressure
- **Weight check** to monitor nutritional status and detect sudden weight gain (which can indicate preeclampsia)
- **Abdominal exam** to measure uterine growth or fundal height (which indicates the baby's growth) and estimate the baby's position
- **Listening to fetal heart tones (FHT)** to help confirm the baby's well-being

Caregivers perform the following assessments only at specific visits, depending on the information gained from them.

- **Pelvic exam** to help confirm pregnancy, estimate the size of the mother's pelvis, check for infection, or perform a Pap smear. In late pregnancy, a pelvic exam reveals cervical changes.
- **Blood test** (at first visit) to confirm pregnancy, determine blood type, test for anemia, and assess exposure to infection. For women with diabetes, caregivers check blood glucose levels periodically throughout pregnancy.
- **Breast exam** to help screen for breast cancer and assess breasts for conditions affecting breastfeeding

For more information on routine exams and screening tests, visit our web site, http://www.PCNGuide.com.

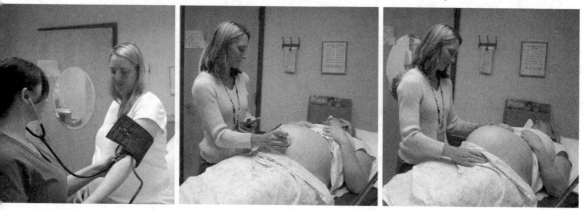

## OTHER EXAMS AND SCREENING TESTS

Caregivers often perform the following exams and tests, but not routinely. Some caregivers don't offer certain tests. If a specific test interests you, talk to your caregiver about your wishes and concerns.

- **Dental exam** (performed by dentist) to check for tooth decay and repair if needed, clean teeth, and check for gum infection, which is associated with preterm labor

## Fact or Fiction?

*Non-medical use of ultrasound, such as at-home Doppler heartbeat monitors and ultrasound videos or photos, are completely safe.* **Fiction.** Although the U.S. Food and Drug Administration (FDA) and the American Institute of Ultrasound in Medicine acknowledge that ultrasound poses no known risks to babies, it can affect the body and the long-term effects of extensive exposure are also unknown. To be safe, health care experts recommend that ultrasound be performed only by a trained provider and only when medically indicated.

- **Fetal movement counts** (kick counts) to help assess your baby's well-being by detecting changes in his normal pattern of movements. This test counts the number of times your baby kicks or moves within a certain period. It's performed by you, not your caregiver. (See page 71.)
- **Ultrasound** to help confirm pregnancy, estimate due date and your baby's size, and detect or rule out complications (See below.)
- **Integrated prenatal screening** to assess the possible risk of Down syndrome and neural tube defects such as spina bifida. This test is a combination of first trimester screening tests (ultrasound and blood tests) and second trimester blood tests. If your test results are outside the normal range, your caregiver will perform diagnostic tests. (See pages 143–145.)
- **Genetic screening** to check for diseases such as cystic fibrosis, Tay-Sachs, thalassemia, and sickle cell anemia. Depending on your family's medical history and ethnicity, your caregiver may offer carrier-screening tests. If these blood or saliva tests reveal a risk, your caregiver may recommend further diagnostic testing.
- **Glucose screening** to detect high glucose levels, which may indicate gestational diabetes (see page 134), between the twenty-fourth and twenty-eighth weeks of pregnancy. After you've had a sugary drink or snack, your blood is drawn. If your blood sugar is high, your caregiver will recommend a glucose tolerance test.
- **Group B streptococcus (GBS) screening** to detect the presence of GBS bacteria in secretions swabbed from the vagina and anus and cultured in a laboratory. See also page 131.

## Understanding Ultrasound

Many caregivers rely heavily on ultrasound to check the baby's heart rate, observe her development within the uterus, and make clinical decisions. Most pregnant women have at least one ultrasound at some point in their pregnancies.

There are two forms of ultrasound: Doppler ultrasound and diagnostic ultrasound scans. *Doppler ultrasound* (or simply Doppler), which monitors the baby's heart rate, uses continuous transmission of sound waves to detect motion of the baby's heart as it beats. Women receive Doppler from a hand-held device at prenatal visits. (See page 252 for more information on monitoring your baby's heart rate.)

*Diagnostic ultrasound scans*, which help caregivers "see" inside the uterus, use intermittent transmission of sound waves for less than 1 percent of the time during the test. For the rest of the test, the equipment receives the echoes of the sound waves, which indicate differences in tissue density. The echoes are converted into a video image that shows the baby's skeleton and organs, amniotic fluid, umbilical cord, placenta, and the mother's womb. Visit our web site, http://www.PCN Guide.com, for more information on diagnostic ultrasound scans.

Studies on diagnostic ultrasound scans have found no evidence that they harm either the mother or baby, and researchers conclude that wise use of ultrasound scans outweigh their possible risks. However, because high exposure may cause unknown side effects, health care experts recommend that pregnant women not receive frequent ultrasound scans or have them for a nonmedical reason, such as to make a keepsake ultrasound video.

The accuracy of ultrasound depends on the quality of the equipment, the skill and experience of the technician and caregiver, and the purpose of the test. In addition, some tests are less reliable than others. For example, using ultrasound scans to estimate the baby's gestational age and weight are less accurate in late pregnancy than in early pregnancy.

Despite the possible risk and inaccuracies, many expectant parents like ultrasound because it allows them to see their babies' faces, fingers, toes, beating hearts, and wriggling bodies. This first sight of their babies inspires many parents to make an effort to have a healthy pregnancy and birth.

## Fetal Movement Counting

During late pregnancy, keeping track of your baby's movements for a short time each day helps you learn more about your baby and his health. Some caregivers ask only those women with high-risk pregnancies to count their babies' movements (see page 71 for instructions), while others suggest that all pregnant women do so. If you're concerned or curious about your baby's well-being, you may decide to count his movements on your own.

Babies who are doing well in the uterus have several active, wakeful periods during the day. They also have quiet periods, when they're sleeping. Even though healthy babies tend to move slightly less often toward the end of pregnancy (because of space restrictions within the uterus), they don't markedly reduce their activity unless they have a problem. If your baby becomes noticeably less active, call your caregiver, who can assess your baby's well-being and take action (for example, early delivery) if necessary.

## Sample Fetal Movement Counting Chart

### Fetal Movement Count

| Date | Starting Time | Record of Movements | Time of 10th Movement | Total Time |
|------|---------------|---------------------|----------------------|------------|
| 8/24 | 7:30 pm | ＴＨＬ ＴＨＬ | 7:53 pm | 23 min |
| 8/25 | 6:00 pm | ＴＨＬ ＴＨＬ | 6:15 pm | 15 min |
| 8/26 | 6:30 pm | ＴＨＬ ＴＨＬ | 6:35 pm | 5 min |
| 8/27 | 7:00 pm | ＴＨＬ ＴＨＬ | 7:25 pm | 25 min |
| 8/28 | 7:15 pm | ＴＨＬ ＴＨＬ | 7:33 pm | 18 min |
| 8/29 | 6:30 pm | ＴＨＬ ＴＨＬ | 6:47 pm | 17 min |
| 8/30 | 9:00 pm | ＴＨＬ ＴＨＬ | 10:05 pm | 65 min |

# Warning Signs of Pregnancy Complications

Because your prenatal visits occur only periodically, you may be the first to notice a change or new discomfort that signals a pregnancy complication. Although most pregnancies are healthy, it's extremely important to know the following warning signs and immediately call your caregiver for an early diagnosis and prompt treatment. Your caregiver also may ask you to report other pertinent signs and any symptom or pain that concerns you. See Chapter 7 for more information on complications in pregnancy.

| Warning Signs | Possible Problems |
|---|---|
| Vaginal bleeding (even a small amount) | Miscarriage (see page 127); placenta previa (see page 139); placental abruption (see page 140); preterm labor (see page 136) |
| Abdominal pain | Ectopic pregnancy (see page 127); miscarriage (see page 127); placental abruption (see page 140); preterm labor contractions (see page 136). May indicate a medical problem, such as appendicitis or gallbladder disease. |
| Continuing, intermittent abdominal cramping or uterine tightening (contractions) | Preterm labor (see page 136) |
| Constant and severe abdominal pain and a hard abdomen, with or without vaginal bleeding | Placental abruption (see page 140) |
| Leaking or gushing of fluid from your vagina | Rupture of the membranes (see page 172) |
| Sudden puffiness or swelling of your face, hands, or fingers | Preeclampsia (see pages 140–142) |
| Severe, persistent headache | Gestational hypertension or preeclampsia (see pages 140–142) |
| Problems with your vision (seeing spots or flashes, blurring, or blind spots) | Preeclampsia (see pages 140–142) |
| Severe and persistent dizziness, lightheadedness | Preeclampsia (see pages 140–142); supine hypotension (see page 89) |
| Noticeable reduction or change in your baby's movement or activity after the 28th week of pregnancy | Fetal distress (see page 69 for fetal movement counting) |
| Painful area in leg, swelling or redness over affected area, or pain in leg when standing or walking | Blood clot in leg or inflammation of vein (venous thrombosis—see page 130) |
| Severe pain in pubic area and hips, with trouble moving your legs | Strain or separation of pubic symphysis joint or sciatica (pain in the lower back from pelvic joint stress) |
| Painful urination or burning sensation, with or without the urgent and frequent need to urinate | Urinary tract infection or UTI (see page 132); sexually transmitted infection or STI (see page 131) |
| Irritating vaginal discharge, genital sores, or vaginal itching | Vaginal infection or STI (see page 131) |
| Fever (temperature over 102°F or 38.9°C) when feeling sick | Infection (see page 130) |
| Persistent nausea or vomiting | Hyperemesis gravidarum (see page 129); infection (see page 130) |

### The Count-to-Ten Method

Any time after the twenty-eighth week of pregnancy, count your baby's movements each day at roughly the same time when he's normally active, such as after dinner. Don't worry if you miss a day now and then, but try to notice if your baby moves every day.

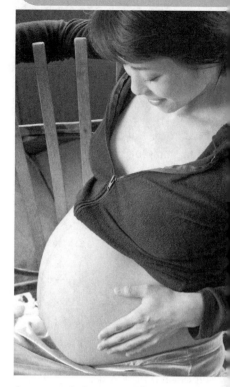

Find a comfortable position and avoid doing anything distracting, then time how long it takes your baby to move ten times. A movement may be short (a kick or a wiggle) or long (a continuous squirming motion). Don't count hiccups. Mark the end of a movement when it's followed by a clear (albeit brief) pause. Record movements on a chart such as the one on page 69. Visit our web site, http://www.PCN Guide.com, to download a template of this chart.

The length of time it takes to complete ten movements varies among babies. Focus not on how your baby's movements compare with other babies', but on whether his activity has slowed down compared to his usual pattern.

If your baby doesn't move at all during the chosen time, he may be asleep. Try waking him with a loud noise, or wait until you feel him move and then begin counting his movements (it may take only a few minutes if you've chosen a time when your baby is usually active). Call your caregiver if your baby clearly takes a longer time than usual to make ten movements or if he doesn't move at least ten times or have an active period within the next twelve hours.

# Reducing Stress during Pregnancy

Few women go through pregnancy without experiencing occasional emotional stress. When you're anxious or feel stressed, your body produces adrenaline and cortisol, stress hormones that signal a "fight or flight" response, causing tight muscles, constricted blood vessels, and elevated heart and breathing rates. In the short term, this response to stress doesn't cause harm and can be beneficial. For example, it may boost your energy level or encourage you to prepare for an upcoming event.

In the long term, however, chronic (continual) stress can constrict blood vessels to the placenta and within it, reducing the amount of blood and nutrients to your growing baby. Constant severe stress may increase your chances of preterm labor or decrease your baby's birth weight even if she's not preterm.[1] High anxiety levels during pregnancy can also affect your baby later in life by increasing her chances of developing behavioral and neurodevelopmental problems, such as attention deficit disorder/hyperactivity, anxiety disorders, and language delays.[2]

Stress can make you feel overwhelmed, out of control, and less productive. Typically, your caregiver can help you manage these effects. Stress, however, becomes detrimental when it makes you extremely anxious or depressed, affects your sleeping and eating schedules, or causes health problems. If you experience any of these harmful effects, contact your caregiver for help immediately. See page 337 for warning signs of postpartum mood disorders (PPMD) that can also occur

## In Their Own Words

During my pregnancy, I had a very demanding job as a nurse and was on my feet for most of every twelve-hour shift. I'd come home at the end of a shift, slump into my chair, and watch reruns of my favorite TV show. After my baby was born, that show's theme song would calm her when she was fussy, just as it had calmed me when she was in utero!

—Amy

during pregnancy. If diagnosed with depression or a mood disorder, you may need the care of a mental health counselor or take medications to manage your stress. You may also want to contact a counselor or an agency that's devoted to the emotional support of pregnant women and new mothers.

## WHAT CAUSES CHRONIC STRESS?

Any situation or event that upsets you can cause chronic stress if left unmanaged. Examples include a demanding job, financial worries, an unstable home life, problems with your partner, a loved one's illness, or violence or danger in your life. (If your partner or your home environment is violent or abusive, your resources and coping skills may be limited. See page 81 for more information on abuse and domestic violence.)

Other ongoing conditions may trigger an excessive stress response to every challenging experience. For example, you may have an extreme reaction to everyday pressures because of unresolved or untreated anxiety from a previous traumatic event (including emotional, physical, or sexual abuse), a chemical imbalance that causes your brain to interpret minor stresses as major ones, or hormonal changes (such as those that occur during pregnancy) that can intensify emotional problems.

## COPING WITH CHRONIC STRESS

To help cope with chronic stress, take these steps:

1. Recognize your stress response. Notice how you feel when you're anxious or stressed; for example, you may feel overwhelmed, have trouble sleeping, or have frequent headaches or bowel problems.
2. Identify the source of your stress. Try to discover which person, situation, or experience is triggering the stress.
3. Try to eliminate that source, if possible. For example, you may decide to quit a stressful job or transfer to another work setting, or you may leave an abusive home environment.
4. Learn better ways to cope with a stressful condition when eliminating the source may be difficult or impossible. The following are steps to help reduce the tension and pressure of stressful situations:
   - To minimize your stress, think of ways to modify the situation. For example, you can stay away from people who trigger a stress response.
   - Take action to reduce your stress. Sometimes, simply attempting to solve the problem diminishes the stress to a manageable level and helps you control your responses to everyday challenges.
   - Try to get enough sleep at night and nap during the day. If you can't sleep, sit or lie down and rest. Remember that fatigue makes everything seem worse.
   - Use the relaxation skills described on pages 216–220. Also use slow breathing (see page 224) while resting, meditating, or listening to soothing music.

- Eat nourishing foods and drink plenty of water and other fluids.
- Exercise regularly to help relieve stress, promote sleep, keep you fit, and improve your health. Walking, swimming, and yoga are great options when pregnant. If you want more vigorous exercise, first check with your caregiver to ensure your exercise regimen is appropriate during pregnancy. (See page 94.)
- Discuss your problems and worries with someone you trust, such as your partner, a friend, a relative, your caregiver, or another health care professional. Sharing your concerns at a support group also may help.
- Nurture yourself by doing something you enjoy. Have a massage, manicure, or facial. Take a walk through a park. Spend time with people who comfort you.

If these steps don't ease your stress or you're unable to use them, you may need to live with the stress—at least for a while. If you're concerned the stress will harm your baby, many counselors suggest regularly talking to your baby to express your love and to reassure him that your troubles aren't his fault. Your baby, of course, won't understand your words, but saying them can lower your stress level and give you a chance to connect with your baby.

# Treating Illness and Discomforts during Pregnancy

If you're in discomfort or feel sick, you may be tempted to take over-the-counter or prescription medications to feel better. During pregnancy, however, talk with your caregiver before taking any medicine; use a medication only if recommended. If possible, try some of the home remedies discussed in the following sections before using medications.

## HOME REMEDIES TO HELP RELIEVE COMMON DISCOMFORTS

These nonmedicinal treatments of common ailments may help you, but if discomforts persist or worsen, consult your caregiver for further treatment.

### Headache

Instead of taking aspirin, acetaminophen (Tylenol), or ibuprofen to relieve a headache, try taking a warm bath, having a massage, or doing tension-reducing exercises (such as shoulder circles) and relaxation techniques. (See pages 216–220.) Heat or cold also may help relieve a headache. Try laying a hot pack across your shoulders or on the back of your neck, or try placing a cold pack on your forehead. Hunger, dehydration, and fatigue can cause headaches. Make sure to eat frequently, drink enough fluids, get more sleep, and arrange for periods of rest and relaxation in your daily routine. Report a severe, persistent headache to your caregiver; it may be a warning sign of a pregnancy complication (see page 70).

### Cold, hay fever, runny nose, or cough

Safe ways to relieve these ailments include getting additional sleep and rest, using a cool-mist vaporizer, using saline nose drops (available at drugstores or made at home by mixing together 1 cup warm water, ⅛ teaspoon salt, and a small pinch of baking soda, and using a neti pot to administer the drops), drinking plenty of liquids, and swallowing a mixture of honey and lemon juice.

**Nausea, vomiting, and heartburn**

See page 119 for nonmedicinal treatments.

**Back pain**

Upper and lower back pain is common in pregnancy, but you can help prevent it by maintaining good posture, using good body mechanics, and doing exercises that strengthen your abdominal muscles and decrease the curve in your lower back. (See Chapter 5.) Treat back pain with rest, massage, warm baths, and hot or cold packs. Avoid taking aspirin, ibuprofen, and muscle relaxants unless your back pain is severe and your caregiver approves or prescribes these drugs.

**Sleeplessness**

Sleeplessness is especially common in late pregnancy because of frequent trips to the bathroom, an active baby, light sleeping, or difficulty finding a comfortable sleep position. (See page 89 for sleep positions.) To help release stress and tension that may prevent sleep, try exercising or taking a brisk walk each day (but not just before bedtime). At bedtime, try taking a warm bath, drinking warm milk, having a massage, or listening to soothing music. If you awaken at night, try reading, writing your thoughts in a journal, or using the relaxation techniques described in Chapter 11. Avoid watching TV or using your computer, which tend to stimulate your brain and make you feel more awake.

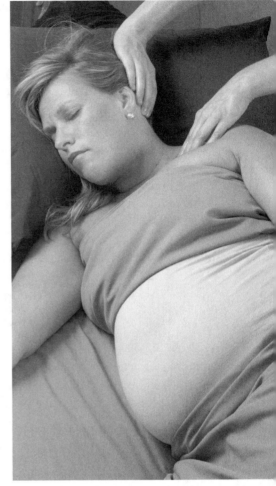

## MEDICATIONS

If home remedies don't make you feel better and your symptoms are troubling, check with your caregiver about over-the-counter medications, which may relieve symptoms but don't treat or cure an illness. If you have a chronic condition or current disease during pregnancy, your caregiver may prescribe prescription medications (such as antibiotics, insulin, antidepressants, anti-seizure drugs, and steroids) because the condition or disease is more harmful than the potential risks of the medications. See the following sections for more information on over-the-counter and prescription medications.

When deciding whether to use a medication, consider the seriousness of your symptoms or condition, the relief the medication may provide, and its possible side effects. To help you weigh a medication's possible risks against its benefits and make an informed decision, ask the following questions:

1. What are the medication's benefits, risks and alternatives? (See page 10 for information about these key questions.)

2. If the benefits clearly outweigh the risks and you decide to take the medication, ask your caregiver or a pharmacist the following questions:
   - What dose should I take and how often should I take it?
   - What's the maximum dose in a 24-hour period?
   - Should I avoid any foods or other drugs while taking it?
   - How long should I take it? Should I stop taking it at any specific time in pregnancy?
3. If the benefits don't clearly outweigh the risks, avoid taking the medication and seek a safer alternative.

## Over-the-Counter (OTC) Medications

When buying any OTC medication, look at its ingredients. Many medications include more than one drug in their pills or capsules. You'll need to learn the benefits, side effects, and possible risks for every drug in the medication. Visit our web site, http://www.PCNGuide.com, to learn current information on some common OTC medications and their effects on pregnancy. You can also find updated information by using the resources listed on page 82.

## Prescription Medications

Some prescription medications are safe to use in pregnancy; others aren't (see below). The safety of many drugs is yet unknown. Some caregivers may feel these medications are safe to take at certain times in pregnancy but dangerous at other times. They may prescribe them only if the benefits clearly outweigh the known risks. Or they may closely supervise their use in certain circumstances when the risks are unclear. When talking to your caregiver about a prescription medication whose safety isn't completely known, discuss other available treatments and their benefits and risks.

## Medications to Avoid

During pregnancy, a few medications are extremely harmful to your baby. Many are teratogens, which are substances that can cause birth defects, deformities, or even death. Some (such as thalidomide and diethylstilbestrol or DES) were prescribed for pregnant women before their severe side effects were known. Now their use has almost disappeared. Research will undoubtedly find more medications that can harm unborn babies. When considering any medication, make sure that all health care professionals working with you know that you're pregnant.

The following are medications known to be harmful during pregnancy:
- Chemotherapy drugs (methotrexate and aminopterin)
- Oral drugs to treat severe acne, such as isotretinoin (Accutane) and vitamin A derivatives (The vitamin A in acne medications differs from the vitamin A found in vitamin pills. Vitamin A in prenatal vitamins is safe to take in pregnancy.) *Note:* Tretinoin, a topical drug, doesn't appear to increase the rate of birth defects, but you may want to avoid it as well.
- Radioactive isotopes (used in imaging studies such as x-ray and MRI)

The following drugs are potentially harmful if taken during pregnancy, but their benefits may outweigh the risks:
- Some medications used to treat hyperthyroidism (such as propylthiouracil, methimazole, or iodide) unless your caregiver recommends their use
- Certain medications used to treat seizure disorders (phenytoin, valproic acid or Depakote, and others), bipolar disorder (lithium), and other conditions—unless your caregiver closely supervises their use

# Substances and Hazards to Avoid during Pregnancy

## Warning!

Research shows that excessive drinking throughout pregnancy may cause severe harm to the baby. The more alcohol a pregnant woman drinks and the more often she drinks during her pregnancy, the more risk her baby has of having problems with growth, development, and mental ability.

Just about everything you consume or are exposed to during pregnancy affects your baby—from common foods and beverages that contain potentially harmful substances, such as caffeinated coffee and herbal teas, to dangerous situations such as abuse and domestic violence. Also included are harmful substances such as some medications, alcohol, tobacco, recreational drugs, environmental agents, and workplace chemicals. (Some of these substances can also affect the reproductive health of men and nonpregnant women.)

With any harmful substance or situation, its effect on your baby and pregnancy depends on the amount and frequency of exposure as well as what trimester of pregnancy you're in when exposed. For example, exposure to a hazardous substance in the first trimester can increase your risk of miscarriage or birth defects; exposure in the second and third trimesters can increase your risk of slowed growth of your baby's body or brain (intrauterine growth restiction, or IUGR) or preterm labor.

In general, the more you're exposed to a harmful substance or situation, the higher are your chances of serious problems for your baby or pregnancy. Harmful consequences may occur even with minimal exposure; however, don't panic if you've already been exposed to an unsafe substance or condition. Babies can be remarkably resilient and some do well despite repeat exposure to harm. Consult with your caregiver for advice to manage your exposure to the following harmful substances or situations.

## DRINKING, SMOKING, AND DRUG USE

When you're pregnant, be extremely cautious about using alcohol or other drugs. Substance abuse can severely harm your baby or pregnancy.

### *Alcohol*

Any alcohol you drink while pregnant crosses the placenta and enters your baby's blood in the same concentration as in your blood, increasing her risk of serious birth defects and long-term problems with her development. The extent that alcohol can harm your baby depends on the amount you drink, how often you drink, and when in pregnancy you drink.[3]

Babies whose mothers drink heavily at any time during pregnancy are at high risk of developing severe problems. In the first trimester, when a baby's organs are forming, excessive alcohol can cause organ defects, facial abnormalities, or miscarriage. Alcohol abuse in the second trimester can affect nerve formation in the brain, and in the third trimester it may interfere with the development of the nervous system. It may also cause preterm labor. Of the babies whose mothers drank heavily while pregnant, 4 percent develop fetal alcohol syndrome (FAS), a cluster of physical, mental, and behavioral disabilities that include growth problems, heart defects, mental retardation, facial abnormalities, and problems with muscle and nerve development.

# Common Questions about Alcohol and Pregnancy

**What if I drank before I knew I was pregnant?**

Alcohol's effects on your baby depend on when in pregnancy you drank and how much you drank. Talk to your caregiver to assess your risk. The important thing to do is stop drinking as soon as you learn you're pregnant. Babies are remarkably strong and resilient. (Consider the high percentage of healthy babies born to mothers who drank alcohol, took medications, or had health problems during pregnancy.) But the earlier you stop exposing your baby to harmful substances, the greater are his chances of healthy development.

**What if I drink just a little only occasionally while pregnant?**

Current studies show that moderate drinking (one standard drink per day) has minimal effect on a baby's risk of birth defects from alcohol exposure. However, research hasn't determined a safe amount of alcohol for pregnant women, because blood alcohol levels vary depending on physical size, genetic factors, the amount of food eaten while drinking, and the amount of time between drinks. For that reason, it's best to avoid alcohol during pregnancy.

**How can I easily avoid drinking alcohol?**

Pregnant women have several reasons to avoid drinking alcohol. Some develop an aversion to alcohol (and to smoking and some foods) during pregnancy. Many avoid alcohol because it's not good for their babies.

At any occasion where alcohol is available, choose a nonalcoholic beverage such as mineral water with a lemon twist, fruit or vegetable juice, or a refreshing seltzer. If offered an alcoholic drink, request something else. You can say that you're pregnant and want to avoid alcohol. Or if you don't want to announce your pregnancy, you can say that you'll be driving home and are already tired.

What's the definition of *heavy drinking*? Some researchers define it as having more than four drinks a day. Other researchers define it as having two or more drinks per day or binge drinking more than three drinks on one occasion. A standard drink is ½ ounce of distilled alcohol (by itself or in a mixed drink), one can of beer, or a 4-ounce glass of wine.

Even light to moderate drinking (one standard drink per day) during pregnancy increases a baby's risk of fetal alcohol effects (FAE), problems that are less severe than FAS but still have subtle, long-lasting neurological and behavioral consequences. When compared to a child whose mother didn't drink any alcohol during pregnancy, a child exposed to alcohol before birth may have a slightly lower IQ, may be less agile or athletic, or may have more trouble with concentration, organizational skills, or impulse control.

Because drinking even a little alcohol may harm your baby, it's best to avoid it during pregnancy—the earlier the better. In fact, avoiding alcohol before becoming pregnant may help you conceive; drinking, especially heavy drinking, may contribute to infertility problems. See above for suggestions on ways to avoid alcohol.

If you find it difficult to quit drinking alcohol, try to avoid occasions, locations (such as bars), and friendships that focus on drinking alcohol. Seek people who support your decision not to drink and, if necessary, consider attending Alcoholics Anonymous (AA) meetings.

## Common Q & A

**Q:** I know I shouldn't smoke during pregnancy, but what can I do to quit?

**A:** Ask your caregiver for information about quitting. He or she may also provide a list of local smoking cessation programs. In addition, you can visit http://smokefree.gov and http://www.cancer.org for helpful tips, as well as other web sites of organizations that help people stop smoking.

One thing *not* to do is use smoking substitutes (nicotine patch, gum, or nasal spray) during the first trimester. They can increase the risk of malformations in your baby if used when his organs and structures are forming.[4]

## Smoking

Cigarette smoke contains numerous toxins that can harm you and directly affect the growth and development of your baby and placenta. These toxins include nicotine, tar, carbon monoxide, lead, and other substances. During pregnancy, the risks of complications from smoking and exposure to secondhand smoke increase with the amount and frequency of exposure.

When compared to pregnant nonsmokers, pregnant smokers have a greater risk of miscarriage, placental abruption, stillbirth, or infant death. If a woman has a family history of clubfoot, cleft lip, or cleft palate, she increases her baby's risk of those deformities if she smokes during pregnancy. In addition, the more a woman smokes while pregnant, the greater is the risk that she may develop placenta previa or have an ectopic pregnancy.

Pregnant smokers often give birth to babies with low birth weight (who tend to have health problems) because of intrauterine growth restriction and *not* prematurity—although smokers also have a higher risk of preterm birth than do nonsmokers.

Smoking also may harm a baby after birth. If a woman smokes during pregnancy, she increases her baby's risk of sudden infant death syndrome or SIDS (see page 391). If her baby lives with smokers, his risk of SIDS increases even more, depending on the number of smokers in the household and the amount of time he's exposed to secondhand smoke.

In addition, smoking during pregnancy and exposure to secondhand smoke after birth increases a baby's risk of respiratory problems later in life.[5]

If you smoke, try to quit (or at least significantly cut back) before pregnancy or as soon as possible during pregnancy.[6] The withdrawal symptoms you'll experience (physical discomfort and psychological stress that last for several days or a few weeks) are difficult. But it takes just a day or so for your baby to benefit from a smoke-free environment. To reduce your exposure to secondhand smoke (and your baby's exposure after birth), stay away from smoky areas and ask friends, colleagues, and relatives not to smoke near you or your baby.

## Illegal Drugs and Prescription Drug Abuse

The most commonly abused drugs are illegal, and most have no accepted medical use. Illegal drugs are often sold on the street, come from unregulated sources, and lack medical supervision. Because most illegal drugs readily cross the placenta to your baby, taking these substances while pregnant can harm not only you, but also your growing baby, depending on the drug you took, how much you of it you took, when in pregnancy you took it, and how often you took it.

If you take an illegal drug in the first trimester, your baby may develop a defect or deformity or you may have a miscarriage. If you take an illegal drug in the third trimester, your baby may have intrauterine growth restriction or IUGR (that is, grow slowly) or suffer the effects of prematurity because of a preterm birth. Each drug has its own harmful effects, and taking a combination of two or more drugs may compound the damage to your baby. Visit our web site, http://www.PCNGuide.com, to learn more about illegal drugs' harmful effects.

Instead of taking illegal drugs—or in addition to taking them—some pregnant women abuse prescription drugs by using them without medical supervision. These women mistakenly believe these substances are safer than illegal drugs and are therefore okay to use during pregnancy. But the effects of prescription drugs can be just as dangerous to babies as the effects of illegal drugs (see page 75). Try to stop using *all* drugs before you're pregnant or as soon as you know you're pregnant, to improve your baby's chances of a healthy life.

# POTENTIALLY HARMFUL SUBSTANCES AND HERBS IN FOODS

Some substances and herbs that are in several common foods and beverages may be potentially harmful to consume when pregnant. During your pregnancy, be careful about consuming the following items.

## Caffeine

Caffeine is a stimulant that can raise your heart rate and blood pressure, constrict blood vessels, affect your ability to sleep, and make you jittery. It's also a diuretic (a substance that makes you urinate more fluid, more often) and increases the amount of calcium you expel in your urine.

Coffee, tea, energy drinks, colas, and other soft drinks contain significant amounts of caffeine. Of these beverages, coffee has the most caffeine, but the amount of the drug in a serving depends on how the coffee is made and the number of ounces in a serving. For example, an 8-ounce serving of brewed coffee may have 65 to 120 milligrams of caffeine; even decaffeinated coffee has 2 to 4 milligrams in an 8-ounce serving. An 8-ounce serving of black or green tea has 20 to 90 milligrams of caffeine.[7] A 12-ounce serving of some sodas has 54 milligrams of caffeine. In addition, several over-the-counter medications include caffeine, and chocolate contains a small amount of a caffeine-like chemical. To learn the amount of caffeine in packaged products, read the labels.

Although researchers haven't found any connections between caffeine and birth defects or delayed childhood development, babies in the womb probably experience the stimulating and diuretic effects of caffeine that their mothers notice. Caffeine can elevate the baby's heart rate and reduce the amount of fluid and calcium available for her optimal growth. The evidence on caffeine's connection to miscarriage, intrauterine growth restriction, and stillbirth is conflicting and controversial. Numerous studies observe a connection, but others don't. Various factors seem to influence results, such as a woman's unique susceptibility to caffeine-related health risks, the amount of caffeine she consumed, and when in pregnancy she consumed the caffeine.

Research suggests that consuming large amounts of caffeine each day (for example, more than eight 8-ounce servings of coffee) at any time in pregnancy may harm your baby. However, consuming more than 200 milligrams of caffeine each day (for example, just two 8-ounce servings of coffee) during the first trimester may increase your risk of intrauterine growth restriction or miscarriage.[8]

Given the potentially harmful effects of caffeine, try to avoid it during your pregnancy or at least reduce the amount you consume.

## Warning!

Just because herbs are considered "natural," they're not necessarily safe. Some herbal preparations and dietary supplements contain potentially harmful ingredients, and most of these can cross the placenta and affect your baby.

## *Herbal Tinctures, Teas, and Capsules*

Traditional healers have used herbal remedies for centuries to help treat or cure various ailments. Pharmacies and specialty shops sell hundreds of herbs and dietary supplements, although little is known about their ingredients. The U.S. Food and Drug Administration (FDA) hasn't tested or approved most of these herbs and botanicals, and their safety is often uncertain. When and how an herb was harvested and processed influence a product's potency, which may range widely from one brand to another and even among different batches of the same brand.

Herbs and dietary supplements affect both the mother and baby during pregnancy. For the mother, caregivers sometimes recommend red raspberry leaf to tone uterine muscles. At the end of pregnancy, some caregivers may recommend herbs that can start labor (such as blue cohosh, evening primrose, and black cohosh); however, women should avoid these uterine stimulants in early pregnancy because they may cause miscarriage. Uterine stimulants can also have potentially dangerous side effects. For example, blue cohosh may cause elevated blood pressure, irritated mucous membranes, and multi-organ injury from lack of oxygen.

During pregnancy, research suggests the potential harm of herbal products on the baby's health stems more from hormonal effects (for example, herbs containing estrogen-like substances) and drug interactions (increasing or decreasing the effect of a prescription medication) than from toxic effects. However, some Chinese herbal medicines, specifically An-Tai-Yin and huanglian, may cause congenital malformations.[9]

To reduce your consumption of caffeine during pregnancy, you may consider drinking herbal teas. But you may experience undesirable side effects to specific herbs. For example, if you're allergic to ragweed and related plants, you may develop allergic symptoms after drinking chamomile tea. In addition, certain herbs have specific side effects when consumed in large amounts. For example, drinking licorice root tea can increase water retention and decrease potassium, and drinking tea with ginseng can cause swollen and painful breasts. For these reasons, be aware of the ingredients in an herbal tea before drinking it.

Because dosages in herbal products and supplements vary and little is known about their risks and benefits, avoid them while pregnant or use them only under the guidance of a naturopathic doctor or other expert. It's also important to consult with your caregiver about any herbal remedies or dietary supplements that you've taken or are considering taking.

## *Mercury and Other Substances in Food That May Cause Harm*

For information on mercury and other substances that can cause harmful illnesses when consumed during pregnancy (such as listeriosis and toxoplasmosis), see page 121.

## ENVIRONMENTAL HAZARDS AND HARMFUL SITUATIONS

The following sections discuss hazardous substances that are present in many homes and workplaces, as well as harmful situations that can affect the health of your pregnancy and baby, such as being in an abusive relationship or having workplace stress.

## Abuse and Domestic Violence

Abuse and domestic violence (any combination of verbal, psychological, emotional, sexual, economic, or physical abuse) can happen to any woman regardless of her age, physical ability, lifestyle, religion, ethnicity, or socioeconomic and educational backgrounds. When you're pregnant, abuse increases your risk of serious pregnancy problems such as high blood pressure, vaginal bleeding, severe nausea or vomiting, urinary tract infections (UTIs), preterm birth, a baby with low birth weight, or a baby who needs intensive medical care.[11] In addition, your risk of being killed by an abusive partner increases during pregnancy.[12]

If you're in an abusive relationship, you are *not* at fault. The goal of abuse is to leave you feeling confused, ashamed, powerless, hopeless, and out of control. Living with abuse is painful, confusing, and stressful. The suggestions for coping with stress on pages 72–73 may be useful. Talking with a trusted friend or relative also may help you cope. You may choose to call your caregiver for information on counselors and local agencies that offer support or resources for abused women. If you decide to leave the relationship, you may require their help. Your caregiver also may suggest further testing to detect any sexually transmitted infections (STIs) or to evaluate you for stress-related pregnancy complications. Childhood sexual, emotional, and physical abuse can also have troubling long-term effects that interfere with your joy in pregnancy. (See page 59.)

National agencies can help you as well. Memorize the phone number for the National Domestic Violence Hotline, 800-799-SAFE (7233), and call if you need to talk to someone or need resources, including help making an escape plan. See also page 362 for more information on abuse and domestic violence.

## Insecticides, Herbicides, and Pesticides

During pregnancy, avoid frequent, sustained exposure to chemicals that kill insects (insecticides), weeds (herbicides), or unwanted insects, bugs, or animals (pesticides). The presence of these chemicals in the air and on food may cause miscarriage, poor growth in the baby, birth defects, and childhood neurobehavioral problems. Because some of these chemicals haven't been tested for their effects on pregnant women and young children, their safety is unknown; however, many governments have banned the use of chemicals that have been proven harmful such as DDT.

To avoid exposure to these chemicals, wash fruits and vegetables well to help remove pesticides and other chemicals. If you need to use a pesticide to remove household pests, plan on leaving your home for at least a day to allow the chemicals to dissipate from the air. Before using the pesticide, close all drawers, cupboards, and other doors to food-storage areas. When you return home, wash counters, tables, and food-preparation surfaces thoroughly.

## Occupational Hazards

Some occupations and workplaces may be more hazardous than others during pregnancy. Studies have shown the potential harm of some workplace chemicals, including anesthetic agents, benzene, cancer treatment (cytotoxic) drugs, carbon monoxide, ethylene oxide, ethylene glycol ethers, formaldehyde, ionizing radiation (x-ray), lead, methyl mercury, organic solvents, polybrominated biphenyls (PBBs), and polychlorinated biphenyls (PCBs). These chemicals can cause severe problems such as miscarriage, birth defects, low birth weight, preterm birth, developmental delays, and childhood cancers. In addition, if you work with any of the medications described on page 75, avoid them as well.

## Internet Resources about Hazards in Pregnancy

**U.S. Food and Drug Administration (FDA)**
http://www.fda.gov
**March of Dimes**
http://www.marchofdimes.com
**U.S. Environmental Protection Agency (EPA)**
http://www.epa.gov/epahome/hotline.htm
**Environmental Working Group (EWG)**
http://www.ewg.org
**U.S. Centers for Disease Control and Prevention (CDC)**
http://www.cdc.gov
**The National Institute for Occupational Safety and Health (NIOSH)**
http://www.cdc.gov/niosh
**U.S. Occupational Safety & Health Administration (OSHA)**
http://www.osha.gov

People who may encounter these chemicals include health care workers (including dental and veterinary offices), pharmacists, battery makers, solderers, welders, radiator repairers, industrial painters, home remodelers, and atomic and electronic workers.[12] In addition, farm workers may be exposed to pesticides.

Researchers are constantly revising the list of substances that are harmful in pregnancy, so ask your caregiver about potentially dangerous chemicals. If you work with any dangerous chemicals, talk with your employer about limiting your exposure to them. Also talk with your employer about limiting your exposure to workplace stress (see page 71 to learn about the harmful effects of chronic stress). Visit the web sites at left for information about occupational hazards.

## Chemicals Used for Hobbies

Many people enjoy hands-on hobbies such as arts-and-crafts projects, furniture refinishing, and auto repair. Several of these hobbies aren't risky during pregnancy, but some require products that may contain dangerous chemicals. If you plan to continue a hobby that uses a potentially toxic product, learn about risks of exposure during pregnancy by contacting the manufacturer or a poison control center, or by getting the product's Material Safety Data Sheets (MSDS) from a store that sells it.

## House Paint

Many people prepare for parenthood by repairing or renovating their homes, which often includes painting. Caregivers generally discourage pregnant women from spray painting (because they can inhale the paint particles), but rolling or brushing house paint onto surfaces is probably safe during pregnancy. However, many brands of paint contain potentially dangerous chemicals (such as ethylene glycol ethers, mercury, formaldehyde, and hydrocarbon solvents) that you may inhale or absorb through touch. Try to avoid using paints that have these chemicals; instead, use low-VOC or no-VOC paints, which contain fewer (or no) harmful volatile organic compounds than standard paint.

When painting, wear gloves and make sure there's ample ventilation. (Better yet, have someone else do the painting!)

If your home contains lead-based paint (which is often found in older homes), don't try to remove it or paint over it yourself. A professional painter can safely handle the toxic paint chips and dust without harm to you or your family.

## Hair Treatments

Women who have their hair colored or chemically treated may worry whether these treatments will harm their babies during pregnancy. Although some studies show a link between chemical hair dyes and an increased risk of childhood brain tumors, the results aren't statistically significant. Other studies find no evidence that dyes cause birth defects. In addition, no direct evidence exists that suggests permanent wave solutions or hair relaxers are harmful in pregnancy.

Most caregivers don't discourage pregnant women from getting chemical hair treatments, but if you have any concerns about their safety, you may choose to wait until after the birth to have your hair treated.

## Saunas, Hot Tubs, and Heat Wraps

During pregnancy, exposure to the extreme heat of saunas, hot tubs, and heat wraps may raise your baby's temperature along with your own. Once overheated, your baby takes much longer than you to cool down. In early pregnancy, high temperatures can cause birth defects or even miscarriage if the exposure is frequent and prolonged, or if it occurs at a critical point in your baby's development. Later in pregnancy, raising your body temperature can produce a fever in your baby and may cause him to develop neurological disorders such as seizures.

To keep your baby safe, avoid using saunas and heat wraps during pregnancy. If you find soaking in a hot tub relaxing, keep your temperature below 102.2°F (39°C). If monitoring your temperature is difficult, keep the water temperature below 99°F (37.2°C) and limit use to ten minutes or less. Keep your shoulders and arms out of the water to promote heat loss and help maintain a safe body temperature. As a safer alternative to using a hot tub, consider taking a warm bath, where your body can maintain a safe temperature because less of it is submerged in warm water.

## Electric Blankets

As with all other electric household appliances, electric blankets emit low-frequency electromagnetic energy, which may harm your pregnancy if exposure is prolonged and close to your body. Although manufacturers have produced low-emission electric blankets that reduce magnetic field exposure, the safety of electric blankets is inconclusive. The few studies on the harmful effects of electric blankets suggest that if health problems occur, they may stem from the heat the blankets generate. Because it's unknown what temperature is too hot for your baby during pregnancy, consider using a down comforter or wool blankets instead of an electric blanket to keep warm.

## Ionizing Radiation (X-rays)

Depending on the dose, radiation may harm your baby during pregnancy. X-rays for medical and dental diagnoses use much less radiation than does radiotherapy for cancer treatment. Because the risk of birth defects from one diagnostic x-ray (about 1 radiation absorbed dose, or rad) during the first four months of pregnancy is tiny, many health care professionals don't consider it dangerous. (See page 144 for more information on diagnostic x-rays.) However, avoid exposure to high radiation levels at work and try to avoid x-rays in the first trimester, when radiation may interfere with your baby's organ development.

## Infectious Diseases

Several infectious diseases may harm your baby before and after birth. Examples include toxoplasmosis, Lyme disease, rubella (German measles), chicken pox, fifth disease (parvovirus B19), listeriosis, hepatitis, and sexually transmitted infections (STIs). See pages 132–133 for more information on infectious diseases.

## THE FATHER'S EXPOSURE TO HAZARDS AND DRUGS

Although little is known about the effects of drugs, environmental and occupational hazards, and other potential dangers on male reproductive health, increasing evidence suggests that a man's exposure to certain hazards during the months before conception may increase the risk of miscarriage, childhood brain tumors, and other problems.[13] Exposure to hazards also may affect a man's fertility (although research results differ about the effects of smoking on male fertility). To increase the chances of producing a healthy baby, men should limit their exposure to the same hazards that are harmful to women in pregnancy.

In addition, fathers and partners can create an environment that supports a healthy pregnancy by controlling their alcohol, tobacco, or drug use. Before and during pregnancy, a woman is more likely to control her use of alcohol, tobacco, or drugs if her partner (male or female) does so as well.

# Traveling during Pregnancy

Being pregnant doesn't mean you can't take a trip, but you may have some restrictions depending on when, where, and how you'll be traveling. Traveling during pregnancy may be more enjoyable if you follow some common precautions and safety tips.

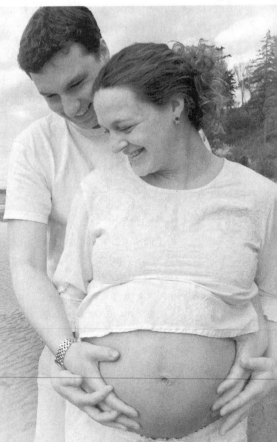

When planning a trip, consult with your caregiver for travel suggestions and any precautions specific to your pregnancy. If you have pregnancy complications, your caregiver may recommend against travel. In the last month of pregnancy, your caregiver may suggest staying within an hour's travel time from home. Even if your pregnancy is healthy, get a copy of your medical history to take with you while traveling.

If you're planning to fly, especially in late pregnancy, find out if your airline has restrictions for pregnant passengers. Some airlines limit travel on domestic flights in the week before a due date, and many have restrictions for international trips. Throughout pregnancy, avoid flying at altitudes above 7,000 feet in small planes without pressurized cabins; the oxygen available to your baby may be reduced.

If you're planning to take a cruise, be aware that some cruise-ship companies also have restrictions for passengers in late pregnancy.

If planning a trip to an international destination, check for any special health concerns or travel warnings. If certain vaccinations are recommended before entering a country, check with your caregiver to learn if you can receive them when pregnant. (Only a few vaccines are considered safe in pregnancy.) For more information on health precautions or recommended vaccinations, contact the U.S. Centers for Disease Control's international travel line at 877-394-8747 or visit http://www.cdc.gov/travel. For information about travel warnings, contact the U.S. Department of State at 202-647-5225 or visit http://www.travel.state.gov.

During pregnancy, long trips by car, bus, plane, or train may limit your movement, which can affect your circulation, increase swelling in your legs, and thereby increase your risk of developing a blood clot in a leg vein. Walking every hour or so and stretching as much as possible can eliminate or minimize this risk. In an airplane, try to sit in an aisle seat or one at the bulkhead to allow for more legroom and an easy exit. Do simple exercises while in your seat to help increase circulation to your legs and arms. (See Chapter 5.) If you have varicose veins, consider wearing support stockings (available at medical supply stores).

In vehicles and airplanes, always wear your seat belt to protect you and your baby in a collision. Fasten the belt low on your hip and below your belly. Use the shoulder strap if available; don't tuck it behind you. If an accident occurs, the seat belt will keep you in your seat, while your muscles and pelvic bones protect your uterus and the amniotic fluid cushions your baby.

Pregnancy discomforts may seem worse while traveling. The constant motion may aggravate morning sickness or nausea. Hours of sightseeing or long business meetings may increase fatigue. Back pain may become more noticeable when your usual comfort measures aren't available. The change in routine may disrupt when you eat, as well as what you eat. Air travel, hot climates, and places with forced air ventilation may increase dehydration if your availability to fluids is limited.

To help minimize pregnancy discomforts when traveling, try to drink lots of fluids, eat well, walk around, and get plenty of rest. Try to use your typical comfort measures as best as you can, or adapt them if possible.

## *Key Points to Remember*

- Throughout your pregnancy, you'll have opportunities to improve your health. By learning about healthy lifestyle choices, knowing potential pregnancy hazards to avoid, and recognizing the warning signs of pregnancy problems, you can make the best choices for you and your baby.
- You can improve your chances of having a healthy, safe, and enjoyable pregnancy by actively participating in your prenatal care. Ask key questions about prenatal tests or procedures so you can make informed decisions about whether to have them.
- Eliminating or reducing your exposure to harmful substances and situations will increase your chances of having a healthy pregnancy and baby. Although your risk of severe problems is small, use caution when considering exposure to environmental hazards or potentially harmful medications, substances, or situations.

# CHAPTER 5

# Feeling Good
# and Staying Fit

To have a healthy pregnancy, it's important to eat well, get enough rest, and avoid hazards. As your body changes to meet your growing baby's needs, it's also essential to exercise regularly, maintain good posture, and move your body with care. Regular exercise helps improve and maintain your overall health and well-being, and it can help prepare you for the physical challenges of childbirth and postpartum recovery. Maintaining good posture helps prevent back pain and reduce fatigue. Moving comfortably and safely reduces the likelihood of becoming injured or exacerbating any existing discomforts.

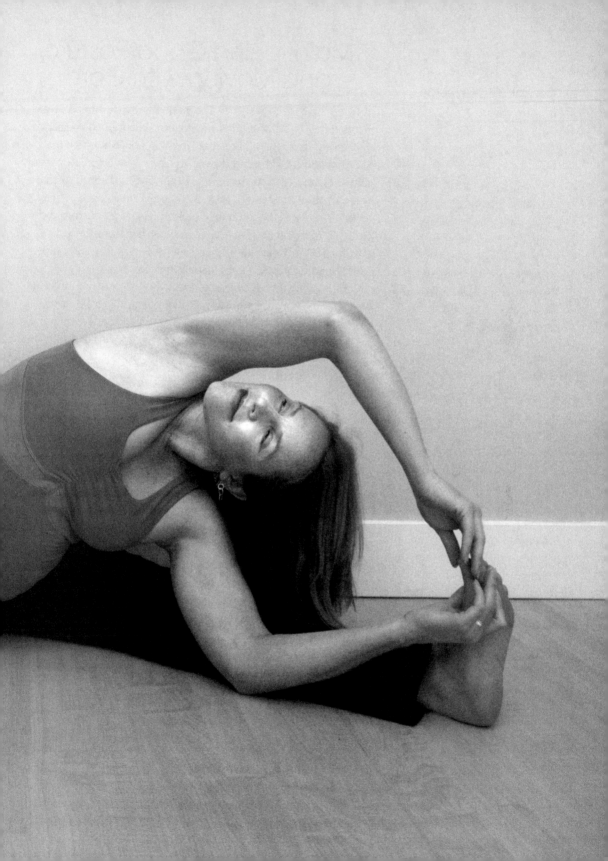

# Maintaining Good Posture and Moving with Care

As your belly grows and your center of gravity shifts forward, maintaining good posture is essential for keeping your balance, preventing back pain, and reducing fatigue. When you're standing, sitting, or lying down, gravity exerts a force on your joints, ligaments, and muscles. Good posture distributes that force evenly throughout your body, preventing excess stress to one or more parts. When someone has good posture, her body is in alignment. That is, if viewing her from the side as she stands, you see that her ears, shoulders, hips, and ankles are in a straight line. (See illustration below.)

As you move your changing body, you protect your muscles, joints, and bones by adjusting how you stand, sit, lie down, lift objects, and so on. Moving with care can reduce fatigue, prevent strain, and minimize common pregnancy discomforts.

## STANDING

To stand with good posture, begin by imagining you're wearing a crown. To keep it in place, position your head so the crown is parallel with the floor. Then use your neck muscles to pull your head back until your ears are in line with your shoulders. Lengthen your spine and let your hips and ankles align with your ears and shoulders. Remind yourself throughout the day to keep the crown on your head.

During late pregnancy, avoid standing for long periods. Prolonged standing may slow blood flow from your legs to your heart and head, making you feel faint or lightheaded. If you must stand for a long time, shift your weight from leg to leg, march in place, rotate your ankles, or rock back and forth.

To help prevent back pain while standing, place one foot on a stool, chair rung, or opened drawer. After a while, switch to your other foot.

## SITTING

When sitting, follow the same directions for standing with good posture to align your ears, shoulders, and hips.

As your belly grows, you may find that sitting in a straight-back chair is more comfortable (and easier to get out of) than sitting in a low, deep chair. For additional comfort, place a small, firm pillow at the small of your back and a low stool under your feet. To prevent straining your back when rising from a chair, move to the seat edge, lean forward, then push against the arm rests or seat and use your legs to raise your body.

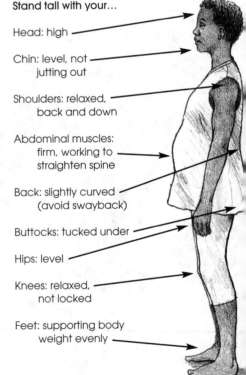

**Stand tall with your...**

Head: high

Chin: level, not jutting out

Shoulders: relaxed, back and down

Abdominal muscles: firm, working to straighten spine

Back: slightly curved (avoid swayback)

Buttocks: tucked under

Hips: level

Knees: relaxed, not locked

Feet: supporting body weight evenly

During late pregnancy, avoid sitting for long periods. Prolonged sitting can affect blood circulation in your legs. If you must stay seated for a long time, shift your position often, rotate your ankles, and avoid crossing your legs at the knees. To help decrease swelling, sit with your feet propped up and calves supported on another chair or ottoman.

## LYING DOWN

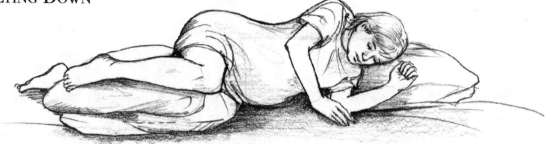

As your pregnancy progresses, staying comfortable while lying down can become more challenging. For example, you may experience heartburn or shortness of breath while lying on your back, especially near the end of pregnancy. To help alleviate these discomforts, lie on your side or use pillows to prop yourself in a semi-reclined position. You can also place pillows or a long body pillow under one shoulder, hip, and leg to tilt your body from the back to one side.

Lying on your back can make you feel dizzy or lightheaded. If this happens, roll to your left side or sit up. For some women, lying on their backs in late pregnancy causes *supine hypotension*, in which the uterus presses on the abdominal vein (inferior vena cava) that carries blood from the legs to the heart and causes a drop in blood pressure. Extended supine hypotension can reduce blood flow to the placenta and restrict oxygen to the baby. For this reason, health care providers recommend that pregnant women lie on their sides after the twenty-sixth week of pregnancy.

When lying on your side, place a pillow between your knees and another under your head to keep your body in alignment. In late pregnancy, you may need to support your abdomen with a small pillow, a wedge-shaped pad, or a long body pillow.

Some women find lying on their sides more comfortable when they roll their bodies slightly forward. To get into this position, place a firm pillow on the side you'll roll toward. As you roll to this side, keep your lower leg straight and bend the knee of your top leg to rest on the pillow. Rest your lower arm behind you and bend your upper arm at the elbow, setting it in front of you so your hand is near your face.

Lying on your side can cause sore hips. To help manage any pain or swelling, apply an ice pack on the sore area. Also consider supplementing your mattress with a deep foam pad or a pillow-top mattress cover.

## GETTING UP AFTER LYING DOWN

Getting up from lying on the floor or in bed also becomes more difficult as your pregnancy advances. Before your belly started to grow, you got up by sitting straight up, then rising. As your pregnancy progresses, however, this movement may strain your abdominal and lower back muscles.

To get out of bed safely, roll onto your side, put your lower legs over the edge of the bed, push yourself to a sitting position, and stand up. To get up from the floor, follow these steps:

1. Roll onto your side and bend your hips and knees. Use your arms to raise your upper body.
2. Get onto your hands and knees. Place one foot on the floor in front of you, while keeping the opposite knee on the floor.
3. Use your legs to stand up. For balance, place your hand on your knee or a stable object.

## LIFTING OBJECTS

During pregnancy, hormones cause your ligaments to relax and soften, and the muscles supporting your posture and core (abdominal, pelvic floor, and back muscles) adapt to your changing shape. As a result of these changes, lifting heavy objects while pregnant increases the likelihood of back injury. To help prevent back injury, avoid heavy lifting whenever possible. For example, teach your toddler to climb into his car seat or onto your lap instead of picking him up.

When lifting any object from a low surface (even a sheet of paper), protect your back by following these guidelines:

1. Get as close to the object as possible.
2. With your feet shoulder-width apart, squat while keeping your back straight and sticking out your buttocks for balance.
3. Grasp the object and hold it close to you. Try not to twist at your waist.
4. As you rise, tighten your abdominal muscles, and squeeze your pelvic floor muscles upward and exhale (instead of holding your breath) to prevent straining your perineum. Use your legs instead of your lower back to raise your body. Keep your back straight.
5. Avoid twisting your spine to turn or set down the object. Instead, move your feet in the direction you want to go.

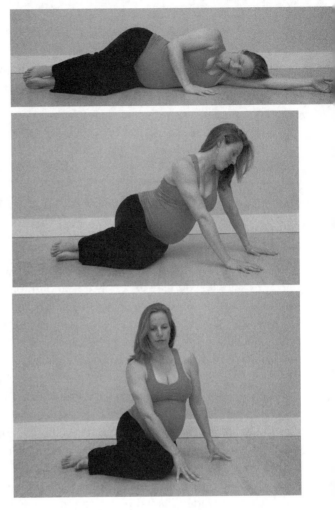

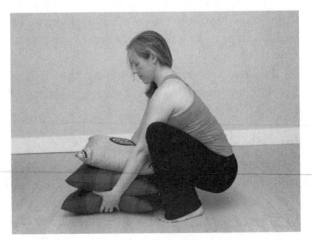

# Exercise in Pregnancy

When pregnancy makes you feel overwhelmingly tired, uncomfortable, and moody, the last thing you want to do is exercise. But exercise can be just what you need to feel energized and healthy.

Regular, moderate physical activity during pregnancy improves or maintains your muscle tone, strength, and endurance. Exercise also protects against back pain, reduces the intensity of common pregnancy discomforts, and boosts your energy level, mood, and self-image. During the last trimester, regular exercise increases your body's production of endorphins (natural pain relievers), which can help you cope with labor.

## HOLISTIC BENEFITS OF EXERCISE

During the childbearing year (from pregnancy through three months after the birth) and beyond, regular physical activity does more than keep your body fit. Exercise also benefits your mental, emotional, spiritual, and social well-being. All these benefits help you meet the demands of pregnancy, childbirth, and motherhood.

### Physical benefits

Appropriate exercise strengthens the muscles most affected by pregnancy and childbirth, including those in the pelvic floor, abdomen, and lower back. Exercise during pregnancy helps maintain good respiration, circulation, and posture. It can also ease common discomforts of pregnancy, such as constipation, heartburn, shortness of breath, leg cramps, fatigue, swollen ankles, and insomnia.

In addition, maintaining your fitness during pregnancy and the postpartum period more easily helps you recover your energy level, strength, and prepregnancy size after the birth.

### Mental and emotional benefits

Regular exercise helps decrease mental stress and fatigue. Aerobic activities release pain-relieving endorphins that improve your sense of well-being, help stabilize hormone-driven mood swings, and can decrease the risk or severity of depression and mood disorders during pregnancy and afterward.

### Spiritual benefits

Whatever your spiritual beliefs, regularly finding time to meditate, relax, or pray lets you clearly and peacefully think about what's important to you, honor the changes you're experiencing, and connect with your baby. An ideal time for meditation, relaxation/visualization exercises, yoga, or prayer is after aerobic exercise, when your body experiences calmness.

### Social benefits

During the childbearing year, you increasingly need others to offer you support and validate your feelings. Taking a prenatal exercise class lets you connect with other pregnant women, and you may learn about pregnancy, birth, the postpartum period, and newborn care through shared experiences.

## FINDING YOUR MOTIVATION TO EXERCISE

Throughout pregnancy, your motivation to exercise may ebb and flow as your energy level rises and falls. At times, you know you *should* exercise, but find any excuse not to. When this happens, reminding yourself of the benefits of physical activity can give you the push you need to keep a regular exercise regimen.

If you need additional help getting your body moving, there are other tricks to try. For example, you're much more likely to do an activity if it's something you enjoy. If you love to dance, consider taking a dance class or dancing at home to some invigorating music.

Find what time of day works best to exercise and schedule that time for physical activity. Depending on what trimester you're in, you may need to work around certain physical symptoms. For example, if you have intense heartburn after eating, choose another time to exercise (or eat a lighter meal and bring antacids with you when you exercise).

Sometimes hearing or reading encouraging words or listening to your favorite music can motivate you. Even an activity you might not enjoy, such as housecleaning, can become a fun exercise session if you play your favorite CD or playlist, warm up with some light dusting, then mop and vacuum vigorously before ending with some gentle stretching. If encouraging words or music motivate you, consider sharing this information with your labor-support team to give them ideas for motivating you during labor.

If you don't want to exercise because you're feeling down or your back aches, remind yourself that exercise can help relieve these and other emotional and physical problems. If you have trouble making time to exercise regularly on your own, consider signing up for a class, hiring a personal trainer, or scheduling a regular appointment to do a physical activity with someone. The extra commitment may prompt you to make the time to exercise.

Visit our web site, http://www.PCNGuide.com, to download a work sheet to record your fitness goals. If you try every trick to get yourself to exercise but are unsuccessful, be kind to yourself and try again the next day.

## EXERCISE OPTIONS

Aerobic exercise is physical activity that increases your heart rate for an extended time, which improves endurance and strengthens your heart and lungs. Anaerobic exercise focuses on strengthening certain muscles and improving balance and flexibility. Both kinds of exercise benefit your health.

How much you should exercise and what kind of activities you should do depend on your general health, the health of your pregnancy, your fitness level, and your usual activity level. Physical changes during pregnancy directly affect your tolerance for exercise. Hormonal changes cause your ligaments to relax and your joints to become more mobile. Your growing belly shifts your center of gravity forward. Changes in your cardiovascular system increase your heart rate more quickly, and your body temperature and metabolic rate (the rate at which you burn calories) are higher.

As you become more aware of these changes, you can better sense when something doesn't feel right and can remedy the problem. For example, if an activity leaves you excessively tired, do it more slowly next time or do a less demanding activity instead. Responding to your body's signals when exercising also prepares you to respond to physical cues in labor and after the birth.

To ensure that an exercise regimen is appropriate for you, consult with your caregiver before starting or continuing to exercise.

### Aerobic Exercise

In general, low-impact aerobic exercise is best for pregnant women because it doesn't involve movements that can strain joints, such as jumping. Low-impact activities include brisk walking, cross-country skiing, cycling, and low-impact aerobics. Dance classes, including belly dancing and Nia (visit http://www.nianow.com for information), can also provide appropriate total-body workouts. Elliptical machines and stationary bikes offer safe workouts as well; however, be aware that spinning classes can quickly elevate your heart rate and body temperature.

Swimming or taking a water aerobics class provides a total-body workout with the lowest possible impact, because the water reduces the force of gravity on your body. In addition, standing or sitting in water that reaches your shoulders reduces swelling (edema) by pushing tissue fluid into your circulation (and eventually out of your body through urination).

Ideally, you should do some kind of aerobic exercise at least three times per week. Aerobic exercise regimens for pregnant women should include the following:

1. At least a five-minute warm-up, consisting of slow, smooth movements and stretching
2. About thirty minutes of aerobic exercise of moderate to vigorous intensity
3. At least a five-minute cool-down (until your heart rate returns to what it was before you began the workout), consisting of mild activity and possibly exercises for strength, flexibility, and relaxation

If you're just beginning an exercise regimen, start slowly and gently. To determine whether you're exercising too hard, take the "talk test."[1] If you can talk without gasping while exercising, your heart rate is at an acceptable level. If you can't talk without gasping, slow down until you can.

## Anaerobic Exercise

The following exercise practices don't increase your heart rate as much as aerobic exercise does, but offer other health benefits.

### Yoga

This practice promotes self-nurturing and harmony of the mind, body, and spirit. Yoga also strengthens core muscles (abdominal, pelvic floor, and back) and postural muscles, and improves flexibility, balance, breathing, and mental focus. (See page 100.)

### Pilates

Pilates is a system of conditioning exercises that strengthens core and postural muscles and improves flexibility and mental focus. During the childbearing year, avoid doing advanced abdominal exercises. They can aggravate or cause abdominal separation. (See page 341.)

### Tai Chi

This system of exercises emphasizes balance, focus, meditation, and smooth, fluid movement.

### Weightlifting

Weightlifting strengthens the targeted muscles and core muscles (when you contract them to stabilize your body). If you lifted weights regularly before becoming pregnant, you can continue working with light weights. If you didn't lift weights before pregnancy and want to begin a regimen, do so only under the direction of a professional trainer knowledgeable about pregnancy.

Gyms, community centers, and even some hospitals offer beginning or prenatal yoga, pilates, tai chi, and weightlifting classes. You can also find many excellent classes on DVD.

## Sports and High-intensity Activities

Pregnancy isn't the time to take up a new sport or activity that requires good balance or sudden movements, or puts you at risk for falling. If before becoming pregnant you played sports such as tennis or softball, or engaged in activities such as vigorous swimming or cycling, you may continue doing them while pregnant for as long as you feel comfortable and if your pregnancy remains low-risk.

In late pregnancy, avoid downhill skiing, water-skiing, snowmobiling, and horseback riding, regardless of your skill level. These activities require excellent balance (which you might not have), and your likelihood of falling increases if you participate in them.

Throughout your pregnancy, avoid potentially dangerous activities such as skydiving, scuba diving, springboard diving, surfing, rock or mountain climbing (especially at elevations higher than 6,000 feet).

To decide whether the benefits of a particular athletic activity outweigh the possible risks, ask yourself the key questions on page 10. If you have further questions about an activity's safety, talk with your caregiver.

# General Guidelines for Safe, Effective Exercise

- Exercise three to seven days per week. Try to do a variety of activities. Always include a warm-up and a cool-down.
- Build your strength and endurance gradually. In the beginning, keep the intensity of your workout low to moderate. As your strength and stamina increase, so should the intensity. Toward the end of pregnancy, decrease the intensity as needed.
- Modify exercises so you can do them safely. If taking an exercise class, let the instructor know you're pregnant and welcome any exercise modifications.
- Lying flat on your back in pregnancy can cause supine hypotension. (See page 89.) If you feel dizzy, short of breath, or lightheaded while on your back, roll onto your left side until you've recovered.
- To prevent dizziness and to avoid increased pressure on your pelvic floor and abdominal muscles, don't hold your breath while exercising.
- Use the "talk test" (see page 93) to ensure you're not exercising too vigorously.
- Eat enough to meet the caloric needs of pregnancy as well as your exercise regimen. Not eating enough can put you and your baby at risk for complications. (See page 117.)
- Drink water before, during, and after exercising to replace fluids lost through perspiration and respiration. Keep a water bottle with you.
- Don't exercise vigorously in hot, humid weather or when you have a fever. Your body temperature shouldn't exceed 101°F (38.3°C).
- Stop exercising if you experience pain, headache, nausea, severe breathlessness, dizziness, blurred vision (or you see spots), vaginal bleeding, or continuing strong uterine contractions. (See below.)
- Be flexible and patient as you work to meet your fitness goals. Pay attention to how your body feels and adapt your exercise regimen accordingly.
- Consult your caregiver if you have questions about exercise.

**When *Not* to Exercise**

Avoid or stop exercising if you have the following conditions:

- Vaginal bleeding
- Persistent Braxton-Hicks contractions
- Increased risk for preterm labor
- Preeclampsia
- Premature rupture of membranes (loss of fluid from your vagina)
- Placenta previa diagnosed after the twenty-sixth week of pregnancy
- A baby with intrauterine growth restriction (IUGR)
- A baby whose movements have noticeably decreased

Consult with your caregiver about exercising if you are pregnant with multiples, are on bed rest, or have high blood pressure, diabetes, chronic heart problems, thyroid disease, or joint disease or injury.

# Core Exercises to Prepare You for Labor

Core muscles include the abdominal muscles, pelvic floor muscles, and back and hip muscles—all of which provide stability, balance, and posture. Giving birth relies on these muscles, and conditioning them during pregnancy prepares them for labor and promotes their speedy recovery afterward.

## CONDITIONING YOUR PELVIC FLOOR MUSCLES

Your *pelvic floor muscles* are attached to the inside of your pelvis and act like a sling to support your abdominal and pelvic organs. These muscles form a figure-eight around your urethra, vagina, and anus.

Regularly exercising your pelvic floor muscles is essential to maintain tone and improve circulation during the childbearing year and throughout your lifetime. During pregnancy, the increased weight of your uterus and the relaxing effect of hormones may make these muscles sag. Hemorrhoids may emerge. Exercising the pelvic floor muscles during pregnancy can reduce the heavy, throbbing feeling you may experience in the area. Exercise (and perineal massage—see page 235) also prepares you to work with the muscles surrounding your vagina as they stretch to let you push your baby out. When these muscles are toned, they can return to their original length after being stretched, which helps with postpartum recovery.

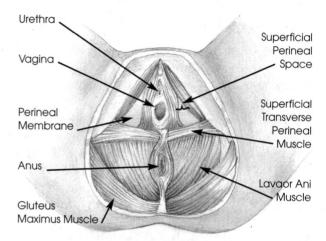

Regular exercise of your pelvic floor muscles may also prevent incontinence (leaking urine or feces) during pregnancy or later in life. If incontinence becomes a problem even after exercising your pelvic muscles, consult a physical therapist who specializes in nonsurgical treatment of incontinence.

As an added benefit, exercising your pelvic floor muscles can increase your ability to control your vaginal muscles, which can make sex more enjoyable for you and your partner.

To check the strength of your pelvic floor muscles, try these exercises:

- While urinating, partially empty your bladder, then stop the flow. If you can't, your muscles are weak.
- Insert one or two fingers into your vagina and tighten your pelvic floor muscles until you feel them squeeze your fingers. The tighter the squeeze is, the stronger your muscles are.
- During intercourse, have your partner tell you how strong your pelvic muscles tighten around your partner's penis or fingers.

If your muscles are weak, don't worry. They strengthen quickly with the following exercises.

## Pelvic Floor Contraction (Kegel or Super Kegel Exercise)

**Aim:** To maintain the tone of your pelvic floor muscles, improve blood circulation in them, decrease the incidence and severity of hemorrhoids and incontinence, and support your uterus and other pelvic organs.
**Starting position:** Any position is fine.
**Exercise:** Without holding your breath, tighten the muscles around your urethra and vaginal opening as if you're stopping the flow of urine. (Try not to tighten the muscles in your buttocks, thighs, or abdomen.) You should feel your pelvic floor lift slightly and become tense. Hold tightly for ten seconds.

At first, you may notice the muscle tension diminishing or fading without your control before ten seconds has passed. If this happens, tighten the muscles again until time is up, then relax and rest for ten seconds before tightening for another ten seconds.

When you can steadily contract the muscles for ten seconds, try a Super Kegel. For this exercise, you hold the contraction for twenty seconds, tightening the muscles when the contraction begins to fade. **Repetition:** Try to do several sets of ten Kegels or Super Kegels throughout the day.

## Pelvic Floor Bulging

**Aim:** To prepare for pushing your baby out (the second stage of labor). Make sure your bladder is empty when practicing this exercise!

**Starting position:** Tailor-sit (sit cross-legged on the floor) or get into any birthing position (see pages 222–223).

**Exercise:** Consciously relax your pelvic floor muscles. Hold your breath and bear down gently as you do when having a bowel movement, letting your pelvic floor muscles further relax and bulge outward. Don't bear down or strain forcefully. (Put your hand on your perineum to help you feel the bulge.) Hold for three to five seconds, then stop bearing down. Inhale, contract your pelvic floor muscles, then exhale and rest. After you can do this exercise while holding your breath, try it while exhaling.

**Repetition:** Do this exercise one to two times per week.

## CONDITIONING YOUR ABDOMINAL MUSCLES

Conditioning your abdominal muscles during pregnancy helps you maintain good posture, keep your core stable, avoid back pain, push your baby out more easily, and recover your abdominal strength after the birth. The four layers of your abdominal muscles work together with other core muscles to bend your body forward or sideways, rotate your core, tilt your pelvis, help with breathing, and stabilize your body when you lift objects.

Because your growing uterus already stretches your abdominal muscles, doing traditional exercises that work these muscles puts you at risk for back and abdominal strains. In late pregnancy, avoid doing double leg lifts or abdominal crunches (traditional sit-ups). The following exercises condition your abdominal muscles without causing excessive strain.

## Transverse Abdominal Contractions

**Aim:** To strengthen your innermost abdominal layer (transverse abdominis), which provides core stability and lets you actively push your baby out. After the birth, this exercise begins flattening your abdomen and closing any muscle separation. (See page 341.)

**Starting position:** Sit upright with your back supported against a straight-back chair or a wall.

**Exercise:** Inhale deeply, letting your abdomen expand. Slowly exhale, bringing your belly button toward your spine. (Put your hand on your belly to ensure you're doing this movement.) Hold the contraction for twenty seconds without holding your breath. *Variation:* During the twenty seconds, pulse the contraction by releasing it slightly as you inhale and tightening it as you exhale. Pulse ten to twenty times.

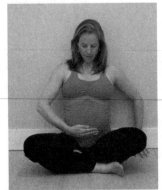

**Repetition:** Begin with two sets of ten repetitions and add repetitions as you become stronger. Expect this exercise to become more difficult in late pregnancy, but make sure to resume it after the birth.

## Pelvic Tilts I, II, and III

**Aim:** To strengthen your abdominal muscles, improve posture, and relieve back pain.

**Starting position:** Lie on your back, get on your hands and knees, or stand. (See following sections for further directions.)

**Exercise:** With an exhalation, tighten your abdominal muscles, and hold the contraction for five to ten seconds. Imagine that these muscles are hugging your baby. Contract your lower abdominals to tilt the front of your pelvis upward. Relax, then repeat.

**Repetition:** Do ten pelvic tilts each day.

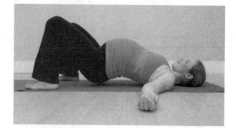

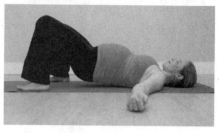

### I. *Pelvic tilt on your back*

**Starting position:** Lie on your back with knees bent and feet flat on the floor. When contracting your abdominal muscles, the small of your back flattens onto the floor. Don't push with your feet or tighten your buttocks. Placing a hand under your lower back may make it easier to feel that the small of your back is flattening. *Note:* If you feel dizzy or lightheaded while on your back, roll onto your left side and try pelvic tilt II or III instead.

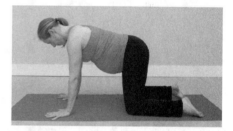

### II. *Pelvic tilt on hands and knees*

**Starting position:** Get on your hands and knees. Keep your back in a neutral position (neither sagging nor arched) and your knees hip-width apart. As you tighten your abdominal muscles, your pelvis curls under and your lower back arches. Your upper back may arch as well.

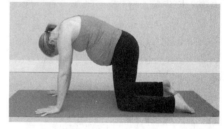

### III. *Pelvic tilt when standing*

**Starting position:** Lean against a wall with knees slightly bent and feet apart and 12 to 15 inches away from the wall. Let your buttocks and shoulders touch the wall. As you contract your abdominal muscles, your back presses against the wall.

After you've mastered the pelvic tilt while leaning against a wall, try it while standing upright. As you tighten your abdominal muscles in this starting position, your pubic bone tilts upward, tilting the top of your pelvis backward. To feel this movement, put your hands on your hips.

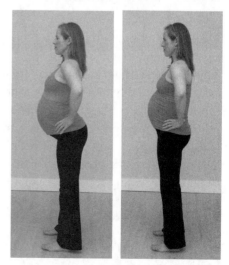

## Common Q & A

**Q:** I know it's good to squat during pregnancy, but I'm having trouble getting up from the position. What can I do?

**A:** To rise from a squat more easily, add an exercise to strengthen your thighs and buttocks, such as wall-sitting. Stand with your back resting against a wall and your feet 12 inches away from the wall. Bend your knees so they're directly above your feet, letting your back slide down the wall. Remain in that position for up to one minute. Try to rise from this position without using your arms. Repeat this exercise five to ten times each day. As you become stronger, place your feet farther from the wall, until you can bend your knees 90 degrees and your thighs are parallel with the floor.

## MOBILIZING YOUR PELVIC JOINTS BY SQUATTING

During late pregnancy, squatting helps condition your pelvic joints. To birth your baby vaginally, the joints of your pelvis need to be flexible enough to allow him to move from your uterus through your vagina. As you approach the end of pregnancy, this exercise becomes even more important. During labor, squatting can be a comfort position for you. (See page 222.) When you push your baby out, squatting can help your baby descend into your vagina.

*Caution:* If you have problems with your hips, knees, ankles, pelvis, or have hemorrhoids, avoid squatting.

**Aim:** To increase the flexibility of your pelvic joints, stretch the muscles of your inner thighs and calves, and increase comfort when squatting.

**Starting position:** Stand with your feet about 2 feet apart.

**Exercise:** Keeping your heels on the floor, squat by lowering your buttocks toward the floor and letting your lower back curve. For better stability and more of a curve in your lower back, distribute your weight

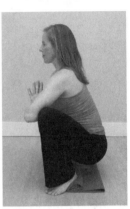

evenly between your heels and toes. Hold the position for as long as is comfortable, then use your legs to rise slowly. As you become stronger, increase the amount of time you hold the position to ninety seconds, which is roughly the length of a long labor contraction.

If you have trouble squatting, try stretching the muscles of your inner thighs by tailor-sitting with your soles touching. If you can't maintain your balance when squatting, hold on to a stable piece of furniture, the doorknobs on either side of a door, or your partner's hands. You can also try this position for stability or if squatting causes pain in your legs or pubic area: Have your partner sit on a chair. Facing away from your partner, stand between his or her knees. Then squat, leaning back with your arms over your partner's knees.

If it's difficult to keep your heels on the floor when squatting or if your feet roll inward, your calf muscles are tight. Try squatting with your feet farther apart, wearing shoes with heels of moderate height, putting a book under each heel, or placing a rolled-up mat or towel under your heels. Many birthing beds in hospitals have bars to grip while squatting.

**Repetition:** Starting at about the thirty-fifth week of pregnancy, squat ten times each day.

# Postural Exercises to Align Your Body

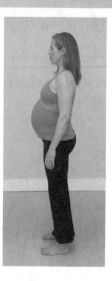

Your postural muscles keep your body in proper alignment. As your baby and uterus grow, your center of gravity shifts forward, which requires you to make an extra effort to maintain good posture. (See page 88.)

The normal changes of pregnancy also stretch your abdominal and upper back muscles and tighten your pectoral (chest) muscles and hip flexors (the muscles in the front of your hips). Strengthening and stretching these muscles helps relieve lower back pain and other discomforts that can arise when your body is out of alignment.

## POSTURE CHECK

To maintain correct postural alignment, prevent back pain, reduce fatigue, and allow your body to function normally, it's important to check your posture several times throughout the day. Follow the instructions on page 88 to ensure good posture when standing or sitting.

### Shoulder Circles

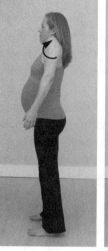
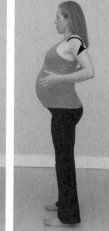

**Aim:** To release tension and put your shoulders into correct postural alignment.

**Starting position:** Stand or sit with your back straight. Keep your arms relaxed and your chin level.

**Exercise:** Raise your shoulders toward your ears, then slowly roll them back and down, then forward and up. Feel the tension release. End with your shoulders in a relaxed back-and-down position.

**Repetition:** Circle your shoulders as many times throughout the day as feels comfortable.

## PECTORAL STRETCH

**Aim:** To lengthen your pectoral muscles, which naturally shorten during pregnancy or with poor posture. This exercise also may help you breathe more deeply.

**Starting position:** Stand with good posture in a doorway.

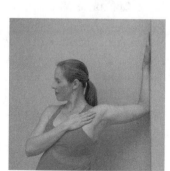

**Exercise:** With your elbow at shoulder level, rest your forearm on the doorframe. While pulling your shoulder blades down your spine, turn your body away from the doorframe until you feel your chest stretch. Breathe deeply, letting your ribs expand with each inhalation. Hold the stretch for fifteen to thirty seconds. Relax, then repeat on your other side.

**Repetition:** Stretch your pectoral muscles twice on each side.

## HIP FLEXOR STRETCH

**Aim:** To stretch the muscles in the front of your hips that naturally tighten in pregnancy.

**Starting position:** Stand with your right leg forward (knee slightly bent) and your left leg back (knee straight). Keep both feet flat on the floor and about hip-width apart. You can hold on to a stable chair for support.

**Exercise:** Contract your left buttock and pull the front of your pelvis upward (as you do with the pelvic tilt—see page 97) until you feel a stretch in the front of your left hip. Hold the stretch for fifteen to thirty seconds. Relax, then repeat with your left leg forward and your right leg back.

**Repetition:** Stretch your hip flexors twice on each side.

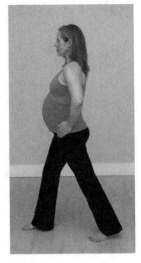

# Yoga Poses to Align Your Body, Mind, and Spirit

Yoga builds strength and stamina, improves flexibility and balance, encourages mindfulness, increases energy, and promotes meditation (which calms the mind and nourishes the spirit).

Unlike many other forms of exercise, yoga focuses on *practicing* movements, not *mastering* them. Even if you practice yoga regularly, you may feel flexible and strong one day and less so the next—and that's okay. Letting go of expectations and self-criticism is essential to the practice of yoga.

This section features yoga poses that especially benefit you during pregnancy and birth. It also includes a sequence of poses that mimics the rhythm of labor, by alternating poses that require exertion with those that call for relaxation.

While doing these poses, make sure you control your movements and pay attention to your body position, mental activity, and emotional reactions. What you learn may help you work with your body in labor. For more guidance, consider taking a prenatal yoga class or following a class on DVD.

If you feel dizzy when in a pose, lie on your left side to recover.

## CAT POSE

**Aim:** To strengthen your abdominal muscles and stretch your back. This pose may help your baby assume a head-down position for birth.

**Starting position:** Get on your hands and knees.

**Exercise:** Inhale and relax the muscles in your back while lifting your tailbone and breastbone. As you exhale, round your mid-back, letting your head, tailbone, and breastbone sink toward the floor. Flatten your mid-back with your next inhalation, making sure your belly doesn't sag.

**Repetition:** Do this pose for five inhalations and exhalations, keeping the movements smooth.

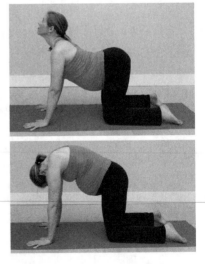

## OPPOSITE-LIMB EXTENSIONS

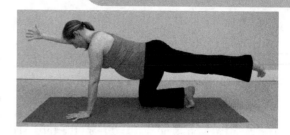

**Aim:** To strengthen your core and postural muscles and help you coordinate your breathing with muscle exertion.

**Starting position:** Get on your hands and knees. In early pregnancy or after the birth, you can lie on your stomach.

**Exercise:** Extend one leg back, with your toes on the floor. Tighten your abdominal muscles to pull your belly button toward your spine. Inhale and tuck your tailbone as you lift your straight leg behind you, then exhale and reach the opposite arm out in front of you. Breathing evenly, lengthen the stretch by reaching toward the wall behind you with your heel and the wall in front of you with your fingertips. Keep your gaze on the floor and your back in a neutral position. Lower your arm and leg after a few breaths, and repeat with the opposite arm and leg.

If you have trouble extending an arm and leg at the same time, extend them one at a time.

**Repetition:** Do this pose five times for each side.

## CHILD'S POSE

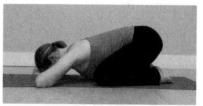

**Aim:** To widen your pelvis, stretch your groin and torso, and provide active relaxation between more challenging poses.

**Starting position:** Kneel on the floor with your knees in a wide V, then rest your bottom on your heels.

**Exercise:** Keeping your torso straight, slowly bend forward from the hips, using your arms to guide yourself forward onto the floor. Fold your arms on the floor and rest your head on your forearms. (If this position causes too deep of a stretch, prop yourself up on bent elbows). If your buttocks have risen, try to return them to your heels. Rest your forehead on the floor and breathe deeply and evenly.

For more of a stretch, rest your forehead on the floor and extend your arms out in front of your head. Use your fingers to pull and lengthen your torso.

**Duration:** Remain in this position for five inhalations and exhalations, or for as long as it takes to relax.

## DOWNWARD-FACING DOG

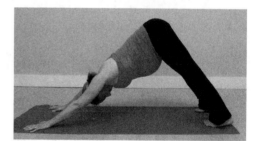

**Aim:** To stretch your calf and hamstring muscles (which become tighter as pregnancy progresses), reduce fatigue, and improve circulation in your legs. This pose also helps relieve tension in your shoulders and spine, and helps improve upper body strength while stretching your chest.

**Starting position:** Get on your hands and knees.

**Exercise:** Spread your fingers wide with the middle finger of each hand pointing straight ahead of you. Tuck your toes under and inhale deeply. As you exhale, make an inverted V with your body by lifting your tailbone toward the ceiling, straightening your legs, and lengthening your spine. Let your head hang and breathe evenly. Position your feet so they're hip-width apart and your toes are facing forward. Try to rest your heels on the floor.

To release the pose, lower your knees or get into child's pose to rest completely.

**Duration:** Hold this pose for five inhalations and exhalations.

# HALF-DOG POSE

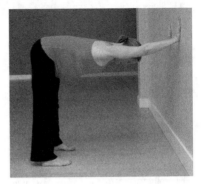

**Aim:** To stretch your back, release tension in your shoulders, and stretch your hamstrings. You can use this pose as an alternative to downward-facing dog.

**Starting position:** Stand facing a wall, then lean forward and place your hands shoulder-width apart on the wall. Walk your feet backward as you bend forward from the hips, sliding your hands down the wall until your back and arms are parallel with the floor. Keep your head in line with your arms and gaze at the floor.

**Exercise:** Inhale and push your hands into the wall. As you exhale, elongate your spine by stretching your tailbone straight out behind you. To keep the natural curve of your spine, rotate your sit bones (the bones you sit on) upward to keep your lower back from flattening.

**Duration:** Hold this pose for five to ten inhalations and exhalations.

# CORPSE POSE

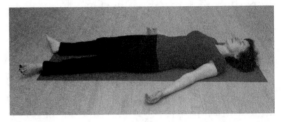

**Aim:** To completely relax while remaining awake and attentive. This restorative pose nurtures the mind-body-spirit connection and helps you connect to your baby.

**Starting position:** Lie on your back with your legs extended, your arms by your side (but not touching you), and your palms up.

**Exercise:** Actively lengthen your body from your heels, through your arms and head. Then relax all your muscles. End the pose by rolling onto your side and into a fetal position. Stay in this position for a few moments, until you feel ready to sit up.

If you become lightheaded, dizzy, or short of breath while on your back (common in late pregnancy), do this pose by lying on your left side and cradling your head with your arms or placing pillows under your head and between your legs.

**Duration:** Stay in this pose for five to ten minutes.

# FIVE-MINUTE MEDITATION

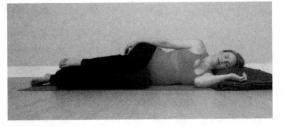

**Aim:** To nurture your mind-body-spirit connection as well your connection to your baby, and create time to release tension and focus on what's important to you. This exercise lets you release your need for control and embrace "going with the flow"—an important mind-set for pregnancy, childbirth, and parenthood.

This exercise can follow or be integrated into corpse pose.

**Starting position:** Because you can do this exercise anywhere, choose a position that works in the moment and one that you can comfortably maintain for five minutes. Options include tailor-sitting, lying on your back or left side, legs-up-the-wall pose (see page 106), sitting in a chair, or lying in a warm bath.

## Yoga Practice for Labor Preparation

This sequence of poses mimics the rhythm of labor (contractions followed by periods of rest) by alternating poses that require exertion with those that call for rest.

1. Tailor-sit with eyes closed while focusing on your breathing, quieting mental distractions, and concentrating on being with your baby.
2. Cat pose
3. Child's pose
4. Opposite-limb extensions
5. Child's pose
6. Downward-facing dog
7. Child's pose
8. Half-dog pose
9. Final pose for relaxation or meditation: Choose corpse pose, side-lying, legs-up-the-wall pose (see page 106), or tailor-sitting.

*Note:* Adapt your yoga practice to accommodate how you're feeling. If at any time you become dizzy or fatigued, rest in child's pose or lie on your left side.

**Exercise:** Quiet any distracting thoughts by focusing on your breathing. With each breath, let your body and mind release any tension and expectations so you can completely relax. Take this time to thank your hardworking body, send your baby loving energy, and honor yourself as well as your partner and family. This exercise can clarify your hopes and fears, and can reveal any gaps in your childbirth preparation or support system. You can also use this time to practice the visualization techniques discussed on page 208.

**Duration:** As the birth approaches, you may want to meditate for longer than five minutes, and you may want to meditate more often.

# Comfort Measures for Common Discomforts in Pregnancy

Even if you consistently maintain good posture, move with care, and exercise moderately, you may still experience discomforts during pregnancy. This section explains the causes of some common discomforts, offers ways you can prevent or minimize them, and suggests treatments to relieve them.

## LOWER BACK PAIN

Over the course of your pregnancy, your abdominal muscles lengthen up to 120 percent. To maintain your balance and alignment, your lower back muscles and hip flexors shorten and tighten, which may cause lower back pain. Here are ways to help prevent lower back pain:

- Maintain good posture. (Poor posture often contributes to back pain.)
- Move with care to prevent straining joints, ligaments, and tendons (which soften and relax from hormonal changes).
- Use positions and exercises that stretch tight muscles and strengthen abdominal muscles.

## Relieving Severe Back Pain

If you have severe back pain, ask your caregiver to refer you to a physical therapist or chiropractor who specializes in perinatal issues. This expert can provide treatment that may include ice packs, heat, hydrotherapy, massage, techniques to mobilize joints, and an exercise regimen designed to address your specific problem. Your caregiver may recommend that you wear a special garment or belt to support your abdomen and lower back.

To relieve pain from muscular tension, use a heating pad or hot-water bottle, or take a warm bath or shower. Use an ice pack to decrease inflammation and relieve pain. For enjoyable relief, get a professional massage or have your partner give you a soothing backrub.

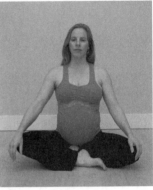

Here are exercises that can relieve lower back pain:

- Half-dog pose, cat pose, or child's pose (See pages 99–102.)
- Pelvic tilt on hands and knees (See page 97.)
- Tailor-sitting (Sitting in this position can keep your lower back relaxed.)
- Squatting (See page 98.)

Another good exercise to try is the **knee-to-shoulder exercise**. Here's how to do it: Lie on your back. Draw one knee toward your chest and hold that leg behind your thigh with one hand, then do the same for your other leg. Keep your knees apart to avoid putting pressure on your belly. Keeping your head on the floor, gently pull your knees toward your shoulders until you feel a slight stretch in your lower back. Hold for a slow count of five, then release without letting go of your knees. Stretch your lower back this way five times. Then lower your feet one at a time. Roll onto your side after you've finished the exercise.

*Notes:* In late pregnancy, you may wish to pull only one leg at a time. If this exercise makes you dizzy or lightheaded, don't do it.

## UPPER BACK PAIN

As your pregnancy progresses, your breasts become heavier and your pectoral (chest) muscles shorten as your upper back muscles lengthen. Your shoulder and neck muscles may try to compensate for these changes by working harder. To prevent or relieve upper back pain, try to maintain proper posture, stretch your pectoral muscles regularly, and do movements to reduce tension in your shoulders, neck, and jaw. Several times a day, take a deep breath, relax your jaw, and roll your shoulders back and down. Massage and the relaxation exercises described in Chapter 11 can also help ease upper back pain.

Shoulder circles (see page 99) and half-dog pose (see page 102) help increase circulation, stretch tense muscles, and decrease back pain. An **upper body stretch** can also help. Here's how to do this exercise: Sit in a chair, tailor-sit on the floor, or stand. Raise your arms (palms down) in front of you to shoulder height. Cross them at the elbows; feel your upper back stretch. While inhaling slowly, raise your hands toward the ceiling and gradually uncross your arms (as if pulling a shirt over your head). Reach upward to feel the stretch in your entire upper body. Keeping your arms extended, exhale as you lower them in an arc along each side of your body until your hands

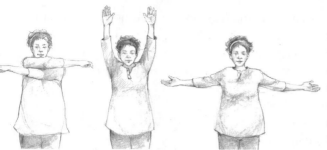

are about 12 inches from each hip. Point your thumbs behind you and tilt your head to look up. Feel the stretch across your chest and upper arms. Maintain this stretch as you breathe deeply, allowing your rib cage to expand. Release your arms to your sides and relax without slumping. Repeat this entire sequence five times.

## TINGLING OR NUMBNESS IN YOUR ARMS OR HANDS

Especially during the night or in the morning after awakening, excess tissue fluid in some pregnant women puts pressure on the nerves and blood vessels, causing tingling or numbness in the arms or hands. If the symptoms are confined to the hands, the condition is called "carpal tunnel syndrome." If symptoms involve the entire arm, it's called "thoracic outlet syndrome."

To prevent or treat the problem, try the following suggestions:
- Lie on your side in a position that supports you without lying on your arm. Or use pillows to support you. (See page 89.)
- Try doing shoulder circles and the upper body stretch. (See pages 99 and 104.)
- Several times a day, stretch one arm upward. Wiggle your fingers for a slow count of five. Lower your arm and repeat with your other arm.
- If you have severe carpal tunnel syndrome, wear a wrist splint to hold your wrist in the best position to prevent tingling and numbness. (Your caregiver can tell you where to get a splint.)
- For thoracic outlet syndrome, try raising your arms to shoulder height, then bending your elbows and placing one hand on top of the other on your forehead. *Note:* Wearing a wrist splint doesn't relieve thoracic outlet syndrome.

## ACHING LEGS, SWOLLEN FEET AND ANKLES, OR VARICOSE VEINS

Hormonal changes and increased body weight often affect the blood circulation in pregnant women, causing aching legs, swollen feet and ankles, or varicose veins. To promote better circulation and ease or prevent these discomforts, try these suggestions:
- Avoid prolonged standing or sitting; sit or walk intermittently.
- Several times a week, take a walk, swim, or use a stationary bike or treadmill.
- When sitting, elevate your feet. If you can't, rotate your ankles and don't cross your legs at the knees. If you plan to sit for a while, try rocking in a rocking chair to exercise the muscles in your legs and feet.
- When resting during the day, lie on your side or elevate your feet.
- Do a pelvic tilt on your hands and knees. (See page 97.) This exercise reduces the weight of your uterus on the blood vessels in the pelvis and abdomen. The rocking movement promotes blood flow.
- Walk (or play) in deep water for an hour every other day. The weight of the water presses on your swollen tissues, reducing swelling and promoting urination to void excess fluid. These benefits last for about forty-eight hours. If you use a hot tub, make sure the water temperature doesn't exceed 99°F (37.2°C).
- Wear support stockings, especially if your job requires a lot of standing. The best time to put on the stockings is before you get out of bed in the morning, because the swelling is at its minimum after you've been in a horizontal position for an extended time.

To decrease swelling while relaxing, you may want to try the **legs-up-the-wall pose**. To do this yoga exercise, place a folded blanket 6 inches from a wall. Sit on the edge of the blanket so your side is parallel with the wall and your hip is touching it. Bend your knees. As you lean back-

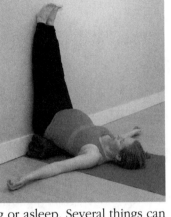

ward, bring your knees to your chest, then extend your legs up the wall as you rotate your body 90 degrees. Your buttocks now should be on the blanket and your legs should be relatively straight. Hold this pose for five minutes. If you like, instead of having your legs straight up the wall, stretch your inner thighs by separating your legs into a V shape.

To get out of this pose, bend your knees, then roll onto your side. Stay on your side for a few breaths before sitting up. *Note:* If you feel dizzy, short of breath, or uncomfortable in this pose, roll onto your left side and remain there until the symptoms disappear.

## LOWER LEG AND FOOT CRAMPS

Cramps in the calves or feet commonly occur when women are resting or asleep. Several things can cause cramps, including pressure on leg nerves, dehydration, impaired circulation, fatigue in calf muscles, or a mineral imbalance in the blood (that is, too little calcium or magnesium, or too much phosphorus, which is found in foods such as soft drinks and processed foods).

To prevent cramps, eat well, drink plenty of water, and avoid pointing your toes or standing on your tiptoes. Right before going to bed, try the following exercises to stretch your calves or hamstrings.

### Relieving Lower Leg Cramps

Stand with your weight on the cramped leg. Step forward with your other foot and bend the knee of that leg. Keeping the knee of your cramped leg straight and the heel on the floor, lean forward to stretch the cramped muscle.

If the cramp is severe, you may need help from your partner. Sit on a chair or bed and have your partner hold the knee of your cramped leg steady with one hand and, while gripping your heel with the other hand, use his or her forearm to gently press your foot and toes up toward your knee.

### Relieving Foot Cramps

A cramp in your foot tightens the muscles of the arch and curls the toes. To relieve the cramp, stretch your toes up and back toward your shin.

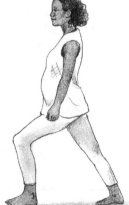

## SUDDEN GROIN PAIN

Round ligaments connect the front of your uterus to each groin, the crease or hollow that connects your inner thigh to your trunk. These ligaments contract and relax like muscles, but much more slowly. When you're in labor, this design is beneficial. As your uterus contracts, these ligaments contract and pull the uterus forward, aligning it and your baby with the vagina for efficient birthing.

Because these ligaments stretch and contract slowly, they work to prevent sudden overstretching. When you stand up quickly or when you sneeze or cough, you may stretch the ligaments too quickly, causing them to contract rapidly (stretch reflex) and causing pain in your lower abdomen or groin.

You can prevent this pain by moving slowly, letting the ligaments stretch gradually. Before sneezing or coughing, try to flex your hips to bring your thighs near your belly to reduce the pull on the ligaments.

## *Key Points to Remember*

- Maintaining good posture and moving with care increase your comfort during pregnancy and promote a faster recovery from birth.
- Regular exercise during pregnancy improves or maintains your muscle tone, strength, and endurance. It also protects against back pain, reduces the intensity of common pregnancy discomforts, and boosts your energy level, mood, and self-image.
- Most pregnant women should do various physical activities three to seven days per week to reap the benefits of moderate exercise.
- Exercises for your core and posture are essential during the childbearing year to condition your muscles for effective birthing and promote a speedier postpartum recovery.
- Align your mind, body, and spirit and connect with your baby through yoga and meditation.
- It's never too late to start an exercise regimen. Set reasonable fitness expectations and celebrate your successes.

# CHAPTER 6

# Eating Well

The quality of the foods you eat before and during pregnancy has a huge impact on your health and on your baby's development and long-term well-being. But which foods should you eat to ensure the best possible pregnancy? How much of them should you eat? How much weight should you gain? What about salt, food cravings, and morning sickness? Over the years, health care professionals have given different answers to these and other nutrition questions. Some advice is based on accurate information; some isn't. This chapter provides the most accurate, up-to-date recommendations so you can make choices that best fit your lifestyle and food preferences.

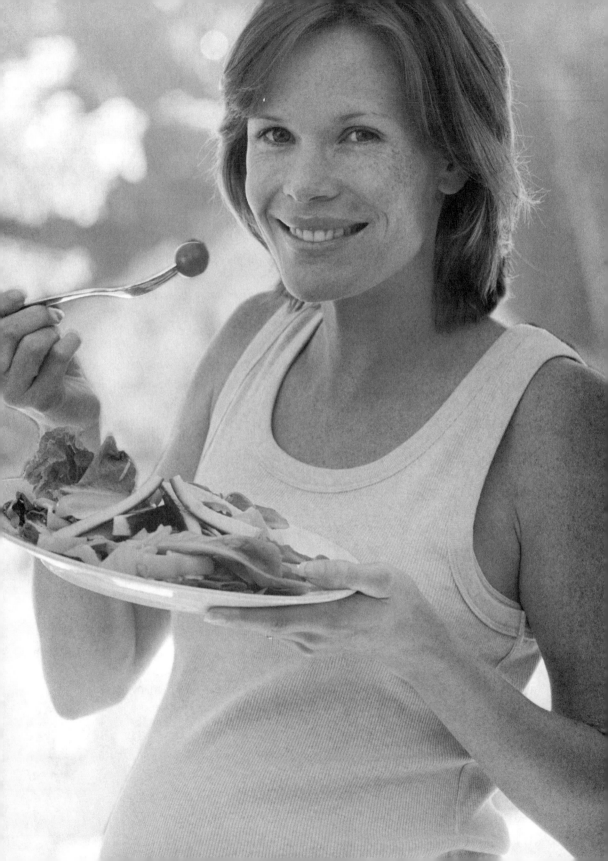

# Good Nutrition during Pregnancy

For good nutrition during pregnancy, your daily diet should be varied and include plenty of fresh fruits and vegetables, whole grains, low-fat dairy products, foods that contain protein, and about 2 quarts of liquids. By eating small, frequent meals each day (for example, three small main meals and three light snacks), you help keep your blood sugar level stable throughout the day, reduce morning sickness in the first trimester, and reduce heartburn in the third trimester.

During the first trimester, you don't need to eat more than you did before you became pregnant. Beginning in the second trimester, however, you need to consume about 200 extra calories each day (assuming you exercise daily for thirty to sixty minutes). Two hundred calories isn't a lot—just two glasses of nonfat milk, one chicken drumstick without skin, or 2 tablespoons of peanut butter.

In the third trimester, you need to consume about 400 more calories than you did before pregnancy. Ideally, these additional calories should come from high-protein, high-calcium, and iron-rich whole foods—not from foods lacking in nutrition, such as chips, cookies, candy, and soft drinks.

Whenever you consider what to eat, make the best possible choice at the time. Don't feel that your diet must always be perfect. Some days, it may be hard to get the healthful food you need. Other days, it may be impossible to resist treating yourself to a favorite junk food. Just be aware of what you eat and try to eat healthfully whenever possible.

Always keep in mind that your baby benefits from any healthy changes you make to your diet. To analyze your diet, visit our web site, http://www.PCNGuide.com, to download a food diary so you can keep track of what you're eating. After recording what you ate for a week, look at the nutritional balance of your food choices and make plans to improve your nutrition for the next week.

## A NOTE TO FATHERS AND PARTNERS

You may be surprised to learn that most of the information in this chapter also applies to you. Even though you're not growing a baby, you can still use these forty weeks to begin eating a well-balanced diet and maintaining a healthy weight and activity level. By making these healthful lifestyle changes, you increase the likelihood that you'll have a longer, healthier life to share with your child. You'll also model the healthful choices you want your child to make.

Although recommendations for specific amounts of nutrients are for pregnant women, this chapter directs you where to find information specific to your needs.

## MYPLATE: RECOMMENDED FOOD GROUPS

In 2011, the U.S. Department of Agriculture (USDA) developed MyPlate (http://www.myplate.gov), a food guidance system designed to provide customized information for specific audiences—including pregnant and breastfeeding women—based on current dietary and physical activity recommendations known to promote health.

ChooseMyPlate.gov

# Sample Daily Menu during Pregnancy

**When you get up for the day**
- Peppermint tea (or other decaffeinated tea)
- 6 whole-wheat crackers (that include 2 grams protein)

**Breakfast**
- Oatmeal (1 cup cooked oatmeal with ¼ cup raisins, ¼ cup chopped walnuts, 1 teaspoon sugar, and ½ cup nonfat milk)
- Orange juice (½ cup)

**Morning snack**
- Mini bagel with low-fat cream cheese
- Water

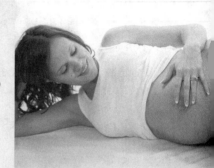

**Lunch**
- Southwestern salad (¾ cup black beans, ½ cup brown rice, ½ cup corn, ½ cup tomato, and cilantro, with 1 tablespoon lime juice and canola oil dressing) served over 1 cup romaine lettuce
- 2 flour tortillas
- Nonfat milk (1 cup)

**Afternoon snack**
- Light microwave popcorn (1 cup)
- Water

**Dinner**
- Stir-fry (4-ounce chicken breast, 1 carrot, ½ cup broccoli, ¼ red pepper, 6 snap peas, and spices), cooked in 1 tablespoon olive oil
- White rice (1 cup)
- Nonfat milk (1 cup)
- Fortune cookie

**Evening snack**
- Smoothie (8-ounce nonfat yogurt with sweetener, 1 banana, 6 frozen strawberries)

To analyze your own daily diet, visit http://www.mypyramidtracker.gov. Enter the foods you've eaten in a day, and the program calculates how many servings you've had in each food group and how much of each nutrient you've consumed.

MyPlate describes five food groups and suggests what to eat each day; for example, "Make half your plate fruits and vegetables." Visit our web site, http://www.PCNGuide.com, to download our food diary so you can track your consumption of foods from each of these groups.

## Grains

This group includes any food made of wheat, rice, oats, cornmeal, barley, or rye. Grains contain iron, B vitamins, minerals, and fiber; some are fortified with folic acid. **Try to make half your grains whole.** Whole grains contain the entire grain and all its nutrients. **Try to limit refined grains**; these grains have been processed, which creates a softer, less chewy texture but removes nutrients. Often, refined grains are enriched (have vitamins and minerals added back in, but not fiber).

Whole grains include brown rice, oatmeal, popcorn, barley, millet, quinoa, spelt, buckwheat, bulgur, and wild rice. Some prepared foods include whole grains; check whether the package ingredients list whole-wheat flour, whole oats, and so on. Refined grains include white rice, white flour, and most prepared grain-based foods (such as bread, tortillas, noodles, crackers, pretzels, cereal, grits, couscous, and pastries).

## Vegetables

Vegetables are rich sources of fiber, vitamins, and minerals. **Try to vary your veggies.** Different vegetables have different nutrients, so eating a variety of vegetables ensures that you and your baby get all the nutrients you need. Here are examples of the different types of vegetables:

*Dark green vegetables*—Bok choy, broccoli, greens (collard, mustard, turnip, chard, and kale), lettuce (dark green leafy lettuce and romaine), spinach, and watercress

*Orange vegetables*—Carrots, pumpkin, squash, sweet potatoes, and yams

*Dried beans and peas (legumes)*—Black beans, black-eyed peas, garbanzo beans (chickpeas), kidney beans, lentils, pinto beans, soybeans and soy products, split peas, and white beans (These foods also belong in the Meats and Beans category; see page 113.)

*Starchy vegetables*—Corn, green peas, and potatoes

*Other vegetables*—Artichokes, asparagus, beets, Brussels sprouts, cabbage, cauliflower, celery, cucumbers, eggplant, green beans, mushrooms, okra, onions, peppers, tomatoes, vegetable juice, turnips, and zucchini

## Fruits

Apples, pears, peaches, plums, bananas, citrus fruits (such as oranges, grapefruit, lemons, and limes), tropical fruits (such as papaya, mango, and guava), melons, berries, and more are rich in fiber, potassium, vitamin C, and folate. **Eat a variety of fruits.**

## Milk (and Milk Products)

Dairy products provide the calcium you and your baby need for strong bones. They're also good sources of protein, potassium, and vitamins A, B, and D. To minimize your saturated fat intake, choose low-fat or nonfat milk products.

## Tips for Choosing and Preparing Fruits and Vegetables

Choose organically grown fruits and vegetables whenever possible. Some types of produce are especially likely to have pesticide residue when conventionally grown. These include apples, bell peppers, celery, cherries, imported grapes, nectarines, peaches, pears, potatoes, red raspberries, spinach, and strawberries.[1] To minimize the amount of chemicals and preservatives you may consume, choose organically grown varieties of this produce, if you can.

Choose fresh local produce that's in season, when it's cheapest and at its peak flavor. The more recently produce was picked, the more nutrients it has. If you can't get fresh produce, frozen is next best, then dried or canned (but avoid those with added sugar and salt).

Raw fruits and vegetables have a higher nutrient content than cooked produce does. If you cook produce, the following methods are ordered from best to worst for preserving nutrients: steaming, microwave cooking, stir-frying, roasting, baking, and boiling.

# MyPlate Food Groups and Servings[2]

| Food Group | What Equals a Serving? | Recommended Daily Servings* |
|---|---|---|
| **Grains** | 1 slice bread; 1 cup dry cereal; ½ cup cooked cereal, rice, or pasta; ½ bagel; 1 pita; 1 tortilla; 1 potato | 9 servings |
| **Vegetables** | 1 cup raw or cooked vegetables; 2 cups raw leafy vegetables; ¾ cup vegetable juice | 3½ servings |
| **Fruits** | 1 cup chopped fruit; 1 orange; 1 apple; 1 banana; ½ grapefruit; ⅛ cantaloupe; 1 handful grapes; 1 cup 100-percent fruit juice | 2 servings |
| **Milk** | 1 cup milk, cottage cheese, or yogurt; 1½-inch cube hard cheese | 3 servings |
| **Meat and beans** | 1 ounce meat, poultry, or fish; 1 egg; ½ cup tofu; ¼ cup cooked beans; ¼ cup nuts or seeds; 1 tablespoon peanut butter | 6½ servings |

These serving sizes are based on the assumption that you're choosing only foods that are low fat and without added sugar. You may also consume up to 330 "discretionary" calories per day from foods that contain **oils, fats, or sugars**. You may choose to eat foods that have a higher fat or sugar content, such as whole milk instead of nonfat, or sweetened cereal instead of unsweetened. Or you may choose condiments or foods that contain mostly fat or sugar, such as salad dressing, jelly, gravy, potato chips, or candy bars.

* Amounts are for a 2,600-calorie diet, appropriate for the second trimester of a 25-year-old, 5-foot 4-inch woman who weighed 160 pounds before pregnancy and exercises 30 to 60 minutes each day. For recommendations customized to you, visit http://choosemyplate.gov.

***If you don't like milk***—Try yogurt and cheese, or you may prefer foods made with milk, such as cream soups, custard, pudding, and ice cream.

***If you're lactose intolerant***—Try lactose-free milk or take a lactase enzyme before eating dairy products. Try cultured forms of milk, such as cheese, yogurt, or acidophilus milk. Your body may tolerate digesting several small servings of dairy instead of a few large servings.

***If you choose not to consume milk products***—Other sources of calcium include canned fish with bones; dark green leafy vegetables; dried beans; nuts and seeds; tofu with calcium sulfate; and calcium-fortified juice, soymilk, or rice milk. Your caregiver may recommend supplements such as calcium, vitamin D, potassium, and magnesium.

## Meats and Beans

Meats and beans contain protein, which builds muscles, skin, enzymes, hormones, and antibodies. They also contain B vitamins, vitamin E, iron, zinc, and magnesium.

***Making healthy choices about meat and fish***—Use food safety practices (see page 120). To minimize your intake of saturated fat, choose the leanest cuts of meat, trim away extra fat, and drain off grease after cooking. When buying prepared meats, check the ingredients label on the package and choose meats that don't include excess salt and fat. Eat fish twice a week. Choose seafood that's low in mercury and high in omega-3 fatty acids. (See page 121.)

***If you choose not to eat meat or fish***—Get the protein you need from eggs, dairy, beans, nuts, seeds, and tofu. You might not get enough iron, calcium, vitamin B12, or zinc unless you closely monitor your intake of those nutrients. If you're vegan, health care professionals typically recommend that you take a daily supplement of at least 1 microgram of vitamin B12.

## Fact or Fiction?

*To ensure you get the best nutrition, you should eat fortified food products that have been scientifically designed to meet all your nutritional needs.*

**Fiction.** Nutrition is an inexact science, and researchers are still learning about the components of a healthy diet. If you consider all the advice that nutritionists have given over the last fifty years, it's amazing to see how much of it was based on faulty reasoning or incomplete information!

The best advice for optimal health is to eat a wide variety of real food that has been processed as little as possible. To learn more about the importance of eating whole foods, read the books *In Defense of Food: An Eater's Manifesto* (2008) or *Food Rules: An Eater's Manual* (2009) by Michael Pollan.

### Empty Calories

Some foods, such as candy and soda, provide calories but no nutrients. Other foods, such as sweetened applesauce, fried chicken, or sugary cereals, contain some nutrients but also contain empty calories from solid fats and added sugars. Minimize your intake, or choose lower-fat, lower-sugar options.

# Nutrients

Certain nutrients are particularly important for ensuring a healthy pregnancy. The following sections discuss these nutrients.

For a complete summary of the functions and sources of all major nutrients, along with recommendations for daily intakes, visit our web site, http://www.PCNGuide.com.

### Protein

Protein builds all your body's cells. During pregnancy, your protein requirement increases to 71 grams (about 23 grams more than your prepregnancy requirement). Your growing volume of blood and amniotic fluid, plus the rapid growth of your placenta, uterus, and baby, are the reasons for the increased requirement.

You should get protein only from food sources. Prenatal vitamins don't supply protein, and protein supplements can lead to nutritional imbalances.

### Fats

Healthy fats are essential for your baby's brain growth, nervous system development, and aiding the absorption of vitamins A, D, E, and K. The healthiest fats are omega-3 fatty acids. Sufficient levels of these essential fatty acids in a pregnant woman's diet may help reduce preterm labor, hypertension, and depression. You can get omega-3 fatty acids only from your diet; your body can't synthesize them. The major sources are flaxseed oil and fish (see page 113). You can also find them in soybeans, walnuts, pumpkin seeds, pecans, hazelnuts, and omega-3 eggs. Omega-3 supplements from fish oil or flaxseed oil are also good sources.

After omega-3 fatty acids, the next best fats are unsaturated fats from plants, such as nuts and vegetable oils (canola, corn, safflower, sunflower, and olive). You can eat these fats in moderation.

Whether you're pregnant or not, your total fat intake each day shouldn't make up more than 30 percent of your diet and shouldn't exceed 85 grams. Limit your intake of saturated fats from animal food sources (such as dairy products and meat) to no more than 28 grams, and avoid hydrogenated fats and trans-fatty acids. These bad fats can elevate cholesterol levels, and they may be linked to other health problems (such as obesity, diabetes, and heart disease).

*Fat substitutes*—Olestra is a fat substitute found in a few brands of chips and crackers. Because olestra depletes the body of the fat-soluble vitamins A, D, E, and K, foods containing olestra are supplemented with those vitamins. Although olestra causes no known risks to the baby, foods containing olestra have few nutritional benefits, and pregnant women should avoid consuming those foods.

## Fluids

During pregnancy, fluids help deliver nutrients to your baby. They also help prevent constipation and urinary tract infections (UTIs). Drinking plenty of fluids doesn't cause swollen ankles; in fact, it helps keep you from retaining too much fluid in your tissues.

Try to drink at least 64 ounces of fluids each day. You know you're drinking enough fluids when your urine is pale yellow.

The healthiest fluid to drink is water, but some of your fluid intake can come from milk, juices, soups, and decaffeinated teas and coffees. Caffeine is a diuretic, which means it increases the amount of fluid in your urine (and decreases fluid retention in your body). As a result, you can't record the entire volume of caffeinated beverages in your daily liquid log. (For example, you can't attribute all the 12 ounces in a 12-ounce caffeinated beverage as part of your 64-ounces daily goal.) For more information on caffeine intake during pregnancy, see page 79.

You may find it difficult to drink enough fluids if doing so isn't a habit. To help make fluids (especially water) enjoyable to drink, find some favorite ways to prepare them. Here are some options to try: over ice cubes, at room temperature, warmed, or with a squeeze of lemon or lime juice. You may also try different ways to drink fluids, such as through a straw or from a water bottle, to discover which ways help you drink more.

### Common Q & A

**Q:** I've heard that bottled water is safer than tap water for me and my baby. Is this true?

**A:** Not necessarily. In the United States, municipal water systems are tightly regulated and monitored, making their water supplies safe for consumption. Bottled water may lack healthful minerals, which were filtered out before the water was bottled. In addition, there's some concern over whether plastic bottles leach harmful chemicals into the water. Unless you're opposed to additives (such as fluoride) or dislike the taste, you may benefit (and save money) from drinking tap water.

## Carbohydrates and Sugars

Carbohydrates (also called "carbs" or starches) are your main source of energy. The 200 grams (or more) of carbohydrates you consume each day make up 45 to 70 percent of your total calories. The majority of your carbohydrate intake should come from foods containing complex carbohydrates. Examples include whole grains, legumes, starchy vegetables, citrus fruits, and nuts. Some of the carbohydrate intake can come from foods containing simple carbohydrates, such as fruit, dairy products, and unsweetened but refined cereal, bread, and pasta.

Minimize your consumption of sugars. Excess sugar may lead to tooth decay, obesity, decreased immune function, diabetes, and osteoporosis. Eat foods with sugar that are lower on the *glycemic index*; they won't rapidly raise your blood sugar level (causing a "sugar rush"). Here's a list of the glycemic load of the various sugars, ordered from best to worst:

1. Fructose, sugar alcohols (sorbitol, xylitol, erythritol, and mannitol)
2. Lactose in milk products
3. Less refined sugars: honey, molasses, maple syrup, date sugar, and fruit juice concentrate
4. Refined sugar (table sugar, brown sugar, turbinado sugar, corn syrup, and glucose syrup)
5. High-fructose corn syrup

**Sugar substitutes (artificial sweeteners)**—You can find low-calorie sugar substitutes in diet soft drinks, chewing gum, desserts, and in individual packets on restaurant tables. The U.S. Food and Drug Administration (FDA) has approved five sweeteners for use in foods: aspartame (Equal and NutraSweet), saccharin (Sweet'N Low), sucralose (SPLENDA), acesulfame-K,

## What about Prenatal Vitamins?

Eating a varied, high-quality diet is the best way to ensure you get all the vitamins and minerals you need. If your diet is excellent, you might not need prenatal multivitamin supplements. However, most caregivers recommend that pregnant women take a daily multivitamin supplement to help ensure they get the required nutrients. This recommendation may be especially important for women who are underweight, have poor eating habits, or avoid many kinds of food.

Talk to your caregiver about prenatal vitamins. If he or she recommends that you take them, choose one that meets all your nutritional needs. Don't take several different kinds of multivitamins—doing so may lead to an accidental overdose of one or more nutrients. During pregnancy, avoid taking more than 100 percent of the recommended daily allowance (RDA) of any nutrient, unless your caregiver specifically recommends you do so.

Visit our web site, http://www.PCNGuide.com, for more information on recommended nutrients.

and neotame. Several extensive studies show that these artificial sweeteners appear safe for consumption by pregnant and breastfeeding women; however, anyone who has phenylketonuria (PKU) should avoid aspartame because it may cause severe health problems.

Although caregivers may prescribe sugar substitutes for women who have diabetes or need to restrict calories, most advise pregnant women to minimize their intake of sugar substitutes as well as sugar.[3]

## Salt

For years, caregivers told pregnant women to restrict their intake of salt, based on the mistaken assumption that salt and water retention caused high blood pressure. Experts now know that gradual, moderate water retention in pregnancy is not only normal, but the extra fluid is necessary for an adequate volume of blood and amniotic fluid.

During pregnancy, consuming an adequate amount of salt helps maintain your fluid balance. Feel free to salt your food to taste.

## Folate and Folic Acid (Vitamin B₉)

Folate is a B vitamin that's found naturally in foods such as leafy green vegetables and some fruits. It's essential for your baby's normal growth, and it's especially important in early pregnancy to prevent certain birth defects. Folate helps form blood cells and promotes the normal development of your baby's brain and spine. Folate that's produced synthetically is called folic acid. Caregivers recommend a daily folic acid supplement of 400 micrograms (0.4 milligram) for all women of childbearing age and 600 micrograms (0.6 milligram) for pregnant women.

## Calcium

Calcium is important for the growth of your baby's bones and teeth. It's especially vital in the third trimester, when your baby requires about two-thirds more calcium than he did earlier in his development. Calcium is also stored in your bones as a reserve for breast milk production. Caregivers recommend that pregnant women consume 1,200 milligrams of calcium each day.

## Iron

Iron is required for the production of hemoglobin, which carries oxygen through your bloodstream to your baby and your cells. During the last six weeks of pregnancy, your baby stores enough iron to supplement her needs for the first three to six months after the birth. Caregivers often recommend that pregnant women take a daily iron supplement of 30 to 60 milligrams. Foods rich in vitamin C (such as citrus fruits and tomatoes) enhance iron absorption, while some antacids and caffeine interfere with it.

Iron supplements can cause nausea or constipation in some women. To relieve these unpleasant side effects, try taking the supplements with food, or try a different brand of supplement that doesn't cause constipation. You may also want to try reducing the dosage of the supplements and taking them more often throughout the day.

## Vitamin A

Vitamin A helps form and maintain healthy teeth and bones, soft tissue, mucous membranes, and skin. It also promotes good vision.

During pregnancy, getting too little vitamin A (less than about 770 micrograms per day) can lead to preterm birth and an underdeveloped baby. However, getting too much vitamin A (more than 3,000 micrograms per day) in the first seven weeks of pregnancy can lead to a higher incidence of birth defects.

# Weight Gain during Pregnancy

A common question women ask during pregnancy is how much weight they should gain. The answer varies because no single amount is appropriate for every woman. The proper amount of weight to gain depends on a woman's prepregnancy weight and height, the quality of her diet before and during pregnancy, her ethnic background, and the number of previous pregnancies she has had.

## RECOMMENDATIONS FOR YOUR WEIGHT GAIN[4]

How can you determine the proper amount of weight to gain during pregnancy? First look at the chart at right to figure out your prepregnancy *Body Mass Index (BMI)*, which takes into account your height and prepregnancy weight to gauge your total body fat. For example, let's say your height is 5-feet 4-inches and your prepregnancy weight was 160 pounds. By looking at the chart, you can see that your prepregnancy BMI is 28. The chart shows the results of a mathematical formula (rounded to the nearest whole number), in which BMI equals weight multiplied by 703 and divided by height in inches squared.

After you've figured out your prepregnancy BMI, look at the table to determine the amount of weight you should gain.

These recommendations are guidelines. Many women gain more or less weight during pregnancy, and they and their babies are fine. However, women who gain too little weight increase their risk of having a premature baby

### Body Mass Index (BMI)
**Weight in Pounds**

| Height in Feet and Inches | 120 | 130 | 140 | 150 | 160 | 170 | 180 | 190 | 200 | 210 | 220 | 230 | 240 | 250 |
|---|---|---|---|---|---|---|---|---|---|---|---|---|---|---|
| 4'6 | 29 | 31 | 34 | 36 | 39 | 41 | 43 | 46 | 48 | 51 | 53 | 56 | 58 | 60 |
| 4'8 | 27 | 29 | 31 | 34 | 36 | 38 | 40 | 43 | 45 | 47 | 49 | 52 | 54 | 56 |
| 4'10 | 25 | 27 | 29 | 31 | 34 | 36 | 38 | 40 | 42 | 44 | 46 | 48 | 50 | 52 |
| 5'0 | 23 | 25 | 27 | 29 | 31 | 33 | 35 | 37 | 39 | 41 | 43 | 45 | 47 | 49 |
| 5'2 | 22 | 24 | 26 | 27 | 29 | 31 | 33 | 35 | 37 | 38 | 40 | 42 | 44 | 46 |
| 5'4 | 21 | 22 | 24 | 26 | 28 | 29 | 31 | 33 | 34 | 36 | 38 | 40 | 41 | 43 |
| 5'6 | 19 | 21 | 23 | 24 | 26 | 27 | 29 | 31 | 32 | 34 | 36 | 37 | 39 | 40 |
| 5'8 | 18 | 20 | 21 | 23 | 24 | 26 | 27 | 29 | 30 | 32 | 34 | 35 | 37 | 38 |
| 5'10 | 17 | 19 | 20 | 22 | 23 | 24 | 26 | 27 | 29 | 30 | 32 | 33 | 35 | 36 |
| 6'0 | 16 | 18 | 19 | 20 | 22 | 23 | 24 | 26 | 27 | 28 | 30 | 31 | 33 | 34 |
| 6'2 | 15 | 17 | 18 | 19 | 21 | 22 | 23 | 24 | 26 | 27 | 28 | 30 | 31 | 32 |
| 6'4 | 15 | 16 | 17 | 18 | 20 | 21 | 22 | 23 | 24 | 26 | 27 | 28 | 29 | 30 |
| 6'6 | 14 | 15 | 16 | 17 | 19 | 20 | 21 | 22 | 23 | 24 | 25 | 27 | 28 | 29 |
| 6'8 | 13 | 14 | 15 | 17 | 18 | 19 | 20 | 21 | 22 | 23 | 24 | 25 | 26 | 28 |

Healthy Weight    Overweight    Obese

Note: This chart is for adults (aged 20 years and older).
**Source: U.S. Surgeon General**

| | Prepregnancy BMI | Total Weight Gain |
|---|---|---|
| Underweight | Less than 18.5 | 28 to 40 pounds |
| Normal Weight | 18.5 to 24.9 | 25 to 35 pounds |
| Overweight | 25 to 29.9 | 15 to 25 pounds |
| Obese | More than 30 | 11 to 20 pounds* |

* For women who are obese when pregnancy begins, some researchers argue for limiting weight gain to just ten pounds.[5]

## Where Does That Extra Weight Go?

Here's a breakdown of the weight distribution in a pregnancy with an average weight gain:

| | |
|---|---|
| Baby | 7 to 8½ pounds |
| Placenta | 1 to 1½ pounds |
| Uterus | 2 pounds |
| Amniotic fluid | 2 pounds |
| Breasts | 1 pound |
| Blood volume | 2½ pounds |
| Fat | 5 to 8 pounds |
| Tissue fluid | 6 pounds |
| **Total** | 27 to 31½ pounds |

or one with low birth weight. Women who gain too much weight increase their risk of developing preterm labor, gestational diabetes, high blood pressure, or macrosomia (large baby that can be difficult to deliver vaginally). These women also find it harder than usual to lose the extra weight after the birth.

Your caregiver will likely monitor your weight gain at each prenatal visit. In early pregnancy, you'll gain weight slowly, typically just 1 to 5 pounds by the end of the first trimester. Beginning in the second trimester, as your baby grows and your amniotic fluid and blood volume increases, you'll gain weight more rapidly—up to 1 pound per week. (An overweight or obese woman may need to gain only ½ a pound per week).

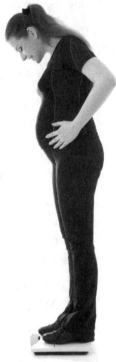

Although a minor increase or decrease in your weight may be a sign that you've eaten more or less than usual, a sudden, excessive change can be a sign of illness or preeclampsia (see page 140), especially if accompanied by other symptoms (such as sudden swelling).

Health care professionals stress that pregnant women should avoid losing weight or overeating; instead, they should concentrate on eating a high-quality diet in appropriate amounts and maintaining an active lifestyle that includes moderate exercise. If you follow that advice, you'll gain weight in the amount that's right for you.

### WEIGHT LOSS AFTER THE BIRTH

You'll lose some of the weight you gain during pregnancy within a few weeks after the birth. By eating sensibly and exercising adequately, some women can lose most of the remaining weight over the following months. For other women, losing the extra weight takes longer.

Breastfeeding promotes weight loss because milk production burns calories. The fat stored during pregnancy provides some of these calories; the food you eat provides the rest. Until your breastfed baby weans, your body may naturally hang on to a few pounds of fat as a way to ensure your baby is well nourished should you experience a food crisis. This extra weight is typically easy to lose after weaning.

# Common Concerns

During pregnancy, normal changes in hormone production, plus the increased size and weight of the uterus, can cause digestive and other problems. The following sections discuss these problems, their causes, and treatments.

## Tips for Managing Nausea

- Eat several small meals a day to prevent an empty stomach and to keep your blood sugar level stable. Include a protein-rich food with each meal.
- Don't drink a lot of fluids with meals. Instead, drink between meals.
- Keep a bland food (such as crackers) by your bed and eat some just before getting up.
- Trust your food preferences. If something sounds good to eat, you'll probably tolerate it.
- Identify and avoid odors that make nausea worse. Try smelling peppermint oil or fresh lemon slices to ease nausea. (Drinking peppermint tea may also help.)
- Caregivers often recommend ginger (but not supplements of dried, powdered ginger root). You can eat ginger in foods, eat candied or pickled ginger, or drink ginger tea or natural ginger ale.
- Increase your intake of foods rich in vitamin $B_6$ (pyridoxine), such as whole grains and cereals, nuts, seeds, and legumes. Vitamin $B_6$ supplements may reduce nausea. Your daily intake should never exceed 100 milligrams; discuss safe amounts with your caregiver.
- Use acupressure wristbands, which are marketed to relieve motion sickness.
- Know that the nausea and vomiting usually passes within 3 to 4 months.

On rare occasions, nausea and vomiting are severe and a woman becomes dehydrated, loses a lot of weight, and can't keep down any food. This condition (called "hyperemesis gravidarum") may require medications (such as Zofran) or even hospitalization. (See page 129.) Because these medications cross the placenta and their safety for the baby hasn't been established, take them only if your caregiver prescribes them.

## NAUSEA AND VOMITING

During pregnancy, nausea is also called "morning sickness." But for many women, morning sickness isn't limited to the morning; they experience nausea at any time throughout the day.

What causes nausea? As production of the hormones that support pregnancy increases, you may feel nauseated until your body adjusts to the increased levels. (Some women also experience diarrhea in early pregnancy, which may be due to hormones or dietary changes.) In the first trimester, nausea is common in women who haven't eaten for several hours, who smell certain odors, or who encounter other triggers. Nausea is neither abnormal nor a sign that you're unconsciously rejecting your baby. See above for tips on managing nausea.

If your nausea leads to vomiting, you may worry about your baby's health. But unless severe and unusually frequent, vomiting doesn't harm your baby. Studies show that a woman who's healthy when she conceives has sufficient reserves to nourish her growing baby, even if she can't eat well for the first several months of pregnancy.

## HEARTBURN

Heartburn is a condition in which you burp up stomach acid, causing a burning feeling in your chest or throat. In late pregnancy, many women experience heartburn. Its cause is a combination of increased pressure from the growing uterus and hormonal effects that relax the muscular opening at the top of the stomach and cause the stomach to empty more slowly. To help ease or prevent heartburn, follow these tips:

- Avoid eating fatty foods, spicy foods, and foods that produce gas or heartburn.
- Eat several small meals a day. Drink only a small amount of fluid with meals.
- Eat slowly and avoid eating just before bedtime.
- To decrease discomfort when in bed, semi-sit rather than lying flat on your back.
- Taking antacids or other medications sometimes controls heartburn, but you should take them only if necessary. Ask your caregiver for recommendations.

## CONSTIPATION

During pregnancy, food moves through your intestines more slowly to let your body absorb more nutrients and water. This slowdown sometimes causes constipation, and pressure from your growing uterus on the large intestine magnifies the problem. Constipation can also aggravate hemorrhoids. Some tips to avoid constipation include the following:

- Exercise regularly and consume plenty of fluids and high-fiber foods, such as fruits and vegetables, whole grains, bran, and prune juice. An easy way to increase your fiber intake is to add a table-spoon of flax meal to your food.
- If proper diet and exercise don't prevent constipation, try an over-the-counter high-fiber product such as Metamucil or Fiberall. Such products are safe and effective; however, avoid taking intestinal stimulants (laxatives). Your body may become dependent on them.
- If you're taking an iron supplement and you think it's causing the problem, ask your caregiver about changing to one that causes less constipation.

## FOOD CRAVINGS AND PICA

Pregnant women frequently crave specific foods in large quantities. Sometimes, women eat foods they rarely ate before pregnancy, such as hot peppers or other spicy foods, one flavor of ice cream, potatoes, or pickles. Although health care professionals don't know why pregnant women crave certain foods, the cravings are usually harmless unless they interfere with good nutrition.

Also common during pregnancy is pica (craving and eating nonfood items). Pregnant women have reported craving ice, baking soda, flour, cornstarch, dirt, clay, cigarette ashes, and other non-food substances. They've also described cravings to smell such substances as gasoline, fingernail polish remover, bleach, and ammonia.

Eating nonfood products and smelling substances can cause mild to severe side effects in both the mother and baby. While many women worry about these side effects, they're reluctant to share their concerns with their caregivers. They may be confused or ashamed by their behavior, or they may worry that their caregivers will advise them not to satisfy the craving.

If you have nonfood cravings, have your caregiver or a counselor help you determine whether satisfying them is harmful to you or your baby. If it is, he or she can help you find ways to cope with the cravings and avoid the harmful substances.

# Food Safety

Some forms of bacteria and environmental contaminants can harm babies' development in the womb. Although the risk of harm is small, pregnant women should take precautions to prevent exposure. The following sections discuss ways you can limit your exposure. For more information on food safety, visit http://www.fda.gov/Food/ResourcesForYou/HealthEducators/ucm081785.htm.

# MERCURY

Mercury is a metallic element that can harm your baby's developing brain and nervous system. It's found in large, long-lived fish, which is regrettable because fish are a great source of essential nutrients, including omega-3 fatty acids. As long as the fish has low levels of mercury, it's better to eat it in moderation than to stop eating fish entirely.

Here are amounts of fish that pregnant women can safely eat, based on mercury levels. The asterisked items are highest in omega-3 fatty acids.

*Up to 12 ounces per week*—Anchovies*, catfish, clams, cod, crab, flounder, herring*, oysters, pollock, salmon*, sardines*, scallops, shrimp, sole, tilapia, and trout*

*Up to 6 ounces per week*—Halibut, snapper, lobster, tuna, and mahi-mahi

*Avoid completely*—Shark, tilefish, king mackerel, swordfish, grouper, marlin, and orange roughy[6]

# FOOD-BORNE BACTERIA

Pregnant women are more susceptible to listeriosis, salmonella, and toxoplasmosis bacteria than other people are. These bacteria can sicken pregnant women and cause miscarriage, preterm labor, and stillbirth. These bacteria live in undercooked meat, fish, and eggs; unpasteurized milk and cheeses; and unwashed fruits and vegetables. Although the chance of exposure is small, the effects can be grave. Use the following food safety practices to prevent exposure. (See page 132 for more information on infections in pregnancy.)

*Keep things clean.*—Before and after handling food, wash your hands thoroughly with warm soapy water. Rinse raw fruits and vegetables thoroughly. Separate raw meat, poultry, and seafood from ready-to-eat foods. After using cutting boards, knives, and plates to prepare raw meat, poultry, or seafood, wash the items thoroughly in hot soapy water before using them to prepare other foods.

*Cook meat, fish, and eggs thoroughly.*—In addition, before eating hot dogs and luncheon meats (such as ham, turkey, bologna, salami), heat them until they're steaming. Cook refrigerated smoked seafood (such as Nova-style lox salmon) before eating.

*Store foods well.*—Set your refrigerator to 35°F to 40°F (2°C to 4.4°C) and your freezer to 0°F to 4°F (-18°C to –16°C). Regularly clean the interior of your refrigerator, and discard all food that's past its expiration date.

*Use the two-hour rule.*—Discard any food that's prone to spoilage if it's been left out at room temperature for more than two hours.

*Be smart about takeout foods, delivered foods, and restaurant leftovers.*—Eat hot foods as soon as possible after purchasing. Eat cold foods within two hours. Refrigerate restaurant leftovers within an hour and eat within two days. Eat delivered foods within two hours.

*Avoid eating unpasteurized foods and some raw foods.*—It's fine to eat foods that contain pasteurized milk, cooked fish, shelf-stable smoked seafood, and canned pâtés and meat spreads. But it's best to avoid eating the following foods:

- Unpasteurized milk products, including soft cheeses made from unpasteurized milk (such as Brie, Camembert, blue cheese, feta, and Mexican fresh cheese)
- Raw fish, especially raw shellfish
- Refrigerated pâtés or meat spreads
- Raw vegetable sprouts (such as alfalfa sprouts and bean sprouts)

# Nutrition for Special Circumstances

In certain cases, having good nutrition is especially important during pregnancy. If one or more of the following sections describe your situation, be particularly conscientious about eating nutritious foods. Seek nutritional counseling from your caregiver or a nutritionist.

## PREGNANT WITH MULTIPLES

If you're pregnant with twins, increase your prenatal vitamin dosages by 50 percent and consume an extra 600 calories each day. You should try to gain 35 to 50 pounds. If you're pregnant with triplets or more, ask your caregiver for nutrition advice.

When pregnant with multiples, it's important to gain at least 24 pounds by the twenty-fourth week of pregnancy to help reduce the risk of preterm birth and babies with low birth weight.

## TEENAGE PREGNANCY

A pregnant teenager needs to eat particularly well to promote her own growth while nourishing her baby. If you're a pregnant teenager, make sure to consume enough calcium, phosphorus, and magnesium.

## PREGNANT WITHIN A YEAR OF GIVING BIRTH

Pregnancy can temporarily deplete your reserves of certain nutrients such as calcium and iron. If you become pregnant within a year of your last birth, you may need extra calories and nutrients. The time needed between pregnancies to correct deficiencies depends on your overall nutritional status and the quality of your diet. Talk with your caregiver about your needs.

## FOOD ALLERGIES

If you have significant food allergies, eliminating problem foods can lead to an inadequate diet. You may need a nutritionist to help you plan a healthful pregnancy diet.

## ANOREXIA AND BULIMIA

If you have a history of anorexia or bulimia, you may have difficulty accepting the weight gain and body changes that occur with pregnancy. In addition, your low weight and poor nutritional status may harm your and your baby's health during pregnancy. Psychological and nutrition counseling may help you, as may anorexia and bulimia support groups.

## HIGH BLOOD PRESSURE

Developing high blood pressure during pregnancy—or gestational hypertension—isn't always preventable. But by eating a healthful diet, drinking plenty of fluids, exercising regularly, and avoiding alcohol and caffeine, you may reduce your risk of severe complications. Although research hasn't yet found a single nutrient that prevents gestational hypertension, several nutrients may reduce the risk, including protein, calcium, magnesium, zinc, vitamins C and E, and omega-3 fatty acids. Make sure your diet includes healthy amounts of these key nutrients. (See page 140 for more on high blood pressure.)

# DIABETES IN PREGNANCY

Whether you have diabetes or are at high risk for developing diabetes, carbohydrates shouldn't make up more than 40 percent of your daily caloric intake. Avoid eating more than 30 to 45 grams of carbohydrates at one meal. Complex carbohydrates are much better for you than simple carbohydrates.

Keep your fat intake to less than 30 percent of your daily caloric intake, and increase your protein intake to 75 to 100 grams. Eat at the same times every day, and eat several small meals each day to keep your blood sugar level stable. (See page 134 for more on diabetes.)

# LOW INCOME

If you're pregnant and have a low income, you may find it difficult to obtain the proper nutritious foods. Here's a list of resources that can help you:

- WIC (Women, Infants, and Children) provides supplemental food and nutrition education to low-income families. To find out if you're eligible for these services, visit http://www.fns.usda.gov/wic.
- You can use government food stamps to purchase food. To find out if you're eligible, visit http://www.fns.usda.gov/fsp.
- Food banks provide supplemental foods. Check a phone book or search online to find a local food bank.

## Key Points to Remember

- Eat a well-balanced diet that includes lots of whole grains, vegetables, and fruits. Choose low-fat milk products, meat, and fish. Eat a variety of beans and legumes. Drink plenty of liquids, and salt your food to taste. Don't try to achieve perfection—just make the best choices you can each day.
- Talk with your caregiver about supplementing your diet with a prenatal vitamin or specific nutrients. (Visit our web site, http://www.PCNGuide.com, for a chart of recommended nutrients.)
- Gain an amount of weight that's appropriate for you by considering your prepregnancy weight and height, and the quality of your diet before and during pregnancy.
- Normal changes in hormone production, plus the increased size and weight of the uterus, can cause nausea, vomiting, constipation, and other problems that can be treated.
- Although the chance of harm to you and your baby from food bacteria and contaminants is small, take precautions to prevent exposure.
- Good nutrition is especially important in certain cases, such as teenage pregnancy or pregnancy with multiples. Seek nutritional counseling from your caregiver or a nutritionist.

# CHAPTER 7

# When Pregnancy Becomes Complicated

Most women have normal and healthy pregnancies. But for some women, a chronic (preexisting) health problem or one that develops during pregnancy can cause complications and make pregnancy challenging, alarming, or stressful. If complications occur in your pregnancy, knowing the warning signs on page 70 will help you detect and report a problem early on. Having good prenatal care and prompt treatment may minimize complications and maximize your chances of having a healthy baby. In this chapter, you'll learn about complications in the order in which they may appear in pregnancy, beginning with conditions that may affect your pregnancy from conception and ending with complications that can arise in the days before the birth.

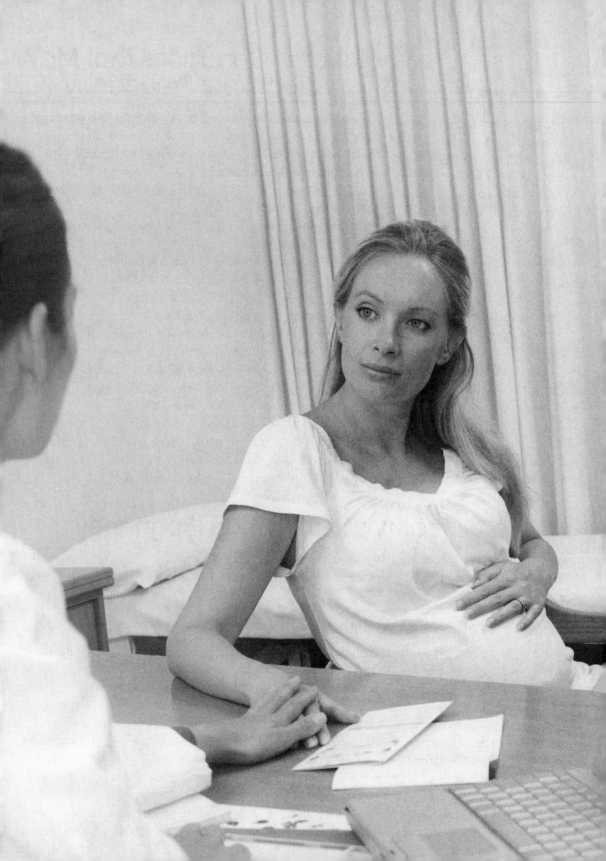

# Chronic Conditions That May Affect Your Pregnancy

If a woman has a chronic condition or illness before becoming pregnant, it might or might not cause problems in pregnancy. With good prenatal care, most women with chronic health problems have healthy babies.

The following is a list of conditions and illnesses that may affect prenatal care:

- Cardiovascular disease (high blood pressure, heart disease, or sickle cell anemia)
- Gastrointestinal illness or nutrition problems (inflammatory bowel disease, phenylketonuria or PKU, Crohn's disease, eating disorders, or gastric bypass surgery)
- Respiratory or lung disease (asthma)
- Hormonal imbalance or disease (diabetes, thyroid disease, polycystic ovarian syndrome or PCOS, or pituitary disorder)
- Autoimmune disorder, in which the immune system harms instead of protects the body (rheumatoid arthritis, lupus erythematosus, and antiphospholipid antibody syndrome or APS)
- Other condition or illness (kidney disease, epilepsy, or physical disability)

If you have one or more of these conditions or illnesses, you improve your chances of having a healthy baby by controlling the symptoms *before* becoming pregnant. Once you're pregnant, talk with both your regular physician or specialist and your maternity caregiver to create a plan for maintaining your health and to learn what you can expect during pregnancy, labor, and the months after the birth.

# Complications That Arise in Pregnancy

Some complications that arise in pregnancy are more serious than others and require medical treatment. Other complications resolve with little or no treatment. The following sections discuss the most common complications.

## VAGINAL BLEEDING IN EARLY PREGNANCY

Spotting or light vaginal bleeding in the first trimester occurs in about 20 percent of all pregnancies. In many cases, the bleeding doesn't harm the mother or baby.

What causes bleeding in early pregnancy? Sometimes, the implantation of the fertilized egg into the uterine wall causes slight vaginal bleeding, usually shortly before the time a woman expects a menstrual period. Other times, cervical tenderness and an increased blood supply to the pelvis can cause spotting after a woman has intercourse. Often, frequent strenuous exercise or a cervical infection causes vaginal bleeding. In rare cases, a condition called molar pregnancy causes brownish vaginal discharge in early pregnancy. In a molar pregnancy, abnormal placental tissue grows into a grape-like cluster; there isn't a baby, even though a pregnancy test is positive.

For about half the women who experience bleeding in early pregnancy, the bleeding stops on its own and many women have no further complications. In other cases, the bleeding is serious and sometimes indicates an ectopic pregnancy or possible miscarriage. (See below.) Women who have continuous moderate or heavy bleeding are more likely to miscarry than those who experience light bleeding only once.

If you experience any vaginal bleeding during early pregnancy, call your caregiver. If you have spotting or light bleeding for only one day, your caregiver may suggest that you rest and avoid strenuous exercise and sexual intercourse. If you experience heavy bleeding along with cramps or abdominal pain, your caregiver may order an ultrasound scan or blood tests to assess your pregnancy.

## ECTOPIC PREGNANCY

About 1 to 2 percent of pregnancies are *ectopic*. An ectopic pregnancy occurs when the fertilized egg implants itself someplace outside the uterus, usually in the wall of a fallopian tube (called a "tubal pregnancy") but sometimes in the cervix, ovary, or abdomen. This type of pregnancy won't result in a live birth, thus parents 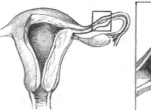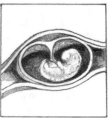 feel a similar sense of loss and grief that a miscarriage evokes (see below).

Symptoms of an ectopic pregnancy usually appear in the first six to eight weeks of pregnancy and may include lower abdominal pain or tenderness (or one-sided pelvic pain) and vaginal bleeding. Additional symptoms include nausea, vomiting, dizziness, or a sharp shoulder pain. An untreated tubal pregnancy causes severe abdominal pain and vaginal bleeding that indicates internal bleeding.

Early diagnosis of the problem and rapid treatment help preserve a woman's future fertility and greatly reduce the risk of death from severe blood loss after a tube ruptures. To diagnose the problem, a caregiver assesses the woman's hormone levels to evaluate the viability of the pregnancy and examines a high-resolution ultrasound scan to discover the implantation site. Surgery may be needed to confirm the diagnosis or to remove the embryo. An intravenous (IV) infusion of a medication called methotrexate may be used to abort the pregnancy or may be combined with surgery to ensure the full removal of pregnancy tissues.

The likelihood of ectopic pregnancy rises for women whose fallopian tubes are damaged by pelvic infection, disease, or surgery. The majority of women who have an ectopic pregnancy can expect to get pregnant again and carry a healthy baby to term.

## MISCARRIAGE

A *miscarriage* (or spontaneous abortion) is the unexpected death and delivery of a baby before the twentieth week of pregnancy. About 10 to 15 percent of known pregnancies end in miscarriage; however, the percentage of early miscarriage (occurring between the first and thirteenth weeks of pregnancy) is probably higher because many women might not have realized they were pregnant before the loss occurred.

Although no one knows the specific cause of most miscarriages, the most commonly suspected reason is random chromosomal abnormalities that interfere with the baby's normal development. Other factors that increase the risk of early miscarriage include a history of infertility and assisted conception, advanced age of the woman (or man), high body temperature, infection, hormonal imbalance, high intake of alcohol or caffeine, smoking, low body weight along with poor diet, frequent high-impact or strenuous exercise, and extreme emotional stress or physical injury.

## Common Q & A

**Q:** My last pregnancy ended in a miscarriage. What can I do to increase my chances of carrying my next baby to term?

**A:** To improve your chances of a healthy pregnancy after a previous miscarriage, try to do the following:

- Have a well-balanced diet.
- Take prenatal vitamins.
- Avoid environmental toxins and infections.
- Don't smoke or use recreational drugs.
- Avoid extremely stressful relationships as much as possible before and during pregnancy.
- Make arrangements for emotional support and medical monitoring, starting early in pregnancy.

Factors that increase the risk of late miscarriages (occurring between the fourteenth and twentieth weeks of pregnancy) include uterine abnormalities such as an incompetent cervix (see page 138), acute infection (see page 132), placental circulation problems (see page 139), uterine fibroids (see page 129), and certain chronic illnesses (such as autoimmune disorders; uncontrolled diabetes; thyroid conditions; and heart, liver, or kidney disease). Treatment of these possible causes can help prevent a miscarriage.

Once a miscarriage starts, it can't be stopped. Signs of a miscarriage include vaginal bleeding and intermittent abdominal pain that often begins in the lower back and develops into abdominal cramping. If you suspect you're having a miscarriage, call your caregiver. He or she may advise you to rest and wait to see if the bleeding stops or may order an ultrasound scan and a blood test to confirm whether you're still pregnant. If you've had a miscarriage and you're Rh negative, you may receive a shot of RhoGAM. (See page 135.)

Sometimes a caregiver discovers that a baby has died before a miscarriage begins. The shock that such a discovery gives expectant parents, combined with waiting for the miscarriage to begin on its own, can be extremely stressful. Some women want an immediate end to the pregnancy by receiving medications to expel the baby or by having surgery to clean out the uterus (dilation and curettage, or D&C). If you're in this situation, discuss the potential risks of these medical procedures with your caregiver. If you decide against them, stay within a thirty-minute drive to the hospital in case you experience heavy bleeding, fever, or strong abdominal pains while awaiting the miscarriage. Be sure to surround yourself with people who can support and nurture you during this difficult time.

It's normal for a woman to feel shock, grief, and sadness after a miscarriage—especially when the pregnancy was wanted, had been achieved by medical or surgical help, or followed a previous miscarriage.

If you experience a miscarriage, you and your partner may need extra rest and support. Even if you hadn't announced your pregnancy to others, seek comfort and help from family and friends as well as from books and support groups on pregnancy loss. Talking about your loss with people who have experienced a miscarriage may be a particularly helpful way to ease your pain. (See also page 303 for useful information.)

Most women who have one or more miscarriages eventually give birth to healthy babies. As you begin planning your next pregnancy after a miscarriage, consider asking your caregiver about medical tests or genetic counseling to determine a possible cause of the miscarriage, to screen for genetic disorders, and to treat a harmful infection or chronic condition. You also may want to seek emotional support to help you manage your fears of another miscarriage, at least until your next pregnancy passes the point at which the miscarriage occurred.

# HIGH BODY TEMPERATURE (FEVER)

Having a high body temperature (an oral temperature over 100.4°F or 38°C) for three to four days may harm your baby, especially in early pregnancy. If you have a prolonged fever, ask your caregiver for advice. Don't take any fever-reducing medication unless your caregiver instructs you to do so. To lower your temperature, drink plenty of liquids and take a lukewarm bath or shower. If your temperature is higher than 102°F (38.9°C), call your caregiver immediately.

Be aware that soaking in hot tubs or taking saunas may raise your body temperature to a level that can be dangerous to your baby. (See page 83.)

# SEVERE NAUSEA AND VOMITING (HYPEREMESIS GRAVIDARUM)

Hyperemesis gravidarum is persistent, severe nausea and vomiting. While nausea and vomiting is the most common complaint of early pregnancy, the intensity of hyperemesis gravidarum far exceeds that of "morning sickness" (see page 40). This serious condition, which affects less than 1 percent of pregnancies, can result in weight loss, dehydration, and changes in blood chemistry.

If you're extremely nauseated and continue to vomit food and fluids for a day or longer, call your caregiver to determine whether the cause is illness or food poisoning. Early management of severe nausea and vomiting may help prevent its progression to hyperemesis gravidarum.

Treatment begins with the same dietary and lifestyle changes recommended for managing morning sickness (see page 119), along with suggestions for helping you keep down foods and fluids. If this treatment isn't effective, your caregiver may prescribe medications to relieve vomiting (antiemetics) and, if necessary, to treat infection. If your vomiting can't be controlled, you may need hospitalization to receive IV fluids. Some women feel nauseated throughout pregnancy and continue to take medications at home.

Sometimes, psychological problems can worsen hyperemesis gravidarum (they may even cause the condition); talking with a trained counselor may help resolve the problems and lessen the nausea and vomiting.

Hyperemesis gravidarum can be debilitating, but it's manageable with treatment and only rarely causes lasting effects on you or your pregnancy. By treating the condition, you'll help prevent dehydration and improve your quality of life.

# UTERINE FIBROIDS

Uterine fibroids are benign (non-cancerous) tumors of the uterine muscle. Up to 75 percent of women develop fibroids (also called "leiomyomas" or "myomas") at some time during their lives, but the fibroids typically don't cause problems. During their childbearing years, less than 25 percent of women with fibroids experience symptoms such as excessive menstrual bleeding, pelvic pain, or infertility; only some have surgery to shrink or remove them.[1]

Although fibroids typically don't cause problems in pregnancy, possible complications include a slight increased risk of miscarriage, preterm labor, or postpartum hemorrhage. Depending on the number, size, and location, fibroids can sometimes complicate birth. Their presence may slow labor progress or interfere with the baby's movement into a head-down position for birth.

If you've been diagnosed with fibroids, your caregiver will likely watch your pregnancy closely and use ultrasound scans to detect changes in the fibroids' size or number and to determine whether they're affecting your baby's growth. If the fibroids are causing abdominal pain or increased pressure, treatment may include bed rest, applying cold or hot packs, and taking pain medications.

## VENOUS THROMBOSIS

Venous thrombosis is a blood clot that typically occurs in a vein in the leg or pelvis. During pregnancy, pressure from your enlarged uterus slows the flow of blood returning from your legs and your blood changes how it clots to help reduce postpartum bleeding. Because of these changes, you have a slightly increased risk of developing blood clots in your legs during pregnancy or soon after the birth.

A clot that develops in a vein close to the skin is called thrombophlebitis, and it causes swelling, tenderness, and redness. Treating thrombophlebitis includes bed rest with the leg elevated, hot packs to the affected area, special support stockings, and a mild pain reliever if needed.

Deep vein thrombosis (DVT) develops in a big vein that's deeper in your body and is much more serious than thrombophlebitis. DVT causes leg or pelvic pain and redness, warmth, or swelling near the affected area. If you have DVT in your calf, you may have increased calf pain when you flex your toes toward your knee.

If you notice symptoms of DVT during pregnancy or after the birth, notify your caregiver immediately. You may be at risk of developing venous thromboembolism (VTE) and possibly a pulmonary embolism, a potentially fatal condition in which a portion of the blood clot breaks loose and travels to a lung. Symptoms of pulmonary embolism include sudden shortness of breath, chest pain, and rapid heart rate. Your chances of developing VTE increase if you're older than thirty, you or your family has a history of blood clots, or you've recently been on bed rest or been sitting for a very long time.

Treating DVT may require pain medication (if leg pain is severe) as well as hospitalization and IV doses of the anticoagulant (blood thinner) Heparin to prevent further clot formation. Heparin doses continue at home until the birth and are administered by self-injection, pump, or IV; then another anticoagulant, Coumadin, is taken orally for six weeks.

## INFECTIONS

Although the risk of acquiring a serious infection during pregnancy is low, some infectious diseases can affect your pregnancy or harm your baby. The potential risks depend on the following:

- What organism (virus, bacterium, or spore) is causing the infection
- Whether you have antibodies to the organism from a prior exposure
- Whether the disease is treatable
- When during pregnancy you acquired the infection

Even if you get an infection during pregnancy, your baby might not become infected—and even if your baby gets infected, he might not be harmed.

The chart on pages 132–133 identifies infections that are harmful during pregnancy, and the following sections provide information on the most serious of them.

# Ways to Avoid Getting Sick

The best way to prevent complications from an infection is to avoid getting sick. Here are a few guidelines to follow:

1. Wash your hands several times each day, especially before eating and after using the toilet. Germs live on doorknobs, handrails, phones, hands, and other surfaces. After touching a germ-covered surface with your hands, you transmit the germs to your food, mouth, nose, and anything else you touch.

2. Stay away from sick people as much as possible, especially if your vaccinations aren't up to date.

3. Update your vaccinations or have your immune status checked before pregnancy, if possible. Health care professionals recommend that women avoid certain vaccines—such as chicken pox (varicella zoster) and measles, mumps, and rubella or German measles (MMR)—in pregnancy or in the month before conception. If you received MMR vaccines as a child, you may be immune to these infections. However, the effectiveness of some vaccines, such as the one for rubella, may diminish over time.

4. Eat safe foods. To avoid food-borne diseases, don't eat certain foods during pregnancy. (See page 121.) Also, wash fruits and vegetables before eating them, adequately cook meats and other foods, and thoroughly clean your food preparation surfaces.

## Sexually Transmitted Infections (STI)

Some STIs (previously called "sexually transmitted diseases" or "STDs") can cause problems during pregnancy, but if treated early, the risks to the baby are minimal. If you've had multiple sexual partners, you're at greater risk for an STI such as chlamydia, gonorrhea, genital herpes, hepatitis B, human immunodeficiency virus (HIV), human papillomavirus (HPV), syphilis, and trichomoniasis. If you have or had symptoms of an STI—such as genital sores, abnormal vaginal discharge, or discomfort or difficulty with urination—see your caregiver to find out if testing and treatment are necessary. Throughout pregnancy, make sure you and your partner practice safe sex to protect against exposure to STIs.

## Group B Streptococcus (GBS)

About 10 to 30 percent of pregnant women are carriers of Group B streptococcus (or are "colonized" with GBS), which means GBS bacteria are present in their bodies but they don't have signs of infection. Without treatment, about 1 in 200 newborns whose mothers are GBS carriers will develop a GBS infection, which can be life threatening. If these mothers receive antibiotic treatment during labor, their babies' risk of infection drops to 1 in 4,000.

Most caregivers follow the GBS detection and treatment guidelines developed by the U.S. Centers for Disease Control (CDC) in 2008,[2] which recommends screening a pregnant woman between the thirty-fifth and thirty-seventh weeks by swabbing her vagina and anus and having the secretions cultured in a laboratory. If a woman is a GBS carrier, her caregiver treats her with antibiotics during labor and watches her baby closely for signs of infection.

Women with the following circumstances may receive antibiotics during labor without prior screening:

- A urinary tract infection (UTI) caused by GBS during this pregnancy (even if she received antibiotics)
- A previous pregnancy with a baby who had severe GBS disease

If a woman hasn't been tested or the results of the culture aren't known when labor begins, she'll receive antibiotics if she has any of the following risk factors:
- Preterm labor (labor that begins before the thirty-seventh week)
- Ruptured membranes for more than eighteen hours before labor begins
- Fever of 100.4°F (38°C) or higher

Antibiotic treatment of all pregnant GBS carriers is controversial. Although only a few babies of GBS carriers develop an infection, all these babies are exposed to possible side effects of antibiotics, such as allergic reaction, creation of drug-resistant bacteria, and yeast infections after birth. Despite the risk of these side effects, most GBS carriers choose antibiotic treatment during labor to reduce the risk of early-onset GBS infections in their babies.

## Bladder and Vaginal Infections

Bladder or vaginal infections increase the risk of preterm labor. Symptoms of a bladder infection (also called "urinary tract infection" or "UTI") include frequent urination, urgency to urinate, blood in the urine, and pain, especially at the end of urination. Symptoms of a vaginal infection include vaginal discomfort or itching and foul-smelling discharge. *Note:* It's normal to have thin, mild-smelling, and whitish vaginal discharge during pregnancy.

If you think you have a bladder or vaginal infection, promptly call your caregiver for treatment.

## Listeriosis

Listeriosis is a form of food poisoning that can harm your baby. While rare, listeriosis affects pregnant women twenty times more often than it affects other healthy adults. The bacteria live in

# Infections during Pregnancy

The following chart describes how certain infections may harm your baby. Because the chart addresses serious potential complications, it may seem scary. But remember: If you get any of these infections, you can minimize the potential risks if your caregiver diagnoses the infection early and you and your baby receive prompt treatment.

### If your baby is infected, the infection increases the risk of:

| Infection | Birth Defects | Preterm Labor | Illness in Baby | Comments |
|---|---|---|---|---|
| Bacterial vaginosis (BV) | | X | | Problems result from prematurity. |
| Chicken pox (varicella zoster) | X | | X | Slight risk of infection affecting one or all of baby's organs. |
| Chlamydia trachomatis | X | | X | Baby not affected before birth, but may have eye infection or pneumonia after birth. |
| Cytomegalovirus (CMV) | X | | X | Risk of brain damage or hearing loss. About 10 percent of babies affected when mother is first infected in first trimester. |

Key: X = Possible   ? = Questionable

| Infection | Birth Defects | Preterm Labor | Illness in Baby | Comments |
|---|---|---|---|---|
| Fifth disease (parvovirus B19) | | | X | May cause severe anemia and related problems for baby. |
| Gonorrhea (Neisseria gonorrhea) | | | X | If baby is infected during birth, infection may cause severe eye infection that may cause blindness. |
| Group B streptococcus (GBS) | X | | X | If baby infected at birth, infection may cause severe disease or death. |
| Hepatitis B (HBV) or Hepatitis C (HCV) | | | X | If baby is infected at birth and untreated, she's at high risk of becoming a HBV carrier, but at low risk of becoming a HCV carrier. |
| Herpes simplex virus (HSV) | | | X | Risk of infection is highest when mother has first outbreak of genital herpes in pregnancy. Any recurrent infection at birth may affect baby. Treatment of outbreaks reduces the chance of infection. |
| Human immuno-deficiency virus (HIV) | | | X | Treatment of mother can greatly reduce the risk of baby's acquiring HIV during pregnancy or at birth. |
| Human papillomavirus (HPV) | | | ? | Low risk of baby's acquiring HPV during pregnancy or at birth. May cause genital warts or cervical cancer later in child's life. |
| Listeriosis (Listeria monocytogenes) | X | | X | May cause miscarriage or infection in baby after birth. |
| Lyme disease | | ? | ? | Bacteria from a tick bite can cross the placenta. Risks are unknown, but may cause miscarriage or stillbirth. |
| Mumps (Paramyxovirus) | | | X | Although the connection is unconfirmed, infection may cause miscarriage. May cause infection in baby after birth. |
| Measles | | ? | X | May cause infection in baby after birth. |
| Periodontal disease (gum disease) | | X | | Severe gingivitis greatly increases risk of preterm birth. |
| Rubella (German measles) | X | X | X | When baby is infected in first half of pregnancy, infection increases risk of problems with hearing, vision, heart function, or brain development. |
| Syphilis (Treponema pallidum) | X | | X | Possible problems with baby's eyes, skin, heart, bones, and nervous system. May cause death. |
| Toxoplasmosis (Toxoplasma gondii) | X | | X | Possible effects on all of baby's organs; may cause death. Problems are more severe if mother is first infected in first half of pregnancy. |
| Trichomoniasis (Trichomonas vaginalis) | | ? | | Problems result from prematurity. Infected mothers often have other infections. |
| Yeast (candidiasis) | | | X | Exposure may occur with vaginal birth, but infection is rare. Chances of infection on mother's nipples or in baby's mouth (thrush) increase if mother had antibiotics near time of birth. (See page 422.) |

Key: X = Possible   ? = Questionable

unpasteurized dairy products, raw or undercooked meats and fish, and in contaminated soil and water. Avoid eating unpasteurized milk and soft cheeses during pregnancy. Don't eat meat, poultry, eggs, or seafood that isn't cooked thoroughly. Wash produce before eating it and carefully clean all food preparation surfaces and utensils. (See also page 121.)

## Toxoplasmosis

Cats are the most common carriers of the *Toxoplasma gondii* parasite, especially outdoor cats that eat rats, mice, and other raw meat. The parasite passes from a cat in its feces, and you can transmit it from your hands to your mouth if you don't wash your hands after handling cats, emptying litter boxes, or working in soil that contains cat feces. You can also ingest the parasite by eating raw or undercooked meat or unwashed root vegetables.

If you've been around cats for many years, you may have become immune to toxoplasmosis, the infection caused by the parasite. However, tests for this immunity are unreliable and aren't usually recommended.

If you get toxoplasmosis for the first time during the first trimester, the infection may cause congenital defects or miscarriage. If you're infected during the third trimester, your baby may be born with the infection. Although you can treat toxoplasmosis with antibiotics, prevention is the best treatment. Wash your hands after touching a cat, have someone else clean the litter box, and wear gardening gloves. Also, cook your meat well and wash vegetables thoroughly.

## DIABETES MELLITUS AND GESTATIONAL DIABETES MELLITUS

Diabetes mellitus (also called "DM" or simply "diabetes") occurs when someone has trouble making or using insulin, a hormone that helps glucose (sugar) pass into cells for the body to use as an energy source. There are two types of the disease. With type 1 DM, the body stops making insulin; with type 2 DM, the body uses insulin ineffectively. Without insulin, blood glucose levels rise dramatically and glucose passes into the urine. DM can cause serious problems in pregnancy if a woman doesn't have proper medical care and nutrition.

When considering getting pregnant, a woman with DM needs to balance her medications with her activity level and diet. She may need to adjust her insulin dose or begin taking injections to control her blood glucose levels. She improves her chances of carrying a healthy baby to term if she controls her blood glucose levels before and during pregnancy.

Gestational diabetes mellitus (GDM), a form of DM that develops or is first recognized in pregnancy, affects about 3 to 5 percent of women. GDM is related to normal changes in glucose metabolism that promote the baby's growth in the womb. Human placental lactogen (HPL) diminishes the effect of insulin and allows more glucose for the baby's growth. In some women, their response to this pregnancy hormone is out of balance, leading to excessively high blood glucose levels.

Early detection and appropriate treatment of GDM can help prevent problems similar to those for a pregnant woman with DM who has high blood glucose levels, such as increased chances of a urinary tract infection (UTI), an overly large baby, preterm birth, stillbirth, and a newborn with hypoglycemia (low blood sugar), jaundice, or breathing difficulties.

Some caregivers use urine tests to screen for glucose in early pregnancy. Most caregivers use blood tests to screen for GDM between the twenty-fourth and twenty-eighth weeks of pregnancy. (See page 68.) If you're at increased risk for GDM, your caregiver may suggest giving you the blood test earlier than the twenty-fourth week. Risk factors include women who have family members with DM, obese women, and those of Hispanic, African, or African American descent.

If your blood test is positive for high glucose levels, your caregiver will order a glucose tolerance test (GTT) to confirm the diagnosis, a process that requires blood tests every hour for three hours. (See page 145.)

If you have GDM, treatment includes a special diet, exercise, and (in some cases) oral medications or insulin injections. The clinic nurse will show you how to check your blood glucose levels. If your caregiver suspects that your baby is overly large or that your placental circulation is affected, he or she may induce your labor near term. After the birth, your blood glucose will probably return to normal levels; however, about half of the women with GDM develop type 2 DM later in life.

## RH (RHESUS) OR RHD BLOOD INCOMPATIBILITY

A characteristic of blood types is the presence or absence of an antigen called the "Rh" or "RhD factor." If your blood type includes a plus sign (such as O+ or A+), the Rh factor is present. More than 85 percent of the population is Rh positive. If your blood type includes a minus sign (such as O- or A-), the Rh factor is absent. About 15 percent of Caucasians, 3 to 5 percent of people of African descent, and few people of Asian descent are Rh negative.

In early pregnancy, your blood is tested for the Rh factor. If your blood is Rh negative, then your baby's father needs to have his blood tested as well. If you're Rh positive and your baby's father is Rh negative, or if both of you are Rh positive or Rh negative, all is well. However, if you're Rh negative and your baby's father is Rh positive, then your baby may be Rh positive—and if so, you and your baby are Rh incompatible.

Although you and your baby don't share blood systems, if you and your baby are Rh incompatible, his blood may enter your bloodstream when you give birth or if you experience a miscarriage or have invasive tests such as amniocentesis or chorionic villus sampling (CVS). As a result, you may become Rh sensitized and start producing antibodies that may cause mild to severe anemia in your baby. Because your body produces antibodies slowly, the first Rh-incompatible pregnancy is usually unaffected. Without treatment, however, a problem can arise in a future pregnancy if that baby is also Rh positive.

Injecting an Rh-negative mother with Rh-immune globulin (RhoGAM) at the twenty-eighth week of pregnancy can prevent Rh sensitization. RhoGAM is also given after a miscarriage or abortion, with any invasive procedure, or if necessary after uterine bleeding or trauma. If a blood test finds that the baby is Rh positive, the mother receives another dose of RhoGAM within seventy-two hours of the birth.

Although RhoGAM has made Rh sensitization rare, if you're Rh negative your caregiver will test your blood for antibodies throughout your pregnancy. If the level of antibodies increases, amniocentesis helps assess how seriously the antibodies have affected your baby. In severe cases of anemia in the baby, treatment may include early birth and a blood transfusion to replace blood cells. Only in extreme cases does a baby need a blood transfusion in the womb.

## VAGINAL BLEEDING IN LATE PREGNANCY

In late pregnancy, heavy vaginal bleeding may suggest problems with the placenta's attachment to your uterus, such as placenta previa or placental abruption. (See pages 139–140.) Call your caregiver immediately if you experience fairly heavy bleeding. Slight spotting in late pregnancy may be a normal sign of labor; however, if your pregnancy is less than thirty-seven weeks, the spotting may indicate preterm labor.

# Preterm Labor

A *preterm labor* is one that begins before the thirty-seventh week of pregnancy, and births that result from preterm labor are called preterm births. About 10 to 13 percent of births are preterm, and their frequency has increased in the United States since the early 1990s. Although no one completely understands why the number of preterm births has risen, some experts speculate that several factors contribute to the cause, including the following: a greater number of women who are delaying pregnancy until their thirties or forties, increased use of reproductive technology that results in more pregnancies with multiples, and a greater number of elective inductions and planned cesareans with incorrect estimates of the baby's gestational age.

Because preterm babies are immature and underdeveloped, they tend to have more health problems than full-term babies do. Very premature babies (born before the thirty-second week of pregnancy) have an even greater risk of life-threatening complications. (See page 392.) Good prenatal care strives to prevent preterm birth by identifying those women most likely to have preterm labor.

## RISK FACTORS FOR PRETERM LABOR

Several factors can increase the risk of preterm labor. Although many women with these risk factors deliver their babies early, many don't. The factors simply mean the women are more likely to have preterm labor than others are—but even women without these risks may have preterm labor.

- Previous preterm labor or birth
- Pregnant with multiples
- Previous abortions
- Abnormally shaped uterus or previous uterine or cervical surgery
- Current infection of the vagina, amniotic membranes, bladder, or mouth and gums (See pages 132–133.)
- Bleeding during pregnancy
- Obese or extremely underweight before pregnancy
- Poor nutrition before or during pregnancy
- Older than thirty-five or younger than sixteen
- Use of reproductive technology to become pregnant
- Heavy smoking or drug abuse
- Disease in baby or birth defects
- Constant emotional stress (domestic violence, extreme poverty, workplace pressures, or other severe stresses)
- High degree of physical stress (heavy lifting, long periods of standing, or very strenuous exercise)

## How to Check for Contractions

1. Empty your bladder and drink two tall glasses of water.
2. Recline with your feet up or lie on your side. Relax.
3. Place your fingertips gently but firmly on your abdomen at the top of your uterus. When you feel your uterus harden, press on it in several places. If your entire uterus doesn't feel hard, you're not having a contraction. (You're probably feeling your baby's back pressing against your abdomen.)
4. Time the contractions for one hour. (See page 175.) Note the length and frequency of them.
5. If you have six contractions during the hour while you're lying down (or four per hour for two hours), call your caregiver. Make sure you tell him or her that you drank two glasses of water and timed your contractions while lying down.

## Signs of Preterm Labor

Because some women without any risk factors deliver their babies early, all pregnant women should know the signs of preterm labor. These signs are common and similar to normal pregnancy sensations, so watch for slight differences or changes. While it's important to be aware of these signs, remember that only about 12 percent of women have preterm labor.

If you have two or more of these symptoms, call your caregiver immediately to help you decide whether you're in preterm labor.

- Uterine contractions that occur every ten minutes, or six contractions in one hour (Contractions come in waves as your uterus alternately tightens and softens; they don't have to be painful. See page 136 to learn how to detect contractions.)
- Continuous or intermittent menstrual-like cramps or pressure in your lower abdomen and thighs (pelvic heaviness)
- Dull ache in your lower back that doesn't go away when you change position
- Intestinal cramping with or without diarrhea or loose stools
- Sudden increase or change in vaginal discharge (watery, blood tinged, or with more thin mucus)
- General feeling that something isn't right

When checking for preterm contractions, think about your typical uterine activity and remember that contractions of irregular length and frequency are normal in pregnancy. Having persistent, fairly regular contractions for two hours (along with other signs) indicates labor.

### PREDICTING PRETERM LABOR

For years, researchers have tried to find a reliable method to predict preterm labor. While a single accurate test isn't yet available, the results of several tests can increase the likelihood of detecting whether a woman at risk for preterm birth will deliver soon. These tests include the following:

- Produced by the baby's membranes, **fetal fibronectin (fFN)** is a protein that increases in the last weeks of pregnancy and during labor. When a test detects fFN in vaginal and cervical secretions between the twenty-second and thirty-fifth weeks of pregnancy, the risk of preterm labor is increased (but not guaranteed).
- A transvaginal ultrasound scan or a vaginal exam can determine **cervical length**, which shows how the cervix is responding to pregnancy. If a woman's cervix shortens (that is, begins effacing) months or weeks before term without labor contractions, the risk of preterm labor increases.
- Other tests may help identify the risk of preterm labor, including **blood tests** for specific biochemical markers and a **saliva test** that looks for an increase of the hormone estriol. (Visit our web site, http://www.PCNGuide.com, for more information on these tests.) However, more research is needed to evaluate the effectiveness of these tests to help prevent preterm labor.

### DIAGNOSING PRETERM LABOR

A caregiver diagnoses a woman with preterm labor if an ultrasound scan or a vaginal exam detects the shortening and opening of her cervix. For women pregnant with multiples, because the babies expand the uterus to a size that may naturally cause these cervical changes, caregivers may use additional tests to help determine the risk of preterm birth. Some caregivers offer these tests to all women with signs of labor to determine whether it's preterm labor. (See above.)

# TREATMENT TO PREVENT PRETERM BIRTH

If you have any symptoms of preterm labor, contact your caregiver immediately. Prompt treatment may help stop labor. If your caregiver determines that you're in preterm labor, he or she may suggest the following measures to try to stop the contractions and prevent a preterm birth:

**Go on bed rest.**

Bed rest ranges from complete bed rest (getting out of bed only when necessary, such as to use the toilet) to a slight decrease in your activity level plus increased rest. Although research doesn't show that bed rest reliably stops preterm labor, many caregivers recommend it to decrease uterine activity—and it often seems to work, possibly because your stress levels may decrease when resting. (The relaxing effects of a warm tub bath may also reduce uterine activity.)

**Monitor uterine contractions.**

If you're hospitalized for preterm labor, electronic monitoring will determine if labor contractions are progressing. If you're at home, your caregiver will ask you to continue checking for contractions by hand and to watch for other labor signs. (Portable electronic monitors were used in the past, but because they don't reduce the rate of preterm birth, their use is rare today.)

**Restrict sexual activity (pelvic rest).**

Orgasm causes the uterus to contract, and semen contains prostaglandins, which can promote preterm labor in women who are at risk. Nipple stimulation may also initiate preterm labor contractions.

**Take medication to help stop or postpone labor.**

Caregivers sometimes prescribe drugs to relax the uterus. If the drugs are successful, caregivers usually stop the treatment when the pregnancy reaches about thirty-six to thirty-seven weeks. These muscle relaxants (tocolytics) include nifedipine, magnesium sulfate, and indomethacin. (See page 292.) They stop preterm labor only occasionally, but may delay the birth for up to seven days, providing time to administer other drugs to improve the baby's health.

Research suggests that progesterone may prevent prematurity when the hormone is injected weekly in women with a prior preterm birth who show signs of cervical changes in the second trimester.

Because certain infections increase the risk of preterm labor, if you have one of these infections, your caregiver may prescribe antibiotics to try to prevent preterm labor contractions.

**Consider cervical cerclage (surgical suturing of the cervix).**

*Incompetent cervix* is when the cervix shortens and opens in mid-pregnancy without preterm labor contractions. This relatively rare condition may occur if the cervix has been weakened by injury or surgery, such as conization or a D&C (see page 128) for an abortion. The cervix may be closed with suture thread in early pregnancy as a preventive measure or in mid-pregnancy (before the twenty-fourth week of pregnancy) if cervical changes occur. The sutures are removed in late pregnancy.

# WHEN PRETERM BIRTH IS UNAVOIDABLE

If treatment doesn't stop the contractions or cervical dilation, caregivers may suggest measures to help increase a premature baby's chances of a healthy life. (See page 292.)

If your baby will be born prematurely, your caregiver may want you to give birth in a hospital with a neonatal intensive care unit (NICU). The survival rate of very premature babies and babies with very low birth weight is greater when they're born in hospitals that provide intensive care. (See page 293.)

## Decreasing Your Risk of Preterm Labor

Although you might not be able to avoid all the risk factors listed on page 136, here are steps you can take to reduce your risk of preterm labor.

1. Attend all prenatal appointments and carefully consider your caregiver's suggestions. Continue treatment for chronic conditions.
2. Eat well during pregnancy and take any prescribed supplements. Try to reach your suggested weight before becoming pregnant and avoid excessive weight gain during pregnancy.
3. Get screened for infections. If any are detected, have them treated.
4. Avoid smoking, secondhand smoke, alcohol, and hazardous substances.
5. Limit strenuous activities and ask others for help when necessary.
6. Decrease job or life stresses as much as possible. Report any abuse and increase your emotional support from trusted friends and family.

# Complications with the Placenta

A few women develop problems with how and where the placenta attaches to the uterus. The following sections discuss the two most common of these placental complications.

## PLACENTA PREVIA

Less than 1 percent of pregnancies develop placenta previa, a condition in which the placenta lies completely or partially over the cervix. Women with placenta previa can't deliver their babies vaginally; instead, they have planned cesarean births, usually after the thirty-sixth week of pregnancy, but before labor begins.

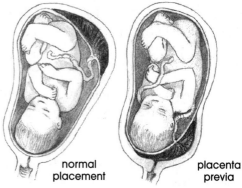

normal placement      placenta previa

In early pregnancy, you may learn from an ultrasound scan that your placenta attached to the lower part of your uterus near the cervix (low-lying placenta). In most cases, as your uterus grows, the site where the placenta attached rises away from the cervix. (If you don't have a low-lying placenta in early pregnancy, you won't develop placenta previa later.) Your caregiver will diagnose you with placenta previa only if a transvaginal ultrasound scan confirms that the placenta continues to cover the cervix later in pregnancy.

Risk factors for placenta previa include: a prior cesarean birth, uterine surgery, or abortion; uterine abnormalities; an age older than thirty-four; many previous pregnancies; and heavy smoking. The most common symptom of placenta previa is painless vaginal bleeding as cervical changes occur in the last trimester. Bleeding is usually intermittent and ranges from light to heavy. As with any vaginal bleeding during pregnancy, notify your caregiver immediately.

Treatment depends on your symptoms and includes measures to prevent heavy bleeding and decrease the risk of preterm birth. If you haven't had any bleeding, your caregiver will avoid doing vaginal exams and will advise you to avoid sex and heavy exertion. You may be put on bed rest. If you've had vaginal bleeding, you may be hospitalized for close observation and, if blood tests show severe blood loss, have a blood transfusion.

## PLACENTAL ABRUPTION

Another rare condition that occurs in about 1 percent of pregnancies is placental abruption, in which the placenta partially or almost completely separates from the uterine wall during the third trimester or during labor. The condition can cause significant blood loss in the mother and can deprive the baby of adequate oxygen. Your risk of placental abruption increases if you have any of the following factors:

- Extremely high blood pressure
- More than five previous pregnancies
- A history of second trimester bleeding
- A prior abruption
- Habit of heavy smoking or cocaine use
- Severe abdominal trauma

Placental abruption may cause any or all of the following symptoms: vaginal bleeding, continuous severe abdominal pain, lower back pain, tender abdomen, and constant tightening of the uterus. Sometimes, vaginal bleeding is absent if the blood collects high in the uterus.

An ultrasound scan may help determine the degree of separation and its effect on blood flow to the placenta. Assessing the mother's blood pressure and the baby's heart rate helps estimate the severity of the abruption and, along with tests to check how well the mother's blood clots, help determine appropriate treatment. When the abruption is small and the baby remains healthy, bed rest and close observation may be the only treatment. If bleeding is severe and the baby's heart rate shows distress (and if the baby's chances of surviving a preterm birth are high), a woman has an immediate cesarean birth and a blood transfusion if necessary.

# High Blood Pressure and Gestational Hypertension

Your activity level, emotional state, and body position can affect your blood pressure. It's usually lower when you're at rest, lying down, or free of emotional stress. It's usually higher when you're active, upright, or stressed. Short-term changes in your blood pressure are normal; however, blood pressure that stays too high can cause health risks at any age.

Someone with high blood pressure (hypertension) has had at least two consecutive readings that are over 140/90. The condition, which affects about 10 percent of pregnant women in the United States, can be chronic or develop during pregnancy. When high blood pressure first appears after the twentieth week of pregnancy and remains high for several readings, it's called *gestational hypertension* or *pregnancy-induced hypertension (PIH)*.

A pregnant woman with high blood pressure is at risk for serious problems with uterine and placental blood flow and possible damage to other internal organs. Reduced blood flow to the placenta can result in less oxygen and fewer nutrients for the baby and may cause growth problems. Both chronic hypertension (high blood pressure present before pregnancy) and gestational hypertension can cause these problems. Gestational hypertension can also develop into a more dangerous condition called preeclampsia.

## PREECLAMPSIA

*Preeclampsia* (previously called "toxemia") is a multi-organ condition with mild to severe symptoms that affects about 5 to 8 percent of pregnancies. It typically occurs after the twentieth week of pregnancy, and the first signs are gestational hypertension and proteinuria (protein in the urine).

Mild preeclampsia developed near term may cause fewer health problems than the possibly serious consequences of severe preeclampsia that begins before the thirtieth week of pregnancy.[3] With early diagnosis and aggressive treatment, complications from preeclampsia are generally minimal and both the mother and baby are typically healthy at birth and afterward.

## Risk Factors for Preeclampsia

Although the causes of preeclampsia aren't well understood, a combination of factors appears to trigger the condition. Some women are at higher risk of developing preeclampsia than others are. The most significant risk factors include the following:

- First pregnancy
- Preeclampsia in a previous pregnancy (or a close family member with it)
- Personal history of chronic hypertension, diabetes, kidney disease, polycystic ovarian syndrome (PCOS), or vascular disease
- Obesity
- Age older than thirty-five or younger than eighteen
- Pregnant with multiples
- African descent
- History of certain autoimmune disorders, such as lupus or rheumatoid arthritis
- Infections during this pregnancy, such as periodontal disease or urinary tract infection (UTI)

Researchers continue to seek ways to evaluate a woman's risk of developing severe preeclampsia. Because it's a complex condition, a complete risk assessment may include a combination of tests, such as blood and urine tests, and uterine blood flow studies.

## Other Signs of Preeclampsia

Two screening tests can detect early signs of preeclampsia. A urine test will show proteinuria, and routine blood pressure checks will discover high blood pressure. A pregnant woman can often notice other signs of preeclampsia. If you have any of the following signs, contact your caregiver immediately.

- Sudden puffiness (edema) in your hands or face
- Rapid weight gain (more than 2 pounds in one week)
- Headache
- Visual changes or problems (flashes or spots before the eyes or blurred vision)
- Pain in your stomach (epigastric pain) or your right side under your ribs, or possible pain in your shoulder or lower back

## Learning More about Pregnancy Complications

To learn more about a specific disease or condition, ask your caregiver for patient-education handouts that describe your condition or disorder. If handouts aren't available, ask where you can get more information.

You can also search the Internet for web sites that provide information about your condition or concern. To ensure the information on a web site is accurate and up to date, check several sites to compare data. Also check the expertise of site authors and find out whether the sources they cite are reliable or biased. Examples of reliable web sites that provide accurate information on a number of pregnancy complications include the following:

- http://www.marchofdimes.com
- http://www.mymidwife.org
- http://www.childbirthconnection.org
- http://familydoctor.org
- http://www.cochrane.org/reviews/en/subtopics/87.html

It's possible—but rare—that a woman with preeclampsia will have high blood pressure and proteinuria and have none of the other symptoms. A particular sign of preeclampsia usually indicates the specific organ system affected. Typically, the more systems that are affected, the more severe the condition is. Severe preeclampsia can cause the following complications:

- Placental abruption (See page 140.)
- The HELLP syndrome (hemolysis, elevated liver enzymes, low platelets), which indicates blood and liver complications
- Eclampsia, which indicates neurological irritability and imminent convulsions
- Seizures, stroke, coma, or even death of mother and baby (in the most severe cases)

## Treating Preeclampsia

If you have preeclampsia, the only cure is the birth of your baby (normal blood pressure usually returns within days or weeks after the birth). However, treatment to avoid further complications is available, based on the severity of the disease and your baby's gestational age and health.

If your symptoms are mild (such as blood pressure over 140/90, proteinuria, and fluid retention), treatment usually includes decreased activity or bed rest, blood pressure checks, and close observation. You may receive medications to lower your blood pressure or to reduce the risk that hypertension will slow your baby's growth.

If you have severe preeclampsia (blood pressure over 160/110 and proteinuria accompanied by liver, blood, or neurological complications), you'll be hospitalized and given drugs, such as an antihypertensive and magnesium sulfate, to reduce your risk of seizures. (Visit our web site, http://www.PCNGuide.com, for more information on these medications.) You'll likely continue to receive magnesium sulfate for at least twenty-four hours after the birth to prevent seizures.

If severe symptoms worsen or don't sufficiently improve with treatment, your caregiver may suggest inducing labor or performing a planned cesarean. If you're concerned how a preterm birth will affect your baby, you may want to postpone induction. If your health or your baby's life isn't in jeopardy, your caregiver may suggest delaying the birth for a day or two so you can receive corticosteroids to promote your baby's lung development before birth.

## REDUCING YOUR RISK OF DEVELOPING PREECLAMPSIA

Research suggests that for women at risk of developing preeclampsia, taking a low-dose aspirin (50 to 150 milligrams) each day helps reduce the risk and may decrease the rate of perinatal death and increase babies' birth weight. Check with your caregiver before taking aspirin.[4] In addition, studies on folic acid supplementation in the second trimester show a reduced risk of preeclampsia in women who took the supplements in this period.[5]

Early detection helps decrease the risk of developing severe preeclampsia and other serious complications. Strive to eat a healthful diet and gain a moderate amount of weight in pregnancy. (See page 117.) Attend all prenatal appointments, have the appropriate screening tests, and work with your caregiver to control high blood pressure and treat other early signs of preeclampsia. If you contract any infection, consult your caregiver for early treatment. Infection may increase your risk of preeclampsia.

# Diagnostic Tests

Caregivers routinely use screening tests in pregnancy to assess the health of the mother and baby. (See page 67 and visit our web site, http://www.PCNGuide.com, to learn more about screening tests.) If a screening test shows a potential problem or if you have symptoms of a specific pregnancy complication, your caregiver may suggest a diagnostic test to confirm that you have a problem and to detect its severity. Because the results from one test might not be completely accurate, your caregiver may order several tests to confirm a diagnosis.

Some diagnostic tests have more risks than others. Asking key questions about a test can help you learn its risks and benefits, and knowing this information will help you decide whether to have the test. (See page 10.)

The following sections describe common diagnostic tests. The tests in each section share a common purpose, and they're discussed by order of frequency, starting with the ones most commonly used. For more information on these and other diagnostic tests, visit our web site.

## Tests to Detect Genetic Defects and Diseases

The following tests can provide helpful information if it's important for you to know in advance whether your baby has a specific genetic problem. However, you may choose not to have these invasive tests because they require penetrating your uterus. Although rare, potential risks of these tests include miscarriage, infection, bleeding, or leaking of amniotic fluid.

### Amniocentesis

Between the fifteenth and twentieth weeks of pregnancy, a laboratory can test a sample of amniotic fluid to help detect Down syndrome, sickle cell anemia, neural tube defects, and other disorders. The results are available in about two weeks. Your caregiver also can use amniocentesis in late pregnancy to assess your baby's lung maturity before a preterm birth.

### Chorionic villus sampling (CVS)

This test examines a small piece from the chorionic villi (the early placenta) to provide information about chromosomal abnormalities in your baby. CVS can be done between the tenth and twelfth weeks of pregnancy.

### Cordocentesis or percutaneous umbilical blood sampling (PUBS)

This test assesses a sample of your baby's blood from the umbilical cord to detect chromosomal defects, blood disorders, and conditions such as infection, anemia, and lack of oxygen. PUBS can be done after the eighteenth week of pregnancy. Because the test carries more risks than amniocentesis, caregivers use it only when they need confirmation of a diagnosis more quickly than amniocentesis can provide.

## Imaging Tests for Your Health and Your Baby's Well-being

The following tests allow a noninvasive look at your baby and uterine structures. Except for x-ray, they pose no significant risks to you or your baby.

### Ultrasound scan

An ultrasound scan helps estimate your baby's gestational age and maturity, locates her organs and structures, and detects her presentation and position in the uterus. It also can determine preterm cervical changes and assess amniotic fluid volume when evaluating your baby's well-being. Caregivers often use ultrasound scans in conjunction with other procedures such as external version of a breech baby, CVS, and amniocentesis. (For information about an ultrasound scan as a screening test, see page 68.)

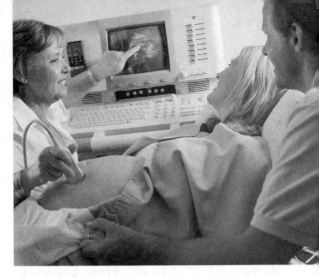

### Magnetic resonance imaging (MRI)

Visual images of the internal structure of your baby can help confirm malformations. MRI also helps assess your internal organs for potential complications. Your caregiver may use MRI when the results of an ultrasound scan are unclear.

### Doppler arterial blood flow studies (velocimetry)

A Doppler ultrasound unit placed on your abdomen provides information about the circulation of blood within and among the uterus, placenta, and your baby. Your caregivers may use this test to identify if your baby is at risk for blood flow complications such as intrauterine growth restriction (IUGR), anemia, and prematurity from severe preeclampsia.

### X-ray

Caregivers rarely use an x-ray on pregnant women. If necessary, however, it can help diagnose problems you may have, such as pneumonia, dental disease, and broken bones.

## Tests for Your Baby's Well-being in Late Pregnancy

Although the following tests help assess your baby's well-being by monitoring his heart rate, their results are sometimes difficult to interpret and may lead to more testing.

### Non-stress test (NST)

By monitoring your baby's heart rate when he's actively moving, your caregiver can better predict his well-being and determine whether a high-risk pregnancy can continue. (See page 252 for more information on fetal heart rate monitoring.) If the results aren't reassuring, your caregiver may use other diagnostic tests to confirm your baby's well-being.

### Biophysical profile (BPP)

To assess your baby's well-being, this test considers information from an NST and uses an ultrasound scan to evaluate amniotic fluid volume and your baby's functions. Your caregiver can use BPP to assess if a high-risk or post-date pregnancy can safely continue or if induction should be considered. Because this test monitors five factors (but not your baby's size), it's a fairly good indicator of his condition.

### Contraction stress test (CST) or oxytocin challenge test (OCT)

For this test, your caregiver induces contractions and monitors your baby's heart rate to predict whether he can withstand the stress of labor contractions (if not, a cesarean may be necessary). It's not usually done unless an NST indicates a problem.

# TESTS TO DETECT POTENTIAL PREGNANCY PROBLEMS

The following laboratory tests offer information that helps your caregiver make an accurate diagnosis and choose appropriate treatment.

**Glucose tolerance test (GTT)**

For this test, you first have your blood drawn, then you drink a sugary beverage and have blood drawn again every hour in a three-hour period. Your caregiver will diagnose gestational diabetes mellitus (GDM) if a screening test suggests the presence of the condition.

**Vaginal or cervical smear**

During a vaginal exam, your caregiver obtains secretions from your vagina or cervical area to detect infectious organisms, premature rupture of membranes, or substances that indicate an increased risk of preterm labor.

## Key Points to Remember

- Most pregnancies don't develop complications, and both the mother and baby are healthy at birth and afterward.
- With appropriate prenatal care and self-care during pregnancy, you can decrease your chances of developing serious problems from a chronic condition or from a complication that arises during pregnancy.
- Promptly contact your caregiver if you see any warning signs of pregnancy complications (see page 70). Early treatment helps minimize the severity of any complication.
- Before making decisions about prenatal tests and procedures, be sure you understand how and why they are being done and the benefits, risks, and possible alternatives. Talk to your caregiver and ask questions until you feel that you can make an informed decision. Also, visit our web site, http://www.PCNGuide.com, to learn more information about a specific test or procedure.

# Planning for Birth and Post Partum

Giving birth can be deeply satisfying when you participate fully in the event and your care is tailored to match your wishes. To help distinguish yourself as an individual with unique needs, it's important to communicate your priorities and preferences for your care. This chapter describes the process of discovering your options, examining your priorities, and discussing your preferences with your caregiver and others providing your care. With this preparation, you'll learn how to create a written plan that effectively communicates your wishes to make your labor, birth, and postpartum period rewarding experiences.

# The Importance of Planning for Birth and Post Partum

The main purpose of planning for your baby's birth and the postpartum period is to establish a line of communication between you and those providing your care, ensuring that they know your priorities and preferences for treatment. If everyone understands and respects your wishes, you're more likely to be satisfied with the care you receive than if your wishes are unrecognized.[1]

If you have only one or two caregivers providing all your care, such as midwives who belong to a small home birth practice or a freestanding (unaffiliated with a hospital) birth center, getting to know one another will occur naturally and easily. The ability to communicate clearly and honestly with one another will strengthen as a personal relationship develops.

If your caregiver belongs to a group practice—and most maternity caregivers in the United States and Canada do—it may be harder to build personal relationships, but establishing good communication is possible. Caregivers who belong to a group practice rotate who's on duty during specific shifts. The caregiver on call attends to all patients from that group practice throughout his or her shift, including those who usually see other caregivers in the group. Nurses and hospital staff assist the on-call caregiver, but you probably won't meet them before arriving at the hospital. This system of rotating shifts ensures that all your care providers have had time off for adequate rest. As long as communication among all staff is good, the system is efficient.

During a shift change in a hospital, the nurse whose shift has ended communicates a patient's clinical status directly with the nurse coming on duty. Nurses also communicate directly with the patient's caregiver whenever necessary.

More important than direct spoken communication is the medical chart. If you're planning a hospital birth, your caregiver electronically records information on your physical and psychological well-bring in your chart at each prenatal visit, and frequently during your hospital stay. This chart becomes a permanent record that's available to you and others caring for you whenever you need medical care in the future.

Some of your priorities and preferences for birth and the postpartum period might not be recorded clearly in your chart, even though you discussed them with your caregiver. This miscommunication can be a problem because your nurses likely won't know much about you before you arrive at the hospital in labor. A birth plan can provide a way to communicate your wishes efficiently and effectively.

# Your Birth Plan

A *birth plan* (also called a "birth preference list," "wish list," or "goal sheet") is a one- to two-page letter you write to everyone attending to your care during labor and birth. In it, you describe your concerns and fears for labor and birth, as well as your wishes for the treatment of you, your partner, and your baby. Although a birth plan lets you express your priorities and preferences, it's *not* a contract that dictates the actions of all your care providers, nor is it a guarantee that problems won't arise that will require a change in your plan. Instead, a birth plan lets everyone know which safe options are most important to you, which in turn increases your chances of receiving personalized care.[2] The goal of the birth plan is to enhance your satisfaction with the birth experience.

# FREQUENTLY ASKED QUESTIONS ABOUT BIRTH PLANS

The following are answers to common questions many expectant couples have about birth plans.

**How does a birth plan help us?**

Preparing a birth plan helps you reflect on how you'll best cope with the unpredictability, stress, and pain of labor and birth. As you learn about the different care options and treatments, think about your needs and preferences to help you decide what kind of care is important to you. Discussing your birth plan with your caregiver is an excellent way to enhance communication, clarify your expectations, and build trust and understanding.

## In Their Own Words

When my cervix was 9 centimeters dilated, I felt that I couldn't handle the pain anymore and asked for an epidural. Our midwife told me that I could certainly have one, but suggested that a bath might help relieve the pain just as much. This was exactly the sort of help I'd requested in my birth plan, so I knew she was respecting my wishes. I got into the bath and stayed until I was fully dilated.

—*Hillary*

Perhaps the most important reason to have a birth plan is to provide a way to introduce yourself and your partner to unfamiliar caregivers, nurses, and hospital staff, and to effectively and efficiently communicate your issues, fears, or concerns to them. By providing a birth plan to read, you free yourself from the need to explain your wishes and expectations each time a new person takes over your care—a clear advantage if you're coping with contractions during a shift change and can't focus on conversation!

**How does a birth plan help my caregiver?**

A birth plan helps your caregiver understand your goals and preferences for labor and birth, and alerts him or her to any misunderstandings or unrealistic expectations you may have. By carefully addressing your priorities and preferences and suggesting alternatives where necessary for safety or practical reasons, your caregiver helps you create a birth plan that reflects the flexibility needed if problems arise in labor or birth.

**How does a birth plan help the nursing staff?**

Because most of the nurses won't have met you before your arrival at the hospital, a birth plan helps them become acquainted with you and individualize your care. It gives them important information about your concerns and preferences, which you expressed before going into labor, when you were calm, comfortable, and able to think clearly. If the nurses know what's important to you, they're better able to meet your needs and help you fulfill your wishes. Studies show that women often feel disappointment, anger, or depression if their desires and expectations about birth aren't met.[3]

**How do caregivers feel about birth plans?**

Reactions to birth plans vary. Some caregivers encourage birth plans and will work with women on them, if asked. Others might not be familiar with birth plans. Still others believe that birth plans are unnecessary. These caregivers argue that they wouldn't administer treatment without the woman's consent; therefore, there's no reason for the woman to express her wishes about treatment beforehand. However, these caregivers might not realize how helpful it is for a woman to know in advance whether her desires for care are realistic and acceptable, or how stressful it can be for her to explain her wishes while coping with contractions.

## Common Q & A

**Q:** What can I do if an intervention is suggested during labor, but it's not in my birth plan?

**A:** If those providing your care recommend treatment that seems to go against your preferences, you or your partner may ask why it's needed. The reason may be that the treatment is the safest way to handle a medical issue that has arisen. Or it's possible that your nurses and unfamiliar caregivers are unaware of your preferences and are following standard protocol. Once they understand your desires and you understand their reasoning for the treatment, you should be able to discuss the matter with them and reach a compromise.

You may need to explain why you're preparing a birth plan. Try to emphasize that you want it to enhance communication and trust among you, your partner, and everyone attending to your care. Let your caregiver know that your plan contains personal information you'd like the staff to be aware of, as well as ways they can best support you.

If your caregiver asks you to prepare a birth plan, he or she believes that it's an essential part of your care. Your caregiver considers your input and collaboration important for building cooperation and trust. Having a strong relationship with your caregiver increases your satisfaction with the birth experience and can provide reassurance if problems arise during labor or birth that lead to necessary changes in your birth plan.

If your caregiver is clearly opposed to a birth plan, you'll gain the valuable knowledge that he or she doesn't want to know what's important to you. You can respond by doing one of the following: Give up your birth plan and do what your caregiver requires, try to negotiate with him or her, or try to find another caregiver. (See page 20.) At the very least, learning about your caregiver's opposition to birth plans will clarify your relationship with him or her, and you won't be confused or surprised in labor when your caregiver provides care that goes against your wishes.

**How do nurses feel about birth plans?**

Some nurses believe that birth plans are guides for providing individualized care. If there's not a birth plan in your chart, these nurses will ask you for one.

Other nurses, however, dislike and resist birth plans. Perhaps in the past they were presented with birth plans that seemed unfriendly, bossy, or unrealistic; as a result, they now believe that birth plans do more harm than good. Perhaps they worry that a birth plan is the woman's attempt to control the staff or keep them from doing procedures that are essential for safety.

To minimize opposition, follow the advice on page 153 when preparing your birth plan. Be clear that you're not trying to tell the nurses the best way to do their jobs. Instead, you're simply trying to introduce yourself and your preferences so the nurses can take them into account when caring for you.

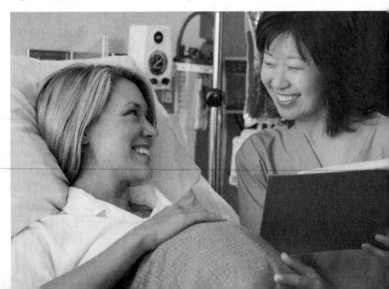

# Preparing Your Birth Plan

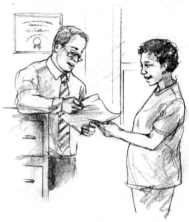

Preparing your birth plan is a task that requires plenty of time; ideally, you should begin working on yours a few months before your due date. To create the most meaningful and helpful birth plan, follow these four steps.

1. Decide what general approach to maternity care you prefer.
2. Learn about specific options available to you if labor progress and birth are normal and if unexpected problems occur. Select the options you prefer.
3. Make a rough draft of your plan and discuss it with your caregiver.
4. Prepare a brief final birth plan that summarizes your priorities and preferences.

## STEP 1: YOUR PREFERRED APPROACH TO MATERNITY CARE

To figure out your preferred approach to maternity care, ask yourself this question: "Of the following two options, which more closely reflects my thoughts about my body, my pregnancy, the kind of care I'm comfortable with, and how I want to participate in my baby's birth?"

**Option A: The self-reliant approach**

I want to actively participate in my labor by using non-medical measures for comfort and labor progress and by taking part in decisions about procedures and other care options. My partner and I are learning about labor and birth, practicing comfort techniques, and attending childbirth preparation classes. We're considering having a doula or another helper with us during labor and birth. I of course will accept medical help if it's truly needed.

**Option B: The caregiver-reliant approach**

I want those providing my care to decide how to manage my labor and relieve my pain. I'm more comfortable with appropriate technology and medical resources than with my own knowledge and non-medical pain-relief techniques. I'll do whatever is asked of me, but I'd like to be kept informed about what's happening to me and my baby and why. I'm not spending much time outside of childbirth classes preparing for labor and birth.

Your preferences may align with one of these approaches, but if they lie somewhere between the two, explain how you'd like to participate and what role you want your caregiver to play. Choose your caregiver based on these preferences (see Chapter 2), or if you already have a caregiver, evaluate the care you're receiving. How does your caregiver respond to your questions? Are you comfortable with his or her answers? Does his or her care match your preferred approach?

It's possible that you chose your caregiver without knowing much about your options. As you learn more about your choices, you may feel happy with your caregiver or you may become uncomfortable with his or her care. If you're uncomfortable, you can take one of the following actions:

1. Continue to accept your current care and give up some of your preferences.
2. Express your discomfort and try to work out acceptable compromises with your caregiver.
3. Change to another caregiver whose care better matches your preferences.

## Two Views on Birth Plans

With this pregnancy, I want to create a simple birth plan that includes only what I feel is most important, and doesn't bother with what I consider "small stuff."
—*Allison*

After my first birth, I didn't get to hold my baby right away, and I regretted that. So for this birth, our birth plan is very basic, but there's a whole paragraph about newborn procedures and how I'd like that first hour to go, assuming all is well with me and my baby.
—*Maria*

## STEP 2: LEARN ABOUT YOUR OPTIONS AND IDENTIFY YOUR PREFERENCES

By reading this book, you can learn about most options and procedures for labor and birth, including key questions to ask about possible risks and alternatives. (See page 10.) Additional resources include other books and web sites, maternity caregivers, friends who have given birth, childbirth preparation classes, and hospital tours. Pay attention to whether the resources you use are evidence based (that is, rely on well-designed research, not on opinions or customs). See page Appendix C for a listing of recommended resources. Your childbirth educator or doula should be familiar with the routine practices of maternity care in your area, and he or she also may be a helpful resource as you prepare and write your birth plan.

As you learn about options, you'll notice those that are natural or low-tech are more compatible with the self-reliant approach, while options that rely on technology and medicine are more compatible with the caregiver-reliant approach. You may discover that you feel strongly about some options; these are good issues to discuss with your caregiver.

To help you choose your preferences, visit our web site, http://www.PCNGuide.com, to download a birth plan work sheet.

## STEP 3: PREPARE A ROUGH DRAFT AND DISCUSS IT WITH YOUR CAREGIVER

Use the following list of topics to prepare a rough draft of your birth plan. (See page 153 for more detailed descriptions of these topics.)

### List of Birth Plan Topics

- Practical information
- Introducing yourselves
- Issues, fears, or concerns
- Care preferences for:
  * Managing labor pain
  * Normal labor and birth
  * Unexpected events, including complications and a cesarean birth
  * Postpartum care
  * Care of a healthy newborn
  * Complications with the newborn

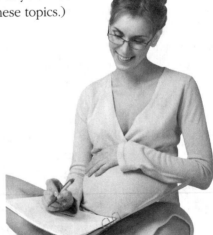

You may need to schedule a longer-than-usual prenatal appointment so you'll have time to discuss your draft with your caregiver and learn whether your plan needs to be revised for clarity, consistency, or safety. This discussion is essential to have because your caregiver may request modifications to better fit with his or her preferred practices, perceptions of safety, and hospital customs. In most cases, you'll probably be able to reach a compromise that satisfies you both.

# Step 4: Prepare the Final Draft

Revise your rough draft into a final draft. Incorporate any suggestions or modifications from your discussions with your caregiver and others. Use bullet points, and don't exceed two pages. A brief yet complete birth plan will be easy for your caregiver and nurses to read and understand. It'll also clearly highlight your priorities and preferences.

Don't include lists of procedures that are acceptable and unacceptable to you. If circumstances change during your labor and birth, some "unacceptable" procedures may become necessary and "acceptable." When expressing a preference about a particular procedure, include phrases such as "unless medically necessary" to indicate that you realize that deviations from your birth plan may become necessary.

After completing your birth plan, read it from a nurse's perspective. Is your plan friendly, respectful, and flexible (that is, does it indicate your awareness that labor isn't always normal or predictable)? Does the tone promote mutual trust and collaboration? If not, revise the language to help ensure that all your care providers will respond positively to your birth plan.

When you're satisfied with your final draft, make copies for yourself, your partner, your caregiver, the nurses, and your doula. Bring extra copies with you when you arrive at the hospital in labor.

## Components of Your Birth Plan

Your birth plan should cover the following topics. Limit your discussion of each topic to one short paragraph or a bulleted list that summarizes just the essential points.

### Practical Information

Give your names, due date, and the names of your caregiver, doula, other support people, and your baby's caregiver. You also may include a statement about the limitations of your birth plan, such as, "We realize our birth plan isn't a contract or a guarantee of an uncomplicated labor. Our highest priority is the health of our baby and me. Thank you for your help."

### Introducing Yourselves

Tell those providing your care a little about yourselves, to help them see the importance of the preferences in your birth plan. For example: "We've been together for six years, and this pregnancy finally happened after three years of trying to conceive. We're hoping for a natural, non-medicated birth, and would value your support."

---

## Issues, Fears, and Concerns about Childbirth

Here are examples of issues, fears, and concerns that couples have included in their birth plans:

*We have a history of infertility and miscarriage, so we tend to worry a lot about our baby's well-being and may need frequent reassurances.*

*I'm terrified of needles and will need someone who's understanding, supportive, and very skilled with inserting needles.*

*I have trouble trusting strangers. Please introduce yourself and talk with me for a while before you begin my care.*

*I'm anxious about labor pain, and worry about losing control.*

*I'm uncomfortable with the idea of being seen without my clothes on; please help preserve my modesty.*

## Preferences for Managing Labor Pain

Here are examples of preferences for managing labor pain that couples have included in their birth plans:

*I'd prefer to give birth without pain medications. My partner and doula will support me using techniques we learned in childbirth preparation class.*

*I'd like to have an epidural as early as possible.*

*As long as my labor is progressing normally and I'm coping, I want to avoid pain medications. However, if my labor is prolonged, if complications arise, or if the pain is too great, I may request an epidural.*

*I feel strongly about avoiding pain medications. Please don't offer them to me; I'll ask for them if needed.*

### Issues, Fears, or Concerns

If you don't have any particular issues, fears, or concerns, you might not need to address this topic. But if you do, here's an opportunity to disclose them. See page 153 for examples.

Your feelings may be influenced by a previous negative experience, such as a miscarriage or a traumatic birth, unpleasant encounters with caregivers or hospitals, or childhood trauma. By disclosing your feelings and the reasons for them, you'll more likely receive treatment that takes your unique needs into account.

### Preferences for Managing Labor Pain

After reading Chapters 10 and 11 to learn about self-help and medical measures for pain relief, describe your preferences for managing labor pain as clearly as possible. This may be a challenge because you don't know how much pain you'll have in labor or how long your labor will last. Use the Pain Medications Preference Scale on page 187 to help you describe your needs for pain relief.

### Preferences for Normal Labor and Birth

Caregivers always recommend some monitoring of the mother and baby in labor, such as checking the baby's heart rate and the mother's temperature, blood pressure, and contractions. When labor and birth proceed normally, few other interventions are necessary to ensure the well-being of the mother and baby.

Some interventions might be routine in hospitals; however, they might not be necessary, especially if there's not an indication of a problem. Examples of such interventions include intravenous (IV) fluids, continuous electronic fetal monitoring, artificial rupture of the membranes, and suctioning the baby's nose and mouth. Other routine interventions exist for the convenience of the staff or caregiver, including the supine (on your back) position for birth and the separation of baby from mother right after the birth for newborn testing and observation. Still other interventions are required by state or provincial governments, such as administering antibiotics to the baby's eyes and conducting newborn screening for various conditions.

Find out which routine interventions you're likely to encounter (along with the reasoning behind them). When preparing this section of your birth plan, mention only the preferences that matter to you. You don't have to express an opinion on every intervention, especially those that usually aren't done in your area. For example, you may say, "I prefer to avoid interventions and procedures, including routines such as IV fluids and continuous electronic fetal monitoring, and I want to discuss any that are being considered, along with possible alternatives."

## Preferences for Unexpected Events, Including a Cesarean Birth

If a problem arises during labor, birth, or the postpartum period, you may need undesired medications or interventions in order to ensure your well-being or your baby's. Under most circumstances, you'll have time to ask key questions (see page 10) such as, "Do we have time to discuss this intervention before you need me to make a decision?" In rare emergencies, however, the need for immediate action may preclude low-tech measures or even explanation and discussion.

When creating your birth plan, consider separating it into a Plan A and a Plan B. Plan A covers your preferences when labor and birth go smoothly. Plan B addresses how you'll want possible complications to be handled. For example, by including modifications to your birth plan that cover a cesarean birth, you can retain some priorities and preferences in your original birth plan in the event you'll require a cesarean birth (see page 328). Although an unexpected cesarean birth can be disappointing, you'll feel better about the experience if you've thought about this possibility, understood your options, and expressed your preferences. By being flexible with your birth plan, you'll increase your chances of having a healthy baby and a satisfying birth.

## Preferences for Your Healthy Newborn's Care

If you and your baby are healthy and doing well immediately after the birth, he'll need little more than skin-to-skin contact with you (with a blanket covering you both) and access to your breasts; later on, he'll also need a warm environment, diapers, and clothing.

Your caregiver will probably want to do routine observations, tests, and procedures on your newborn to discover serious congenital disorders or to prevent potentially serious illnesses. When considering the options listed on pages 370–371, balance concerns for your baby's comfort and well-being with the potential benefits and risks of each procedure. Some one-time common routines and procedures are now unnecessary or even harmful. For example, feeding sugar water or formula to healthy breastfed babies was once routine, but now pediatricians and lactation consultants consider the practice unnecessary or harmful.

## Preferences for Unexpected Problems with Your Newborn

You may worry about prematurity, illness, birth defects, birth trauma, or even stillbirth. To help manage your concerns, consider in advance how you'll want these misfortunes handled. This way, if a problem does arise, your forethought will prevent having to make such decisions when you're upset and unable to think clearly. Your birth plan can reflect your consideration of these rare possibilities, which increases the likelihood that you'll receive treatment tailored to your preferences. (See page 303.)

# Sample Birth Plans

The following are two examples of birth plans. While both plans cover many of the same topics, each is written in a style that reflects the personality of the writer.

## Birth Plan for Pat Rosen

- My primary caregiver is Dr. Sally Doe, and my due date is July 5.
- My support people will be my husband, Ken; a doula; and perhaps a friend.

### Who We Are
- Ken and I are both originally from the South, so we feel it's a little exotic to have a kid born on the West Coast! This is our first baby, and we don't know if it's a boy or girl. We figured, why spoil one of life's big surprises?

### Issues, Fears, Concerns
- As a child, I had minor surgery involving my urethra, and I remember it as painful and quite frightening. So I have lingering anxiety around vaginal exams and interventions (for example, needing a catheter). Not very convenient when giving birth, I know, and I've tried to get around the anxiety, but it does crop up.

### Preferences for the First Stage of Labor
- Controlling pain: I'd like to use natural coping techniques (breathing, focused relaxation, comfort positions) to a point, but expect I'll want pain meds in active labor. Please let me know when it's okay to have an epidural.
- Medical interventions: I'd like to avoid interventions; delay them until I get the epidural or if a problem comes up.

### Preferences for the Second Stage of Labor
- Positioning: I hope the epidural will be light enough that I can try different positions in the bed to help the birth.
- Pushing efforts: I'd like to labor down, barring any complications, and have help knowing when and how long to push.
- Medical or surgical interventions: I'd like to avoid an episiotomy, and will work very hard to avoid a forceps delivery or a vacuum extraction.

### Preferences for Unexpected Labor Events
- Complicated labor or problems with my baby: We'd like to make informed decisions, so please keep us informed if you have concerns about our baby's well-being or mine.
- Cesarean surgery: I'd like to have at least two of my people with me.

### Preferences for My Postpartum Care
- I plan to breastfeed and would like a visit from a lactation consultant. I have inverted nipples and anticipate needing a little extra help.

### Newborn Care Plan
- Immediately after the birth: Bonding time is very important to us. We'd like to have our baby placed naked on my chest as soon as possible after the birth, unless there's a medical reason not to do so.
- Newborn procedures: Please delay newborn procedures until after the first hour.
- Feeding: We plan to breastfeed exclusively and on cue. We'd like advice from the lactation consultant, as this is all new to us!
- Vaccinations: Please don't give our baby a hepatitis shot. We'll have the pediatricians give vaccinations when recommended.
- If our baby is sick: We absolutely want our baby to have help if needed, and ask that you include us in the decision-making process so we can do all we can for our baby. We wish to stay with our baby so we can hold and feed him or her as much as possible.
- Visitors: We'd like our baby's grandparents brought in to see us and meet him or her as soon as possible after the birth; other friends can come as well, provided we have the energy to visit with them.
- Our educational needs: Because this is our first baby, we need all the advice and help we can get about baby care and feeding!
- Discharge: We hope to stay in the hospital for as long as our insurance policy allows.

## Birth Plan for Jane Smith

**Due date:** April 12

**Support people:** Joe, my husband; Mary Jones, doula (or her backup, Carla Davis)

**Our baby's caregiver:** Dr. Jim Adams, Seattle Pediatric Services

**Introducing Ourselves:** We've selected the midwives at Metro Hospital because we're interested in a safe and natural birth process. We've struggled for years with infertility issues and are very excited to, at long last, welcome our first child to our family through the help of in vitro fertilization.

**Issues, Fears, Concerns:** I'm a private person and am sensitive about my modesty. I'll be more comfortable if you knock before coming into my room, and if only essential people come in. I want to be kept covered, including while in the tub.

**Preferences for Managing Pain:** On the Pain Medications Preference Scale, we're at -7, which means we prefer a natural birth to avoid side effects of medications to me, my labor, or my baby. I'll be disappointed if I elect to use pain medication. Please don't suggest it to me. If I get discouraged, please suggest comfort measures and encourage me. My code word is *pumpernickel*. If I say that word (and *only* if I say it), you should stop encouraging me to go without pain medication, and help me get an epidural or other effective pain medication.

**Preferences for Normal Labor and Birth:**
*First stage of labor*
- Prefer to avoid routine interventions and wish to discuss any being considered, such as IV fluids, continuous electronic fetal monitoring, and so on.
- Desire freedom of movement.
- Prefer intermittent monitoring of my baby.
- Plan to use breathing, shower, bath, and other comfort measures.
- Want to drink clear juices, Popsicles, and eat light snacks.

*Second stage of labor*
- Use upright positions or positions suggested by my midwife.
- No episiotomy–please take steps to avoid tearing (warm compresses, controlled pushing, and support of my perineum).
- Let my baby's cord stop pulsating before being cut. (Joe to cut the cord.)
- After my baby's birth, immediate skin-to-skin contact and breastfeeding

*Third stage of labor and the first hours after the birth*
- Delay all routine procedures until an hour after the birth or the first feeding.
- Decline hepatitis B shot; decline circumcision.
- Keep my baby in my room at all times unless otherwise requested or required.
- Breastfeeding only, no supplements unless needed

**Preferences for Unexpected Labor Events:**
*Prolonged labor and induction*
- If induction is necessary, I'll try self-help measures and acupuncture first.
- If pain is too intense, I desire input from staff for relaxation, pushing techniques, and other ideas to help me avoid taking medication.
- I strongly prefer to avoid (but understand the possible necessity for) the following interventions: Epidural or narcotics for exhaustion or specific medical procedure such as vacuum extraction or cesarean surgery. Please explain the reasons for any suggested procedure.

*Cesarean surgery*
- Prefer regional anesthesia
- Please explain everything during surgery.
- Joe and Mary (doula) to be present.
- Prefer to have the screen lowered at the time of the birth.
- Prefer for immediate contact between my baby and Joe.
- If my baby must go to nursery, Joe goes with her; Mary stays with me.

## *Preferences for the Postpartum Period in the Hospital*

If giving birth in a hospital, your postpartum stay will likely last one to three days. Because the length of your stay is limited, carefully plan how you'll use the time. For example, will you want friends and relatives to visit, or will you prefer to rest and focus on your baby? Will you want help with breastfeeding or formula feeding, diapering, dressing, or bathing your baby? Before leaving the hospital, find out your options for follow-up help with feeding and baby care. See below for more information on creating a postpartum plan.

## A FINAL WORD ABOUT BIRTH PLANS

You'll need time for research and thought as you prepare your birth plan. Decisions you make in advance, when you're calm and able to concentrate, will help guide everyone when you need to devote all your energy to coping with labor and birth. When you've finished writing your birth plan, you'll have a fairly complete idea of what you can expect for your care during labor, birth, and the immediate postpartum period. By communicating your priorities and preferences for care both under normal circumstances and if complications arise, you can receive treatment that's modified with your wishes in mind.

# Your Postpartum Plan

A postpartum plan is quite different from a birth plan in that it's designed for you, your friends, and your family to ensure that the needs of you and your baby are met in the days or weeks after the birth. You don't need to create a formal document, as you did with your birth plan, but be sure to discuss your wishes with your partner and any friends or relatives who will be helping you after the birth.

These first weeks almost surely will be more challenging and stressful than you expected (but also more wondrous). You'll appreciate the help from family, friends, support groups, and professionals such as lactation consultants and doulas. Your postpartum plan will ensure that everyone knows and understands your needs during this time.

## DECISIONS TO MAKE FOR YOUR POSTPARTUM PERIOD

To help ease the transition into parenthood, identify your postpartum needs in advance and plan for how they'll be met. Here are some questions to get you thinking:

- Whom will you want to see after the birth? How will you restrict visitors if you're tired and frazzled and are trying to figure out breastfeeding?
- What resources are available to help you in the first weeks after the birth, such as classes, support groups, books, and DVDs? Visit our web site, http://www.PCNGuide.com, to download a form that helps you keep track of the resources you've found.
- Will your baby be breastfed or formula-fed? (See Chapter 18.) What help will you need with feeding?
- What help will you need with transportation, housework, meal preparation, shopping, and child care for older children?
- Who will help you? Your partner, relatives, friends, a postpartum doula, or a mother's helper? (See page 26.)
- If you're feeling overwhelmed or depressed, whom can you call? Make a list of family, friends, and counselors who can help if necessary. (See Chapter 16.)

- What equipment, supplies, and preparations will you need for your baby? (See page 160 for a list of useful baby items.)
- Will you use cloth or disposable diapers or both? Will you use a diaper service? (See page 374.)
- Will you work outside your home after the birth? If so, when will you start? Will you work part-time or full-time? Who will provide child care when you and your partner are at work? Can you and your partner share some or all child-care duties? (See page 28.)
- Will you continue to breastfeed while working? Is there a private, comfortable place at work where you can pump your breast milk? (See page 431.)
- How will your financial situation change after the birth? Plan and follow a budget, if necessary, to avoid excessive spending and ensure that you can meet expenses.

Develop your postpartum plan from the answers to these questions and from information you've gathered from friends and relatives with experience parenting a newborn.

## YOUR POSTPARTUM RESOURCE LIST

After the birth, you'll thank yourself many times over if you take the time now to gather the contact information of people who can help with postpartum care. Visit our web site to download a template that you can complete. Make several copies of this list for yourself and your partner. Post one on your refrigerator door, stash another in your purse, set a copy by your landline phone, and program the list into your cell phone. For help preparing your list, consult your caregiver, a postpartum doula, lactation consultant, or your childbirth or parent educator. You can also search the Internet for resources that may help.

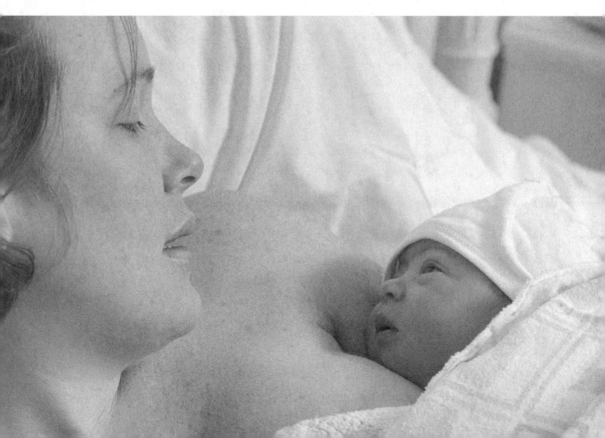

# EQUIPMENT AND CLOTHING FOR YOUR NEWBORN

If you've ever browsed through a baby boutique or big-box store, you may be overwhelmed by the amount of stuff that's advertised as necessary for proper baby care. However, the number of essentials you'll need is modest. Use the following guide to help you acquire the necessary newborn equipment and clothing before your baby's birth. Visit our web site, http://www.PCNGuide.com, to download a checklist of this guide.

### Bed
- A safe sleep space in your bed or your room
- Bassinet, co-sleeper, crib, or hammock bed
- 2–4 sets of bed linens for the crib or bassinet
- 3–6 lightweight blankets
- 1–2 blanket sleepers for warmth
- Special swaddling blanket (optional)
- 2–4 waterproof pads for your baby's sleep space, your lap, and diaper-changing areas

### Diapers
- Ask the retailer or diaper service how many diapers to purchase or order for the diaper system you've chosen. (See page 374.)
- 6–8 waterproof wraps or pants for use with cloth diapers
- Changing table (optional)
- 3–6 washcloths, or diaper wipes, to clean your baby when diapering
- Diaper pail (if using cloth diapers)
- Diaper rash ointment (Ask your caregiver what to use.)

### Bath
- 2–4 hooded towels or soft towels
- 6–8 baby washcloths
- Mild soap and shampoo
- Baby bathtub (optional)
- Cotton swabs for the umbilical cord

### Baby clothing (Some babies are born too big for newborn-size clothing.)
- 1–2 sweaters or jackets (depending on the season)
- 4–8 undershirts or "onesies"
- 3–6 gowns or stretch suits with feet
- 2 blanket sleepers (depending on the season)
- 1–3 pairs of booties or socks
- Hats: 1 knit hat for a newborn and 1 appropriate for the season (sun hat for summer, warm hat for winter)

### Travel
- Car seat
- Diaper bag

### Baby equipment (These are optional, but come in handy.)
- Thermometer that's safe and accurate for babies (see page 388)
- Dresser
- Baby carrier or sling
- Carriage or stroller
- Birth ball (inflatable exercise ball)
- Blunt-tipped nail scissors or baby nail clippers
- Massage oil
- Mobile
- Baby swing

# Key Points to Remember

- Preparing a birth plan will help you and your partner learn about your caregiver, birthplace, and safe care options for normal and complicated labor and birth. Begin preparing your birth plan a few months before your due date.
- By providing a birth plan, you better ensure that everyone can understand your priorities and preferences for care.
- A complete birth plan includes practical information about you; issues, fears, or concerns you may have; and your preferences for managing labor pain, normal labor and birth, unexpected events, postpartum care, and newborn care.
- Think about what assistance and support you'll need during the early weeks and months after the birth. Seek helpful resources for the postpartum period, and use them to prepare your postpartum plan.

# When and How Labor Begins

In the last month or so of your pregnancy, your baby begins gearing up for life outside your womb. She's grown strong and mature enough to handle physiological functions on her own, such as breathing, eating, and regulating her temperature. Sometime between the thirty-seventh and forty-second week of pregnancy, your baby signals to your body that she's ready to be born. At that point, labor begins. This chapter describes the events and changes that occur in you and your baby during the shift from late pregnancy to labor.

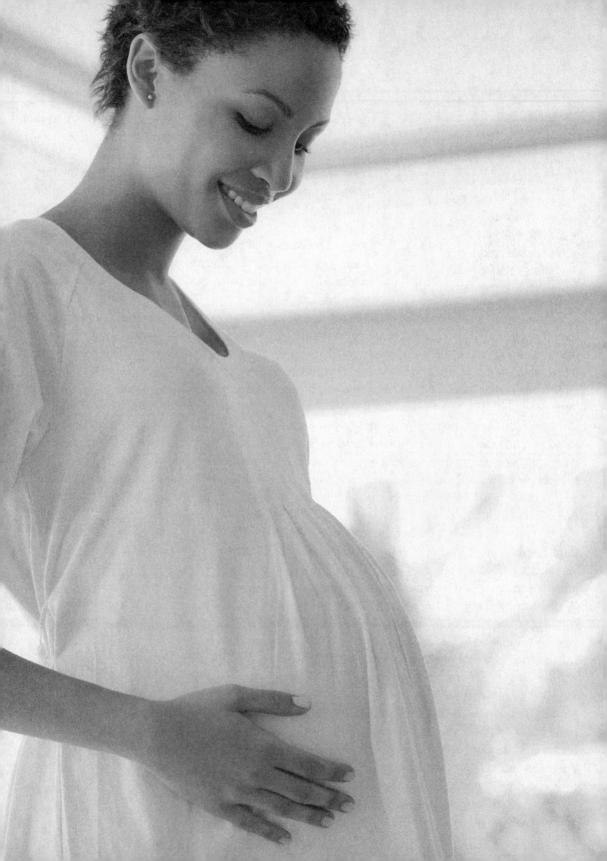

# The Last Weeks of Your Pregnancy

As you near the end of pregnancy, you may wish for it to be over. You may feel awkward, tired, fat, hot, and uncomfortable. You and your partner are probably eager to meet your baby and ready to enter the next stage of your lives. If your pregnancy passes your due date, try to remember that labor likely hasn't begun because your baby isn't ready to be born.

Most normal, healthy births occur after the thirty-seventh week of pregnancy but before the forty-second week. However, some preexisting conditions can override the physiological interaction among the baby, mother, and placenta, leading to births that aren't "on time." Examples of such conditions include illness or infection in the mother, heavy smoking or other drug use, extremely stressful life circumstances, as well as unknown factors. About 12 percent of births occur before the thirty-seventh week of pregnancy, and between 5 and 10 percent of births would occur after the forty-second week if labor weren't induced.[1] (See Chapter 10 for more information on the effects of labor induction, which bypasses the intricate hormonal processes of normal birth.) See Chapter 13 for further discussion on premature and post-mature births.

During the last weeks of pregnancy, your entire body and your baby undergo many changes to prepare for the birth. Your breasts produce more *colostrum* (first breast milk). Your uterus contracts more often and more strongly. You may have contractions when you exercise, sneeze, bump your belly, or for no apparent reason. You may swear that you're in labor only to have the contractions stop. Along with your changing hormones, these contractions are helping your body prepare for labor.

Your pelvic joints relax, allowing room for your baby to descend into your birth canal. You produce more cervical mucus, and your vaginal wall becomes more elastic. Even though you aren't yet in labor, you're making good progress.

Your baby is rapidly storing iron, enough to meet his needs for the next six months (along with the iron he'll consume from your breast milk). He becomes chubby and able to regulate his own temperature. His lungs mature, preparing him to breathe without difficulty after the birth.

As your placenta ages, the membrane between your baby's bloodstream and yours becomes more permeable, permitting large molecules such as *antibodies* to reach your baby. These protect him against diseases to which you're resistant or immune, and the protection lasts for months. If you breastfeed your baby, such protection will continue for as long as you nurse him.

When your baby is ready to survive outside your body, his body and yours initiate labor.

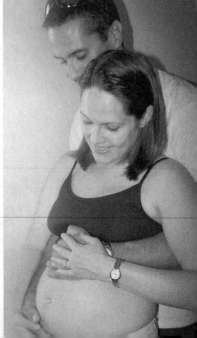

## Events of Late Pregnancy

During the last 6 to 8 weeks of pregnancy, numerous complex interrelated events take place among your baby, your body, and the placenta. A change in one of these three components triggers changes in the other two. This process typically leads to the birth of your mature, capable baby and prepares you to nourish and nurture her. Here's a breakdown of the events of late pregnancy.

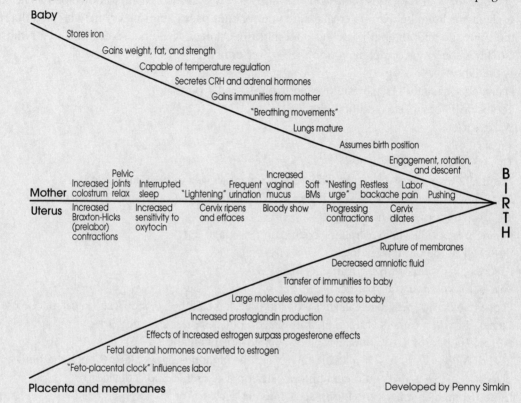

Developed by Penny Simkin

# Preparations for Your Baby's Birth

In the final months of pregnancy, there are many things you can do to prepare for your baby's birth. If you're planning to give birth in a hospital or birth center, use the following lists to help you get organized. If planning a home birth, many of these tasks are still relevant, but ask your midwife what additional preparations you should make in your home, such as what food and beverages to have available for everyone and what birth supplies to have on hand.

1. Prepare a birth plan and review it with your caregiver. (See Chapter 8.) When preparing your birth plan, consider consulting with your childbirth educator or doula, who can answer questions you may have. Make sure your birth plan reflects your priorities and preferences.

2. Tour your hospital, or backup hospital if you're planning to give birth at a birth center or at home. (See page 13.)

3. Preregister at the hospital. (Preregistration may be unnecessary for an out-of-hospital birth.) Sign admission forms, including a general consent form. During labor, you may need to sign additional consent

forms for specific procedures. Try to read these forms before you arrive at the hospital in labor, and ask for clarification of information that you don't understand or that makes you uncomfortable.

4. If you have other children, arrange for their care while you're in the hospital or birth center. If you have pets, also arrange for their care while you're away (and for the first few days after you bring your baby home).

5. Pack three bags for the hospital or birth center: one bag for labor, one for the postpartum stay, and one for your baby. Visit our web site, http://www.PCNGuide.com, to download a checklist of the items listed below. Also make sure your partner packs items he or she will need during the labor and after the birth, such as a toothbrush, changes of clothes, pajamas, and a swimsuit (so he or she can accompany you in the shower or bath).

## Items for labor

- Hairband, headband, or barrette (to keep your hair off your face)
- Toothbrush, toothpaste, and lip balm
- Warm socks
- Massage oil
- This book
- Two nightgowns or long T-shirts (if you don't want to wear a hospital gown)
- Hot water bottle (or fill a sock with uncooked rice, tie off the open end, and heat it in a microwave for three to five minutes)
- Rolling pin or other item to relieve back pain (See page 231.)
- Birth ball (if the birthplace doesn't have one)
- Favorite juice, tea, or frozen fruit juice bars
- Snacks for you and your partner
- Phone numbers of people to call after the birth (Check the birthplace's policies on cell phone use.)
- Camera or video camera (Check the birthplace's policies on recording births.)
- Personal comfort items (your own pillow, photos, blanket, and so on)
- iPod or MP3 player, CDs of relaxing music, and headphones or speakers (Check the birthplace's available audio equipment and policies on listening to audio devices.)
- Laptop computer (Check the birthplace's Internet access.)

## Items for your postpartum stay

- Nightgowns or pajamas that you can nurse in
- Robe and slippers
- Cosmetic and grooming aids
- Nursing bra
- Clothes for the ride home (You won't return to your prepregnant size immediately after giving birth, so make sure the clothes are a comfortable size.)
- Other personal items

## Items for your baby

- Cloth diapers and waterproof diaper cover, or disposable diapers
- Undershirt or "onesie"
- Nightgown or stretch suit
- Receiving blanket
- Warm blanket and cap (for the ride home)
- Car seat (properly installed in your vehicle before labor)

# Key Vocabulary for Late Pregnancy and Labor

During late pregnancy or early labor, your cervix changes so it can dilate, and your baby assumes his birth position (usually head down). To describe and assess these changes and developments, your caregiver may use a special vocabulary. The following sections define terms that you may hear during labor and birth.

## PARITY

*Parity* describes the condition of having given birth. *Primigravidas* are women who are pregnant for the first time, *nulliparas* have never given birth, and *primiparas* have given birth once (this term is often wrongly used to refer to nulliparas). *Multiparas* are women who have given birth more than once.

## PRESENTATION AND POSITION

Babies can situate themselves in the uterus in several ways, some more suitable for an easy birth than others. *Presentation* or *presenting part* describes the part of your baby that's lying over your cervix and will emerge from your body first. The most favorable and most common presentation (95 percent of births) is *vertex,* in which the top of your baby's head is down over your cervix. Other presentations are the frank breech (buttocks down), breech (one or two feet down), complete breech (buttocks and feet down), and shoulder, face, or brow presentations. (See Chapter 13 for further discussion of these rare presentations that may cause labor difficulties.)

   *Position* refers to the direction toward which the back of your baby's head (the *occiput*) or other presenting part lies. The possible positions are *anterior* (toward your front), *posterior* (toward your back), and *transverse* (toward your side).

Here are the most common descriptions of presentation and position:

**Occiput anterior (OA)**
The back of your baby's head is pointing toward your anterior (front).

*Left (or right) occiput anterior (LOA or ROA)*
The back of your baby's head is toward your left (or right) front.

**Occiput posterior (OP)**
The back of your baby's head is directly toward your back.

*Right (or left) occiput posterior (ROP or LOP)*
The back of your baby's head is toward your right (or left) back.

*Right (or left) occiput transverse (ROT or LOT)*
The back of your baby's head is toward your right (or left) side.

Your baby's position may change during labor among OA, OT, and OP, although by birth most babies are OA.

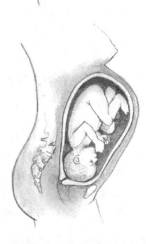

## Six Steps to Birth

The following six steps occur before a vaginal birth. The first three steps usually begin days or weeks before labor starts (prelabor), and the last three steps happen during labor.

1. Your cervix moves forward.
2. Your cervix ripens.
3. Your cervix effaces.
4. Your cervix dilates.
5. Your baby's head rotates and tucks (chin to chest).
6. Your baby's head molds, descends through your pelvis, and is born.

## STATION AND DESCENT

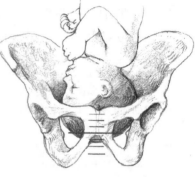

*Station* refers to the location of the top of your baby's head (or other presenting part) within your pelvis. It's measured in centimeters, in relation to the middle of your pelvis (the ischial spines), which is referred to as 0 station (see illustration). For example, if the top of your baby's head is at 0 station, it has descended to the middle of your pelvis. If her head is still "floating" above the level of your pubic bone, it may be as high as a -4 (minus four) station (4 centimeters above the middle of your pelvis). If her head is at a +1 (plus one) or +2 (plus two) station, it's 1 or 2 centimeters below the middle of your pelvis. When her head is at your vaginal opening and on its way out, it's at a +4 station.

The downward movement of your baby into your pelvis is called *descent*. During late pregnancy and birth, your baby moves from the highest station (-4) to the lowest station (+4) and is then born. For primigravidas, some descent—either gradual or sudden—usually takes place several weeks before the onset of labor. These women may begin labor at a -1 or 0 station. For multiparas, it's common for labor to begin with their babies still "floating." Most descent, however, takes place during pushing in late labor.

Other terms associated with your baby's descent before labor include *lightening* and "dropping." These terms refer to the decreased pressure in your chest and upper abdomen, and the increased pressure on your bladder. *Engagement* describes the condition in which the top of your baby's head (or other presenting part) is "engaged," or at 0 station, and fixed in your pelvis. It can be determined by palpating your abdomen or by a vaginal exam.

## CERVICAL CHANGES

Changing levels and interactions of hormones cause your cervix to change gradually, beginning before labor and ending just before your baby's birth. Your caregiver can assess these changes during a vaginal exam and evaluate your body's readiness for labor as well as the progress of your labor.

Because these cervical assessments are subjective, they may vary if more than one person examines you. You may become

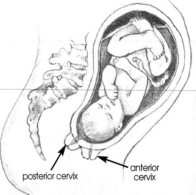

posterior cervix            anterior cervix

confused or discouraged if examined within a short time by two people whose assessments differ. If the same caregiver checks your cervix each time, you can rely on his or her assessment of your progress.

The following describe the changes your cervix undergoes during the labor process.

**Your cervix moves forward.**

Usually weeks before labor begins, your cervix is high and posterior (pointing toward your back); as labor approaches, your cervix gradually moves down to an anterior position (pointing toward your front). See illustration on page 168.

See illustration on page 168.

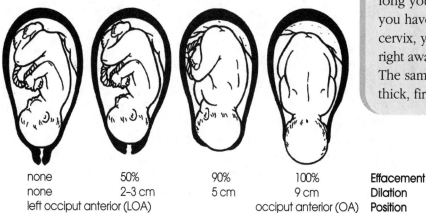

| | | | | Effacement |
|---|---|---|---|---|
| none | 50% | 90% | 100% | Effacement |
| none | 2–3 cm | 5 cm | 9 cm | Dilation |
| left occiput anterior (LOA) | | | occiput anterior (OA) | Position |

**Common Q & A**

Q: Will a vaginal exam tell me when I can expect labor to begin?

A: While a vaginal exam can provide information about the present state of your cervix, it can't predict when you'll go into labor or how long your labor will last. If you have a very ripe, effaced cervix, you may go into labor right away or in several weeks. The same is true if you have a thick, firm cervix.

**Your cervix *ripens* (softens).**

During pregnancy and prelabor, when your cervix is still firm, it doesn't change during Braxton-Hicks (or practice) contractions. However, once your cervix begins to ripen, other cervical changes begin. Your cervix may begin to ripen weeks before labor begins or just a few days before. This variation in the timing of ripening helps explain why some women's cervixes dilate in late pregnancy, while others don't even with strong, frequent contractions.

**Your cervix *effaces* (thins or shortens).**

The cervix of a primigravida usually effaces a lot before it dilates. The cervix of a multigravida typically effaces and dilates at the same time.

Effacement is measured either as a percentage or as a length in centimeters. Zero percent effacement means that your cervix is 3 to 4 centimeters long and hasn't begun to thin. Fifty percent effacement, or 2 centimeters, means that your cervix has thinned about halfway; 100 percent effacement, or "paper-thin," means that your cervix has thinned completely. Make sure you don't confuse the centimeters of effacement with centimeters of dilation!

**The cervix *dilates* (opens).**

Although your cervix usually dilates before labor begins (1 to 2 centimeters in primigravidas or up to 4 centimeters in multigravidas), most dilation occurs during labor. Dilation is measured in centimeters. When your cervix has opened the width of a fingertip, it's 1 centimeter dilated; when fully dilated, it's about 10 centimeters.

## Hormonal Interactions That Start Labor

If you've had a normal pregnancy, labor typically begins when your baby has grown enough to thrive outside your body and has needs that the placenta can't meet. At that time, a complex interplay of biochemical events signals to both your body and your baby that it's time to start labor. Here's a breakdown of the interactions that lead to your baby's birth.[2] (See also page 242.)

1.  In your baby's brain, the hypothalamus (the main control center of the autonomic nervous system) secretes corticotrophin-releasing hormone (CRH), which sets in motion a cascade of hormonal interactions.

2.  The CRH goes to the pituitary gland (which influences hormone secretion) in your baby's brain, stimulating the gland to secrete adrenocorticotropic hormone (ACTH), which makes his adrenal glands secrete large amounts of the steroid hormone androgen into his blood-stream and onto the placenta.

3.  In the placenta, androgen is converted into *estrogen*, which overrides the calming effects of the hormone *progesterone* on your uterus. Estrogen also causes your uterus, membranes, and placenta to produce *prostaglandins*, which may lead to cervical ripening and uterine contractions. It further causes changes to your uterine muscles, increasing the number of *oxytocin* receptors by 100 to 200 percent. This greater number of receptors makes your uterus more sensitive to oxytocin, which increases the frequency of your contractions.

4.  As your uterus contracts, it places pressure on your cervix and causes it to stretch. Nerve fibers carry impulses from your cervix up your spinal cord to your pituitary gland.

5.  The stimulation of your pituitary gland causes it to release more oxytocin, further increasing the frequency of your contractions.

6.  The process thus gains momentum, and your contractions intensify and speed up throughout labor.

# How to Distinguish between Prelabor and Early Labor

As you near the end of pregnancy, one of your biggest challenges is figuring out whether you're in labor or still in prelabor. For most women, the shift from prelabor contractions (Braxton-Hicks contractions that intermittently tighten your uterus) and labor contractions (ones that dilate your cervix) is subtle and gradual. For a few women, this shift is obvious if their membranes rupture (bag of waters breaks) with a gush before contractions begin, or if their contractions begin suddenly and intensely.

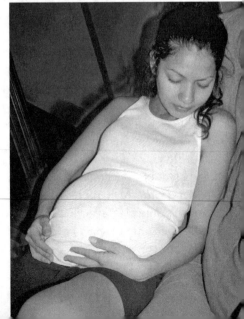

# Prelabor

During *prelabor*, contractions can last thirty to forty seconds each and occur ten to twenty minutes apart, or they may last up to two minutes each and occur five minutes apart. Some women barely notice prelabor contractions, while others need to use distraction, slow breathing, tension release, and other comfort techniques to get through them (see Chapter 11).

The distinguishing feature of prelabor contractions is that they're nonprogressing; that is, they change very little in length, frequency, and intensity over time. They may even subside for a while and resume later. See page 241 for more tips on distinguishing between prelabor and labor contractions. Prelabor may last for a few hours to a day; if it lasts longer than a day, it's considered a *prolonged prelabor*, which can be tiring and discouraging. (See page 245.)

As puzzling and frustrating as prelabor contractions may be, try to recognize that they're getting your cervix ready to dilate by moving it forward and helping it ripen and efface. While some women's cervixes undergo these changes without noticeable contractions, others (especially those of first-time mothers) need the help of contractions to change. Both situations are normal.

You may wonder why it matters whether you're in prelabor or labor. You have to deal with its contractions, whatever it's called! From a clinical viewpoint, the status of your labor determines when you can be admitted to the hospital or birth center. For a normal pregnancy, maternity care providers consider prelabor and early dilation no different than the events of late pregnancy. If you arrive at your birthplace with prelabor contractions and a cervix that hasn't yet dilated to 3 or 4 centimeters, you'll likely be sent home with instructions on when to return. For a home birth, your midwife probably won't stay with you if you're in prelabor, although his or her birth assistant may.

If you're not admitted to the hospital or birth center because you're still in prelabor, you may feel embarrassed, disappointed, or upset. To overcome these negative feelings, try to focus on helpful ways to get through prelabor. See page 243 for practical suggestions on restful, distracting, and pleasant activities to make both prelabor and early labor positive experiences.

## A Note to Fathers and Partners

The events of prelabor can be difficult to understand, making this time challenging for everyone. But prelabor can be a pleasant experience with support, guidance, and the right attitude. Join your pregnant partner in distracting activities and try to remain patient, cheerful, and attentive. If you become confused or frustrated, contact your doula or a friend who has been through labor. He or she can offer support, reassurance, and companionship.

## Signs of Labor

Recognizing the signs of labor is the best way to ensure that you don't mistake prelabor contractions for labor contractions. The signs of labor are divided into three categories: *possible signs, prelabor signs,* and *positive signs.* You might or might not experience all categories of signs.

Possible signs of labor occur in late pregnancy and may indicate that the hormonal changes described on page 170 are underway (but cervical changes aren't yet occurring). These signs occur intermittently for days or weeks, but they don't indicate labor.

Prelabor signs of labor indicate that your cervix is probably moving forward, ripening, or effacing. These signs may progress into positive labor signs the same day they begin, or they may simply alert you that labor will begin in a few days or weeks.

Positive signs of labor include contractions that become longer, stronger, and more frequent (*progressing contractions*), and the *rupture of membranes* in a gush of amniotic fluid (that is, your bag of waters bursts, not leaks). These are the *only* reliable signs that labor has begun and (with few exceptions) your cervix is dilating. Although most labors start with progressing contractions but without the rupture of membranes in a gush of fluid, about 6 percent of labors start with the latter sign. If this happens to you, you'll almost certainly begin having contractions within minutes or hours of the rupture.

*Caution:* If you're at least thirty-seven weeks pregnant, these are all normal healthy signs of labor. However, if you're less than thirty-seven weeks pregnant and have two or more possible signs along with six contractions in an hour (or eight contractions in two hours), whether or not the contractions are progressing, call your caregiver. You may be in preterm labor. Your caregiver may ask you to try resting, taking a bath, or drinking water to stop your contractions. If they don't stop, you'll probably be asked to go to the hospital for further assessment. (See page 249.)

## Possible Signs

### Restless back pain that comes and goes

This vague, nagging back pain is often accompanied by a feeling of uneasiness or restlessness. You're unable to be comfortable in any position for long. This pain differs from the postural back pain that you may feel after standing or sitting for a while. It may resemble the back pain you feel before a menstrual period and may occur off and on for days. If restless back pain is the only symptom you have, don't get too excited. By itself it doesn't indicate labor or even prelabor.

### Mild to moderate abdominal cramping

These cramps may be similar to menstrual cramps and may be accompanied by discomfort in your thighs. With time, they may progress into distinct contractions, or they may stop.

### Frequent, soft bowel movements

This sign may be accompanied by intestinal cramps or an upset stomach. It's probably due to increased levels of prostaglandins, which cause your lower digestive tract to clear itself in order to make room for your baby as she descends.

### Nesting urge

In this sudden burst of energy, you focus on getting your "nest" ready. Whether you scrub every floor in your home, shop extensively, tie up all loose ends at work, or spruce up your baby's room, you do it with a sense of urgency. Your behavior may seem reasonable to you at the time, but it may surprise others. In fact, you might not recognize it as a nesting urge until after the birth.

Think of the extra energy as a sign that you'll have strength to handle labor, but try to avoid doing exhausting activities.

## Prelabor Signs

### Nonprogressing contractions

These contractions occur regularly and may continue for hours without changing in intensity, frequency, or duration. They don't dilate your cervix, but probably prepare it for dilation. (See page 170 for more information on prelabor contractions.) Although nonprogressing contractions can be strong, long, and frequent, they're most likely to be mild and occur eight to twenty minutes apart. They may last for a short time or continue for hours before they disappear or begin to progress. Try to be patient and maintain normal activity—eat, drink, and alternate between resting and doing distracting activities.

**Bloody show**

Throughout pregnancy, your cervix contains thick mucus, which may be loosened and released when your cervix begins effacing and dilating. Sometimes this loosened mucus appears as a sticky plug. More often, the mucus becomes thin and liquid (*leukorrhea*). It may be tinged with blood from small blood vessels in your cervix that broke as your cervix thinned and opened. Bloody show can appear before any other labor sign or it might not appear until hours after contractions have begun. You continue to pass bloody show throughout labor.

You may wonder how much blood to expect. In general, if the bloody show is more mucus than blood, you're fine. However, if it's more blood than mucus or your vagina is dripping blood, you may have a larger broken blood vessel or a more serious problem. In that case, call your caregiver immediately.

In late pregnancy, you may pass brownish, bloody discharge within twenty-four hours after a vaginal exam or sexual intercourse, both of which can cause harmless cervical bleeding. It's easy to mistake this discharge for bloody show. If you're unsure, note the appearance of the blood. If it's pink or bright red and mixed with mucus, it's bloody show. After an exam or intercourse, it's usually brownish, like dried blood.

**Leaking of amniotic fluid**

Your membranes (bag of waters or amniotic sac) may begin to leak before labor. Leaking amniotic fluid before labor occurs in about 10 percent of pregnancies. (In more than half of those cases, it's a gush of fluid rather than a trickle—see page 172). Leaking may mean that you've developed a small hole in the bag high in your uterus and amniotic fluid is seeping out. Your underwear feels damp and you notice leaking when walking or changing position. Let your caregiver know about the leaking. He or she may want to confirm that it's amniotic fluid. (It may be urine or liquid mucus.) If your caregiver knows or suspects that you have Group B streptococcus (GBS—see page 131), he or she may want to give you antibiotics after your membranes have ruptured or begin to leak.

## Positive Signs

**Progressing contractions**

The purpose of progressing contractions is to dilate your cervix and push your baby down and out of your uterus. Unlike nonprogressing contractions, over time these become longer, stronger, and more frequent (or at least two of these three changes)—regardless of whether your prelabor contractions were twenty minutes apart and lasted thirty seconds each, or they were five minutes apart and lasted a minute each. The point is, these contractions become stronger and harder to manage than your earlier contractions.

In early labor, your contractions probably feel like abdominal tightening with some back pain. As labor advances, your contractions likely become painful. (See page 241 for further description of contractions.) If you've given birth before, you may have contractions that come and go for several hours until their pattern becomes continual and progressive. These intermittent contractions can make it difficult to determine whether your contractions are progressing. To help you decide, time your contractions and keep a written record. (See page 175.)

## Rupture of membranes with a gush of amniotic fluid

Also known as "when your bag of waters breaks," the rupture of membranes (ROM) doesn't occur in most pregnancies until the active phase of labor or later. However, some labors begin when ROM occurs with a gush of ½ to 1 cup of amniotic fluid. If ROM occurs this way, you may think you've wet yourself. You may even hear a popping sound before feeling the wetness. Contractions usually start within hours of ROM. If your membranes rupture before you have contractions, follow these guidelines:

1. Note the time and the color and odor of the fluid. Describe the amount of fluid (a trickle or a gush). Amniotic fluid is normally clear and practically odorless. A strong foul odor may mean infection. Brownish or greenish fluid is a sign that your baby has experienced stress. (See page 253.)

2. Notify your caregiver or call the hospital immediately. Your caregiver may recommend inducing your labor soon after ROM, if it occurs at term and especially if you tested positive for GBS (see page 131). See page 10 for the key questions to ask about induction. Also see page 277 for information on side effects of induction.

   Or your caregiver may wait to see if you go into labor spontaneously or if you can get labor to start. (For suggestions, see page 278). If ROM occurs before term, your caregiver may take steps to try to prevent labor.

3. After ROM, don't put anything into your vagina (such as tampons or fingers); doing so increases the risk of infection. Vaginal exams also increase the risk of infection, so try to limit the number of exams you have after ROM. It's fine to take a bath for comfort or pain relief after ROM. Research hasn't found that vaginal exposure to bath water causes infection.[3]

   If you've tested positive for GBS or you're at risk of the disease, you'll probably receive antibiotics to prevent an infection in your baby. (See page 131.)

   *Caution:* On rare occasions (fewer than 5 in 1,000 pregnancies), the baby's umbilical cord prolapses (slips through the mother's cervix into the vagina) when the membranes rupture with a gush. This event requires immediate medical intervention because the baby may press against the cord and cut off his oxygen supply. (See page 302 for further information on prolapsed cord.)

## Changes in your cervix confirmed by vaginal exam

Your caregiver or nurse will check you for changes in cervical position, ripening, effacement, or dilation (more than 4 centimeters typically indicates labor). After ROM, your caregiver should postpone this exam until there are clear, positive signs of active labor (see page 173), in order to reduce the chance of infection.

## Signs of Labor

### Possible Signs
- Restless back pain (See page 172.)
- Cramps
- Diarrhea
- Nesting urge (See page 172.)

### Prelabor Signs
- Nonprogressing contractions
- Bloody show (See page 173.)
- Leaking or trickle of amniotic fluid

### Positive Signs
- Progressing contractions*
- Cervix dilated more than 4 centimeters
- Rupture of membranes in a gush of amniotic fluid

* See the Early Labor Record on page 175 for instructions on determining whether your contractions are progressing.
*Note:* Visit our web site, http://www.PCNGuide.com, to print out complete descriptions of these symptoms.

## Sample of an Early Labor Record

Contractions on _____(date)

| Starting Time | Duration (in seconds) | Interval or Frequency (minutes since beginning of last contraction) | Comments |
|---|---|---|---|
| 1:54:10 AM | 40 seconds | — | Bloody show noted at 6 PM. |
| 2:03:00 AM | 45 seconds | 9 minutes | Can't sleep |
| 2:10:15 AM | 45 seconds | 7 minutes | Loose BM, back pain |
| 2:17:30 AM | 50 seconds | 7 minutes | Stronger! |

# Early Labor Record

To help you decide whether you're in labor, keep an Early Labor Record. See above for a sample, and visit our web site http://www.PCNGuide.com to download a template. You can also search the Internet to find online programs for recording your contractions, such as http://contractionmaster.com/.

Keeping track of your contractions also helps you decide when to call your caregiver or when to go to the hospital or birth center. (See page 244 to learn about the 4-1-1 or 5-1-1 rule.) Many women begin timing contractions when they can't walk or talk through one or when they need to use slow or light breathing (see pages 224 and 225).

Either you or your partner can time your contractions. If you're timing them manually, you need a watch or clock with a second hand. When a contraction begins, write down the time (hour, minutes, seconds) in the appropriate space. When the contraction ends, write down how long it lasted in seconds (duration). Note the length of time from the beginning of one contraction to the beginning of the next (interval or frequency). This information tells you how often your contractions are occurring. You can also include comments about the intensity of contractions, your appetite and the foods you've eaten, breathing rhythms used, bloody show, status of your membranes (have they ruptured?), and so on.

Time five to six contractions in a row. Then stop timing them until their pattern seems to have changed (this may take many hours or just a few), at which time you can resume timing. If your contractions are progressing, you're probably in labor. If they're not progressing, you're probably still in prelabor.

## *Key Points to Remember*

- Your baby and your body play key roles in the complex interplay of factors that trigger labor.
- It can be difficult to determine whether you're in labor. Recognizing the signs helps you figure out if you're in labor or still in prelabor.
- The most reliable signs of labor to look for are progressing contractions (ones that become longer, stronger, and more frequent over time) and the rupture of your membranes in a gush of amniotic fluid. To confirm that you're in labor, your caregiver may also check for cervical dilation.

# CHAPTER 10

# Labor Pain and Options for Pain Relief

When new mothers were asked to describe the sensations of childbirth, some used words that depicted a positive experience, such as *exhilarating, empowering,* and even *orgasmic*; others used words that portrayed a negative experience, such as *painful, exhausting,* and *traumatic*. For still other women, childbirth wasn't a particularly transformative event, and they used words such as *tedious, uncomfortable*, and *manageable* to describe the experience.

The preparations you make during pregnancy can influence the kind of birth experience you'll have. You're more likely to have a positive birth experience if you learn about your pain relief options, practice a variety of coping techniques,* and arrange for continuous labor support from people who respect your preferences for pain relief. This chapter describes labor pain and provides an overview of your options for coping with it so you can have the best possible birth experience.

* See Chapter 11 to learn specific skills you can practice in pregnancy and use in labor.

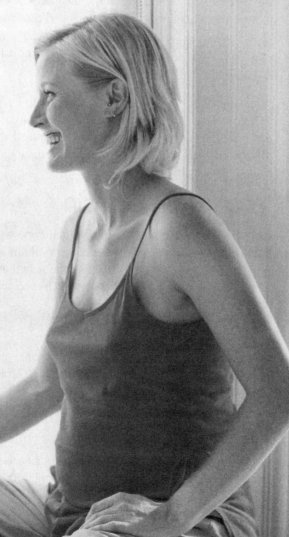

# Why Labor Is Painful

In almost all pregnancies, labor begins with mild contractions that come and go. As labor progresses, the contractions occur more frequently and their intensity increases. Although a few women have reported experiencing little to no pain during labor, the process is painful for most women. The following physical changes contribute to labor pain:

- Reduced oxygen supply to the uterine muscle during contractions, which creates a buildup of waste products, such as lactic acid, that in turn causes pain (The pain disappears as soon as the contraction stops.)
- Stretching of the cervix as it dilates
- Pressure of the baby on nerves in and near the cervix and vagina
- Tension and stretching of the ligaments of the uterus and pelvic joints during contractions and the baby's descent
- Pressure of the baby on the urethra, bladder, and rectum
- Stretching of the pelvic floor muscles and vaginal tissues during the birth

Although these changes can hurt, the pain isn't a sign of harm. Instead, it's an expected side effect of the normal labor process that lets women efficiently and effectively push their babies out into the world. For this reason, labor pain is often called "pain with a purpose."[1]

# Your Perception of Pain

Simply understanding the physical reasons for labor pain helps many women cope with it. They're able to acknowledge that labor pain is normal and temporary, which allows them to work with their bodies and prevent the pain from overwhelming them. By changing the way they think about the pain, these women alter their perception of it and reduce its severity. The following sections describe two theories about other factors that influence pain perception.

## THE GATE CONTROL THEORY OF PAIN

The Gate Control Theory of Pain helps explain why people feel more pain in some cases and less pain in others, and why some people feel more or less pain than others do. You've probably had some of the following experiences with pain:

- A headache that goes away when you're watching an exciting movie, but returns when the movie ends
- A stubbed toe that hurts less when you dance around
- A bruise, acquired while playing a sport, that goes unnoticed until the game is over
- The pain of physical exertion that's eased when you focus on silently creating a rhythm (counting, chanting, or singing a song in your head)
- The pain from dental work that's eased when listening to music through headphones

Although the pain stimulus never goes away in any of these examples, your awareness of it decreases when your brain receives other stimuli that are non-painful or pleasant (*pain modifiers*). This theory states that the balance between painful and non-painful stimuli that reach your consciousness determines your perception of pain and its severity. This explains why distractions help relieve pain. Your brain is so busy processing the non-painful stimuli that it can't pay as much attention to painful sensations.

You can make pain more manageable during labor by increasing pleasant stimuli (such as massage, music, cold packs, a heating pad, or other distractions) and focusing on them.

## THE NEUROMATRIX THEORY OF PAIN

The Neuromatrix Theory of Pain is an expansion of the Gate Control Theory of Pain and takes into account all possible factors that can influence how pain is felt and interpreted.[2] It has been applied to help explain why women differ in their reactions to labor pain, and why some women find comfort measures more helpful to relieve pain than other women do. The theory acknowledges that the painful and non-painful stimuli a woman receives in labor aren't the only factors that affect her perception of the pain. Past experiences of pain or trauma are also factors, as are preexisting factors such as chronic pain or painful medical conditions, anxiety, personality or temperament, physiological factors such as the central nervous system's and endocrine system's reactions to stress, and cultural or familial attitudes toward pain. Some of these factors are genetically determined; others are formed earlier in life.

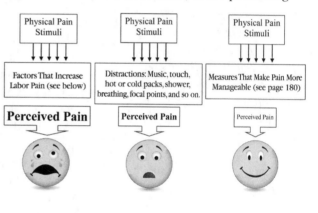

## *Factors That Increase Labor Pain*

**Physical factors**
- Hunger or thirst
- Fatigue
- Muscle tension
- Full bladder
- Discomfort from staying in the same position for too long

**Emotional or mental factors**
- Fear, anxiety, loneliness, or feeling watched or judged (All of these emotions can cause the release of excessive stress hormones and make labor longer or more painful than usual.)
- Lack of confidence and preparation
- Ignorance or misinformation about labor and birth
- Unsupportive staff or relatives
- Feeling powerless to make decisions, or feeling that your decisions aren't being respected

**Variations during labor**
- Frequent long contractions, or coupling contractions (occur in pairs with little break between the first and second contractions)
- Baby that's malpositioned (See page 285.)
- Prolonged, tiring labor; exhaustion
- Rapid intense labor, with little break between contractions
- Expectations for labor and birth that don't match the actual experience
- Hospital policies, procedures, or interventions that limit mobility or ability to use coping techniques

## Different Views on Labor Pain

When asked to describe the pain experienced in labor, new mothers had many different responses. Here are a few examples:

*I'd first feel cramping in my back, then it'd move around to my front and my whole belly would tighten. Later in labor, I could feel the cramping even in my thighs.*

*The pain is hard to explain. The contractions were just really intense. My body demanded my complete attention, like it does when I sneeze, orgasm, or vomit. The contractions were all my body would let me think about right then.*

*The best way to describe labor pain is that it's like the kind of aching pain you get when you do something that requires a lot of effort such as doing a chin-up or holding an advanced yoga pose for a long time. Your muscles burn as they get tired. That's what my uterus felt like.*

### Measures That Make Labor Pain More Manageable

To minimize the factors that increase labor pain, be aware of them in advance, make plans to manage them, and ensure that your support people are aware of them and work to minimize their impact on you. The following are examples of ways to counteract the pain-increasing factors listed on page 179:

- Eat and drink enough to stave off hunger and thirst.
- Dim the lights and arrange for minimal interruptions to increase your sense of privacy.
- If past trauma has made you fearful, get counseling before the birth to help you learn skills to manage the fear. Visit our web site, http://www.PCNGuide.com, to download a work sheet to help with this process.

Throughout your life, you've learned ways to make pain and anxiety more manageable. To help you prepare for coping with labor pain, ask yourself these questions and brainstorm as many answers as you can.

- What comforts you when you're sick?
- When you were a child, what did your parents do when you were sick that made you feel better? (Or what do you wish they had done?)
- What do you do during heavy physical exertion to help you keep going?
- What soothes the pain of a headache or sore muscles?
- What helps you feel safe in an unfamiliar situation?
- What calms you when you're stressed or scared?
- What kind of support from others best helps you? Do you want a shoulder to cry on? Someone to cheer you on? Empathy and gentle guidance? Reassurance and a calm, quiet presence? Distracting chatter and entertaining activities? Your answers to these questions will give you clues about what you'll find most helpful in labor. Visit our web site to download a work sheet to help track your observations.

A number of other comfort measures are also particularly helpful in labor, such as massage, relaxation techniques, breathing techniques, positions and movement, and pain medications. See Chapter 11 for more information on non-medicated comfort measures.

## PAIN VERSUS SUFFERING IN LABOR

While pain is a natural part of the labor process, suffering certainly isn't. *Pain* is a mildly to severely unpleasant physical sensation that might or might not be associated with physical damage. *Suffering* is a debilitating emotional state that might be associated with pain or with another cause such as grief, humiliation, or defeat.

You can have pain without suffering. For example, during a strenuous workout, you may experience the pain that accompanies exertion. You know why your body hurts, but you also associate the pain with improved physical conditioning, which makes the pain manageable. In the same way, you may experience intense pain during labor but not feel as though you're suffering, because you associate the pain with normal labor progress.

Despite the fact that pain in labor doesn't necessarily lead to suffering, some women nonetheless do suffer. Suffering includes any of the following experiences:

- A perceived threat to your body or psyche
- Helplessness and loss of control; distress
- The inability to cope with a distressing situation
- Fear of dying or the death of the baby[3]

The Neuromatrix Theory of Pain (see page 179) helps explains why some women suffer in labor while others don't, even though all experience pain. If you don't receive enough stimuli that help reduce your perception of pain (such as massage, movement, baths, and encouraging words) or if you have too many factors that increase your perception of pain (such as fear, loneliness, ignorance of what's happening, immobility, unkind or insensitive treatment, and anxiety or depression), you're more likely to be overwhelmed by the pain and feel as though you're suffering.

## *Rating Your Intensity of Pain and Your Ability to Cope*

In many hospitals, the staff use a very helpful tool called a pain intensity scale to assess how much pain a patient is experiencing during a medical procedure or postoperative recovery. By rating the intensity of pain, the patient can alert staff of potential problems that are then treated with pain medications. During labor, however, pain is a normal and expected part of the process, and women have a range of preferences for how they want to manage the pain, which don't always include pain medications.

**Pain Intensity Scale**

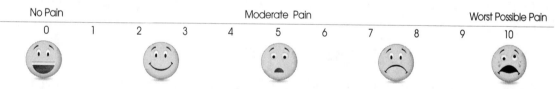

Another way to assess labor pain is by using a pain coping scale. This scale focuses not on how much pain a patient is experiencing, but rather on how well she's coping with the pain. If you're asked to rate your pain on the pain intensity scale, do so, but then also rate how well you're coping. Let the staff know whether you find the pain manageable or overwhelming.

**Pain Coping Scale**

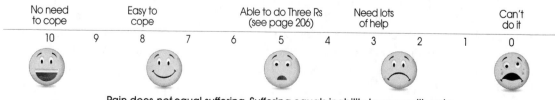

Pain does *not* equal suffering. Suffering equals inability to cope with pain.

## CONTROL IN LABOR

For many pregnant women, the possibility of losing control of themselves during labor is the most upsetting part of childbirth. They worry that the pain will be so intense, they'll do or say things they'll regret later. They've seen movies or heard stories in which a laboring woman panics, screams, or says hurtful things to those around her. To avoid becoming "that woman," some expectant mothers plan to dull labor pain with anesthesia to prevent themselves from behaving in a way that's socially unacceptable.

Normal behavior in labor, however, isn't the same as normal behavior in everyday life. Childbirth is an emotionally transformative and physically demanding experience that compels your body to work hard and requires your complete attention to seeking comfort, maintaining the Three Rs (see page 206), and expressing yourself freely. As long as you're coping well in labor, the idea of whether your behavior is socially acceptable shouldn't be a concern to you or to those attending to you.

### Releasing Control versus Losing Control

Although you can't consciously control your contractions any more than you can control digestion, you can control how you respond to them. For example, during pregnancy you may prepare for labor by practicing a certain breathing technique and making sure you'll have access to a bathtub. When labor begins, however, you may find yourself breathing in a different, unplanned rhythm and needing to walk rather than soak in the tub.

Instead of forcing yourself to follow your plans, you *choose* to give them up—that is, you release control and allow yourself to discover new ways of coping that help you work in harmony with the labor process. Releasing control is a matter of responding to your labor in the moment, as it unfolds.

Conversely, losing control in labor comes from feeling overwhelmed and helpless when labor doesn't go as expected, or from feeling that you're being excluded from the decision-making process. To help avoid feeling discounted, passive, or powerless in your care, learn about your options for childbirth well before labor begins (see Chapter 2), ask your caregiver the key questions on page 10 for any interventions you're considering, and make sure your decisions are reflected in your birth plan (see Chapter 8).

# Options for Pain Relief

While some women want a drug-free birth, others can't imagine giving birth without pain medications. Most women's opinions fall in between these two extremes: They want to minimize the amount of strong pain medications they receive during labor, yet they don't want the pain to overwhelm them. The information in this section will help you form your own opinions on pain-relief options.

To effectively manage labor pain, it's essential to have a "toolbox" of coping options. During pregnancy, you can read books on childbirth and take childbirth preparation classes to help you stock your toolbox with options such as the following:

- Coping skills you've used throughout your life to comfort yourself when you're sick, tired, worried, in pain, or physically exerting yourself (See page 180.)
- Self-help skills that you can practice during pregnancy to lessen labor pain or help you cope with it, such as breathing techniques, relaxation techniques, and visualization and attention-focusing (see Chapter 11) as well as positions that enhance comfort and labor progress (See pages 221–223.)

- Comfort items that you can use at the birthplace, such as your own pillow or clothes, snacks and beverages, heating pads and cold packs, birth ball, and shower or bathtub (See page 212.)
- Hands-on support from your partner or doula, such as massage, gentle stroking, and acupressure (See pages 213 and 214.)
- Changes to the environment to make it more comfortable, such as dimming the lights, playing music, using pleasing scents or aromatherapy, and asking for minimal disruptions
- Pain medications, including intravenous (IV) narcotics (see page 194) and epidural or spinal analgesia (see page 196).

Before labor, you may think you know which coping techniques will work best for you. During labor, however, you may discover that those options don't work as well as expected. This is why it's important to learn a variety of coping techniques: The technique you never imagined you'd use may be the one that helps you the most!

## AVAILABILITY OF PAIN-RELIEF OPTIONS

Your options for pain relief depend on where you plan to give birth. If you'll give birth at home or in a freestanding (unaffiliated with a hospital) birth center, you can use most non-drug coping techniques, but you won't have access to pain medications such as epidural analgesia. If you'll give birth in a hospital, medications will be available. Hospital policies, care practices, and available equipment might or might not support various comfort techniques such as eating in labor, mobility, baths and showers, birth balls, acupuncture, and aromatherapy.

To learn what pain-relief options are available at your birthplace, ask the questions on page 10 during your prenatal care appointments, hospital tour, and childbirth preparation classes. If you're considering using pain medications, ask your caregiver which ones are typically available, which can be given by your caregiver or nurse, and which require an anesthesiologist. Also ask about the availability of the anesthesiologist. Some hospitals have anesthesiologists on call at all times; others don't. Lastly, make sure to discuss the risks and benefits of pain medications with your caregiver (see page 193) so you can better make an informed decision about using them.

## EFFECTIVENESS OF VARIOUS PAIN-RELIEF OPTIONS[4]

The following table summarizes the effectiveness of various pain-relief options. The ratings are based on reports given by women who were surveyed in the first year after giving birth.

| | Percent Who Used the Option | Percent Who Said the Option Was Very Helpful | Percent Who Said the Option Was Somewhat Helpful |
|---|---|---|---|
| Epidural or spinal analgesia | 76% | 81% | 10% |
| Immersion in bathtub or pool | 6% | 48% | 43% |
| Hands-on techniques (such as massage) | 20% | 40% | 51% |
| IV narcotics | 22% | 40% | 35% |
| Birth ball | 7% | 34% | 33% |
| Shower | 4% | 33% | 45% |
| Application of heat or cold | 6% | 31% | 50% |
| Mental strategies (such as relaxation) | 25% | 28% | 49% |
| Position changes | 42% | 23% | 54% |
| Changes to environment (such as dimming lights) | 4% | 21% | 57% |
| Breathing techniques | 49% | 21% | 56% |

This table shows that the majority of women received epidural or spinal analgesia to help cope with labor pain, and most found the medications to be very helpful. However, this option wasn't the only one that effectively relieved or reduced labor pain. Of the other options included in the survey, all proved somewhat to very helpful for most of the women who used them. For example, the total percentage of women who found pain relief from immersion in a bathtub or from hands-on techniques (such as massage) equaled the total percentage of women who found pain relief from epidural or spinal analgesia (91 percent).

If non-drug measures were found to help relieve pain, why didn't more women use them? For example, less than 10 percent tried making changes to their environment or used the tub, shower, birth ball, or applications of heat and cold. The overall effectiveness of these pain relief options was rated between 67 to 91 percent. The reason these measures weren't used as often is probably because most of the women surveyed either didn't know about them or hadn't learned how to use them—which is unfortunate, given their safety and effectiveness for pain relief.

Although pain medications—especially epidural analgesia—can effectively minimize or eliminate labor pain, they're also expensive and carry risks and disadvantages that may complicate labor and birth. See pages 193–197 to learn about the potential tradeoffs, side effects, and risks of pain medications.

Conversely, non-drug methods for pain relief are free (or inexpensive) and easy to use, have few side effects, can be easily discontinued or replaced by other measures, and allow you to work with your body and take an active role in childbirth. See the chart below for a more complete comparison between a non-medicated labor and a medicated one.

As you think about pain relief for your labor, consider trying various non-drug methods *first*, to see if they can help you manage the pain effectively. See Chapter 11 for information on comfort techniques. Remember that you can increase overall effectiveness of these methods by using several at any one time and shifting to others whenever you desire. If you find that these methods aren't helping you cope as labor progresses, you can always request pain medications at that time.

Even if you're planning to receive an epidural or use pain medications in labor, it's still wise to learn the comfort techniques in Chapter 11, because you'll need ways to cope with contractions before heading to the hospital or while waiting to receive an epidural or pain medications at the hospital, or if the drugs turn out to be ineffective for you. Some comfort techniques—such as relaxation, breathing patterns, massage, and some movements—are more effective if you practice and adapt them well before labor begins.

## Non-medicated Labor versus Medicated Labor

The following chart compares a labor that's managed by using non-drug coping techniques with one that's managed with medications. This comparison helps you see how your labor may differ based on the choices you make.

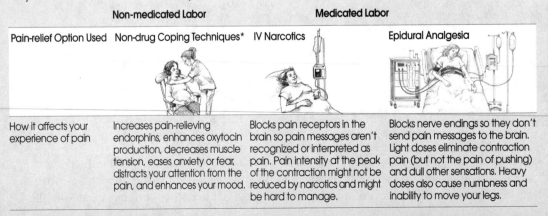

| | Non-medicated Labor | Medicated Labor | |
|---|---|---|---|
| Pain-relief Option Used | Non-drug Coping Techniques* | IV Narcotics | Epidural Analgesia |
| How it affects your experience of pain | Increases pain-relieving endorphins, enhances oxytocin production, decreases muscle tension, eases anxiety or fear, distracts your attention from the pain, and enhances your mood. | Blocks pain receptors in the brain so pain messages aren't recognized or interpreted as pain. Pain intensity at the peak of the contraction might not be reduced by narcotics and might be hard to manage. | Blocks nerve endings so they don't send pain messages to the brain. Light doses eliminate contraction pain (but not the pain of pushing) and dull other sensations. Heavy doses also cause numbness and inability to move your legs. |

| Pain-relief Option Used | Non-medicated Labor | Medicated Labor | |
| --- | --- | --- | --- |
| | Non-drug Coping Techniques* | IV Narcotics | Epidural Analgesia |
| Feedback from women who used it | "It was really challenging to handle the contractions. I finally discovered that if I got on my hands and knees and rocked and roared, I could do it. It was as though I'd found my inner tiger!" | "I felt really fuzzy-headed and slept between contractions. During a contraction, I'd wake up, cry out, and rock back and forth while my husband rubbed my back. Then I'd crash again." | "After I got the epidural, it was great. No more pain! But then it seemed as though labor took forever, and we were sitting around watching TV—it wasn't quite what I thought birth would be." |
| How it affects your mental state | You're fully focused on coping with the contractions and are less aware of surroundings. | You're relaxed, drowsy, foggy, or disoriented. You may hallucinate. | You return to your normal, everyday mental state. You may be chatty or may sleep through much of labor, if tired. |
| How it affects your mobility | You're fully mobile to find comfort: You can walk, rock, sway, sit, and so on. You may need to keep moving in order to cope with pain. | Mobility may be limited by policy, by equipment, or if you're unsafe standing because you're dizzy or groggy. | You're rarely allowed out of bed. Movement in bed is limited by equipment and lack of sensation. You may need assistance to move at all. |
| What you'll need from your support people | You'll need their continuous presence; active, hands-on assistance with massage, movement, and positions; encouraging words; and more. | You'll need some assistance with movement and mental reorientation (if you're foggy) and help coping at the peak of contractions. | You'll need companionship to help pass the time, manage anxieties, identify contractions, and guide pushing. |
| Equipment and precautions required | None (However, you may choose to use the bathtub, shower, birth ball, rocking chair, cold packs, or heating pads. In addition, you'll have periodic monitoring of your baby, contractions, blood pressure, and vital signs.) | Intravenous (IV) fluids, electronic fetal monitors (EFM) to continuously check your baby's heart rate; equipment to frequently monitor your blood pressure, respiration, and vital signs; oxygen supply and mask. | Epidural catheter and pump; IV fluids; EFM to continuously monitor your baby's heart rate; equipment to frequently monitor your blood pressure, respiration, and vital signs; oxygen supply and mask; pulse oximeter; bladder catheter. |
| Impact on labor progress | Usually promotes labor progress. | May slow normal labor.** | Likely to slow normal labor progress (may require Pitocin).** |
| Timing | Can be used at any time during labor and birth. | Best used in active labor. Effects last 45 to 90 minutes. Can be repeated. Not used if birth is expected to occur within 2 hours. | Can be used at any time except if birth is anticipated within 30 to 60 minutes. Once started, the medications usually stay in effect until after your baby is born. |
| Availability | Anytime, anyplace | All hospitals, anytime | Some hospitals, anytime; other hospitals, limited hours and an anesthesiologist must be called in at night. Not available in 3 percent of U.S. hospitals.[5] |
| Possible risks to you | None (But you'll still have labor pain.) | Some (See page 195.) | Some (See page 197.) |
| Possible risks to your baby | None | Some (See page 195.) | Some (See page 197.) |
| Cost | Free or inexpensive | Moderate | Expensive |
| Best option for you if… | You're committed to a non-medicated labor or want to delay use of medication, have a supportive staff, have made necessary preparations, and have recruited a support team. | You want only an hour or two of moderate pain relief, or feel that you're coping well at the peak of contractions but want to feel as though you have a longer rest between contractions. | You want to experience the least amount of pain, and are willing to have more medical interventions to minimize the adverse side effects of the epidural and to maintain labor progress; or you require painful interventions for safety or progress. |

* It's assumed that you'll use a variety of techniques from among those listed on pages 182–183 and described in Chapter 11.
** Deep-seated fear, stress, and pain-related anxiety can slow labor. If you experience a prolonged labor due to these causes, pain medications may speed up progress by lowering stress hormones.

## Two Views on Managing Labor Pain

I wanted to be able to use pain medications. But Ben was worried about the side effects. We talked with our caregiver about how to minimize the possible side effects and risks, and created a plan that we were both comfortable with.
*—Ann*

Ashley really wanted to have a "natural" labor. But I knew it'd be hard for me to see her in pain. I worried that I'd talk her into getting drugs. Luckily, we have a friend who had given birth without pain medications. She came with us to the hospital and helped us both cope with natural labor.
*—Nick*

# Determining Your Preferences for Pain Relief

The following are factors that help determine whether you'll use or avoid pain medications in labor.

**Your preference for pain medications**

Do you prefer to give birth without drugs, or do you prefer to use medications? How strongly do you feel about this preference? Your views may be influenced by past experiences with pain, your expectations about how challenging labor will be, your confidence in your ability to cope with pain, and whether you want to rely on your own resources or prefer to turn over management of your labor to others. (See the Pain Medication Preference Scale on page 187 to help clarify your preferences.)

**Preparation**

You're better able to cope with labor pain if you have complete information on all available options for pain relief, and have had opportunities to learn, practice, and adapt non-medicated comfort measures. Without such preparation, you're likely to need pain medications.

**Support**

You're more likely to avoid, postpone, or minimize your use of pain medications if you have the following:

- A partner or doula (see page 190) who encourages you and helps with self-help comfort measures
- Support staff who are skilled in comfort measures
- A caregiver who's patient and encouraging

**Luck**

The nature of labor affects the use of medications. The more uncomplicated your labor is, the better your chances are for a non-medicated birth. If your labor is prolonged, complicated, or includes the use of potentially painful interventions (such as Pitocin, forceps delivery, vacuum extraction, or cesarean section), you're likely to need medications.

## DEFINING YOUR PREFERENCES WITH THE PAIN MEDICATION PREFERENCE SCALE (PMPS)

Even though it's impossible to know how painful labor will be for you, the PMPS lets you determine how strongly you feel about medications and under what circumstances you'll use them. Whatever your preferences, address them in your birth plan (see Chapter 8) and remind your caregiver and hospital staff of them during labor.

### Using the PMPS with Your Labor Support Partner

During pregnancy, review the PMPS with your partner to help discover whether you have different preferences for pain medications. First, read the statements under "Your Preference" and find the one that best describes how you feel. Keep your selection to yourself. Next, have your partner read these statements and mentally choose the one that's closest to what he or she wishes you'd choose. Then, reveal your selections to each other and discuss them to clarify how you'll work together to achieve your goal. Also discuss the tips in the third column to plan how your partner can help you cope with labor and support your preferences for pain relief. If your partner is uncertain about his or her ability to support you, consider having an additional support person at your labor.

## Pain Medication Preference Scale (PMPS)

| Rating | Your Preference | How Your Partner, Doula, and Others Can Help You |
|---|---|---|
| +10 | I don't want to feel any pain. I prefer to be numb and to get anesthesia before labor even begins (typically not possible). | • Discuss your wishes and fears with you.<br>• Explain that you'll have some pain, even with anesthesia, and plan how you can cope.<br>• Promise to help you get medications as soon as possible. |
| +9 | I want as much medication as I can have. I fear labor pain and don't want to experience any pain and stress. | *Same as for +10 rating, plus:*<br>• Help you write a birth plan that expresses your fears and preferences.<br>• Review circumstances when an epidural may be delayed and how to cope while waiting.<br>• Ensure that someone will always be there to help you. |
| +7 | I want pain medications as early in labor as my caregiver will allow, and definitely before labor becomes painful. | *Same as for +9 rating, plus:*<br>• Help you learn the policies on timing of doses.<br>• Help you use relaxation techniques and comfort measures to cope in early labor, and while waiting for the anesthesiologist. |
| +5 | I want epidural analgesia in active labor (cervix dilated 4 to 5 centimeters). I'll try to cope until then, perhaps with narcotic medications. | *Same as for +7 rating, plus:*<br>• Help you with relaxation techniques and comfort measures in early labor.<br>• Suggest medications when you're in active labor. |
| +3 | I want to use some pain medications, but I also plan to use self-help comfort measures for as much of labor as I can. | *Same as for +5 rating, plus:*<br>• Help you with self-help measures.<br>• Help you get medications if you decide you want them. |
| 0 | I have no opinion on pain medications or preference for or against them (a rare attitude among pregnant women, lthough not rare among partners). | • Help you become informed about labor pain, comfort measures, and medications. |
| -3 | I'd like to avoid pain medications if I can. If I find labor too painful, I'd like to use as little medication as possible, but won't feel guilty for taking it. | • Emphasize coping techniques.<br>• Avoid suggesting pain medications.<br>• Avoid trying to talk you out of medications if you request them.<br>• Suggest half doses of narcotics or a light epidural. |
| -5 | I really don't want to use pain medications so I can avoid their side effects on my baby, my labor, and myself. I'll accept them only if labor is complicated or long. | *Same as for -3 rating, plus:*<br>• Prepare to play a very active role in your labor support.<br>• Practice comfort measures with you.<br>• Avoid suggesting drugs, even if you appear to be having trouble coping. Suggest other non-drug options instead.<br>• Be aware of your code word (see page 189), which alerts your partner that you want him or her to stop suggesting other options.<br>• Help you accept pain medications if you're exhausted, can't keep a rhythm during contractions (see page 206), or if none of the comfort measures help. |
| -7 | I strongly desire a non-medicated childbirth because of its benefits to my baby and my labor, and the gratification of meeting the personal challenge. I'll be disappointed if I use drugs. | *Same as for -5 rating, plus:*<br>• Help you enlist the support of your caregiver and request a nurse who will help with natural birth.<br>• Plan and rehearse ways to get through discouraging times. |
| -9 | I definitely don't want pain medications. If I ask for them, I want my support team and the staff to refuse and insist I continue without drugs. | *Same as for -7 rating, plus:*<br>• Explore with you the reasons for your feelings.<br>• Explain that if you change your mind, staff can't deny your requests for medications.<br>• Reinforce that it's your decision to use or avoid pain medications. |
| -10 | I want no medication, even for a cesarean section (an impossible extreme). | *Same as for -9 rating, plus:*<br>• Help you gain a realistic understanding of the risks and benefits of pain medications.<br>• Explain that there are situations in which pain medications are required, and plan how you can cope if such a situation arises. |

## BEING FLEXIBLE WITH YOUR PLAN FOR PAIN RELIEF

While it's helpful to plan for pain relief, it's also important to be flexible with your plan in case labor doesn't go as expected and your preferences are no longer possible or necessary. For example, if you planned to use medications, you may find that labor is easier than anticipated and you don't need drugs. Or your labor may progress faster than expected, leaving no time for medications—or you may be one of the unlucky few for whom medications don't provide adequate pain relief, in which case you'll need to try non-drug comfort techniques instead. (This is why it's important to learn and practice these techniques even when you're planning for a medicated labor.) If you planned for a non-medicated birth, you may find labor to be more challenging than expected, or you may have unexpected interventions that make it difficult or impossible to give birth without pain medications.

Most women have particular times in labor when they doubt their ability to cope (see page 189). If you begin to doubt yourself, your partner can remind you of these predictable challenges to help you regain confidence. If your doubt turns into dismay and you ask for pain medications, your partner should remember your pain medication preferences and act accordingly. If you'd said you wanted pain medications, he or she should help you get them. If you'd planned to delay receiving medications, he or she should suggest trying another coping technique for four or five contractions before helping you get drugs if the technique is ineffective. If you'd planned to continue striving for a non-medicated birth, he or she should continue to encourage you to cope unless you say your code word (see page 189).

# Preparing to Labor without Pain Medications

If having a drug-free labor is your goal, the following suggestions can help you avoid pain medications or minimize your need for them:

- During pregnancy, confirm that your partner agrees with your goal and feels capable of helping you achieve it. If he or she doesn't, ask someone who does to accompany you both in labor to provide support.
- Choose a birthplace that supports non-medicated birth and has non-medical tools available to provide pain relief and comfort (such as birth balls and large bathtubs). Choose a caregiver with experience supporting women who labor without pain medications. Ask both the birthplace and the caregiver what percentage of their clients use pain medications. If most women do, the staff may have little skill or experience supporting women who don't.
- Learn the comfort techniques in Chapter 11. Practice the relaxation and self-help comfort techniques with your partner or support person.
- Take childbirth preparation classes that focus on learning and practicing comfort techniques.
- Consider hiring a birth doula to guide and reassure you and your partner. (See page 190.) Studies show that a doula's presence and guidance reduce a laboring woman's need for pain medications.[6]
- State your wishes in your birth plan (see Chapter 8). Ask hospital staff to avoid offering you pain medications and instead provide you with encouragement, advice for labor progress, and ideas for comfort measures. (You will, of course, receive medications if you ask for them.)
- Avoid or minimize interventions that can increase labor pain (such as induction and augmentation) or that limit your mobility (such as continuous electronic fetal monitoring and IV fluids).

- Consider having a *code word* to communicate that you've changed your mind and you no longer want to labor without medications. Women with a strong desire for a non-medicated birth (rating a -5 to -7 on the Pain Medication Preference Scale—see page 187) often use a code word so they're free to complain, vocalize, cry, or curse without others misunderstanding their actions as a plea for pain medications. For example, one woman told her support team that if she said, "I can't" or "This is too hard," she was really saying, "I need more support." But if she said her code word *uncle*, her partner knew to help her get pain medications.

  If you want to use a code word, make sure it isn't one that's commonly said in a childbirth setting or associated with pain or pain relief, such as *drugs*. That way, you'll avoid having others mistakenly believe you want pain medications if you happen to say the word during labor. Instead, choose a word that's unrelated to childbirth, such as *pumpernickel*. Let everyone attending to your labor know what your code word is as well as its purpose.

- Know the predictable challenges of labor and prepare for ways to manage them without medications:

  * As you move from early labor to active labor (when your cervix dilates from about 3 to 5 centimeters), your contractions will become painful but you'll realize you still have a long way to go before your baby is born. You may feel that labor is beyond your control. Try to adapt your breathing, movements, or activities in whatever way will help you cope. (See Chapter 11 for ideas.) You may find that if you can release control, you'll spontaneously discover new ways of coping.

  * When your cervix has dilated to 6 to 7 centimeters, your contractions may become very intense. Don't expect to feel peaceful and relaxed during contractions. If you can relax *between* contractions and can maintain a rhythm in your breathing, movements, or activities during contractions, you'll be coping well. Remember that as labor intensifies, progress speeds up. (See the graph on page 284.)

  * As you move from active labor to transition, when your cervix dilates to 7 or 8 centimeters, you may need to rely heavily on your support team to help you keep your rhythm. Your partner can remind you that your contractions are about as painful as they'll become (although they may occur closer together). If you can cope at this time, you can probably manage the rest of your labor without pain medications—as long as you want to do so and your labor continues to progress normally.

If you begin to struggle with the pain at any point in labor, you and your support team should have a contingency plan for coping. See page 191 for more information.

## A Note to Fathers and Partners

It's easy to neglect your own needs when caring for a woman in labor, especially one who's laboring without pain medications. By taking care of yourself, you can help your partner meet the demands of labor. Stay hydrated and keep up your energy by eating nutritious snacks. Conserve your strength when physically supporting your partner (for example, sit or lean against something whenever possible, rather than standing), use good body mechanics (for example, lift with your legs, not your back), and work within your body's limitations (visit our web site, http://www.PCNGuide.com, for more information). If others want to provide support, let them if you need the rest. Maintaining your stamina will help you provide the invaluable contribution that only you can make during the birth of your baby.[7]

# The Invaluable Birth Doula

When considering options for pain relief, don't overlook the important services that a birth doula can provide. Unlike the nursing staff, who must concentrate on completing clinical tasks while providing care, a doula can focus solely on you and your partner, making sure you're both coping well.

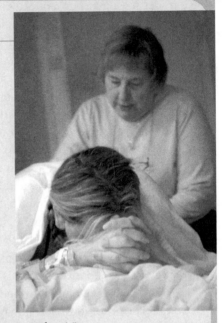

This person (usually a woman) knows all the comfort measures and when to use them. From her meetings with you before the birth, she'll know your birth plan (see Chapter 8), your pain medication preferences, your likes and dislikes, and your hopes for birth. She'll know what to say and do to comfort and encourage you—and what not to say and do. For example, one woman told her doula, "Don't tell me 'you're doing great' when I'm clearly not. Please acknowledge what I'm feeling by saying, 'I can see that it hurts, and I know it's hard, but we can do this together.' "

Women hire doulas for many reasons. One woman without a partner hired a doula to be her primary support person and to help her ask the caregiver or staff important questions. Another woman, whose mother had died, hired a doula because she wanted a mother figure with her during labor. One woman wanted the feminine energy of someone who had given birth and had supported many women through labor. Another wanted someone to help her and her partner with comfort measures so she was less likely to use pain medications.

Some couples hire a doula just as much for the partner as for the laboring woman, especially if the partner isn't completely comfortable with the demands of labor support and needs a guide or helper, or wants someone else to take over the role of primary support person. If the partner has personal concerns, he or she may find that hiring a doula is a good idea. For example, a doula can provide backup support if the partner has a medical condition such as hypoglycemia (which necessitates getting regular food and rest), becomes queasy at the sight of blood, has physical limitations, or simply wants to avoid the pressure of having to learn and remember all the comfort measures.

A doula can also do necessary tasks for the partner, allowing him or her to focus on providing primary support. For example, the doula can run errands and fetch food, beverages, and comfort items such as ice packs. She can take photos of the labor and birth. She can report progress and developments to the couple's friends and family. She can massage the woman's back while her partner helps her maintain a rhythm. She can continue support so the partner can eat, get some air, or take a much-needed nap. For more information on doulas, see page 23.

*Notes*: Doulas might not be available in every area; see page 23 for information on finding a doula in your area. Furthermore, not all birthplaces welcome doulas; see page 13 for questions to ask potential birthplaces. If a doula isn't available or allowed in your birthplace (or you don't want one), trusted relatives or friends can do many of the things a doula can do, especially if they attend childbirth preparation classes with you and your partner.

## CONTINGENCY PLAN

What if you plan to give birth without pain medications, but begin to have second thoughts during labor? If you truly don't want to labor any longer without drugs, you can say your code word (see page 189) and your support people should help you ask for pain medications. However, if you're struggling to cope but still don't want to receive drugs, here are ideas to try:

- Change your environment. Take a walk or a shower, dim the lights, or put on some relaxing music.
- Change your ritual or your breathing techniques. (See pages 207 and 223.)
- Consider contacting another supportive friend or relative to be with you.
- Eat something or drink a sugary beverage. Sometimes all you need for pain relief is a quick energy boost.
- Find out how far your cervix has dilated. Labor may be difficult because you're making rapid progress!
- Don't base your decision to use pain medications on your experience with just one hard contraction. First try a new comfort technique (see Chapter 11 for ideas) for four or five contractions in a row. During this time, your endorphins may kick in and labor may feel manageable again. (See page 242 for more information on endorphins.)

If your labor is still too intense after trying all these suggestions, you may choose to receive pain medications. If you do, try not to feel disappointed in yourself or feel that you've failed in some way because you didn't reach your goal. Take comfort in the fact that many women in this situation have reported feeling better about their decision because they'd first tried everything possible to manage without drugs, but were wise enough to change their minds when the pain led to suffering.

# Preparing to Labor with Pain Medications

It's wise to learn about pain medications during pregnancy, whether or not you plan to use them during labor. That way, if the need for medications arises in labor, you'll already have some knowledge about them and can make an informed decision about their use.

Because both you and your baby are affected if you take pain medications, you and your caregiver should evaluate all possible risks and benefits of a drug. You should also be informed of extra precautions or interventions that may accompany pain medications to ensure their safety, as well as any acceptable alternatives to the drugs.

## WEIGHING THE RISKS AND BENEFITS OF PAIN MEDICATIONS

The benefits of pain medications include an increased ability to relax and sleep, and the reduction or elimination of pain. If pain medications are used judiciously and with current methods, the side effects are often mild, manageable, and familiar to hospital staff.

However, as with all interventions, pain medications have potential risks. Examples include decreased blood pressure in the mother, prolonged labor, forceps delivery or vacuum extraction, fever in the mother and baby, and variations in the baby's heart rate. While these risks are typically moderate, they may require additional interventions that have their own potential side effects. If you use pain medications in labor, your caregiver will be aware of all potential risks and take measures to either prevent or manage them.

## Epidural Birth versus Natural Birth

Here's one woman's account of her birth experiences, one with an epidural and one without:

*For my first birth, I'd planned to labor without drugs, but in transition I panicked and accepted an epidural. Soon we were cracking jokes and watching for my next contraction on the monitor. I didn't feel any pain, but almost immediately after Hannah was born, I just wanted to sleep.*

*For my next birth, I again planned to cope naturally. When contractions got intense and I felt that I couldn't possibly do it, my support people encouraged me that I could—and I did. I felt so alive afterward. Some friends still think I was crazy for not having an epidural. My only response is that I've given birth with drugs and without, and nothing compares to the euphoria I experienced with a drug-free birth.*

As you consider the risks and benefits of laboring with pain medications, keep the following factors in mind:

- While medications can minimize pain or even eliminate it for some portion of your labor, they generally can't prevent you from experiencing *any* pain throughout your entire labor.
- Any medication you receive affects your baby. Because his liver and kidneys are immature, the effects of some drugs last longer for him than for you. A medication's effects depend on the drug, the amount received, how and when it's given, and other factors. (Visit our web site, http://www.PCNGuide.com, for more information.)
- Pain medications affect your labor progress. They often slow contractions and may increase your need for other medical interventions. However, if labor progress is abnormally slow, drugs may speed up progress by letting you relax.
- Special precautions are required with most pain medications to prevent, minimize, or treat side effects that may interfere with labor progress or harm you or your baby. For example, the following interventions are necessary more often when pain medications are used than when they're not: restriction to bed, restriction of eating and drinking, IV fluids, Pitocin augmentation, administration of oxygen, frequent monitoring of blood pressure and blood oxygen levels, bladder catheterization, continuous electronic fetal monitoring (EFM), vacuum extraction, and cesarean section.
- Several factors influence which medication is right for you, including the nature of your pain, stage of labor, allergies or medical conditions, other medications you use regularly, unusual anatomical conditions of your spine or lower back, and availability of anesthesia services at your birthplace. Tell your caregiver if you've ever had an allergy or adverse reaction to medication.

## KEY VOCABULARY OF PAIN MEDICATIONS

Each drug has specific characteristics that make it safe and effective for pain relief in particular phases of labor. The following describe key terms for medications that can relieve labor pain:

### Route of administration

How you receive a medication is its route of administration. *Oral medication* is a pill or liquid you swallow; *inhalation medication* is a gas you breathe. *Intramuscular (IM) medication* is a shot given into muscle, while *intravenous (IV) medication* is an injection into a vein, often through an IV catheter (see page 250). Lastly, *neuraxial medications* are drugs that are injected into the space surrounding the spinal cord (neuraxis), such as epidurals and spinal blocks. How quickly a medication takes effect depends on the route of administration.

# Questions to Ask Your Caregiver about Pain Medications

During a prenatal visit, ask your caregiver the following questions about pain medications so you can make an informed decision about them before you're in labor or in an emergency situation, when you're in pain and clear thinking may be impossible.

- What medications are most commonly used for pain relief? How is each medication given?
- How does each medication relieve pain? How effective is it?
- What are the potential risks or undesirable side effects of the drug on me, my baby, or labor progress? What precautions do you take to prevent, control, or treat side effects?
- What are my alternatives to pain medications?

Be aware that the answers you receive may vary depending on whom you ask. For example, an anesthesiologist and a home birth midwife may give very different answers to these questions. An anesthesiologist, who is trained in the best pharmaceutical solutions to relieving pain, will likely believe that the side effects of recommended pain medications are manageable and their benefits outweigh any potential risks. A home birth midwife who's familiar with non-drug coping techniques may recommend them first because they're low-cost, low-risk, and can be done anywhere.

Keep any potential biases in mind when listening to your caregiver's answers, and supplement the information you learn from him or her with the knowledge you've learned from research-based sources of information (such as this book and our web site, http://www.PCNGuide.com). This way, you can better make an informed decision about pain medications.

**Area of effect**

Medications may be *systemic* (affecting your entire body), *regional* (affecting a large area of your body), or *local* (affecting a specific, relatively small part of your body). In general, you need more medication to get the desired results with a systemic medication than with a regional or local medication.

**Type of effect**

*Analgesia* is any effect that reduces your perception of pain. In this chapter, this term refers specifically to medications that act on the brain so you don't recognize pain stimuli or don't interpret them as pain. *Anesthesia* indicates a loss of sensation, including pain sensation. Anesthetics block nerve endings from sending pain impulses to your brain.

## SYSTEMIC MEDICATIONS

Systemic medications come in many forms, including pills, injections, and gases. All are absorbed into your bloodstream and affect your entire body. The desired effect is to reduce your pain, but there may be side effects.

Because systemic medications are carried in your bloodstream, they may affect your baby as well, because the placenta can't screen them out. The magnitude of effects depends on the type and amount of medication used and the time between the last dose and the birth. Other factors include your baby's maturity, health, and response during labor. If a healthy, full-term baby and a premature, ill, or distressed baby were each exposed to the same amount of medication during labor, the healthy baby would show fewer side effects than the baby with problems.

## Two Views on Narcotics

Initially, fentanyl made me feel as though I were drunk. I was a little dizzy, and I don't think I was mentally all there. The contractions were still very painful, but more manageable, especially in the hot tub. About an hour later, my cervix was dilated to 6 centimeters, and I got another dose of fentanyl. The pain continued getting stronger, and I got a third dose, which unfortunately wasn't effective at all.

—*Sami*

Within two hours of being admitted, I asked for drugs because the pain was making me very anxious. The Nubain helped me relax and focus on my breathing for the next wave of contractions. I completely lost track of time as I found myself instinctively using rhythm to cope. My cervix was checked ninety minutes later, and it had dilated to 7 centimeters. I was assured that an epidural was still an option, and the anesthesiologist was called.

—*Jennifer*

The medication or its byproducts might not disappear from your baby's bloodstream for hours or days, and neurobehavioral changes may be present during the first few days after birth (visit our web site, http://www.PCNGuide.com, for details). These changes may be obvious, or they may be noticeable only to professionals who use highly sensitive tests to examine your baby.

*General anesthesia* is a systemic medication that causes a total loss of sensation and consciousness. It's used for only a small percentage of cesarean births. (Visit our web site to learn more about this and other systemic medications such as sedatives, tranquilizers, and nitrous oxide.) Intravenous (IV) narcotics are the systemic medications used most commonly in labor, although intramuscular (IM) narcotics are sometimes given.

### IV Narcotics or Narcotic-like Medications

*Narcotics and narcotic-like drugs* reduce the transmission of pain messages to the pain receptors in your brain.

**Benefits**

The analgesic effect is often described as "taking the edge off the pain." It may take you longer to notice that a contraction has started, and it may seem to fade away sooner. The peak of a contraction, however, may still be intense enough that you feel the pain despite the narcotics.

Narcotics may work well for you if you're handling the pain at the peak of a contraction but want to feel as if you have a longer break between contractions so you can rest. You may even be able to doze between contractions and wake up to manage the peak.

*Note:* Narcotics might not work well for you if you can't handle the pain at the peak of a contraction, or if you can handle the pain only if you can feel the onset of the contraction and can begin using a coping ritual before the peak occurs. If you do use narcotics and doze between contractions, your partner or doula can help you prepare for the pain by noting the onset of the contraction (as indicated by a monitor or by your wincing or moaning), awakening or alerting you, and guiding you to use rhythmic breathing (see page 223) before the peak.

**Tradeoffs**

IV fluids, continuous electronic fetal monitoring (EFM), and restriction to bed may be necessary when narcotics are used. Narcotics may cause sleepiness or lethargy, and they may cause a hazy feeling, disorientation, or euphoria. Some women find the sensation relaxing or pleasant, while others feel out of control, which may make it difficult to use self-help techniques.

### Possible side effects

Common side effects include itching, nausea, and vomiting. Narcotics may slow labor and cause variations in your baby's heart rate. You can receive a drug called a narcotic antagonist to reduce these side effects, but it'll reduce pain relief. After the birth, the narcotics in your baby's bloodstream may cause her to breathe slowly and have poor muscle tone. She can receive a narcotic antagonist if needed. See page 448 for more information on possible side effects.

### Timing

The effects of narcotics last for sixty to ninety minutes. Narcotics are used in early to active labor, when it's believed that the birth is at least two hours away. This timing allows the narcotic effects on your baby to fade before the birth.

## LOCAL AND REGIONAL ANESTHETICS

Local or regional anesthetics (often called "blocks") cause reduced feeling or numbness in a particular area of your body. When an anesthetic drug is injected near specific nerves, it blocks the transmission of sensations along them. It also affects muscle control, blood flow, and temperature in the affected area to a degree. Lower doses of an anesthetic eliminate or dull pain while allowing some muscle control. Higher doses remove both sensation and the ability to use your muscles. Local and regional anesthetics don't affect your mental state. Most anesthetic drug names end with the suffix "-caine," such as lidocaine and bupivacaine.

## *Local Anesthetics (Perineal Block)*

Local anesthetics block sensation in a small area near nerve endings. They're injected into the skin, mucous membranes, or muscles. During labor, they're typically injected in the perineum (perineal block). They can be injected in the cervix (paracervical block) or the vagina (pudendal block), but these blocks aren't often used.

### Benefits

Because a perineal block numbs the perineum, it's necessary for the repair of an episiotomy or lacerations. It may also be used to numb the perineum before an episiotomy or a forceps delivery. (See pages 289–290 for information on these procedures.)

### Tradeoff

The injections may be painful.

### Possible side effects

If a perineal block is given during the repair of an episiotomy or lacerations, the side effects are minimal (barring an allergic reaction). If it's given early in the second stage (which is rare), the medication may affect the baby's heart rate during labor or his reflexes at birth. See page 449 for more information on possible side effects.

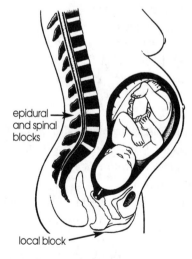

epidural
and spinal
blocks

local block

### Timing

Local anesthetics are given during the second stage if an episiotomy or forceps delivery is necessary. They're given in the third stage for the repair of an episiotomy or lacerations.

## Common Q & A

**Q:** Is it ever too late for an epidural?

**A:** You may have heard that it's best to receive an epidural in early labor because you won't be able to receive one in late labor. It's true that if your labor is progressing quickly and birth is anticipated within thirty to sixty minutes, your caregiver may recommend against an epidural. However, if labor progress is slow, it's possible to receive an epidural even during transition or the second stage.

If comfort techniques are helping you cope, don't feel that you have to get an epidural in early labor because you fear it'll be your only chance to get one. Keep using comfort techniques for as long as they help you manage contractions. If you decide later that you want an epidural, it's very likely that you'll be able to get one.

## Regional (Neuraxial) Analgesia and Anesthesia: Epidural and Spinal Blocks

*Neuraxial medications* are injected in your lower back near nerve roots in the spinal column. The medications affect the region of your body to which these nerves and their branches go. The region can be as small as your abdomen and lower back, or as large as the area from your chest to your toes. The medications are often a combination of an anesthetic medication (see page 193) and a narcotic-like drug such as fentanyl, which enhances the overall numbing effect. A *spinal block* is an injection that takes effect quickly and lasts for an hour or two. An *epidural catheter* is a tube through which medication is given for as long as it's needed.

### Benefits

The American College of Obstetricians and Gynecologists (ACOG) and the American Academy of Pediatrics (AAP) have stated that among all options for medicated pain relief, the epidural is the most effective for reducing pain, while allowing the woman to stay alert and actively participate in her labor.[8] Among women who receive epidural pain medications, almost all (98.8 percent) have significant pain relief for at least some of their labor. (See page 202 for information about the possibility that an epidural may fail to provide effective pain relief for a woman during her entire labor.) Once the epidural takes effect, the medications typically continue to provide relief for the rest of labor.

Because of the locations of the injection sites, much smaller amounts of neuraxial medications can be used than are needed for either local anesthesia or systemic analgesia. With neuraxial medications, women typically have fewer mental and respiratory side effects, and have a higher level of satisfaction than with other pain medication options. At birth, their babies are more alert, breathe better, and have better muscle tone than babies born with higher doses of systemic narcotic-like medications.[9]

### Tradeoffs

To minimize the side effects of neuraxial medications, various additional precautions and interventions must be used to maintain safety. For example, an epidural is accompanied by IV fluids, a bladder catheter, and continuous monitoring of blood pressure, contractions, and your baby's heart rate. Eating and drinking are restricted and you're confined to bed. Along with the effects of the medications, the accompanying medical equipment significantly reduces mobility (you might not be able to move your legs or change positions in bed without assistance) and contributes to the feeling that the birth has become a medical event.

## Possible side effects

The most common side effects include decreased blood pressure, a longer labor, a longer pushing stage, and fever. These effects may lead to further interventions (such as Pitocin augmentation, vacuum extraction, or forceps delivery) and secondary side effects on both you and your baby (such as uterine hyperstimulation or variations in your baby's heart rate). The narcotics in the epidural can also cause itching and nausea. Some women worry that an injection near the spinal cord may carry the risk of paralysis or even death; however, these outcomes are so rare, they're nearly nonexistent. See pages 450–451 for more information on the possible side effects of neuraxial medications.

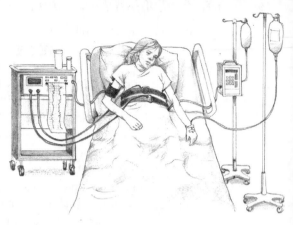

Current methods of epidural analgesia focus on finding a balance between maximizing pain relief and minimizing side effects. Caregivers and nurses are trained to recognize and treat side effects when they occur. With an "ideal" epidural, your pain is significantly reduced, you and your baby experience few side effects, you have at least a slight urge to push, and you can move your legs and change positions with assistance.

Whether you'll have few or many side effects can't be predicted or controlled, and your experience won't depend solely on the skills of the anesthesiologist who administers the epidural. Many other factors will influence your experience, including your and your baby's physical state and well-being as well as how your body reacts to medications.

A postpartum side effect of epidural analgesia may be a shortened duration of breastfeeding. Compared to a woman who had a non-medicated birth, a woman who had an epidural is more likely to stop breastfeeding sooner, partly because she might have taken longer after the birth to begin holding and nursing her baby, and partly because of a mistaken perception that she might not make enough milk.[10] These problems can be overcome by early and frequent skin-to-skin contact between the mother and baby, and by starting breastfeeding within the first hour after the birth. The earlier a woman initiates breastfeeding and the more often she nurses, the more milk she makes and the more likely she is to have breastfeeding success. (See Chapter 18 for more information on breastfeeding.)

## Timing

Some caregivers recommend (or require) that a woman be in active labor (4 to 5 centimeters cervical dilation and strong, regular contractions) before receiving an epidural. This recommendation is based on past research that indicated epidurals given in early labor were likely to slow or stall labor. Other caregivers allow a woman to receive an epidural at any point in labor, a practice based on conflicting research that doesn't show early epidurals prolong labor. Still other caregivers use a *combined spinal-epidural (CSE)*: that is, spinal narcotics early in labor and an epidural later on.

## Procedure for Epidural and Spinal Blocks

If you decide to receive an epidural or a spinal block, here's the procedure you can expect:

1.  As you wait for the anesthesiologist, who might or might not be immediately available, you cope with contractions that may be especially intense and require you to rely on extra support to manage them.

2.  You may receive IV fluids to help reduce the risk of a drop in blood pressure and to allow for administration of additional medications, if needed. This procedure can take ten to twenty minutes. If you have an IV in already, your nurse can increase the flow to give you ¼ to 1 liter of fluid quickly.

3.  When the anesthesiologist arrives, you're asked to either lie curled on your side or sit up and lean forward to curve your back. The anesthesiologist then cleans your lower back with an antiseptic and numbs your skin with a shot of local anesthetic. This preparation, along with the delicate placement of the epidural catheter or spinal needle, can take ten minutes or longer. You may need extra support to help you sit or lie still during contractions. If you can't stay still during the peak of a contraction, the anesthesiologist can pause until the pain subsides.

4.  Where and how the anesthesiologist places the needle or catheter in your back depends on the type of block.

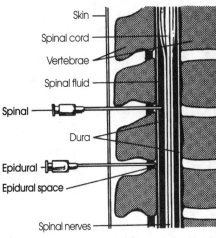

**Spinal block**

A single injection of an anesthetic or narcotic is given with a needle that's inserted through the dura (the tough membrane that surrounds your spinal cord) into the *intrathecal* space, which is filled with cerebrospinal fluid. (See the illustration at right.) Drugs given in this location and in this way are called intrathecal medications. A spinal block takes effect within minutes and lasts a few hours.

**Epidural catheter**

A needle is inserted into the epidural space, just outside the dura. A thin plastic tube (catheter) is threaded through the needle, the needle is removed, the catheter is taped to your back, and a test dose of medications is given through the catheter to ensure you don't react poorly to the drugs. The catheter is attached to a pump device that steadily releases small amounts of anesthetic or analgesic.

Within a few minutes, tingling and numbness are noticeable; within fifteen minutes, you're likely to be completely numb from the top of your uterus to your pelvis or even from your chest to your toes. (The effects sometimes take longer to be felt, and the catheter may need to be repositioned to yield the best effects.) The catheter remains in place and pain relief continues throughout the rest of your labor. You may receive medications by continuous drip, from a series of doses (a method that's becoming uncommon), or from doses that you administer when you need them (*patient-controlled epidural analgesia, or PCEA*—see page 200 for more information).

**Combined spinal-epidural (CSE)**

The epidural needle is inserted, then the smaller spinal needle is inserted through it and into the intrathecal space for the administration of a spinal narcotic. The spinal needle is then removed and the epidural catheter is inserted. No medication is added to the epidural at this time. The effects of the spinal narcotic last a few hours or until your cervix has dilated to 4 to 6 centimeters and the intensifying contractions cause you to feel pain. When you need more relief, the epidural medication is given through the catheter.

5. Your temperature, blood pressure, pulse, and blood oxygen levels are checked frequently, and your contractions and your baby's heart rate are closely monitored. You may also have an electrocardiogram (EKG) to monitor your heart function.

6. Many women receive excellent pain relief with epidural analgesia and don't experience any side effects beyond the tradeoffs described on page 196. However, if monitoring indicates that you or your baby are reacting poorly to neuraxial medications, then more interventions may be necessary.

For example, if your blood pressure drops signifcantly, your baby's heart rate will also decrease. To improve your oxygen levels and increase your baby's heart rate, your nurse or caregiver will turn you onto your side, place an oxygen mask on your face, and ask you to breathe deeply. While the oxygen mask may concern you and your partner, it almost always corrects the problem quickly. If not, you may also be given medications or additional IV fluids to raise your blood pressure.

Managing side effects often causes a "cascade of interventions," in which the use of one intervention leads to additional side effects that necessitate even more interventions. For example, if epidural medications cause your contractions to slow down, you may receive Pitocin to stimulate them—which may overstimulate your uterus, which can lead to variations in your baby's heart rate, which may increase your need of a cesarean section. To be able to make an informed decision about any pain relief option, you need to acknowledge the possibility of this type of outcome.

Any side effects you experience can also have an impact on your baby. For example, your chances of fever increase when you have epidural anesthesia, because the medications alter your ability to regulate your temperature. The longer the epidural is in place, the higher your risk of fever is. When you have a fever, your baby's heart rate may increase to a worrisome level, a problem that may require an intervention such as a cesarean section to resolve. In addition, although an epidural won't cause an infection in your baby, it may increase the chance she'll need to be treated for one. The reason is because if you have a fever during labor, your baby may have one at birth. If she does, her fever can't be assumed to be a result

## Different Views on Epidurals

When asked about epidurals, new mothers had many different responses. Here are a few examples:

*For me, taking fentanyl and getting in the hot tub weren't much help, so I just rested on my side in bed for a while and did my breathing exercises. Some time later the epidural came—relief at last! I even slept. I think the epidural slowed things down, but the pain relief was very helpful.*

*I had twenty hours of labor with a great support team and without drugs. I was coping with the pain okay, but I was exhausted. So I got an epidural and slept. My son was born by vacuum extraction ten hours later, after four hours of pushing. I was glad to get the epidural, but the birth was definitely a much more medical experience than I'd expected.*

*I'd hoped the epidural would take away all my pain, but it didn't. I was pretty numb overall, but this one spot on my belly hurt a LOT. It was almost harder to cope with that window of pain than it'd been to cope with regular contractions. Luckily, James remembered all the comfort techniques we learned, and helped coach me through the contractions.*

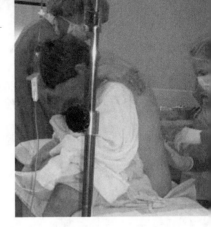

of the epidural, because fever is also associated with infection. Your baby will be checked for infection with blood tests and possibly a spinal tap. She may be kept in the special care nursery and given antibiotics for two days, until her test results are known. Although the testing and preventive treatment will separate you from your baby and can be worrisome, test results will likely show that your baby is fine.

See the chart on pages 450–451 for more information about the effects and side effects of regional medications.

## Options for Epidurals

The types of epidurals offered vary among hospitals. Ask your caregiver about the availability of the following options, and whether he or she recommends them. Side effects of the medications may be reduced for some options; however, because side effects can still occur, all precautions and safety procedures that accompany an epidural must still be used (see page 196).

**Patient-controlled epidural analgesia (PCEA)**

PCEA allows you to press a button attached to your epidural pump to give yourself more medication when you need it. When women are allowed to control their dosage, they tend to use less medication and are more satisfied with the epidural experience than when the dosage is controlled for them. Although you have some control over the flow of medication with PCEA, the device has a timer that limits the number of doses, which are carefully measured so you can't overdose. (*Note:* Patient-controlled analgesia, or PCA, may also be available for IV narcotics.)

**Combined spinal-epidural (CSE)**

CSE uses a spinal narcotic in early labor (which may allow for more mobility), then an epidural later in labor, when you need more pain relief.

**Light or late epidural**

You can reduce some side effects by delaying an epidural until you're in active labor (late epidural) and requesting a low concentration of the medications (light epidural).

Policies for managing labor with an epidural also vary among hospitals. Ask your caregiver about the following measures:

*Movement*

Ask whether you'll be able to move with an epidural and whether movement in bed is encouraged.

*Food and drink*

Many hospitals allow women with epidurals to consume only ice chips; however, the American Society of Anesthesiologists recommends allowing women to drink clear fluids. Ask what you'll be allowed to consume.

*Delayed pushing (also called passive descent or laboring down)*

Rather than pushing as soon as your cervix is fully dilated, you may wait to push until your baby's head is visible at the vaginal outlet. Delayed pushing has been proven to reduce vaginal tears, forceps delivery, vacuum extraction, and the need for a cesarean section. It also won't harm your baby. Ask whether delayed pushing is common practice.

*Lowering the dosage or discontinuing the epidural*

By slowing or stopping the flow of epidural medications at the beginning of the second stage of labor, you may be able to bear down more effectively. (However, labor pain may be intolerable when it returns.)

## A Note to Fathers and Partners

When your laboring partner has an epidural, the shift from intense effort and pain to complete physical relaxation may be sudden. At that point, you may think that she no longer needs your constant support. You may begin thinking about taking a nap, going for a walk, or turning on the TV; however, your job isn't done. Even though your partner may be more comfortable physically, she still needs your emotional support. If you shift your attention away from her once the epidural has taken effect, she may feel as though you're abandoning her.

To reassure your partner that you'll continue to provide support, stay with her and relax together. Do things that soothe her such as holding her hand or brushing her hair. An epidural may leave your partner feeling disconnected from her body and the birth experience; talk with her about the labor and your baby to help her reconnect with events. (Resist the temptation to turn on the TV, post status updates online, or text everyone you know!) If she's worried or anxious, listen to her fears, acknowledge them, and reassure her. Help her change positions as much as possible; if she has a light epidural, she may even be able to get on her hands and knees with assistance and if you remain by her side to help keep her steady. If she falls asleep, she'll probably be restless. She'll be reassured by your staying awake or at least staying in the room so she can wake you if she needs anything.

There are occasional challenges with epidurals. Your partner might not initially receive sufficient pain relief, she might experience "windows" of pain, or the pain might return after initial relief. (See page 202 for more information.) Be sure to alert the staff if any of these situations occur. They may be able to fix it by adjusting the epidural or by having her change positions. If your partner is among the few women for whom an epidural doesn't provide effective pain relief, even after multiple attempts to correct the problem, she'll need your support to help cope with the pain and to deal with the disappointment that the epidural failed her.

Your partner may also experience discomforts that are caused by the medications, such as itching, nausea, and feeling overheated or chilled. Make her more comfortable by giving her a massage, helping her change positions, covering her with a warm blanket, placing a cool cloth on her forehead, or giving her ice chips or sips of water (if allowed). Do *not*, however, place heating pads or ice packs on any part of her body that's affected by the epidural. The medications will affect her sense of temperature, and she might not be able to tell if a heating pad or cold pack is damaging her skin.

Be aware that some side effects of epidurals may lead to other interventions or may require a decision from your partner on how to manage the problem. Try to stay calm and supportive so you can help her make decisions that are best for her.

Even with pain relief, your partner may experience intense pressure or burning during the pushing stage. Reassure her that these sensations are normal and signal that your baby will be born soon. If you're holding up one of her legs as she pushes, be careful not to pull it back too far. Think about her hips' normal range of motion, and don't force her leg beyond that point so you avoid straining her hips, thighs, or lower back. (Your partner will be unable to tell you when her muscles are straining because the medications will have numbed all sensation.)

After the birth, help your partner get lots of early skin-to-skin contact with your baby so breastfeeding can begin in the first hour.

# THE IMPORTANCE OF LEARNING COMFORT TECHNIQUES WHEN PLANNING FOR AN EPIDURAL

If your Pain Medication Preference Scale rating is +5 or higher (see page 187) and you're planning for an early epidural, you may think you don't need to learn self-help techniques to relieve pain. Keep in mind, however, that it's likely you'll have at least a few painful contractions before the epidural takes effect. It's also possible that even if your epidural is effective, you'll still feel strong, painful sensations deep in your pelvis when pushing. For these reasons, it's wise to know how you'll cope with the pain.

## Failed Epidurals

Although epidurals are very effective for most women who use them, they can pose challenges for some women. Twelve percent of epidurals don't provide complete pain relief when first inserted, while 7 percent may provide good pain relief initially but fade over time. Some epidurals provide only minimal pain relief; others allow for "windows" of pain, in which most of the area is numbed but one spot still has sensation and the woman can fully feel the pain in that area.[11]

If you have a problem with your epidural, the staff may be able to fix it by changing your position, increasing the medication, or repositioning the epidural catheter. These measures have resulted in good pain relief for nearly all women with epidurals (98.8 percent). However, while the staff works to correct the problem, comfort measures can help you cope.

When you're unprepared to manage labor pain, your inability to cope can make you feel that you're suffering, which in turn can create a very unhappy memory of what should be one of the best days of your life. Learn self-help techniques in Chapter 11 so you can manage these challenges and have a more satisfying birth. As a bonus, these techniques can help you deal with other challenging or painful situations at other times in your life.

# Key Points to Remember

- Labor pain is a physical sensation that many women can manage by using coping techniques and receiving continued respectful support. Suffering is an emotional response that includes feelings of helplessness, fear, and panic. No one should suffer in labor.

- Well before the birth, learn about your pain relief options and discuss your preferences with your caregiver to help you and your support team plan how to meet your needs in labor.

- Many non-drug techniques can reduce labor pain. Learn and practice them during pregnancy so they're effective in labor.

- The goal of using medications is to relieve pain without compromising the well-being of your baby or labor progress. The side effects to you or your baby are influenced by the medications used, total amount received, route of administration, your response to the drugs, and your baby's condition during labor. To learn more information about pain medications, see pages 193–200 and visit our web site, http://www.PCNGuide.com.

- Be flexible with your plans for pain relief. Have a contingency plan in place, in case your labor proceeds differently than you expected.

# Comfort Techniques for Pain Relief and Labor Progress

As your due date approaches, you may wonder how you'll cope when your contractions become intense, or what you can do if your labor becomes slow or extra challenging. Comfort techniques such as rhythmic breathing, body positions, and relaxation exercises can help you cope with labor pain and maintain progress with less need for intervention.

This chapter describes how you and your partner can practice and adapt comfort techniques during pregnancy so they can help you effectively manage the pain and stress of labor. Instead of using pain medications, you may use these techniques to keep your pain at a manageable level. Or you may use them along with pain medications to enhance your comfort and reduce the amount of medication you need. In either case, comfort techniques can help make the birth of your child a rewarding, fulfilling, and joyful experience by allowing you to participate in the event more fully.

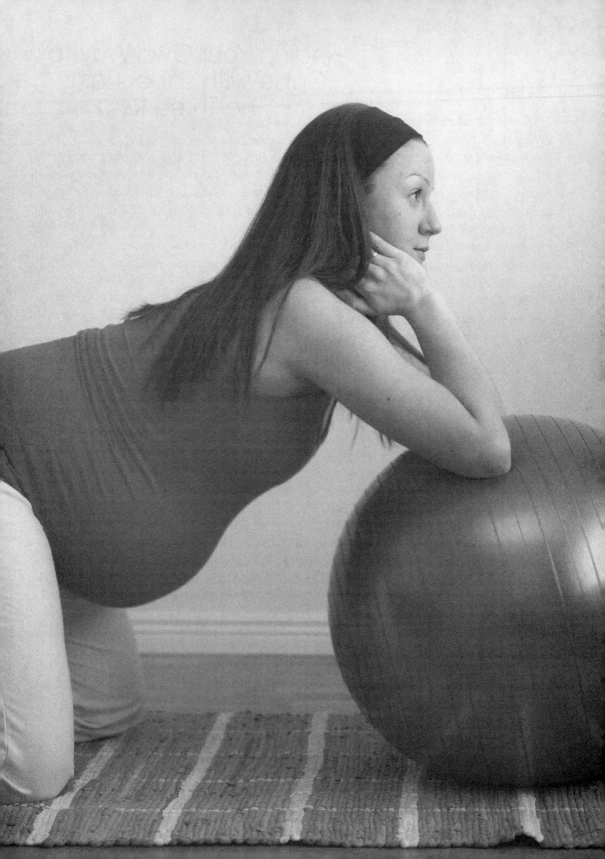

# Finding Your Own Way to Cope with Labor Pain: The Three Rs

Every woman responds to labor pain in her own way. Your response will depend on the nature of your labor, your coping style, your goals and expectations, and how prepared you feel for labor.[1] Although you can learn about labor from other people and resources, such as your caregiver or childbirth preparation classes, only you can develop your own approach to handling labor pain. You have your own learning style, values, and ways of dealing with change, stress, and pain. With the help of your partner and others on your support team, you can adapt the following comfort techniques to suit your labor and modify them to match your personality and preferences.

## THE THREE RS: RELAXATION, RHYTHM, AND RITUAL

*relaxation    rhythm    ritual*

Although every woman responds to labor differently, those who cope well have three behaviors in common: relaxation, rhythm, and ritual. These Three Rs describe the instinctual coping behaviors observed in hundreds of women who were managing labor well.

## Relaxation

Women who cope well in labor use relaxation in various ways. They may move about between contractions and let their muscles relax during contractions. They may become active during contractions (for example, swaying, rocking, and stroking their bellies) and relax only between contractions. Or they may remain quiet and unresponsive to their surroundings during and between contractions for all or part of labor. (For more information on relaxation techniques, see page 216.)

## Rhythm

Women who cope well in labor rely on *rhythm* in various forms. Rhythmic activity calms the mind and lets a woman work well with her body. For example, she may rhythmically breathe, moan, or chant during contractions. She may rhythmically tap or stroke something or someone. She may rock, sway, or dance in rhythm. She may even curl her toes in rhythm!

A partner's (or doula's) role is to enhance the rhythm and reinforce it through contractions. For example, if you're breathing and swaying in rhythm, your partner can follow the same rhythm when rubbing your back. If you start to lose the rhythm during a contraction, your partner can help you find it again. If you aren't coping well, your partner can help you find rhythm by dancing with you or directing you to breathe rhythmically.

## Ritual

In labor, *ritual* is the repetition of a meaningful rhythmic activity during contractions. Relaxation, breathing (see page 223), and attention-focusing (see page 208) are common rituals that childbirth educators teach expectant women and couples. These planned rituals help women in early labor establish an effective coping style.

As labor progresses and intensifies, most women spontaneously adapt their planned rituals to increase their ability to cope, instead of struggling to maintain the planned ritual. That is, if they feel uninhibited and are free to move (change positions, walk, sway, rock, and so on), they'll spontaneously adapt a ritual or find a new one to help them cope with labor pain.

A partner's behavior and actions can influence the effectiveness of a ritual. If your partner is part of your ritual, he or she must not do anything to change it. Given the anxiety and uncertainty of labor, having someone act in the same way during each contraction will be enormously reassuring to you. Your partner's job may include maintaining eye contact with you; holding, touching, or stroking you; swaying with you; repeating the same words or phrases; or counting your breaths through each contraction. If your coping style is to focus inward, your partner's job simply may be to remain close by and do little but protect you from interruption.

Although it's difficult to know beforehand exactly what you'll do or need in labor, expect to change your ritual from time to time. If you begin to feel overwhelmed and can't carry on with a ritual, look to your support team for help. Your partner, doula, or caregiver may be able to help you reestablish a ritual or create a new one.

If you plan to give birth in a hospital, be aware that it may be difficult to find your own ritual if hospital policies, routine procedures, or medical interventions limit your options or interrupt your rhythm. For this reason, make sure to practice a rhythmic activity that you can maintain during disturbances, such as self-talk (silent or vocal), tapping, or stroking. Your partner or doula can help you focus by maintaining the rhythm you established before the interruption, or by using the Take Charge Routine (see page 256).

## Unplanned Rituals

The following are examples of unplanned rituals discovered by women in labor:

- Rocking in a rocking chair in rhythm with her breathing
- Silently repeating, "Be still like the mountain; flow like the river"
- Having her partner stroke her lower leg up and down in rhythm with her breathing
- Having her partner softly count her breaths and point out when she has probably passed the halfway point of the contraction
- Having her partner continuously repeat a word or phrase with her during contractions (One couple said, *"Ruuussssh!"* together through many hours of labor.)
- Having her partner move with her in a way that she finds comforting (One couple walked everywhere during labor—in the park, grocery store, and hospital. With every contraction, they'd stop, embrace, and sway until the contraction was over.)

# Comfort Techniques for Labor

Most pain is associated with injury, illness, or stress. Labor pain, however, is associated with a normal, healthy body function. Recognizing that labor pain is a productive part of the birthing process is key to keeping the pain manageable.

As you prepare for labor, remember the Three Rs (see page 206). Think about what helps you relax, such as listening to music, having a massage, hearing soothing voices, taking a warm bath or shower, meditating, praying, chanting, humming, recalling pleasant places and activities, or visualizing empowering images. Then think about the people and objects that help you feel safe and comfortable, such as your partner, mother, sister, friend, or doula, as well as your pillow, nightgown, pajamas, or favorite photo. Plan to use these activities, people, and objects to help you relax or feel secure.

When rehearsing your response to contractions, try the following comfort techniques. You'll probably prefer some more than others, but be ready to try more than one if a particular favorite loses its appeal during labor. Visit our web site, http://www.PCNGuide.com, to download a checklist of comfort techniques; use it to record the ones you prefer.

## TUNING IN AND TUNING OUT

To cope with labor, you may find it most helpful to tune in to the pain by focusing on it, accepting it, and tailoring your response to it. Or you may prefer to tune out the pain by using distraction techniques, concentrating on outside stimuli, or performing mental activities.

## ATTENTION-FOCUSING

During contractions, focus your attention to calm yourself and help keep your mind from wandering to pain or anxiety. (See page 178 to learn why distraction can help women cope with labor pain.) The following sections describe attention-focusing techniques that laboring women have used. Some techniques were planned before labor began, but many were unplanned.

### Visualization

Closing your eyes and visualizing an encouraging or empowering image can help you cope with labor pain by "seeing" a goal or a positive way to interpret the labor process. Here are suggestions:
- Picture your uterine muscle contracting and pulling your cervix open. Visualize your baby pressing your cervix open.
- Imagine calm, pleasant places or recall happy, peaceful events.
- Like a gull soaring above choppy waves, picture yourself as lightly breathing above your contractions.
- Visualize each contraction as a hurdle to clear, a steep hill to climb, a race to run, or a wave to ride.

### Cognitive Attention-focusing

By focusing on a mental activity, such as thinking or saying the words of a song, poem, verse, or prayer, you can direct your attention to the activity and away from the labor pain. You may plan this activity in advance. One woman imagined herself in labor as the "Little Engine That Could" and planned to say to herself as each contraction built to a peak, "I think I can, I think I can."[2] As each contraction subsided, she planned to repeat, "I thought I could, I thought I could."

Conversely, you might not think of doing this activity until you're in labor and find yourself choosing a word or phrase to use on the spot. One woman began rhythmically stroking her belly and chanting, "Keep stirring and you won't boil over." The day before she went into labor, she had become distracted while making fudge and had allowed the ingredients to boil over, so repeating this phrase seemed an appropriate way to prevent herself from becoming overwhelmed by her contractions.

Some women combine cognitive attention-focusing with physical activity. For example, they'll rhythmically count along with rocking, swaying, walking, dancing, tapping, or stroking.

## Visual Focus

Instead of closing your eyes to visualize a positive image, you may prefer to focus on an image within your sight. Here are some suggestions:

- Look at your partner's face, a picture or design, a reminder of your baby (perhaps a toy or a bootie), a flower, or the view from your window. One woman chose to stare at a hole in her pillowcase—not an inspiring image, but it worked for her!
- Focus on a line, such as the edge of a window casing, and visually follow that line around the object during each contraction.

## Sounds

Many laboring women use sounds as a way to focus their attention. To use this technique, try listening to your favorite music, your partner's soothing voice, repeated rhythms, or a recording of rhythmic environmental sounds such as a pounding surf, rainfall, or babbling brook. Or you can make your own rhythmic sounds by moaning, sighing, counting your breaths, singing, reciting poems or prayers, or chanting. In the past, maternity care experts disapproved of vocalizing during labor and birth, but today many recognize its usefulness. Rhythmic moaning (or vocal breathing) isn't the same as screaming in fear or panic. If you make rhythmic low-pitched sounds, like moaning, you're using an effective technique for maintaining a sense of control while releasing tension. If your sounds are high-pitched, frantic, or nonrhythmic, your support team should guide you to make low-pitched rhythmic sounds instead.

## BATHS AND SHOWERS

At most birthplaces, using baths and showers for pain relief and relaxation is an available option. A long soaking bath, whirlpool bath, or shower can be a marvelous comfort measure during labor. The warmth and buoyancy of the bathwater or the gentle massage provided by the showerhead or whirlpool jets can help your body relax.

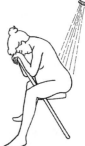

If you take a bath during labor, you may get instant relief or it may take up to twenty minutes before you feel relaxed. (Try to stay in the water for at least this long before giving up and trying another pain relief option.) When in the water, you can lean back against a bath pillow or folded towels. If the tub is large enough and you're uncomfortable sitting up or lying on your back, try kneeling and leaning over the side of the tub (especially helpful for relieving back pain) or lying on your side with your head elevated on a bath pillow.

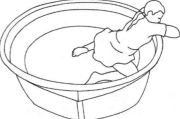

Be sure the water temperature stays around your normal body temperature: 98°F to 99°F (36.7°C to 37.2°C). This temperature is warm enough that you can comfortably stay in the water for an extended period (possibly up to ninety minutes), but not so warm that you become overheated and need to

## Advice from the Authors

If you're planning a home birth, be aware that long showers or soaks in a large tub may use up your regular hot water supply before you're ready to get out of the water. To ensure you'll have enough hot water during labor, turn up the temperature on your water heater in advance. As a precaution against burns, leave a note that warns of the hot water temperature by each faucet in your home, and make sure to keep small children away from faucets.

get out of the water to cool off. If you let your body temperature rise, you'll increase your baby's temperature, which will cause her heart to beat too rapidly.

If you take a shower, lean against the shower wall or sit on a towel-covered stool or birth ball so you can rest. Direct the spray where it best relieves tension. (Directing it against your lower back helps immensely to relieve back pain.) If you like (and if there's room), your partner can accompany you in the shower or tub to provide additional comfort measures such as massage. (If you'll be birthing in a hospital or birth center, make sure he or she packs a swimsuit.)

In the past, maternity care experts believed that letting a woman bathe after her membranes had ruptured would lead to infection; however, the results of several studies show that this belief is false.[3] Rather, in addition to relieving pain, taking a bath or shower may lower blood pressure if it's elevated and can affect labor progress. For example, taking a warm bath in early labor may slow down your contractions,[4] which is helpful if your labor progress has been slow and you need to rest. As a result, however, you may need a medical intervention such as the medication Pitocin to speed up labor later on. If you don't want to slow down contractions in early labor, take a shower and use other comfort measures instead of taking a bath. In active labor, taking a bath often speeds up labor while delaying the intensity of the pain.[5]

## FOODS AND FLUIDS

To keep up your energy in early labor, eat high-carbohydrate foods that appeal to you, such as fruit, pasta, toast, rice, and waffles. Also eat and drink easy-to-digest foods and beverages, such as soup, broth, and herbal tea. As labor progresses, you may become less interested in food; however, hunger (or low blood sugar levels) may decrease your tolerance for pain. You may lose your appetite when you begin active labor, but your need for fluids will continue. If labor progresses normally, you can sip clear broths, suck on Popsicles, or drink water, tea, juice, or sports drinks to quench your thirst and keep your body hydrated. Because a full bladder may slow labor and increase pain, be sure to empty your bladder often.

If you're planning to give birth at home or at a freestanding birth center, your caregiver will probably encourage you to eat and drink during labor. If you'll be giving birth in a hospital, find out the policy on eating and drinking during labor, so you'll know what to expect in advance. Some hospitals have no restrictions against eating and drinking in labor. Other hospitals restrict eating throughout labor or after active labor begins, but permit drinking fluids. A few hospitals don't permit women to eat *or* drink in labor, in case they need a cesarean section or require general anesthesia; however, this policy is controversial. A recent review of the research found no clear advantages or disadvantages of eating or drinking during labor for women at low-risk of needing general anesthesia. It concluded that women should be free to eat and drink in labor as they wish.[6]

If your caregiver won't permit you to drink fluids in labor, your labor is prolonged, or you're vomiting, you'll probably receive fluids intravenously to prevent dehydration. A rolling intravenous

## Water Births

The idea of water birth appeals to some expectant parents as a relaxing and gentle way to bring a baby into the world, and they seek out a birthplace and caregiver that support this option. Many caregivers who attend births at homes and at freestanding birth centers (unaffiliated with a hospital) are comfortable with water births.

Sometimes a woman who hadn't planned ahead for a water birth discovers during labor that a bath is so relaxing and helpful for relieving pain, she doesn't want to leave the water when she's ready to push. If she's giving birth in a hospital, however, she might not have a choice. Although laboring in the bath is common in most U.S. and Canadian hospitals, few have policies that allow women to give birth in water. Many hospital administrators (and caregivers) have the following objections to water births:

- Concerns about the baby's safety
- The caregiver's need to master new techniques to facilitate birth positions and to protect the woman's perineum
- The physical agility needed by the caregiver to deliver the baby
- Extra difficulty managing a difficult or complicated birth
- Other practical concerns, such as extra precautions for infection control (for example, shoulder-length gloves for caregivers and nurses) and insufficient room around the tub for access to the woman

Although these concerns can be addressed, few U.S. and Canadian hospitals do so. If you're interested in learning more about water birth, visit http://www.waterbirth.org.

(IV) unit allows you to move around, walk, and shower or bathe while receiving fluids. You may develop a very dry mouth; sucking on ice chips, a Popsicle, or a sour lollipop will help moisten it. You may also try brushing your teeth or rinsing your mouth with cold water or mouthwash.

## HEAT AND COLD

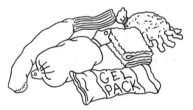

An electric heating pad or hot-water bottle on your lower abdomen, back, groin, or perineum relieves labor pain. Another soothing heat source is a cloth bag or sock filled with uncooked rice or other grain and heated in a microwave. You can also soak washcloths in hot water, wring them out, and apply them wherever you need relief. Wrapping these warm compresses in plastic retains their heat longer. If you'll be birthing in a hospital, check whether there are any restrictions on heating devices brought from home. (If so, only warm compresses will be allowed.)

A cold pack on your lower back can relieve back pain, too. (Ice packs may also soothe your perineum immediately after the birth.) Examples of cold packs include a cool wet cloth, a bag of ice cubes or frozen peas, frozen wet washcloths, cold cans of soda, or frozen gel packs used to treat athletic injuries (preferably those with straps so you can move about while wearing one). When using a cold pack, wear a warm robe or use a blanket to avoid feeling chilled.

## Two Views on Comfort Measures

By the time we reached the hospital, my contractions were quite stunning! I was 3 centimeters dilated. I used the birth ball, but it seemed to increase the pain. The whirlpool tub saved me! I spent an hour in there, which helped me relax. When I got out of the tub, I'd dilated to 10 centimeters, so I could push.
—*Clarissa*

Once labor began, it felt natural and empowering to use the tub, birth ball, and breathing and vocal rhythms to process the pain. Thanks to those comfort measures and my doula's and my husband's gentle coaching, I was very aware throughout labor.
—*Susan*

During labor, your tolerance for heat and cold might be affected, and you might not notice that a compress is too hot or cold for your skin. To prevent injury, have your partner test the heat source or cold pack before applying it to your skin. He or she should be able to hold it in his or her hand for several seconds without pain. Have one or more layers of cloth between your skin and the heat source or cold pack to protect your skin and to let you adapt to the temperature change gradually. If you're given pain medication that causes loss of sensation (such as epidural anesthesia), avoid using heat or cold on numbed areas to prevent skin damage.

## COMFORT ITEMS

The following is a list of items that can provide comfort during labor. You may already have some; most others are easy to find.

- Rolling pin or rolling massage devices, plus other massage aids (for back pain—see page 231)
- Gardener's foam knee pad (for kneeling on the bed, floor, or in the tub)
- Shawl or rebozo (for abdominal lift—see page 229)
- Warm blanket and socks (Hospitals typically provide only light cotton blankets.)
- Fan (Labor is often hard, sweaty work.)
- iPod or MP3 player (Listening to favorite music or motivating dialogue can provide encouragement and comfort.)
- Transcutaneous electrical nerve stimulation (TENS) unit (See page 231.)
- Birth ball (See below.)

You may have other objects in mind, but these items provide a good foundation for comfort and pain relief in labor.

### *Birth Ball*

A *birth ball* is the same thing as a physical therapy or fitness ball: a large inflatable plastic ball that provides a soft yet firm place to sit comfortably. Because the ball forces you to have proper posture when you sit on it, it can help decrease muscle strain.

When in labor, you can use a birth ball to help with positioning and relaxation. For example, to help relax your trunk and perineum, sit on the ball and sway your hips from side to side during and between contractions. Or to help relieve back pain and adjust your baby's position, place the ball on your bed, then either kneel on the bed or stand next to it and lean over the ball. Sway your hips from side to side or from front to back. The ball allows such movement to be comforting and almost effortless—a definite advantage when you're tired from the hard work of labor.

Many hospitals and birth centers provide birth balls, but you may wish to own one. You can inflate it to your desired firmness and use it at home for comfort and for prenatal or postpartum exercises. (You can also use a birth ball after the birth to soothe your baby by bouncing gently on the ball while holding him.) Birth balls are available at many chain discount retailers such as Target and Walmart, hospital physical therapy departments, sporting goods stores, and birth supply companies.

Birth balls come in different sizes. A ball with a 65-centimeter diameter is best for a woman of average height (63 to 70 inches). A much shorter woman may require a ball with a 55-centimeter diameter, and a much taller woman may require a ball with a 75-centimeter diameter. Make sure the ball is strong enough to hold your weight without bursting; a ball strength of at least 300 pounds should be adequate for most women.

Practice using a birth ball before your labor begins. Put one hand on the ball as you carefully lower yourself onto it. Use your other hand to hold on to someone or a stable object. With practice, you'll be able to use the ball without support. Because the ball may get sticky or pick up germs from being on the floor, cover it with a towel before sitting or leaning on it.

## MASSAGE AND TOUCH

Massage and touch are two of the most effective ways to direct your attention away from labor pain. Being massaged or touched in a manner that you find enjoyable can convey encouragement, reassurance, support, and love. Having someone firmly stroke, rub, or knead your neck, shoulders, back, feet, or hands can be soothing and relaxing. Having someone lightly stroke your back or thighs can also help with relaxation and pain relief. You may find relief if someone presses firmly on tense areas such as your hips, thighs, shoulders, hands, or lower back. Other tactile ways to focus your attention away from pain include tightly embracing your partner or directing the spray from a hand-held showerhead onto tense areas.

To relax and relieve pain by yourself, try lightly and rhythmically stroking your belly, following the lower curve of your uterus, imagining that you're stroking your baby's head. Or stroke your belly in circles with one or both hands. To make your hands slide more easily on your skin, dust your palms with cornstarch or baby powder. Breathe slowly as you massage your belly, matching your movements with your breaths.

### Crisscross Massage

The crisscross massage can ease back pain and relax your lower back muscles during or between contractions. Here's how you and your partner can practice this technique in pregnancy so it's most helpful during labor.

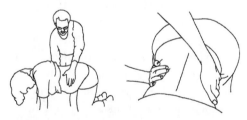

Kneel forward on your hands and knees or over a birth ball, or lean forward onto a counter, chair, or birth ball. Flex your hips so your thighs are about 90 degrees from your spine. Your partner stands or kneels next to you, facing your side. He or she then places a hand on each side of your body at the narrowest part of your waist, with the fingers on the far hand pointing down and the fingers on the near hand pointing up. (See illustration.)

Next, your partner firmly presses into your sides, then moves each hand up and over your back, following your waistline with each hand passing the other as it continues to the other hand's starting place. Your partner then uses the same firm pressure to return the hands to their original starting positions. Have your partner repeat this motion for as long as you like, trying to match the movements with the rhythm of your breathing or moaning.

## Acupressure for Comfort and Progress in Labor

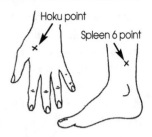

Hoku point

Spleen 6 point

By pressing a finger or thumb on a certain acupressure point, you or your partner may reduce your pain and speed up labor. The two most popular points are Hoku and Spleen 6. The Hoku point is on the back of your hand, in the V formed where the bones extending below your thumb and index finger come together. The Spleen 6 point is on the inner side of your leg, about the width of four fingers above your inner anklebone.

Press your thumb steadily into the point for ten to sixty seconds, then rest for the same length of time before pressing again. Repeat this pattern three to six times whenever you want during labor. Be aware that these spots are sensitive and may hurt a bit when pressed.

## Warning about Acupressure

Maternity care experts advise against pressing on the Hoku and Spleen 6 points before your due date, because doing so can cause contractions and may increase the risk of preterm labor. During your pregnancy, have your partner find these points on his or her body but not press them on your body until after your thirty-eighth week of pregnancy.

## A NOTE TO FATHERS AND PARTNERS

Practicing comfort measures and relaxation techniques during pregnancy not only allows you and your pregnant partner to adapt them to your own style, but it also increases the likelihood that you'll remember how to do them when under the stress of labor.

Here are suggestions for how you can practice together. Many of these tips will also be useful in labor.

- To signal the beginning of a practice contraction, your partner says, "Here it comes," or begins to breathe rhythmically. You both practice coping techniques for the next thirty to sixty seconds, until she says, "It's over." Take turns starting the contractions so you both get used to beginning a coping technique whether you're ready or not.
- To understand the effectiveness of a comfort measure, try this experiment: Each of you holds an ice cube in one hand for a minute while breathing rhythmically or using another comfort measure. Then switch the ice cube to the other hand and hold it for another minute without using the comfort measure. You'll probably be surprised and reassured to discover how much better you tolerated the cold when using the comfort measure.
- If the above experiment helps your partner realize the effectiveness of a comfort measure, suggest that she hold ice cubes to simulate contractions as you practice other comfort measures together. It may help her determine which techniques are most effective.
- While practicing, try to detect any tension your partner is holding. Help her relax by touching or massaging her, talking to her, reminding her to move around, breathing with her, or steadying her breathing with a visual cue such as by moving your hand as though conducting an orchestra to keep a rhythm.
- Be aware of your facial expressions, tone of voice, and way of touching your partner. You'll convey anxiety by having a troubled expression, speaking loudly or worriedly, and rubbing your partner brusquely or distractedly. You'll convey reassurance and encouragement by having a confident expression, speaking soothingly, and massaging your partner smoothly and slowly.

# Relaxation and Tension Release

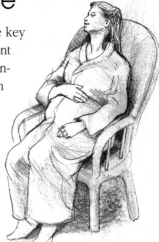

Relaxation is the art of recognizing and releasing muscle tension; it's the key to finding comfort during labor. Remaining relaxed is especially important during early labor, when contractions are usually manageable. If you consciously release muscle tension during early contractions, you'll establish a habit of keeping relaxed during the intense contractions of active labor and transition. Conversely, if you tense up during early contractions, you'll have trouble relaxing in later labor.

Here are just some of the benefits of relaxation during labor:

**Conserves energy and reduces fatigue**

If you don't consciously relax your muscles during contractions, you'll probably unconsciously tense them. Tension wastes energy and increases pain and fatigue.

**Calms your mind and reduces stress**

A relaxed body leads to a relaxed state of mind, which in turn reduces stress. Anxiety, anger, or fear causes stress in labor, which produces excessive *catecholamines* (stress hormones) such as epinephrine (adrenaline) and norepinephrine (noradrenaline). High levels of these hormones can prolong your labor by decreasing the efficiency of your contractions and can harm your baby by decreasing the blood flow to your uterus.[7] (See page 242 for more information on stress hormones.)

**Reduces pain**

Relaxation allows more oxygen to reach your contracting uterus, which may decrease pain because a working muscle becomes painful when deprived of oxygen. In addition, consciously releasing tension focuses your attention away from the contractions and reduces your awareness of pain.

## RECOGNIZING MUSCLE TENSION

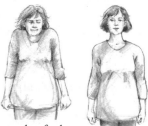

In order to release muscle tension, you first need to be able to recognize it. Try this exercise to practice recognizing muscle tension:

1. Sit on a chair or the floor.
2. Make a tight fist with your right hand. Pay attention to how hard the muscles in your forearm feel. Touch them with your left hand.
3. Relax your right hand, letting it droop. Notice how soft the forearm muscles feel.
4. Raise your shoulders toward your ears and tense up. Notice how tight you feel when your shoulders are tense.
5. Lower your shoulders and relax. Then relax even further. Do you notice an additional release? You can often release residual muscle tension when you become aware of it.

## PRACTICING TENSION RELEASE WITH YOUR PARTNER

As you become aware of muscle tension and learn how to relax, your partner also can learn how to recognize when you're tense and when you're relaxed by using the following methods:

- Observation (How do you look when you're anxious, uncomfortable, calm, content, or asleep?)
- Touch (How do your muscles feel? Hard or soft?)
- "Floating a limb" (Your partner lifts one of your arms or legs, and moves the joints, feeling for the looseness and heaviness that signal relaxation.)

Help your partner practice spotting muscle tension by deliberately tightening the muscles of your arm or leg and having your partner locate the tense limb. If your partner assesses your body calmly and gently, you'll develop confidence in his or her ability to help you relax in labor.

Once your partner has located the tension, find out what releases it. Your partner may touch or massage the area, place a warm compress on it, or simply remind you to let those muscles relax. You may explore other options together to determine what techniques best release your tension. See below for a discussion on relaxation techniques.

As you practice together, you'll learn which muscles you tense most often (and thus may be the most difficult to relax). You may discover that you frequently tense your shoulders, forehead, mouth, jaw, or fists. These areas, or *tension spots*, should receive special attention as you practice relaxation and especially during labor.

# Relaxation Techniques

Once you can recognize muscle tension in your body, the next step is to learn how to release that tension. By focusing on different parts of your body and consciously releasing the tension in them, you can relax both your body and mind.

Some women are able to relax more easily than others, but almost anyone can learn to relax with practice. The following sections describe several relaxation techniques. Try them all at least once, but practice only those that appeal to you and seem to best relax you.

When you first begin practicing a relaxation technique, lie on your side with plenty of pillows supporting you, or sit in a comfortable chair with your head and arms supported. After you've mastered the relaxation technique in this position, practice it while sitting up (or lying down, if your first position was sitting), standing, and walking. You'll use various positions during labor, so you'll need to be able to relax in any position.

Begin practicing a relaxation technique in a quiet, calm area. As you master the technique, progress to practicing it in louder, more active surroundings. Especially if you'll be laboring in a hospital, you'll need to be able to relax in a noisy, busy environment.

When you're done practicing a technique, stretch your arms and legs and rise slowly (if seated or lying down) to avoid becoming lightheaded or dizzy.

## PASSIVE RELAXATION

This exercise calls for your partner to guide you through steps to relax your entire body, while you rest in a comfortable position. (If your partner is unavailable, use a relaxation CD to guide you. Consider playing pleasant, relaxing music each time you practice this technique. Playing the same music will help create a familiar and relaxed environment that you'll find comforting when you use this technique during labor.

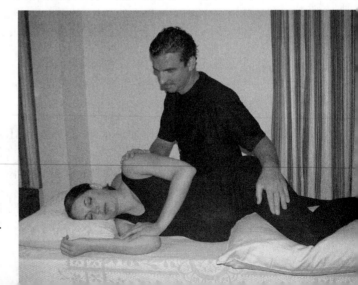

## *Practicing Passive Relaxation*

To get into position for this exercise, lie on your side or sit in a semi-reclined position with the floor or bed supporting your head and limbs. Take your time getting comfortable. You may want to put pillows under or between your knees, beneath your head, or under your belly to increase comfort and support.

To practice this exercise, begin breathing slowly, easily, and fully. This is how you breathe as you fall asleep: Your body and mind release tension and thought, your breathing slows, and you pause slightly at the end of each inhalation and exhalation. (To see this process in action, observe the way someone else's breathing gradually slows as he or she falls asleep.)

Next, have your partner read the following script in a calm, relaxed voice.

## Script for Passive Relaxation

Have your partner read the following script calmly and slowly, letting you focus on releasing the tension in each area of your body. Take a couple of breaths after you release each area.

1. Yawn or exhale completely.
2. Focus on your toes and feet. Feel how warm and relaxed they are.
3. Think about how floppy and loose your ankles are. They're relaxed and comfortable.
4. Now focus on your lower legs. Let those muscles become loose and soft. Good.
5. Now focus on your knees. They're supported and relaxed—you're not holding your legs in any position. Wiggle them to see how relaxed they are.
6. Think about your thighs. Their large, strong muscles are soft and relaxed, and they're fully supported. Good.
7. And now think about your buttocks and perineum. This area needs to be especially relaxed during labor and birth, so just let it become soft and yielding. When the time is right, your baby will travel down the birth canal, and the tissues of your perineum will spread to let your baby make her way out. You'll release, letting your perineum relax and open for your baby.
8. Focus on your lower back. Imagine that someone with strong, warm hands is giving you a lovely backrub. It feels so good. Your muscles are relaxing, and your lower back is comfortable. Notice the tension leaving your back.
9. Let your thoughts turn to your belly. Let those muscles relax. Let your belly rise and fall as you breathe in and out. Good. Now focus on your baby within your uterus. She's floating or wiggling and squirming in the warm water of your womb—a safe place where you're meeting all your baby's needs for nourishment, oxygen, warmth, movement, and stimulation. Your baby hears your heartbeat, your voice, my voice, and other interesting sounds. What excellent care you're giving your baby.
10. Now focus on your chest. As you inhale, your chest swells easily, making room for the air. As you exhale, your chest relaxes to help the air flow out. Breathe easily and slowly, letting the air flow in and flow out, almost as though you're asleep. Good.

    Now try inhaling through your nose and exhaling through your mouth—slowly and easily, letting the air flow in and out. At the top of an inhalation, notice just a little tension in your chest, which you can release with an exhalation. Listen as you exhale. Your breath sounds relaxed and calm, almost as if you were asleep. Every exhalation is relaxing. Use your exhalations to breathe away any tension. Good. *Continued on the next page*

*Script for Passive Relaxation, continued*

11. Focus on your shoulders and upper back. Imagine you've just had them massaged. Let those muscles release. Feel the warmth as the tension slips away.

12. Now focus on your arms. As you exhale, let your arms go limp—from your shoulders, all the way down your arms, to your wrists, hands, and fingers. Let them become heavy, loose, and relaxed.

13. And now your neck. All the muscles in your neck are soft because they don't have to hold your head in any position. Your head is either comfortably balanced or completely supported, so just let your neck relax. Good.

14. Focus on your lips and jaw. They're slack and relaxed. You're not holding your mouth closed or open. It's comfortable; no tension there.

15. And now your eyes and eyelids. You're not keeping your eyes open or closed. They're the way they want to be. Your eyes are unfocused and still. Your eyelids are relaxed and heavy.

16. Focus on your brow and scalp. Think about how warm and relaxed they are. You have a calm, peaceful expression on your face, reflecting a calm, peaceful feeling inside.

17. Take a few moments to enjoy these feelings of calmness and well-being. You can relax this way anytime—before bedtime, during an afternoon rest, or during a quiet break. This is how you'll want to feel in labor. Of course, during labor, you won't lie down all the time. You'll walk, sit up, shower, and change positions. But whenever a contraction comes, you'll let yourself relax all the muscles you don't need to hold a position, and you'll let your mind relax, giving you a confident, peaceful feeling. This feeling will help you yield to contractions, letting you focus on breathing and finding comfort through each one.

18. Now it's time to end the exercise. Gradually open your eyes, stretch, tune in to your surroundings, and slowly rise. Take your time. There's no need to rush.

## RELAXATION COUNTDOWN

Once you've learned to recognize muscle tension and have mastered passive relaxation, use the following technique to release tension quickly. This exercise uses your breathing to create a wave of relaxation that passes from your head to your toes. It's particularly helpful when you want to fall back to sleep, when you're stressed, or when you're trying to relax after a contraction.

### Practicing the Relaxation Countdown

Inhale through your nose. As you exhale through your mouth, release muscle tension in the following order. By the time you count down to one, you'll be fully relaxed.

5. Head, neck, and shoulders
4. Arms, hands, and fingers
3. Chest and abdomen
2. Back, buttocks, and perineum
1. Legs, feet, and toes

At first, use five slow breaths (one for each of the five areas) to count down to total body relaxation. Then try to relax all five areas while slowly exhaling one deep breath (rapid relaxation countdown).

During labor, you can use the first or last breath of each contraction as a rapid relaxation countdown to maximize tension release and reduce discomfort or pain.

# TOUCH RELAXATION

For this technique, you relax or release tension in response to your partner's comforting touch. During pregnancy, this exercise is a pleasurable way to practice relaxation. During labor, you'll use your partner's touching, stroking, or massaging as a cue to relax.

To begin this exercise, lie on your side or sit in a comfortable position. Next, contract a set of muscles (for example, stiffen one arm or leg) and have your partner use a firm yet relaxed hand to touch the tense area, molding his or her hand around the muscles. Release the tension and relax into your partner's hand. Imagine the tension leaving that part of your body.

Have your partner try the following types of touch. Tell him or her which types you prefer, but be sure to practice all of them. Your preference may change during labor.

**Still touch**

Your partner places a relaxed hand on the tense area while you release the muscle tension until you're relaxed.

**Firm pressure**

Your partner firmly presses on the tense area, then gradually relaxes the pressure as you release the tension.

**Stroking**

Your partner lightly strokes the tense area as you let the tension flow out. If stroking your arms or legs, he or she strokes in the direction of your fingers or toes. When stroking your belly, your partner may make circles.

**Massage**

Your partner firmly rubs or kneads your tense muscles. Give feedback on the amount of pressure that feels best to you.

Whenever your partner uses a touch relaxation technique, he or she should always keep one hand in contact with your body. When your eyes are closed, it'll be hard for you to relax if your partner's touch disappears, leaving you to wonder where and when it'll reappear.

## *Practicing Touch Relaxation*

Practice contracting the following muscle groups, then releasing them in response to your partner's touch.

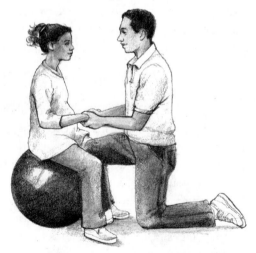

- Brow and eyes
- Jaw
- Neck
- Shoulders
- Arms and hands
- Abdomen
- Buttocks
- Legs and feet

# ROVING BODY CHECK

Sometimes you may think you're entirely relaxed, but you're still retaining tension in one or more areas of your body. This exercise helps you systematically release tension throughout your entire body, allowing for deeper relaxation.

## *Practicing the Roving Body Check*

Get into a comfortable position and begin breathing slowly, rhythmically, and easily, inhaling through your nose and exhaling through your mouth. Focus on one area of your body with each breath. As you inhale, notice any tension in that area. As you exhale, deliberately release that tension. Then focus on another area. Note any tension as you inhale and release it as you exhale. Repeat, moving your attention from one area to another in the following order:

1. Brow, eyes, and eyelids
2. Jaw and lips
3. Neck and shoulders
4. Right arm and hand
5. Left arm and hand
6. Upper back
7. Lower back
8. Buttocks and perineum
9. Right leg and foot
10. Left leg and foot

Use the roving body check during or between labor contractions to make sure you're releasing tension throughout your body. Your partner can help by telling you which area to relax with each exhalation, or by touching or stroking a different area with each exhalation. You may prefer to have your partner focus only on those areas you know are tense.

### RELAXING IN DIFFERENT POSITIONS AND WHILE ACTIVE

During labor, you'll use various positions and frequently move around to find comfort and to help your labor progress. For this reason, it's important to practice relaxation techniques when you're not lying down and inactive. Different positions require different muscle groups to support you, and your aim is to completely relax the muscles you don't need to use while in a position. For example, you can't relax your legs while standing, but you can relax your shoulders, arms, and face. Relaxing these muscle groups will help you achieve the same relaxed mental state you have while practicing passive relaxation (see page 216).

# Movement and Positions for Labor

Moving around and changing positions allow you to discover ways to be comfortable during labor. Using different positions may speed up a slow labor by changing the shape of your pelvis and by using gravity, both of which help your baby rotate and descend into your birth canal. Changing positions can also affect your mind-set during labor. For example, being in an upright position may give you a greater sense of control and active involvement in your labor than when you're lying down.

The following chart describes positions and movements that you can use during the first and second stages of labor. You may also find swaying from side to side, rocking, or making other rhythmic movements to be comforting. Plan to change positions at least every thirty minutes, especially if your labor progress is slow.

## Positions and Movements for the First Stage of Labor

| Position or Movement | What This Position or Movement Does | |
|---|---|---|
| Standing | • Takes advantage of gravity.<br>• Makes contractions less painful and more productive.<br>• Helps your baby descend by lining him up with the angle of your pelvis.<br>• May speed up labor if you've been lying down.<br>• May increase your urge to push during the second stage of labor. | |
| Walking | *Same as standing, plus:*<br>• Causes rhythmic shifts in the shape of your pelvis, nudging your baby to rotate and descend.<br>• Can tire you if you walk for too long. | |
| Standing and leaning forward on your partner, bed, or birth ball | *Same as standing, plus:*<br>• Relieves back pain.<br>• Is a good position for a back rub.<br>• May be more restful than standing.<br>• Encourages your baby to rotate if he's occiput posterior (OP—see page 285). | |
| Slow dancing | *Same as walking, plus:*<br>• Enhances your sense of well-being, because a loved one is embracing you.<br>• Increases comfort through rhythm and music.<br>• Is a good position for your partner to give back pressure. | |
| Lunge (See page 230.) | • Widens one side of your pelvis.<br>• Encourages your baby to rotate if he's OP.<br>• Can be done while standing or kneeling. | |
| Sitting upright* | • Is a good resting position.<br>• Uses gravity (to a degree). | |
| Sitting or rocking in chair | *Same as sitting upright, plus:*<br>• May speed up your labor because of the rocking movement.<br>• May increase your comfort. | |
| Sitting, leaning forward with support | *Same as sitting upright, plus:*<br>• Relieves back pain.<br>• Is a good position to receive a back rub. | |
| Open knee-chest position (See page 229.) | If your baby is OP and you use the position in early labor, gravity will encourage your baby to back his head out of your pelvis and rotate.<br>• Helps in early labor to relieve back pain and encourage cervical dilation.<br>• In later labor, reduces pressure on your cervix if it's swollen. | |
| Semi-prone* | *Same as side-lying (see page 222), plus:*<br>• May help your baby rotate into a position better suited for birth. | |

For more information on labor positions, see pages 229–230.
* Can be used if you receive epidural anesthesia (although you may need support).

## Positions and Movements for Either the First or Second Stage of Labor

| Position or Movement | What This Position or Movement Does |
|---|---|
| Sitting on toilet or commode* | *Same as sitting upright, plus:*<br>• Helps with effective pushing and prevents holding back (because of the position's association with bearing down to have a bowel movement). |
| Semi-sitting* | *Same as sitting upright, plus:*<br>• Is an easy position to get into (on the bed or delivery table).<br>• Is a common birthing position.<br>• *Disadvantages:* May increase back pain and does not allow expansion of the pelvis. |
| Hands-and-knees* | • Helps relieve back pain.<br>• Helps your baby rotate if she's OP.<br>• Allows for pelvic rocking (see page 229).<br>• Takes pressure off hemorrhoids.<br>• May reduce premature urge to push.<br>• May slow a rapid second stage of labor because the position neutralizes the effects of gravity. |
| Side-lying* | • Is an excellent resting position.<br>• May reduce back pain.<br>• Helps lower your blood pressure.<br>• Is a safe position if you've received pain medications.<br>• Neutralizes the effects of gravity, making the position useful for slowing a rapid labor.<br>• Takes pressure off hemorrhoids.<br>• In the second stage, allows your sacrum to shift to create a wider opening for your baby's descent. |

## Positions and Movements for the Second Stage of Labor

| Position or Movement | What This Position or Movement Does |
|---|---|
| Squatting | • May relieve back pain.<br>• Takes advantage of gravity.<br>• Widens your pelvic outlet (but may diminish your pelvic inlet, which is why this position is best to do in the second stage and not the first).<br>• May enable your baby to rotate and descend in a difficult birth.<br>• Is helpful if you don't feel an urge to push.<br>• Allows you the freedom to shift your weight for comfort. |
| Lap squatting | *Same as squatting, plus:*<br>• Reduces strain on your knees and ankles (when compared to squatting).<br>• Allows more support and requires less effort (ideal if you're exhausted).<br>• Enhances your sense of well-being, because a loved one is embracing you.<br>• *Disadvantage:* If you're much heavier than your partner, this position might not be possible. |

For more information on labor positions, see pages 229–230.
* Can be used if you receive epidural anesthesia (although you may need support).

## Positions and Movements for the Second Stage of Labor

| Position or Movement | What This Position or Movement Does |
|---|---|
| Supported squat | • Allows greater mobility of pelvic joints than any other position, and eliminates external pressure (from the bed, chair, and so on).<br>• Takes advantage of gravity.<br>• Lengthens your trunk, allowing more room for your baby to maneuver into position.<br>• Allows your baby's head movements to change the shape of your pelvis.<br>• *Disadvantage:* Requires your partner to have strength enough to support you for long periods. |
| Dangle | *Same as the supported squat, except your partner sits so his or her legs are braced and well supported, making this position easier to sustain.* |

For more information on labor positions, see pages 229–230.
\* Can be used if you receive epidural anesthesia (although you may need support).

# Breathing Techniques as Comfort Measures

When you swim, run, practice yoga, sing, or play a musical instrument, you need to regulate your breathing to perform effectively and efficiently. In this way, labor is no different from any other activity that requires physical coordination and mental discipline. Each childbirth preparation method focuses on some form of breath awareness because of the following benefits:

• Enhances relaxation.

• Helps reduce pain by supplying your muscles with oxygen.

• Provides a focus to calm you and distract you from pain. Breathing won't make labor pain completely disappear, but it'll help make pain more manageable.

The rhythm you'll use to breathe during labor depends on your preferences and on the nature and intensity of your contractions. In early labor, you'll likely use slow breathing for as long as it relaxes you. You may continue to breathe slowly for your entire labor, or you may switch to light breathing or some variation in late labor.

During pregnancy, try to master the breathing techniques described in the following sections, even though you might not use them all. You can't be sure that your favorite techniques *before* labor will be the same *during* labor. Practice rhythmic breathing in the positions shown on pages 221–223. Use the illustrations accompanying the descriptions of the breathing techniques as a visual guide to the typical length and intensity of contractions.

You can combine rhythmic breathing with other comfort measures, such as moaning, movement, massage, tension release, hot or cold packs, bath, shower, and so on. Through practice, experimentation, and adaptation, you'll discover how best to use and adapt the techniques to help you relax in labor.

## AVOIDING HYPERVENTILATION

When you breathe too deeply or too quickly (or both), you exhale too much carbon dioxide, which alters the balance of oxygen and carbon dioxide in your blood and may cause *hyperventilation* (overbreathing). While rarely serious, hyperventilation makes you feel lightheaded or dizzy, or it can make your fingers, feet, or the area around your mouth tingle. If you've mastered rhythmic breathing before labor begins, you're unlikely to hyperventilate during contractions. Without even thinking about it, you'll adapt the pace and depth of your breathing to your changing needs in labor.

If hyperventilation occurs, try these suggestions to correct it:

- Breathe into your cupped hands, a paper bag, or a surgical mask (available if you're in a hospital).
- Hold your breath after a contraction until you feel the need to inhale. This will allow carbon dioxide levels in your blood to normalize.
- Relax and reduce tension and anxiety, which can lead to hyperventilation. Taking a shower or bath, having a massage, using touch relaxation (see page 219), or listening to music may help you relax.
- Breathe with a slower rhythm or breathe more shallowly. Your partner can help you pace your breathing with a visual cue (such as by moving a hand as though conducting an orchestra to keep a rhythm), by talking to you in time with your breathing, by using rhythmic stroking, or by breathing with you. (*Note:* If your partner hyperventilates, he or she should use any of these measures to correct it.)

## SLOW BREATHING

In labor, slow breathing can help calm you. The keys to the technique are keeping an even rhythm and trying to release tension during exhalations. Begin using slow breathing when your contractions become so intense that you can't walk or talk through them or can't be distracted from them. Use slow breathing for as long as it comforts you—probably until you're well into the first stage of labor and possibly throughout your entire labor. Shift to light breathing or a variation if you strain to keep your breathing slow at the peaks of contractions.

### *Using Slow Breathing in Labor*

Here are the steps that explain how to use slow breathing in labor.

1. As soon as a contraction begins, inhale fully and easily and sigh as you exhale, releasing all tension. Use this as your "organizing" breath or as a signal to your partner. If your partner is timing contractions (see page 175), he or she will note the time.

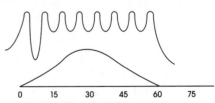

2. Focus your attention. (See pages 208–209.)
3. Inhale slowly through your nose and exhale completely through your mouth. Pause for a moment before you inhale. Take about five to twelve breaths per minute (this is about half your normal breathing rate).
4. Inhale quietly, but keep your mouth slightly open and relaxed when exhaling so someone nearby can hear your breath. In labor, you may also vocalize or moan as you exhale.
5. Keep your shoulders down and relaxed. Relax your chest and belly so they can swell as you inhale. Your partner should touch you, move around you, and talk to you in rhythm with your breathing.

6. Signal to your partner as the contraction ends or take a final deep breath. You may prefer to yawn to mark the end of a contraction.
7. Completely relax, change positions, sip liquids, and do whatever you need to feel comfortable.

## Rehearsing Slow Breathing for Labor

Rehearse slow breathing until you're confident in your ability to use the technique for sixty to ninety seconds at a time (the typical length of a contraction). Practice it while in different positions. With each exhalation, focus on relaxing a different part of your body (see page 219 for the Roving Body Check) so you can relax every muscle that's not required to maintain your position.

While practicing slow breathing, you may find it uncomfortable to inhale through your nose and exhale through your mouth. If this is the case, you can breathe only through your nose or mouth. You may find that you prefer letting your belly expand first, then your chest, as you inhale deeply (belly breathing). Or you may prefer letting only your chest expand as you inhale (deep chest breathing). However you practice slow breathing, make sure it's rhythmic, calming, and relaxing.

## LIGHT BREATHING

Light breathing helps you manage labor pain when you can no longer relax during contractions, when the contractions are too painful with slow breathing, or when you instinctively begin speeding up your breathing. Many women feel the need to switch to light breathing when contractions are close together and intense. When you're in active labor, let your responses to contractions help you decide when to begin using light breathing. If your partner notices that you're losing your rhythm, tensing, grimacing, clenching your fists, or crying out at the peak of a contraction, he or she may suggest switching to light breathing.

## Using Light Breathing in Labor

Here are the steps that explain how to use light breathing in labor.

1. As soon as you feel a contraction begin, take a quick, shallow inhalation and signal to your partner that the contraction has begun. Exhale quickly to release all tension—go completely limp.
2. Focus your attention. (See pages 208–209.)
3. Take short, light, and shallow breaths, inhaling and 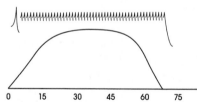 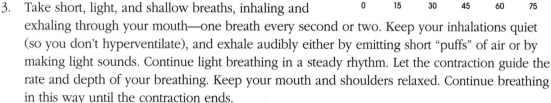 exhaling through your mouth—one breath every second or two. Keep your inhalations quiet (so you don't hyperventilate), and exhale audibly either by emitting short "puffs" of air or by making light sounds. Continue light breathing in a steady rhythm. Let the contraction guide the rate and depth of your breathing. Keep your mouth and shoulders relaxed. Continue breathing in this way until the contraction ends.
4. When the contraction ends, use your last exhalation to "sigh" the contraction away. Then tell your partner that the contraction is over.
5. Completely relax and do whatever you need to feel comfortable, such as change positions, sip liquids, and so on.

Advice from the Authors

**Tips for Partners When Using Breathing Techniques**
During a one-minute practice contraction, interject encouraging words or phrases as you count your pregnant partner's breaths. For example, say, "One, okay. Two, good. Three, let go. Four, just like that. Five, great...." During labor, the number of breaths she'll take to get through a contraction won't vary significantly from one contraction to the next.

This means you'll be able to figure out when a contraction is at its peak and half over. When counting her breaths, point out when she has passed the halfway point—information she'll be encouraged to receive. As one woman recalled, "Having my partner tell me when a contraction was half over seemed to cut its intensity in half. I knew that when I had passed the peak, I could make it the rest of the way."

## Rehearsing Light Breathing for Labor

When you first begin practicing light breathing, you may feel that the technique isn't right for you. It may make you tense, or it may make you feel as though you're not getting enough air. With practice, however, light breathing will become second nature and you'll be able to work with your body much more easily during labor.

Also keep in mind that light breathing will come more naturally as your labor becomes more intense. Just as running makes you breathe faster to meet your oxygen needs, the rising intensity and frequency of contractions will increase your need for oxygen, which will naturally guide your breathing rate during labor.

Begin practicing light breathing by taking one breath every second or two, for ten seconds. If you take between five and ten breaths in that time, you're doing the technique correctly. Continue breathing at this rate for thirty seconds to two minutes. When you can do light breathing effortlessly for two minutes, try the adaptations described in the following sections.
*Notes:*

- If you become lightheaded or dizzy while doing light breathing, try to focus on your exhalations, perhaps by making small sounds while exhaling, such as "hee-hee-hee" or "puh-puh-puh." By doing so, your body will naturally inhale as much air as it needs.
- Breathing lightly through an open mouth may cause dryness. To help moisten the air that you breathe, try touching the tip of your tongue to the roof of your mouth just behind your teeth, or hold a moist washcloth near your mouth. During labor, you may also try sipping water or other fluids between contractions, or sucking on ice or a Popsicle. Brushing your teeth or rinsing your mouth occasionally may also help relieve a dry mouth.

## ADAPTATIONS TO BREATHING TECHNIQUES

The following are ways to adapt rhythmic breathing by combining slow and light breathing patterns. During labor, try switching to one of these techniques to help you cope if you become overwhelmed or exhausted, can't relax, or begin to despair. You may even discover a spontaneous rhythmic pattern of your own in labor.

### Vocal Breathing

This technique combines slow or light breathing with vocalization. As you exhale with each rhythmic breath, you moan, sigh, count, sing, recite poems, recite affirmations, chant, or make or say other sounds or words. For example, one woman found that repeating, "One, two, three, *Max*!" (her baby's name) let her maintain a rhythm and keep a sense of control during contractions. Another woman chanted, "Epidural, epidural" during contractions because she felt that as long as she could say the word, she didn't need the epidural.

If you make sounds when vocal breathing and you're coping well, they'll probably be rhythmic low-pitched moans. Loud high-pitched sounds, especially if you've lost your rhythm, may indicate suffering or fear.

If your sounds are high-pitched and not rhythmic, your partner can ask, "Are the sounds you're making helping you?" If they aren't, then your partner can help you lower the pitch by moaning with you and maintaining your rhythm with the Take Charge Routine (see page 256). Of course, if making rhythmic high-pitched sounds helps you cope, then no one should try to make you change what you're doing! Your support team should keep doors closed so you can make sounds without worrying about disturbing others.

## Contraction-tailored Breathing

For this technique, use the intensity of the contraction to guide the rate and depth of your breathing. If your contractions are peaking slowly, breathe slowly when each contraction begins. As the contraction intensifies, quicken and lighten your breathing past the peak. As the contraction subsides,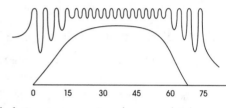
gradually slow and deepen your breathing. Think of each exhalation as a way to relax completely.

If your contractions are peaking quickly, slow breathing won't help you cope. Instead, use light breathing throughout each contraction.

## Slide Breathing

Some women, especially those with a respiratory condition such as asthma, find that the quicker pace of light breathing makes them uncomfortable and tense, regardless of how often they practice the technique. If you can't master light breathing after several practice attempts (see page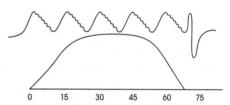
225), slide breathing is a good alternative. To do this technique, inhale deeply and slowly, then exhale with three or four light puffs of air. Pause, then repeat this process. To help guide your breathing, say "in" to yourself as you inhale, drawing out the word to match the length of your inhalation, then say "out" with each puff of air you exhale. Although the deep inhalations make slide breathing similar to slow breathing, the change in rhythm provides a different focus.

## Variable Breathing

Because variable breathing combines light, shallow breathing with a longer or more pronounced exhalation, it's sometimes called "pant-pant-BLOW" or "hee-hee-HOO" breathing. Just as with slide breathing, variable breathing is an option for women who feel uncomfortable or short of breath when using light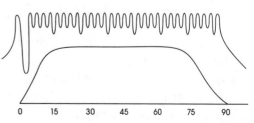
breathing. It's also helpful for women who prefer their breathing patterns to have structure.

With variable breathing, use light breathing for two to four breaths, then take another light inhalation followed by a long, slow, emphasized exhalation (the "blow"). This last exhalation helps you steady your rhythm and release tension. Some women emphasize it by making a drawn-out "hoo" or "puh" sound.

Find a comfortable pattern and then repeat it throughout the contraction. To help keep your rhythm, your partner can count your breaths: "One, two, three, BLOW!" Or you can count your breaths to yourself as a way to focus your attention.

## *Rehearsing Breathing Adaptations for Labor*

When practicing breathing techniques, include your favorite adaptations and practice them while in various positions. Relax for only thirty seconds or so between practice contractions to prepare for the brief rest you'll experience between contractions during the late first stage of labor. In this stage, contractions may last two minutes or they may occur in pairs with little break between the first and second contractions (coupling). During labor, you'll need to be prepared to use light breathing or its adaptations for up to three minutes without losing your breath.

## USING BREATHING TECHNIQUES TO AVOID PUSHING

During labor, you may have an early urge to push at the peak of a contraction. This urge is considered premature if it occurs before your cervix is completely dilated. If you have an urge to push and you don't know if your cervix is completely dilated, alert your nurse or caregiver. He or she will confirm dilation by vaginal exam. If dilation isn't complete, you'll be asked to resist the urge to push. To avoid pushing, lift your chin and either breathe deeply, pant, or blow lightly until the urge subsides. You may find it helpful to say or sing "puh, puh, puh" or "hoo, hoo, hoo" with each exhalation. When the urge to push passes, resume rhythmic breathing for the rest of the contraction. Changing positions can also help reduce the premature urge to push (Try hands-and-knees, side-lying, and open knee-chest positions.)

These breathing techniques won't take away your body's urge to push. Instead, they'll help you keep from holding your breath and bearing down with the urge.

## *Rehearsing Breathing Techniques to Avoid Pushing*

When rehearsing breathing techniques, occasionally practice a premature urge to push. Hold your breath or grunt as you breathe to signal to your partner that you have an urge to push. He or she can remind you how to resist the urge until it passes. Rehearsing this technique can be silly and fun, but it's also good preparation for avoiding premature pushing during labor.

# Comfort Techniques for Back Pain, Slow Labor, or an Extra Challenging Labor

Certain circumstances may make it challenging to cope with contractions. For example, your contractions may begin to couple (occur in pairs with little break between the first and second contractions) or become irregular. Your labor may become prolonged. Your baby's position in your womb may give you back pain. See page 285 to learn more about the possible positions your baby can assume, such as occiput posterior (OP) and occiput anterior (OA), and the effects each position can have on your labor.

The following sections describe measures that can help you cope with back pain or a slow or extra challenging labor.

# POSITIONS AND MOVEMENT

To reduce the pressure of your baby's head on your back or to help speed up a slow labor, use positions that encourage your baby to rotate into a better position, or use movements that decrease back pain.

## Open Knee-chest Position

Get onto your hands and knees, then lower your head and chest to the floor or bed. Move your knees back enough so your hips are high in the air. (See illustration on page 221.) Try to remain in this position for thirty minutes. Your partner can help support you, if necessary. This position is best used during prelabor or very early labor to help eliminate back pain and possibly reposition an OP baby.

## Leaning Forward

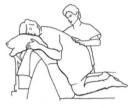

Positions that allow you to lean forward may help rotate your baby into the OA position and help keep him there. Examples include leaning over a birth ball, the labor bed, or a counter (while kneeling, standing, or sitting). The hands-and-knees position is also effective. These positions also relieve back pain by easing the pressure of your baby's head against your sacrum.

## Pelvic Rocking

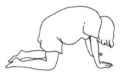

While kneeling and leaning forward over a birth ball or a chair seat, rock your pelvis forward and back or move your hips in a circle. The motion helps ease your baby up out of your pelvis, and the position encourages her to rotate out of the OP position.

## Abdominal Lift

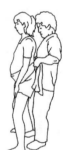

While standing, interlace your fingers and place your hands palms up, beneath your belly and against your pubic bone. During contractions, bend your knees (to tilt your pelvis slightly) and use your hands to lift your abdomen up and slightly in. This movement often relieves back pain while improving the position of your baby.

Because the abdominal lift can be hard work for you, your partner can do it using a woven shawl or rebozo. Fold the shawl so it's about 5 inches wide, then position it around your waist and below your belly (the same place that you'd put your hands). Have your partner stand behind you and cross the ends of the shawl behind your back. During the contraction, your partner will pull on each end of the shawl to lift your belly. Adjust both the shawl and the strength of your partner's pulling so the lift feels good.

*Caution:* If your baby wiggles a lot during the abdominal lift, he may be experiencing uncomfortable pressure. Discontinue the abdominal lift and use another comfort technique.

## Standing, Walking, Slow Dancing, and Stair Climbing

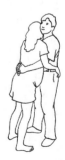

These movements take advantage of gravity and help align your baby with the upper part of your pelvis (pelvic inlet) and encourage her descent into the birth canal. Moving also allows your pelvis to change shape slightly, which encourages your baby to rotate.

## *Asymmetrical Movement and Positions: Lunge, Side-lying, and Semi-prone*

The lunge, side-lying, and semi-prone are considered *asymmetrical* because one side of your body is doing something different from the other side. Try them on both sides of your body. If you're more comfortable on one side than on the other, use that side to lunge or be in a side-lying or semi-prone position. If you have no clear preference, alternate sides.

### Lunge

The lunge is usually done during contractions. Find a sturdy armless chair that won't move when you lean against it. Stand in front of the chair, facing to the side. Lift the foot that's closest to the chair and set it on the seat, with your toes pointing toward the back of the chair (so they're at a 90 degree angle from the direction your body is facing). Remaining upright, slowly and rhythmically lunge sideways toward the chair (by further flexing your knee) and return to the starting position. You should feel a stretch in both inner thighs. Lunge throughout the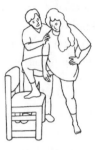
contraction, then rest when the contraction is over. Repeat this exercise for five to seven contractions. If lunging is uncomfortable with one leg, try using the other leg during the next contraction. Continue lunging with the leg that feels best to you.

### Side-lying

Lie on your side with your hips flexed and your knees bent. Place a pillow between your knees. (See illustration on page 222.) Try switching sides about every thirty minutes whenever you're awake, for as long as your baby's heart rate is normal.

### Semi-prone

Lie on your side with your lower arm behind you and your lower leg out straight. Flex the hip of your upper leg and bend the knee, resting it on a doubled-up pillow. Roll slightly toward your front. (See illustration on page 221.) Alternate this position with side-lying when you must remain in bed.

## A NOTE TO FATHERS AND PARTNERS ABOUT RELIEVING BACK PAIN

The following measures can help reduce your laboring partner's back pain and make her more comfortable. If any measure causes her more pain or doesn't help her, discontinue it and try another comfort measure.

## *Counterpressure*

Throughout each contraction, use your fist or the heel of your hand to steadily press on your partner's lower back. Use as much pressure as she wants. You can give counterpressure while she's in various positions. For example, when she's in the hands-and-knees position or an upright position, hold the front of one of her hips with one hand (to help keep her balance) and press steadily and firmly in one spot on her lower back 4 to 6 inches below her waist,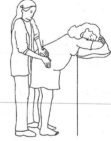
slightly away from her spine. The exact spot will vary over the course of the labor; she'll let you know where to press to give her the best relief. Between contractions, rest or massage the area you pressed.

## Double Hip Squeeze

Have your laboring partner kneel and lean forward on a birth ball or chair seat, or get on her hands and knees on the bed or floor. (If on the floor, place a pillow or pad beneath her knees.) During a contraction, stand close behind her, then press on the roundest part of each buttock with your palms. Apply steady pressure (instead of pressing and releasing repeatedly) as you try to press her hips together to relieve pelvic pressure and ease back pain. Try other places on her hips to press and apply as much pressure as she needs.

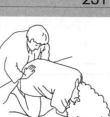

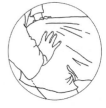

If another person is available to help, the two-person double hip squeeze is easier to do than the usual technique. Instead of standing behind your pregnant partner, you and the other person stand on opposite sides of her, facing each other. You each place one hand on the roundest part of the closer buttock, then together press on her buttocks. Be sure to coordinate timing and amount of pressure. Ask your partner if the pressure feels even, and adjust accordingly.

## Knee Press

Have your laboring partner sit upright in a chair that won't slide when you press your weight against it. If necessary, elevate her feet so her thighs are parallel to the floor. Kneel in front of her and cup a hand over each knee. Lean toward her so your hands press straight back toward her hip joints. Keep the pressure steady throughout the contraction.

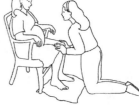

# OTHER COMFORT MEASURES TO REDUCE BACK PAIN

Heat and cold (see page 211) are excellent comfort measures to relieve back pain, as are baths and showers (see page 209). The following sections describe additional measures that you may want to try.

## Rolling Pressure

Have your partner move a rolling pin over your lower back. This is a soothing way to relieve back pain and muscle tension during and between contractions. You may find additional relief if your partner uses a can of frozen juice, a cold can of soda, or a hollow rolling pin filled with ice, because the cold helps numb the area. If the rolling object is cold, make sure there's a layer of cloth on your back so the object isn't in direct contact with your skin.

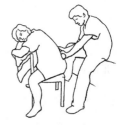

## Transcutaneous Electrical Nerve Stimulation (TENS)

TENS relieves back pain during contractions by creating tingling, buzzing, or prickly sensations on your skin. According to the Gate Control Theory of Pain (see page 178), TENS reduces your awareness of pain by increasing your awareness of pleasant or distracting stimuli. Another theory to explain the effectiveness of TENS is that it gradually increases endorphin production in the area where it's applied. Endorphins are your body's natural pain relievers that block transmission of pain signals. If TENS begins in early labor, the level of endorphins in the lower back will increase by the time labor intensifies. Many women find TENS helpful for relieving back pain, but some don't.

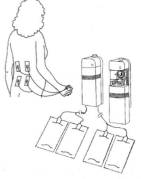

TENS devices are simple to use. Four stimulating pads are placed on the back, then connected to a small hand-held battery-operated generator that produces tingling, buzzing, or prickly sensations. Models vary but all have controls to regulate the intensity of the sensation and to switch the pattern of the stimulation between a continuous mode and an intermittent burst mode.

Either you or your partner can hold and control the device. Between contractions, set the intensity to the level that feels comfortable and set the stimulation to burst mode. When the contraction begins, change the stimulation to continuous mode. When the contraction ends, switch it back to burst mode. As your back pain increases, increase the intensity.

Specially designed maternity TENS devices are widely available in Canada and the United Kingdom, but are hard to find in the United States. You may be able to learn more about TENS from a physical therapist who uses it to treat numerous pain conditions. If you plan to hire a birth doula (see page 23), she may be trained to use TENS and have a device to loan you. You can purchase a maternity TENS device online at a retailer such as http://www.bodyclock.net.

Although there are no known harmful side effects of TENS, be sure to check with your caregiver before using it.

# Comfort Techniques for the Second Stage of Labor (Pushing)

Many of the comfort techniques used during the first stage of labor are also helpful during the second stage. Here are some ideas specific for helping you find comfort when pushing out your baby.

## WORKING WITH THE URGE TO PUSH IN LABOR

Around the time your cervix becomes completely dilated, your breathing rhythm will change and you'll feel pressure on your pelvic floor as your baby moves deep into your pelvis. These developments will cause you to have an irresistible urge to push. At first, you may mistake this urge for the need to have a bowel movement. (See page 255.)

*Note*: If you have an epidural, you'll feel the urge to push much less clearly or you might not feel it at all. See pages 233–234 and page 259 for more information on directed or delayed pushing with an epidural.

## SPONTANEOUS BEARING DOWN

Your responses to contractions during the second stage will depend on the sensations you feel. You'll probably feel several strong surges (irresistible urges to push) during each contraction. Each surge will last a few seconds.

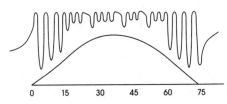

During a surge, you'll use *expulsion breathing*. Simply breathe using whatever technique suits you, until you have an urge to push and your body begins bearing down (a spontaneous reaction to the urge). Bear down for as long as you feel the urge. Then breathe lightly until either you feel another urge or the contraction ends. Expect to bear down three to five times per contraction, with each effort lasting about five to seven seconds. Between contractions, rest and relax.

How hard you bear down in response to an urge is similar to how hard you sneeze in response to an irritant in your nose. Both sneezing and spontaneous bearing down are involuntary reflexes. Sometimes you need one tiny sneeze to clear an irritant; other times, you need several explosive

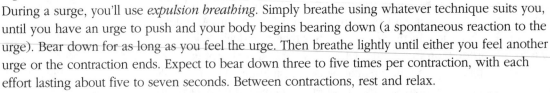

sneezes. Sometimes you need to gently bear down; other times, you'll feel compelled to push with all your strength.

Spontaneous bearing down is recommended if labor is progressing normally and you haven't had anesthesia. If you have anesthesia, you'll use delayed pushing (see page 259) or directed pushing (see below). Anesthesia diminishes the pushing sensations and the effectiveness of your ability to spontaneously bear down.

## Using Spontaneous Bearing Down in Labor

Here are steps that explain how to use spontaneous bearing down in labor.
1. As the contraction begins, start slow or light breathing (see pages 224 and 225).
2. Focus on a positive image, such as your baby moving down and out of your uterus.
3. Breathe rhythmically as the contraction intensifies. When you can no longer resist the urge to push, bear down or strain while holding your breath or while slowly releasing air by grunting or vocalizing, whichever feels best. *Relax your pelvic floor!* (See page 96.) Your partner may need to remind you to relax your perineum.
4. Exhale when the urge passes (usually after five to seven seconds) and breathe rhythmically for several seconds until you feel another urge to push. Then, bear down again. The urge to push will come in waves during the contraction, giving you time to "breathe for your baby" (that is, to oxygenate your blood to provide enough oxygen for your baby between urges).
5. When the contraction ends, slowly lie or sit back (or stand up if squatting) and take one or two relaxing breaths.

## Rehearsing Spontaneous Bearing Down for Labor

When practicing comfort techniques for the second stage of labor, bear down just enough to feel your pelvic floor bulge. (See page 96.) Don't bear down forcefully. To practice more effectively, use different positions and imagine what will be happening when you're pushing in labor. Visualize your baby descending and rotating into your birth canal. Remind yourself that contractions are proof that your baby is working to be born and it's important to relax and bulge your pelvic floor.

## DIRECTED PUSHING

Unlike with spontaneous bearing down, when you push in response to an urge, directed pushing is bearing down when someone tells you to do so. You'll use this type of pushing in the following circumstances:

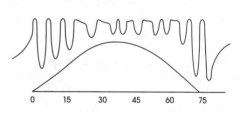

- You've had an epidural and don't feel contractions.
- You don't have an urge to push or you're not pushing effectively when spontaneously bearing down, even after trying gravity-enhancing positions such as squatting, sitting, dangling, lap squatting, or standing upright (see pages 221–223).
- Directed pushing is routine for your hospital or for your caregiver.

Directed pushing is typically more forceful than spontaneous bearing down, which means it may be more stressful for both you and your baby. For this reason, many caregivers reserve this type of pushing for births that may require forceps delivery or vacuum extraction. Before the birth, check whether directed pushing is routine for your caregiver or birthplace. If it is, find out when and under what circumstances it's used.

## Using Directed Pushing in Labor

Here are the steps that explain how to use directed pushing in labor. Your caregiver, nurse, or partner will tell you when, how long, and how hard to push. You can use various positions to do directed pushing.

1. At the beginning of a contraction, take two or three breaths. When you're told to push, inhale and hold your breath. Curl forward, tucking your chin on your chest, and bear down, tightening your abdominal muscles.
2. Relax your pelvic floor muscles. Bear down for five to seven seconds. Quickly exhale as directed, then take another few breaths.
3. Repeat steps 1 and 2 until the contraction subsides.
4. When the contraction ends, slowly lie or sit back (or stand up if squatting), rest, and breathe normally.

*Note:* Directed pushing will continue for each contraction until your baby's head is almost out. At that point, your caregiver may tell you to stop pushing to allow your baby's head to pass slowly through your vaginal opening. Relax and exhale completely to decrease your risk of developing a vaginal tear.

## Rehearsing Directed Pushing for Labor

Because with directed pushing you'll be told when and how hard to push, you need to practice this technique only enough to coordinate holding your breath with bearing down and bulging your pelvis (see page 96), as your partner coaches you through the contractions as described above. You may find it helpful to occasionally hold your breath and bulge your perineum during perineal massage (see page 235).

## PROLONGED DIRECTED PUSHING

In labor, prolonged directed pushing requires you to hold your breath and push hard for ten seconds. For those reasons, caregivers generally don't recommend the technique, but some circumstances may require it. (See page 289.) Because you'd use prolonged directed pushing only under your caregiver's guidance, there's no need to practice it before labor.

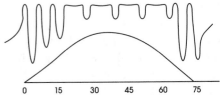

## POSITIONS FOR THE SECOND STAGE OF LABOR

Just as moving around and changing positions can help with labor progress and pain relief during the first stage of labor, these comfort measures can help you during the second stage. Until you're in labor and ready to push your baby out, you won't know which positions will feel right. Try to practice spontaneous bearing down (see page 232) in all the positions shown on pages 221–223 so you're prepared to effectively bear down while in any of them.

If your baby descends rapidly, you might not have the time or desire to change positions; however, if your second stage progresses slowly, you'll have a chance to try many positions.

Other factors may influence the positions you can try during the second stage, such as your caregiver's preferences or your willingness and freedom to change positions. Some procedures and equipment may impair your mobility, including electronic fetal monitors, catheters, anesthetics, IV equipment, and narrow beds. But with help and encouragement, you can safely work around these obstacles.

Discuss birthing positions when preparing your birth plan (see Chapter 8). Although some caregivers are comfortable with any birthing position a woman chooses to use,[8] most are confident only with the supine (woman lying on her back) or semi-sitting position for delivery. Ask whether you can use other positions that allow the pelvic outlet to open fully during the beginning of pushing, until your baby is close to being born.

## PERINEAL MASSAGE

Prenatal *perineal massage* stretches the inner tissue of your lower vagina. It teaches you to respond to pressure in your vagina by relaxing your pelvic floor muscles. In this way, it's a rehearsal for responding to the sensations of vaginal stretching during birth.

Perineal massage is also thought to enhance the hormonal changes that soften connective tissue during late pregnancy, which can reduce your chances of needing an episiotomy (see page 289) or developing a serious tear during birth.[9] Massaging your perineum five to seven times a week during the last five to six weeks of pregnancy may help you avoid an episiotomy or serious tear.

Some caregivers aren't familiar with the benefits of perineal massage, and don't recommend it. Even if their caregivers recommend perineal massage, some women find it distasteful and don't want to do it. Others, however, feel the massage is worthwhile if it can reduce the chances of an episiotomy or a serious tear. Some even find it enjoyable, especially after they've learned to relax while it's done.

*Note:* If you have vaginitis, a genital herpes sore, or another vaginal problem, perineal massage may worsen the condition. Wait until the problem is completely gone before beginning perineal massage.

## *How to Do Perineal Massage*

You or your partner can do this massage with clean hands and short fingernails. If either of you has rough skin, consider using disposable vinyl or latex gloves. If doing the massage yourself, you may want to use a mirror at first, to help you see your perineum.

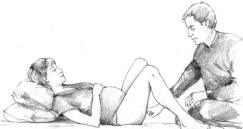

1.  Get into a semi-sitting position (if your partner is doing the massage—see page 222 for a description of the position) or stand with one foot on the side of the tub or a chair (if doing the massage yourself).
2.  Use a squeeze bottle to squirt vegetable oil on your thumb or partner's index finger(s). (Dipping your fingers into the oil can contaminate it.) Wheat germ oil has a high vitamin E content, which may be soothing on your skin. You can also use another vegetable oil or a water-based lubricant such as K-Y Jelly. Don't use baby oil, mineral oil, petroleum jelly, or hand lotion—many women who used these products reported that their skin didn't tolerate them well.
3.  Place your thumb, or have your partner place an index finger (one at first, then both as you become comfortable), well inside your vagina (up to the second knuckle). Do a few Kegel exercises (see page 95)

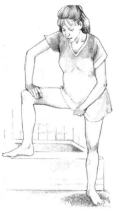

so you can feel your pelvic floor muscles tense. Relax the muscles. Curl your thumb, or have your partner curl his or her finger, and gently pull it outward and downward toward your anus, then rhythmically move it within your vagina in a U motion. Focus on relaxing your pelvic floor muscles. Do this massage for about three minutes. At first, your vaginal wall will feel tight. After a few days of practice, it'll relax and stretch more easily.

4.   Concentrate on relaxing your muscles as you feel the pressure and stretching. As you become comfortable with the massage, increase the pressure just enough to make the tissue begin to sting or burn slightly. (The same sensation will occur as your baby's head is being born.)
5.   If you have questions after trying the massage, ask your caregiver, childbirth educator, or someone who's familiar with this technique for advice.

# Practice Time as a Rehearsal for Labor

When taking the time to practice these comfort techniques with your partner, try to think of it as a rehearsal for labor. Discuss when you may use the techniques and why. Review what you've learned about the emotional and physical events of labor. (See Appendix B.) Most importantly, learn how to work together to use the techniques effectively and adapt them to fit your needs.

## AMOUNT OF PRACTICE TIME

You don't have to practice every day to master comfort techniques, especially if you and your partner attend childbirth preparation classes together. Practice enough so you're completely comfortable with each technique and have time to figure out any adaptations you may want to use. Then, review them periodically so they become familiar and easy.

## SUGGESTED PRACTICE SEQUENCE

The following sequence will help you master the techniques discussed in this and other chapters. (Visit our web site, http://www.PCNGuide.com, for an additional practice guide.) You may choose to take a few months to complete the sequence, or you may decide to begin closer to your due date and finish it in a few weeks. Either way, practicing these exercises, breathing rhythms, and relaxation techniques will increase your confidence in your ability to handle labor and birth.

1.   Conditioning exercises (see pages 95): Continue practicing these exercises until the birth.
2.   Comfort measures for discomforts (see page 103): Use as needed.
3.   Body awareness exercises (see page 215)
4.   Passive relaxation (see page 216)
5.   Relaxation countdown (see page 218): At first, use several breaths to relax, then work toward relaxing with one breath.
6.   Perineal massage (see page 235): During the last five to six weeks of pregnancy, do five to six times a week.
7.   Slow breathing (see page 224)
8.   Touch relaxation (see page 219)
9.   Roving body check (see page 219): Practice this exercise by yourself and with your partner's direction.
10.   Slow breathing with roving body check (see pages 224 and 219)
11.   Attention-focusing (see page 208)
12.   Crisscross back massage (see page 213)
13.   Possible positions for the first stage of labor (see pages 221–222): Practice slow breathing in each position.

14. Light breathing (see page 225): Experiment with the depth and rate of your breathing to find what works for you.

15. Adaptations of slow and light breathing—contraction-tailored, vocal, slide, and variable breathing (see pages 226–227)

16. Variety of positions for the first stage of labor (see pages 221–222) while practicing breathing adaptations

17. Ways to decrease back pain in labor (see pages 229–232): Practice the double hip squeeze, counterpressure, abdominal lift, open knee-chest position, knee press, and lunge. Combine these techniques with breathing patterns.

18. Ways to avoid pushing (see page 228)

19. Spontaneous bearing down and directed pushing (see pages 232–234): Practice gently bearing down and incorporate the bulging exercise (see page 96). Occasionally, practice panting to avoid pushing in the middle of a practice contraction.

20. Positions for the second stage of labor (see pages 222–223): Try the positions while practicing spontaneous bearing down (expulsion breathing).

21. Labor rehearsal: Practice all the coping techniques during a series of pretend contractions. Your partner can help by observing you and helping you fully relax in all positions.

# Key Points to Remember

- Every woman responds to labor differently, but those who cope well use the Three Rs: They **relax** during or between contractions; they move, breathe, and vocalize in **rhythm**; and they have a **ritual** during which they repeat the same rhythmic activities through many contractions.

- Figure out which comfort techniques may be most effective in labor by practicing them with your partner during pregnancy. Have pretend contractions while practicing techniques to make each practice session a rehearsal for labor.

- Mastering several comfort techniques and adapting them to suit your needs will increase your confidence and ability to cope with labor pain.

- When you're in labor, be prepared to discover and use unplanned coping techniques and rituals.

# CHAPTER 12

# What Childbirth Is Really Like

When your labor begins, all the information you've gathered and the plans you've made will suddenly merge with the reality of childbirth, a physical and emotional experience that's often unpredictable and uncontrollable. You'll be glad you took the time during pregnancy to learn about giving birth and to figure out your preferences and needs. This chapter describes the sequence of events that occurs in a normal, healthy labor and birth. It also discusses steps you can take to respond to any variation in labor, from a rapid labor to a prolonged one.

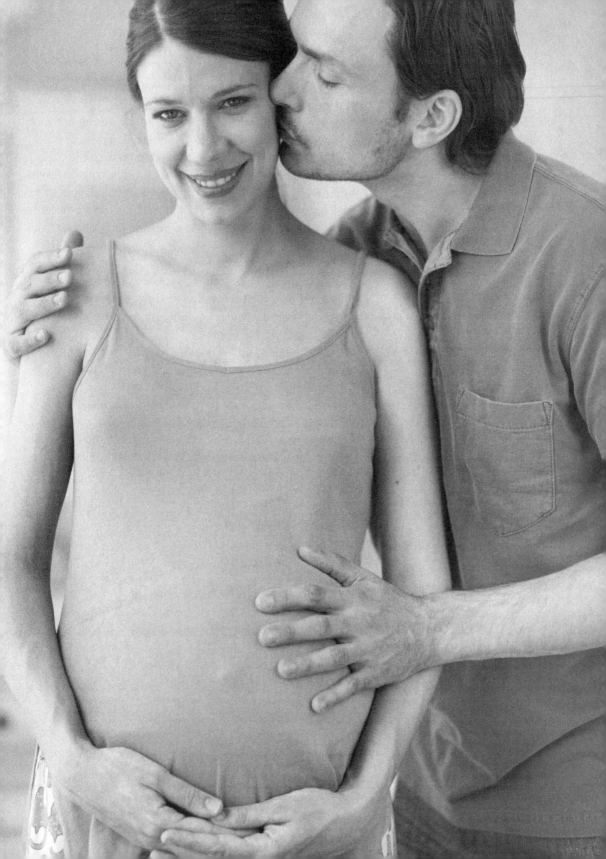

# Stages and Phases of Labor

Labor marks your baby's transition to an independent existence and your transition to parenthood. Even before labor begins, changes occur that prepare your body for it. During prelabor, which may last for days or weeks, your cervix moves forward, ripens (softens) and effaces (thins or shortens).

Over the course of labor, your uterus contracts, your cervix continues to ripen and efface and begins to dilate, your baby rotates and moves down your birth canal, and you give birth to your baby, placenta, umbilical cord, and amniotic sac. The entire process (excluding prelabor) can take anywhere from a few hours to a day or longer.

Labor is divided into four stages, each of which marks a sign of progression. The first and second stages are further divided into phases, which represent more subtle changes than the stages.

The *first stage of labor* (dilation) begins with contractions that are becoming longer, stronger, and more frequent (that is, progressing) and ends when your cervix is completely dilated. It has three phases: early labor, active labor, and transition. The *second stage of labor* (birth of your baby) begins when your cervix is fully dilated and ends when your baby is born. The *third stage of labor* (delivery of the placenta) begins with the birth of your baby and ends with the delivery of the placenta. Lastly, the *fourth stage of labor* (recovery) begins after the placenta is delivered and ends one to several hours later, when your condition has stabilized.

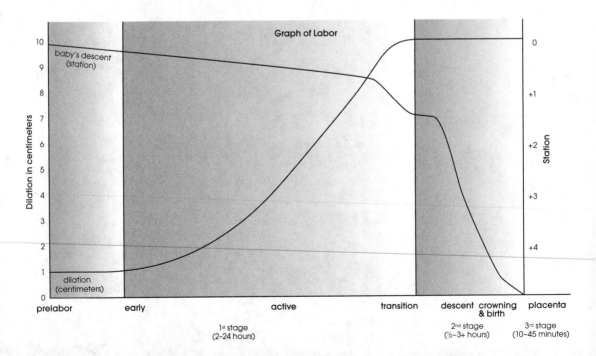

# First Stage of Labor: Dilation

When your contractions are progressing and your ripening, effacing cervix begins to dilate, you're in the first stage of labor. Dilation increases with each phase of this stage, until your cervix is about 10 centimeters in diameter. In early labor, your cervix dilates to 4 or 5 centimeters. In active labor, it further dilates to 8 centimeters, and in transition, it completely dilates to 10 centimeters. As labor progresses, each successive phase usually becomes shorter and more intense than the previous phase. Each phase has recognizable characteristics that present unique physical and emotional challenges.

The first stage typically lasts between two and twenty-four hours. For a first-time mother, the average length of the first stage is twelve and a half hours. For a woman who has given birth before, the first stage usually lasts half that amount of time (if labor wasn't induced).

For some women, the first stage may be much slower or quicker than average. See pages 245 and 247 to learn more about handling the challenges of a prolonged labor or a rapid labor.

## Common Q & A

**Q:** My mother said labor went by pretty quickly when she gave birth to me. Will my labor progress as fast as hers did?

**A:** It might—or it might not. The answer depends on many variables, including whose body build and other characteristics you inherited, your overall health, and characteristics that your baby inherited from his father.

## LABOR CONTRACTIONS

Throughout the phases of the first stage, your contractions become increasingly intense. But what exactly is a labor *contraction*? By the end of your pregnancy, your uterus has become the largest and strongest muscle in your body. When it contracts, it hardens and bulges like any other muscle does, and the muscle fibers shorten and pull your ripe, effaced cervix open. The sensation you feel during this process may be mild and uncomfortable or it may be intense and painful.

Contractions are involuntary; you can't control them. Each contraction follows a wavelike pattern: It builds to a peak, then gradually disappears, allowing your uterus (and you) to rest. The frequency of contractions increases until your cervix is completely dilated.

In early labor, contractions usually feel like dull lower back pain or abdominal cramps. Very early contractions are usually short and mild, lasting thirty to forty seconds, and the time between them may be as long as fifteen or twenty minutes. These contractions may make it difficult to tell whether you're in labor or still in prelabor. (See Chapter 9.)

As labor progresses, contractions become markedly stronger and longer. By the end of the first stage, contractions usually are very intense and last as long as ninety seconds to two minutes. When trying to cope with the intensity of labor, it helps to remind yourself that every contraction has an end. The time from the beginning of one contraction to the beginning of the next may be as short as two or three minutes, allowing you just a brief rest between contractions.

## Hormones in Labor

Before, during, and after labor, your body produces several hormones, including:

- *Oxytocin*, the "love hormone," which plays a major role in orgasm, breastfeeding, and childbirth. In labor, it causes contractions and helps with progress.
- Stress hormones (*catecholamines*), which counteract oxytocin and can slow contractions, leading to a prolonged labor.
- *Beta-endorphins*, your body's painkillers, which are secreted when you experience pain, stress, and physical exertion. They help you transcend pain and enter a trance state that's sometimes called the "birth zone."
- *Prolactin*, which is produced after the birth. It's necessary for milk production, and it calms and elevates your mood.

To decrease stress hormones and increase oxytocin and beta-endorphins during labor, the following are essential: confidence, a sense of safety, privacy, quietness, familiar places and faces, supportive interactions with others, and feeling loved (and reciprocating that feeling) through touch, massage, kissing, and caressing. Conversely, the following increase stress hormones and decrease oxytocin and beta-endorphins: anxiety, fear, anger, decision-making, frequent disturbances, and feeling watched or judged.

For more information about hormones and optimal hormonal interactions, read *Gentle Birth, Gentle Mothering: A Doctor's Guide to Natural Childbirth and Gentle Early Parenting Choices* by Sarah Buckley and Ina May Gaskin (2008).

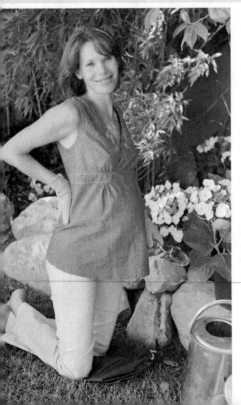

# First Phase: Early Labor

*Early labor* or the *latent phase* is usually the longest phase in the first stage, often because contractions are further apart, shorter, and less intense than they'll be later in labor. During early labor, your cervix becomes fully effaced and dilates to 4 or 5 centimeters. You'll probably spend most of this phase at or near home, keeping busy or relaxing if it's daytime and resting if it's nighttime. Because this is the "waiting and wondering" phase, review Chapter 9 and use the Early Labor Record on page 175 to help you decide whether you're in early labor or still in prelabor.

The best way to cope with early labor is to ignore the phase until your mind or body no longer lets you. At that point, use coping techniques, such as those discussed on page 243, to help you enter a confident, optimistic state of mind. This mind-set can influence the interactions of hormones in a way that optimizes labor progress (see above).[1]

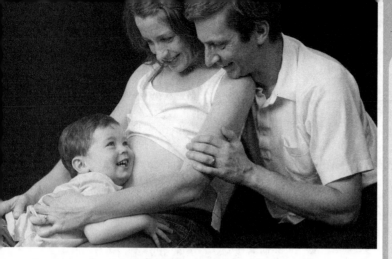

## *Getting through Early Labor*

When you begin early labor, you may feel excited and a bit nervous. You'll probably want your partner near so he or she can provide support, now that labor feels real to you. The key to coping with this phase is to avoid assuming your labor is progressing much faster than it really is. Try not to focus too much on each contraction. In fact, if you can ignore these early contractions, do so! Becoming preoccupied with early contractions often has the unwelcome effect of making your entire labor seem longer than you were anticipating.

During early labor, rest if you're tired or if it's nighttime. Otherwise, try to keep busy doing activities that are fun, calming, or distracting (but not exhausting). Here are some activities that may appeal to you in early labor:

- Pack your bag to take to the hospital or birth center (see page 166) or prepare your home if you're planning a home birth.
- Meditate or use guided visualization.
- Have a massage. During contractions in early labor, it's natural to tense specific areas of your body, or *tension spots*. Tension increases your perception of pain, so releasing tension with early contractions gets you into the habit of relaxing your muscles for later phases, when contractions will be more intense. See page 215 to learn how you and your partner can recognize and release muscle tension.
- Take a long shower (but not a bath—see page 210).[2]
- Consume easy-to-digest foods and drinks that appeal to you, such as soup, broth, and herbal tea, as well as high-carbohydrate foods such as fruit, pasta, toast, rice, and waffles.
- Go for a walk, visit with friends, listen to music, write in your journal, e-mail relatives, watch a movie, dance, or play cards or other games.
- Do a preplanned "early labor project," such as working on a hobby, gardening, laundering and sorting your baby's clothes, preparing one-dish meals to freeze and enjoy after the birth, or baking a birthday cake to welcome your new arrival.

## Two Views on Getting through Early Labor

The first contraction woke me at 3:25 AM. For most of that day, I had a contraction every ten minutes or so. The pain was mild, so my husband and I thought it was best just to go about our business as though it were any other day. We returned a rented DVD, ran errands, ate a nice meal, and napped. It was a relaxing time.

—*Joy*

My first contractions weren't very strong or frequent. To take my mind off the contractions, I took a shower, walked my dog, watched a movie, and just tried to relax. That night, after an entire day with little change in my labor, I tried to slow down the contractions with a bath so I could sleep. The bath helped, and I slept off and on for several hours.

—*Katie*

# When to Go to Your Birthplace or Call Your Midwife

At some point, as early labor progresses, you'll begin thinking about going to the hospital or birth center, or calling your midwife to come to your home. Because you may have trouble determining your progress, during your last month of pregnancy your caregiver will tell you when and whom to call if you think you're in labor. Depending on your caregiver and birthplace, you may call the hospital maternity unit (especially at night), an answering service, or your caregiver's direct line.

Your caregiver probably will recommend that you use the following guidelines when deciding whether to call:

- If this is your first baby, call when your membranes rupture (or may have ruptured), or follow the *4-1-1 or 5-1-1 rule*. This rule means that your contractions are intense enough to require you to focus and breathe rhythmically, and are *four or five* minutes apart, each lasting at least *one minute* for a period of *one hour*. Whether you follow 4-1-1 or 5-1-1 depends on your caregiver's advice and how long it takes you to get to your birthplace or for your midwife to come to your home.
- If you've given birth before, call your caregiver or hospital maternity unit when your membranes rupture or when you're having progressing contractions and other signs of labor (for example, you have bloody show, soft bowel movements with contractions, and so on). Because you've given birth before, you're likely to quickly shift from early to active labor. Consequently, you don't necessarily need to wait for 5-1-1: You may be advised to go to the hospital or birth center as soon as your contractions are five minutes apart.
- If you have a condition that requires hospital observation during early labor, call whenever you suspect labor. Examples of such conditions include positive Group B streptococcus (GBS), a herpes sore, and any high-risk condition. See Chapter 13 for more information on these potential complications.
- Regardless of the status of your labor, you may always call your caregiver or the hospital maternity unit if you're anxious, have questions, live far from the birthplace (or your home birth midwife lives far from you), or have received specific instructions to call before labor is established.

When you do call, be ready to report the following information that you've noted in your Early Labor Record (see page 175):

- How long your contractions last (duration)
- How many minutes apart they are, from the start of one to the start of the next (interval or frequency)
- How strong the contractions seem (intensity)—can you talk through them or do you need to use your planned ritual?
- How long your contractions have been like this
- Status of your membranes—have they ruptured? Is there a color or strong odor to the fluid?
- Presence of bloody show
- Other information that will help your caregiver (or the on-call caregiver) know about you and your pregnancy

The nurse or caregiver who takes your call uses this information to determine whether to tell you come to the hospital or birth center, or recommend that you stay home until further changes have occurred (for example, until your membranes have ruptured or your contractions become longer or occur closer together). If you're having a home birth, your midwife uses this information to decide whether to come to your home immediately or later, when your labor has further progressed.

## *The Three Rs: Relaxation, Rhythm, and Ritual*

After several hours (or even a day or longer) of prelabor and early labor, you'll at last reach a point when you're unable to ignore your contractions. You can't walk or talk through a contraction without having to pause at its peak. Activities are no longer distracting or fun. This point marks a shift in your coping strategy. Instead of using distracting activities to cope with contractions, you instead begin using the *Three Rs: relaxation, rhythm, and ritual*. See page 206 for a full discussion on the Three Rs.

## *A Note to Fathers and Partners*

Early labor is an exciting time for you as well. Try to spend it constructively. Contact your laboring partner's caregiver and doula. If the birth will occur in a hospital or birth center, make sure her bags (and yours) are packed and stowed in your vehicle, and check that there's enough fuel in the tank. If you're planning a home birth, make sure you have the birth supplies that the midwife requested, as well as enough food and beverages for everyone. Have comfort items ready and accessible. Tidy up your home so your partner and the midwife can move about during labor without having to navigate around messes and clutter. Make sure your vehicle has enough fuel, in case a transfer to the hospital is necessary.

Help your partner through early labor contractions by following her lead. If she becomes quiet and uncommunicative during contractions, you should also become quiet. Don't ask her questions and try not to act more excited than she is. However, if she becomes chatty, active, and excited between contractions, respond to her in kind.

Be aware of how she's coping during contractions, but don't hover or stare at her—this may have the unintended but annoying effect of making her feel watched. If you notice that she's tensing any area of her body during a contraction, alert her of the tension by firmly touching the tense area, or by telling her about the tension between contractions in a gentle, nonjudgmental way. For example, you may say, "I noticed you seemed to tense up in your shoulders with that contraction. With the next one, try to breathe away any tension in your shoulders with each exhalation."

In general, look for rhythm in her breathing and movements during contractions, and try to match her rhythm with your touch, movements, and voice. Remind her to sip water after every contraction or two. See Appendix B for suggestions on ways you can help your partner throughout labor, and see Chapter 11 for more information on relaxation techniques and comfort measures. Working with your partner during early labor contractions will pay off later, when her contractions become more challenging.

## PROLONGED PRELABOR OR EARLY LABOR

Sometimes, labor is *prolonged*; that is, it takes a long time to get started. If early labor seems slow, you may wonder whether you're truly in that phase yet. It can be difficult to distinguish between a long prelabor (in which your contractions aren't progressing and your cervix isn't dilating) and a slow early labor (in which contractions and cervical dilation are progressing slower than usual for this phase).

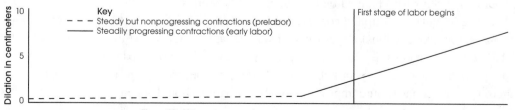

Key
- - - Steady but nonprogressing contractions (prelabor)
——— Steadily progressing contractions (early labor)

First stage of labor begins

Dilation in centimeters: 0, 5, 10

Time (12–48 hours or more)

How much time must pass before early labor is considered prolonged? One theory claims that early labor is prolonged if regular contractions continue for longer than twenty hours.[3] However, many caregivers believe that if early labor is taking a physical or psychological toll on the woman, it's prolonged—regardless of the amount of time that has passed in the phase.

If your early labor is prolonged, you may become tired and discouraged, but don't assume that your entire labor will be slow. Prolonged early labor is *not* a labor complication. In most cases, labor progresses normally as soon as it reaches the active phase.

In a prolonged early labor, it's important to figure out the cause so that you, your partner or doula, and your nurse or caregiver can take action (if possible) to speed up your progress. The following are the most probable causes for a prolonged early labor:

- Your contractions have begun before your cervix has moved forward, ripened, or effaced—the changes that prepare it for dilation. (See page 169.)
- Your cervix is scarred from a previous surgery, cone biopsy, or another cervical procedure. For your cervix to dilate, it may require many frequent and intense contractions to overcome the resistance caused by the scar tissue.
- Your baby is malpositioned, such as occiput posterior (see page 285) or with a raised chin. You may also have back pain. Your contractions may seem irregular or they may couple (occur in pairs, with a short break between the first and second contractions).
- You're tense, anxious, or distressed, all of which increase the levels of stress hormones that can hinder labor progress (see page 242). Several factors can cause stress, including a previous unresolved emotional or physical trauma, a previous difficult birth experience, grief from a miscarriage or abortion, a stressful relationship (with your partner, caregiver, or relatives), and fears about your or your baby's well-being.

## What You Can Do

If early labor is prolonged, the following are suggestions to help you cope mentally and physically as you wait for your labor to progress.

- When you have a vaginal exam, ask your caregiver whether your cervix has moved forward and is ripe; also ask how much it has effaced. If your cervix hasn't changed much, you need patience and stamina to allow early contractions to complete these changes before they can dilate your cervix.
- Try not to become discouraged or depressed by your slow progress. Visualize your contractions bringing your cervix forward, then ripening and effacing it. Try to accept a prolonged early labor as temporary and appropriate for your body at this time.
- Nurture yourself with food, drink, and loving support.
- Alternate doing labor-stimulating activities with restful, distracting activities (see page 243).
- Don't time every contraction. Instead, time six contractions in a row, then wait until the pattern of your contractions has changed before timing another series.
- If you have irregular or coupling contractions (occur in pairs with a short break between the first and second contractions) or back pain, assume that your baby isn't in an ideal position for birth. Use the techniques described on pages 229–232 to relieve back pain and move your baby into an ideal position. Once your baby is in a better position, back pain should dissipate, your pattern of contractions should improve, and labor progress should speed up.

- If you're worried or tense, talk with your partner, caregiver, or other supportive person. He or she may be able to help you put your concerns into perspective. If all else fails, having a good cry—in private or with a compassionate companion—can help release any overwhelming sadness or anxiety.

*Note:* If you know or suspect that you'll be very worried or tense in labor, talk with your caregiver, doula, counselor, or childbirth educator during pregnancy to help you identify and address any potential sources of stress. Together, you can plan ways to cope with the stress during labor, such as using relaxation techniques and slow breathing to calm yourself (see Chapter 11).

## Medical Care for a Prolonged Early Labor

Despite your best efforts to cope with a prolonged early labor, if you become exhausted or have made little or no progress for more than twenty-four hours, you and your caregiver may need to decide whether to turn to medical interventions. There are two major approaches to speeding up a labor medically:

1. Using medications to stop contractions or to help you rest. Your caregiver may recommend drugs such as tranquilizers, sedatives, uterine relaxants, morphine, or alcohol.
2. Using medications or procedures to stimulate more effective contractions. Your caregiver may suggest stripping your membranes, mechanically ripening or dilating your cervix, breaking your bag of waters, ripening your cervix with prostaglandins, or inducing labor with Pitocin. (See pages 279–283.)

These medications and procedures can affect your baby and have undesired side effects for you, so they shouldn't be used without good reason. To help you make an informed decision, ask your caregiver the key questions about the risks and benefits of these options (see page 10). Your decision depends on your stamina and your willingness to continue. If you and your baby are doing well and you feel you can continue coping on your own, let your caregiver know. However, if you feel too exhausted or discouraged to continue on your own, request medical help.

If scar tissue on your cervix is causing a prolonged and very painful early labor, you likely need medical help. Your caregiver may quickly massage your cervix open a few centimeters. If this procedure is successful, your cervix begins dilating, and your labor progress may then continue normally. The procedure is painful, and you may need to follow the Take Charge Routine (see page 256); if it's unsuccessful, you may need narcotics or other pain medications.

## RAPID LABOR

Some women—especially those who've given birth before—have rapid labors. These labors begin with contractions that are only three or four minutes apart, and become increasingly stronger, longer, and more frequent than usual. If your labor progresses this quickly, see page 301 for more information on what to do.

### In Their Own Words

After ten hours of mild contractions that were six minutes apart, I called the hospital to see if I could come in for medication to help me sleep. An examination showed that my cervix was 3 centimeters dilated and 100 percent effaced. My midwife gave me three options: get a morphine shot and go home to sleep, get the shot and sleep in an unused room upstairs, or be admitted and get an epidural. I chose to get the shot and go home, where I was able to sleep for a couple hours. When I woke up, contractions were strong, so I headed to the hospital. My cervix was 6 centimeters dilated, so I was admitted.

—*Carrie*

# Second Phase: Active Labor

When your cervix is dilated to 4 to 5 centimeters, your contractions usually reach the 4-1-1 or 5-1-1 pattern (see page 244). At this point, you're shifting from early labor to *active labor*. During this phase, dilation usually speeds up, contractions typically become painful (but manageable), and labor progresses with each contraction. Most expectant couples go to the hospital or birth center in this phase, or await the arrival of their home birth midwife.

## Getting through the Active Phase

Active labor may be emotionally challenging for you. Your contractions have intensified and require your full attention to manage. You may feel discouraged when you think about how long it's taken your cervix to dilate just halfway and may assume it'll take the same amount of time for your cervix to dilate to 10 centimeters. (It won't; dilation typically speeds up in active labor.) You may feel trapped, as you realize that your contractions are beyond your control and will continue to intensify until your cervix is fully dilated. You may weep because you feel overwhelmed. These reactions to this demanding phase are normal.

Although active labor can be challenging, you're *not* doomed to suffer through it. You can manage this phase (and cope better afterward) if the following are true:

- You're allowed to labor in an environment that fosters privacy, preserves your modesty, and minimizes disturbances. When you're undisturbed, you can focus inward and find your *spontaneous rituals* (see page 207) to help you get through contractions.
- You have support people who unconditionally accept your coping style and assist you whenever needed. In this phase, you become serious, quiet, and preoccupied. During contractions, you require your partner and others to focus on you—they shouldn't talk among themselves or to you, unless you request a response. (If you feel that someone isn't acting in a way that contributes to your emotional well-being, ask that he or she leave the room.)
- You have the freedom to move about and seek comfort in whatever ways you find helpful.

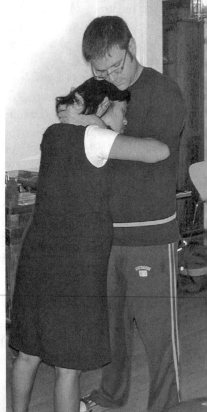

If giving birth in a hospital or birth center, traveling to the site during active labor creates a major disturbance in your coping strategy. A good way to prepare for this disruption is to practice comfort techniques (see Chapter 11) in noisy, busy environments *before* labor. That way, you may be able to continue coping during the ride and the admitting procedures as best as you can (see page 249 for suggestions), then return to your ideal focused state once you're settled in your room—assuming, of course, you're not being watched, judged, or told how to behave.

## A Note to Fathers and Partners

Figure out how to help your laboring partner by following her lead. Just as in early labor, be attentive to her in active labor, but don't disturb her. If she wants silence during contractions (or all the time), keep quiet. Match her mood. Observe and support her ritual during contractions (see page 207). She may want you to help her cope by slow dancing or walking with her, stroking her, moaning with her, matching her rhythm by swaying or by moving your hand or head, keeping eye contact with her, or counting her breaths. Or she may be so inwardly focused that she wants only your calm presence, perhaps allowing you to hold her hand or offer her sips of a beverage between contractions. See Appendix B for suggestions on ways you can help your partner throughout labor.

If she seems disappointed with her progress, encourage her to be patient and trust that she's doing well. If you're discouraged with her progress, take her caregiver or doula aside (so you're out of your partner's earshot) and ask about her well-being. Once labor progress speeds up, you'll both feel encouraged.

## In Their Own Words

After a nurse examined me, she said I was still in early labor and told my partner and me to go home and rest. When we got home, I couldn't sleep and found many tasks to complete around the house. I'd later regret not taking the advice to rest, but keeping active did allow my labor to progress, and I was admitted to the hospital just four hours later.

*—Jennifer*

## ARRIVING AT THE HOSPITAL OR BIRTH CENTER

After you've called to report the information in your Early Labor Record (see page 175) and are told to go to the hospital or birth center, make sure you have your bag, your birth plan (see Chapter 8), and any last-minute items (for example, a towel if your bag of waters is leaking) and head to the birthplace. Do *not* drive yourself; have your partner drive. If you know beforehand that your partner might not be able to drive you, recruit someone else.

The ride to the birthplace may be challenging and uncomfortable. You'll probably be more aware of every bump and pothole than ever before! Your partner should drive carefully and not speed. Try to think of the trip as a way to confirm whether you need to be at the birthplace. Focus your breathing on something in the vehicle to give you a rhythm to follow. For example, your partner can nod his or her head in rhythm with your breathing or count your breaths.

If giving birth in a hospital, find out ahead of time which entrance to use. If you arrive in the middle of the night, the emergency room may be the only open entrance. Once you're in the hospital, walk to the maternity unit or use a wheelchair if necessary.

When you arrive at the birth center or the hospital's maternity unit, an admitting nurse should greet you, then take you either to a birthing room or the *triage* (observation) area, where she or he assesses your condition, your pattern of contractions, your dilation (with a vaginal exam), and your baby's well-being. This information helps the nurse decide whether to admit you. If you think your bag of waters has broken, the nurse may give you a sterile speculum exam to obtain a sample of your amniotic fluid for diagnosis. (See page 173 for information on the leaking of amniotic fluid.)

If the nurse decides that you're still in very early labor, he or she may suggest that you leave the hospital or birth center until your labor pattern changes. You should follow this advice. If you stay at the birthplace, your labor progress is likely to dominate your thoughts, which can make your entire labor seem extremely long. If you leave the birthplace, you can keep busy at home until your labor pattern changes. Also, your labor is likely to progress more readily when you're in an environment that feels safe, secure, and familiar.

It's natural to become discouraged when learning that you can't be admitted to the hospital or birth center, especially if you're tired and are finding your contractions uncomfortable and difficult to cope with. You may feel concerned, angry, ignored, or frustrated. You may worry that you won't return to the birthplace in time. If you feel this way, tell the admitting nurse. He or she may be able to reassure you, help you with coping strategies, give you medication to help you rest, or suggest other options if you don't want to return home (such as taking a walk near the birthplace or going to the cafeteria). As you wait for your labor pattern to change, focus on ways to relax or distract yourself during contractions and on ways to rest between contractions. (See Chapter 11 as well as pages 245–247 for a discussion on prolonged prelabor.)

When you meet the criteria for admission to a hospital's birth center or maternity unit, you're taken to your birthing room, where you meet your labor nurse. He or she may assess you in the same way that the admitting nurse did, as well as make other assessments, including taking your medical history, getting urine and blood samples, and checking your baby's heart rate and position. You change into a hospital gown (or your own) and get an identification bracelet. You may have an *intravenous (IV) catheter* inserted at this time. The nurse begins monitoring your contractions and your baby's heart rate (see page 251) for twenty to thirty minutes, typically with an external electronic fetal monitor (see page 252) or possibly with a hand-held Doppler.

In some ways, admission to a freestanding birth center (unaffiliated with a hospital) is similar to admission to a hospital birth center or maternity unit. You're assessed in the same way; however, your midwife makes the assessments, not a nurse. You also wear your own clothing and don't receive an identification bracelet.

## IV Fluids in Normal Labor

In some hospitals, it's routine to insert an IV catheter in all laboring women shortly after they're admitted. In other hospitals, an IV catheter is inserted only if needed—for example, if you need medications such as Pitocin or antibiotics, if you choose to take pain medications, or if you're unable to keep down enough fluids to stay hydrated.

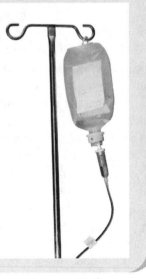

IV catheters carry a few mild risks; visit our web site, http://www.PCN Guide.com, for more information. In addition, an IV catheter can limit mobility in labor because you're connected to a wheeled pole that holds the bag of fluids. During a prenatal appointment, ask your caregiver if IV catheters are routine or used only when needed. If they're routine, ask whether you can instead have a *Heparin Lock* (or Hep-Lock), which involves inserting an IV catheter, but doesn't require hooking it to an IV bag and pole until IV fluids are needed.

## INITIAL PROCEDURES FOR A HOME BIRTH

After you've called your midwife and he or she has decided your labor progress warrants coming to your home, your midwife assesses your progress in a way that's similar to how an admitting nurse makes assessments (see above). Your midwife then brings medical implements, medications, and other essential equipment (such as an oxygen tank) into your home. Depending on your labor progress, he or she may remain with you or may leave your home for a while (but stay within a reasonably close distance). Your midwife may work with an assistant, who remains with you if your midwife leaves for a time during early labor.

## WORKING WITH YOUR LABOR

After your labor nurse finishes assessing you, make yourself as comfortable as possible. Continue your ritual or begin a spontaneous one (see page 207) to help find your best way to cope. Use comfort measures as appropriate, such as placing pressure and cold packs on your back or hot compresses on your lower abdomen and groin. Empty your bladder every hour or so; a full bladder increases discomfort and can slow labor. Make sure to keep yourself hydrated by sipping water after a few contractions or by sucking on a Popsicle or ice chips.

Try not to lie in bed throughout your labor. Keeping immobile in this position may increase the pain of your contractions and slow labor progress.[4] Unless you need to rest or your contractions are coming so fast that you can't move, try to periodically move about in bed or take advantage of gravity by standing and walking in your room and in the hall. (See pages 221–223 for a discussion of ideal positions for labor.) *Note*: If you choose to receive pain medications, your mobility may be limited. (See Chapter 10.)

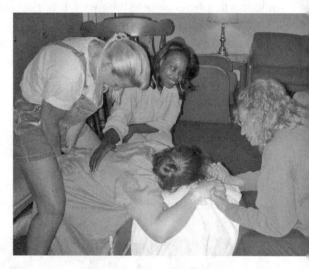

Continue slow breathing (see page 224) for as long as it helps you relax. Switch to light breathing or one of the adaptations (see pages 225–228) if your breathing begins to feel labored, if you can't keep your breathing rate slow, or if you can't maintain your rhythm, even after renewed efforts and active encouragement from your partner. Light breathing may be better suited for demanding contractions than slow breathing, just as short, quick breaths are better suited for demanding physical exercise than long, deep breaths are. By tuning in to your contractions, you can adapt your breathing rhythms as needed.

## MONITORING YOU AND YOUR BABY DURING NORMAL LABOR

Whether you labor in a hospital, birth center, or at home, expect your caregivers to monitor you and your baby closely, watching for signs of potential problems that may require medical intervention. As long as your labor is normal and your baby is doing well, you don't need medical procedures. Visit our web site, http://www.PCNGuide.com, for descriptions of techniques used if monitoring indicates that a complication has developed in labor.

### *Monitoring You*

Throughout labor, your nurse or caregiver regularly checks and records your blood pressure, temperature, pulse, urine output, fluid intake, activity, and emotional state. He or she may also perform vaginal exams periodically to determine the effacement and dilation of your cervix and the station, presentation, and position of your baby. These results are recorded on a chart that shows your labor progress. Your nurse or caregiver observes the frequency and intensity of your contractions either by hand or by an electronic monitor (see below). These assessments are all your nurse or caregiver needs, provided that no problems develop in either your labor or baby.

## Monitoring Your Baby with Fetal Heart Rate Monitoring

During labor, many things influence your baby's heart rate: your contractions, his activity (fetal movements), medications, your body temperature, your position, and other factors. The normal fetal heart rate (FHR) range is between 120 and 160 beats per minute. FHR varies within this range in response to changes in the amount of oxygen that's available. If your baby is handling labor well, he has a "reactive" heart rate, which naturally slows down to compensate for the temporary reductions in oxygen during a contraction and speeds up between contractions. This fluctuation indicates that he's compensating well to the normal variations in oxygen flow.

Depending on the maturity and health of your baby, his ability to compensate varies. If a lack of oxygen continues over time, his reserves may become exhausted. He might no longer be able to compensate and might become distressed (fetal distress, also known as *nonreassuring fetal heart rate* or *fetal intolerance of labor*). When FHR is nonreassuring, close observation and further testing help caregivers identify those few babies who aren't tolerating labor well and may need immediate medical intervention.

Your baby's heart rate can be monitored either by *auscultation* or by *electronic fetal monitoring (EFM)*. With auscultation, your nurse or caregiver listens to your baby's heartbeat during and between contractions with a Doppler, a hand-held ultrasound stethoscope. (Some caregivers may use a fetal stethoscope.) At the same time, he or she may place a hand on your abdomen to feel your contractions, then count your baby's heartbeats, noting whether they speed up or slow down and recording the findings.

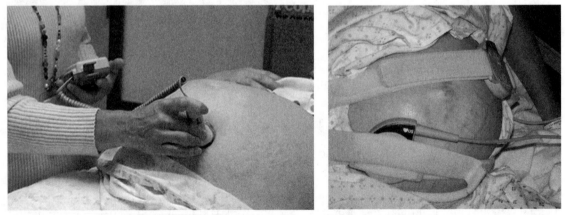

There are two types of EFM. The commonly used external EFM uses belts to place two sensors on your abdomen, and the rarely used internal EFM uses two sensors placed inside your uterus. (Caregivers use internal EFM only if external EFM isn't picking up adequate signals.) One sensor picks up your baby's heartbeat; the other picks up changes in your uterine tone or pressure (that is, your contractions). These sensors may be connected to video screens in your room or at the nurses' station. The screen displays two graphs that indicate your baby's heart rate and the intensity of your contractions. A printout of the data may also be produced. All data are stored electronically. Your caregiver checks the video screen or printout to assess your baby's well-being and your contraction pattern.

Studies that compare auscultation and EFM (continuous or intermittent) report that each method has similar newborn outcomes. Most caregivers at hospitals, however, prefer EFM because it lets nurses monitor many women at the same time from the nurses' station (an advantage when the nursing staff is overextended) and frees them from having to record a baby's heart rate by hand. Plus, electronically storing the data saves paper.

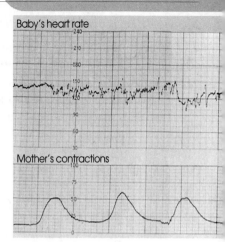

Baby's heart rate

Mother's contractions

Continuous EFM may limit your contact with your nurse and may keep you in bed. By comparison, auscultation may feel more personal because your nurse focuses on you—not a screen—to monitor you and your baby, and it may work better with your coping strategy because you're not restrained from moving about by the EFM device.

Caregivers generally prefer to use continuous EFM for women with high-risk pregnancies. If you and your baby are healthy and low-risk, you shouldn't have to be monitored continuously. Twenty minutes of EFM when you're first admitted to the hospital, followed by fifteen minutes of EFM each hour, is an accepted protocol as long as your baby's heart rate remains normal. Obstetrical associations in the United States and Canada also endorse the protocol of auscultation for one minute during and after a contraction every fifteen to thirty minutes in the first stage, and every five to fifteen minutes during the second stage.

During pregnancy, check whether your caregiver or hospital uses continuous EFM and under what circumstances. If continuous EFM is routine for all laboring women, check whether the hospital offers wireless (or telemetry) EFM, which allows staff to monitor you continuously while you're out of bed, walking around, or even in the bathtub.

For more information on the different types and techniques of monitoring, visit our web site http://www.PCNGuide.com.

## Evaluating Your Amniotic Fluid

When your membranes rupture, the appearance of your amniotic fluid can indicate your baby's condition. Normal fluid is clear and has a slightly fleshy odor. If your fluid has the strong odor of old fish, you may have an infection. If your fluid is green or dark, your baby has expelled meconium (first waste) from her bowels, which may indicate that she's stressed. The presence of meconium in amniotic fluid isn't uncommon; it occurs in 20 percent of all labors. If your fluid shows signs of meconium, your caregiver will observe your baby's heart rate frequently to assess her well-being.

When researching your caregiver and birthplace during pregnancy, ask about the protocol for treating a newborn who has expelled meconium during labor. Many caregivers suction the baby's nose, mouth, and trachea (windpipe) when the head is born and before the first breath. The belief is that suctioning prevents the baby from inhaling meconium, thereby preventing breathing problems or a rare type of pneumonia called meconium aspiration syndrome. Other caregivers choose not to suction a baby who's vigorous at birth, instead letting her breathe immediately. Research hasn't found that aggressive suctioning prevents meconium aspiration syndrome.[5] Instead, suctioning seems to cause abrasions in the membranes of the baby's nose and mouth.

## *Monitoring Your Baby's Well-being with Fetal Scalp Stimulation and Other Tests*

If FHR monitoring raises concerns, your caregiver may further assess your baby's well-being by fetal scalp stimulation. This test is reliable, simple, inexpensive, and can be repeated easily. During a vaginal exam, your caregiver presses or scratches your baby's scalp. If your baby's heart rate speeds up, he's likely fine. If his heart rate slows down, he might not be tolerating labor well.

Fetal scalp blood sampling is another test that may be used to monitor your baby's condition. It involves taking blood from your baby's scalp and analyzing it for changes in blood chemistry caused by a lack of oxygen. Although this test is helpful, it's rarely used because it's invasive to the baby, takes longer to analyze, and is uncomfortable for the mother.

# Third Phase: Transition

As its name suggests, you *transition* from the first to the second stage of labor during this phase. Your cervix is reaching complete dilation, and your baby is beginning to descend into your birth canal. At this time, your contractions are longer (ninety seconds to two minutes) and closer together (two to three minutes apart). Although your labor is still technically in the first stage, your body shows some signs of the second stage. Your emotions and physical sensations are intense. You feel tired, restless, irritable, and totally consumed by your efforts to cope. You may lose your ritual (see page 207). Your body begins secreting high levels of adrenaline, which may lead to a "fight or flight" response (temporary fear, nausea, vomiting, agitation, hot flashes, chills, and trembling), but the hormone is beneficial because you become more alert and have renewed strength and energy just when you need to push out your baby.[8]

Involuntary spasms (precursors of bearing down) may stimulate your diaphragm, causing you to hiccup, grunt, or belch. You may find yourself holding your breath and straining or grunting during each contraction; this reaction is the urge to push. (See page 258 for more information.) Your back or thighs may ache. Increased pressure may cause your legs or even your whole body to tremble, and it may also cause heavy vaginal discharge of bloody mucus. Despite the intensity and pain of contractions during transition, you may doze between contractions, as though your body is conserving all energy for managing them.

Transition often lasts less than an hour (usually between five and twenty contractions).

## GETTING THROUGH TRANSITION

During transition, you become focused only on your labor; nothing else matters. The intensity of your labor may frighten you. You may feel that transition will last forever and you can't cope much longer. In this phase, the encouragement and support from your partner, doula, and caregivers are essential.

Your responses to transition (such as fear, nausea, trembling, despair, crying, dependence on others, and difficulty maintaining your ritual) are natural and unique to your labor. Your goal at this

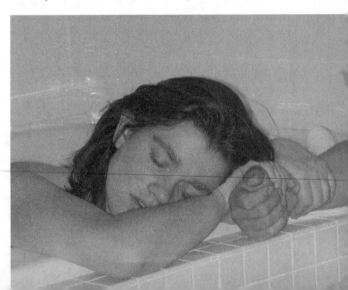

time isn't necessarily to remain calm, still, and relaxed during contractions. Instead, your aim is to maintain a coping ritual, with the help of your partner or doula if necessary (see page 256). You may rhythmically sway from side to side, tap your fingers or feet, stroke your belly, or rock back and forth. Or you may want your partner to stroke you or murmur rhythmically in your ear. You may find that moaning during contractions helps release tension. Or you may remain still and quiet during your contractions. Between contractions, try to relax and rest, if only for a few seconds.

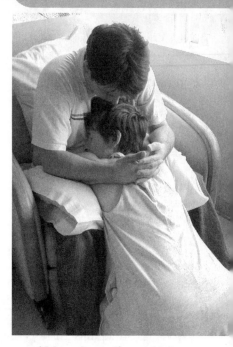

You might like your partner to hold you close, or you might not want to be touched. You may want your partner to provide only eye contact and verbal encouragement. You may find hot, damp towels on your lower abdomen soothing. If you're sweating, your partner can fan you or wipe your face, neck, and chest with a cool, damp cloth. If you're able to doze between contractions, your partner can help you focus and begin breathing rhythmically as soon as the next contraction begins so the intensity doesn't overwhelm you.

If you recognize that you're in transition, you can cope better with this phase. If you think your cervix is only 5 or 6 centimeters dilated, you may become discouraged and worry that you have hours of demanding contractions to go. However, when you and your partner recognize the signs of transition described on page 254, your progress can hearten you. You can see that the challenges of transition lead to the second stage of labor, when your mental state will improve as the birth of your baby draws closer.

## Pain Medications during Transition

You can get through transition without pain medications, especially if you have the following: a desire for a non-medicated labor, knowledge of what to expect and how to cope in this phase, good support, and a labor that's progressing normally. Some women, however, find that transition is too much for them to handle; the pain is too great, they're exhausted, or they lose control or panic. If this happens to you, pain medications are usually an option. (See Chapter 10.)

While there's no shame in wanting medical help during this phase, don't take pain medications just because you fear that the intensity of your labor is abnormal. Remember that strong emotional responses and challenging contractions are completely normal in transition. Before deciding on pain medications, first find out how far your labor has progressed. Because transition typically lasts less than an hour (ten to twenty contractions), you may decide that pain medications are unnecessary.

## Urge to Push in Transition

In this phase you may develop an urge to push, which may feel as though you need to have a bowel movement (because your baby's head is pressing against your rectum). You may also start catching your breath and grunting (that is, making "pushing sounds"). When you first feel an urge to push, let your nurse or caregiver know. Try not to push until he or she can assess you. If your cervix isn't completely dilated or is almost dilated except for one thickened area (a "lip" of cervix), you may be asked not to push.

## In Their Own Words

It's hard to watch your girlfriend be in pain and know there's *nothing* you can do. I just stayed strong for her and let her know I wouldn't leave her side. Observing the confidence in the staff and seeing my girlfriend smile when our son was born let me know that everything was fine.

—*Tom*

While it's usually okay to bear down in labor, doing so isn't worthwhile before your cervix is fully dilated. In fact, pushing too early may cause your cervix to swell and slow your labor progress. You may find it difficult and uncomfortable to keep from pushing when the urge is strong. If you're asked not to push, try blowing or panting to keep from holding your breath. (See page 228.) You may be able to relieve a premature urge to push by changing positions, such as to the hands-and-knees, side-lying, or other positions that neutralize the effects of gravity. See page 258 for more information on the urge to push.

### A Note to Fathers and Partners

Transition is probably the most difficult challenge that you'll ever see your laboring partner experience. Her pain and discouragement may trouble you, but remember that her intense sensations and emotions are normal. She and your baby are all right. Nonetheless, you both need reassurance and encouragement from your doula, nurse, or caregiver at this time. See Appendix B for suggestions on ways to help your partner throughout labor.

Your job during this phase is simple: Help her keep a rhythm (see page 206). Listen closely for whatever rhythm she may have and help her maintain it. It's very likely she may need you to give her a rhythm to follow. (See the Take Charge Routine below.) Don't mistake rhythmic moans, groans, or other intense sounds for cries of agony. If they're rhythmic, she's coping.

If she begins catching her breath and grunting (making pushing sounds), she may have an urge to push. Call her nurse or caregiver. She may be in the second stage of labor and ready to push!

## Take Charge Routine for Partners

Use this routine when your laboring partner is in despair, weeping, crying out for help, or ready to give up. Also use this technique when she's overwhelmed with pain, can't relax, and can't regain her coping rhythm or ritual.

- Keep your composure. Your touch should be firm and confident. Your voice should be calm and reassuring. Give simple, concise directions. Don't ask her questions.
- Stay close to her. Remain by her side with your face near hers.
- Anchor her. Hold her hand or cradle her in your arms.
- Make eye contact. Tell her to open her eyes and look at you or at your hand. This helps her focus.
- Give her a rhythm to follow with her breathing; move your hand or head to set a pace for her to follow (about one breath per each second or two). If she loses the rhythm, say, "Breathe with me; follow my hand. That's the way, just like that." Nod your head in time with her breathing to reinforce the rhythm.
- Encourage her. Acknowledge that labor is difficult, but not impossible. Remind her that she's made a lot of progress and that her baby will be here soon. Tell her to look at you the moment she feels the next contraction so you can help her. Immediately set a rhythm for her to follow.
- Repeat yourself. She might not be able to do what you tell her for more than a few seconds, but repeating your instructions will help her continue.

# Short, Fast Labor

Occasionally, a woman's entire labor lasts only six hours or less and leads to a *precipitate birth*. In this type of labor, contractions may have started only three or four minutes apart, lasted a minute each, and were already so intense that the woman couldn't cope with them. A labor this fast is rare among first-time mothers, but a few may have labors that are as short as three hours. Short, fast labors are much more common for women who have given birth before. If your labor progresses quickly and a precipitate birth is imminent, forget the 4-1-1 or 5-1-1 rule (see page 244)—call your caregiver!

Although a quick labor may sound appealing, it presents its own challenges. Early labor may pass unnoticed or so quickly that you suddenly find yourself in active labor without time to prepare psychologically. Your first noticeable contractions may be long and painful. You may feel confused, unprepared, and even panicky, especially if you think what you're experiencing is prelabor or early labor. You may quickly lose faith in your ability to handle the rest of labor.

If you've planned a hospital birth, you may hurry to the hospital, all the while trying to cope with strong, almost continuous contractions. At the hospital, you're probably met by unfamiliar caregivers, who spark a flurry of activity. You may feel anxious and alone if your partner is unable to accompany you. Even if he or she is with you, you may want to give up and take any medication available to you to make the pain disappear or at least become manageable. Your partner is probably caught off guard and shocked by the sudden intensity of your labor, especially if he or she also believes you're experiencing early labor.

## *What You Can Do If Your Labor Is Rapid*

If it's clear that your baby will be born quickly, don't give up on your ability to cope. Try not to tense up during contractions and use slow breathing (see page 224). If slow breathing doesn't help you, use light breathing (see page 225). Moan or bellow rhythmically, if doing so is helpful. Consent to a vaginal exam before making any decision about pain medication; your cervix may have already dilated to 8 or 10 centimeters. If your labor has progressed this rapidly, anesthesia may be unnecessary or may take effect too late to provide relief before your baby's birth. Rely on your partner, doula, and staff to help you cope with contractions and to reassure you that you and your baby are doing well.

In a rapid labor, contractions are intense and effective, and you may have the urge to push before staff is ready. If this happens in your labor, lie on your side and pant or gently bear down. Doing so gives your birth canal and perineum more time to stretch, decreasing the likelihood of vaginal tearing.

After the birth, you'll probably be relieved that you and your baby are safe, but stunned that the entire event passed so quickly. You may also feel disappointment because you weren't able to fully appreciate the experience, to use all the breathing and relaxation techniques you learned, or to share the birth with your partner as you'd planned. You may need to discuss the sequence of events with your caregiver and partner so you can process the birth and come to terms with it.

Although less than 1 in 1,000 babies are born on the way to the hospital or birth center,[7] in the unlikely event that you start to give birth before you leave home or en route to the birthplace, or before your home birth midwife arrives, you and your partner should know how to safely catch your baby. See page 300 for more information on rapid birth without medical help.

# Second Stage of Labor: Birth of Your Baby

As soon as your cervix has dilated completely, you're in the second stage of labor. A new sequence of events begins: Your baby gradually leaves your uterus, rotates within your pelvis, descends through your vagina, and is born.

The second stage typically lasts between fifteen minutes to more than three hours. For a first-time mother, the average time for this stage is ninety minutes to two hours. For a mother who has given birth before, the second stage is usually faster than it was for her first birth.

## SIGNS OF THE SECOND STAGE

During the second stage, the pain of your contractions lessens and the interval between them increases. You calm down and can think clearly again. You experience renewed energy and become optimistic and aware of those around you. Now you can collect yourself for pushing your baby out.

### Urge to Push

The *urge to push* is the most significant sign of the second stage. It's a combination of forceful sensations and reflex (involuntary) actions caused by the pressure of your baby in your vagina during contractions around the time your cervix is fully dilated. The urge to push occurs several times within a contraction and indicates that your uterine muscles are pushing your baby downward. When you have the urge to push, you experience a compelling need to grunt or hold your breath and bear down. It may feel like a strong urge to have a bowel movement.

Whether you have an urge to push immediately at this time or after a brief rest depends on the degree and speed of your baby's descent, her station and position within your pelvis, your body position, and other factors. Ask your caregiver to check the dilation of your cervix. If it's fully dilated, you generally can begin pushing when you feel the urge. If it's not fully dilated but is very ripe and effaced, you may be asked to bear down only enough to satisfy the urge. If your cervix isn't completely dilated, you may be asked not to push (see page 228). Because the urge to push is involuntary, resisting it may postpone pushing, but only temporarily.

For many women, responding to the urge to push is one of the most satisfying aspects of the birth experience; some women even orgasm when giving birth. Others find pushing painful and exhausting, while many are simply relieved to be able to start pushing.

*Note:* Some women don't feel a strong (or any) urge to push in this stage. Usually, time or changing to an upright position can strengthen the urge to push. Also, if you receive pain medication, especially epidural anesthesia, you might not feel the urge to push or it might be a vague sensation.

## THREE KEY CONCEPTS FOR THE SECOND STAGE

During the second stage, the following three key concepts should guide you and your caregiver: *Don't rush. Push when you have an urge. Use different positions.*

### Don't Rush

Although you and your caregiver are anxious to have your baby born, it's best not to rush the birth. Bear down or push spontaneously as the urge demands and allow time for your vagina to stretch open gradually, which decreases the likelihood of vaginal bruising or tearing.[8] Don't use prolonged pushing (see page 258). You also use your energy more efficiently if you don't rush. By holding your breath and bearing down only when you can't resist the urge, you're working with your uterus and not wasting effort.

## *Push When You Have the Urge*

The following are descriptions of the different ways to push under certain circumstances in labor.

### Expulsion breathing and spontaneous bearing down

Use when you have an urge to push (see page 258). With *spontaneous bearing down*, you naturally bear down or strain for five to six seconds at a time and take several breaths between efforts. This type of pushing makes more oxygen available to your baby than if you hold your breath and bear down for as long as possible.[9] Spontaneous bearing down also allows your vagina to stretch gradually, reducing your risk of tearing.

### Delayed pushing (passive descent or laboring down with an epidural)

When you have an epidural, you probably don't have an urge to push until your baby is close to being born. Your uterus continues pushing your baby down and into a good position, but you don't feel the need to push in response.

With *delayed pushing*, try to rest and refrain from pushing until your baby's head can be seen at your vaginal opening (crowning) or until you feel the urge to push. This way, if your baby is occiput posterior (see page 285) or his head is tilted (either a likely occurrence if you have an epidural), you avoid forcing him too deeply into your pelvis before he can reposition himself. Delayed pushing usually means a longer second stage, but as long as your baby is doing well, research shows that waiting an hour or two before pushing with an epidural gives your baby time to gradually reposition until his head is visible.[10] Delayed pushing is also much less tiring for you. It greatly improves your chances of a spontaneous vaginal birth (one that doesn't require vacuum extraction or forceps delivery) and greatly decreases your chances of needing a cesarean.

When it's time to push, your nurse or caregiver will probably tell you when and how long to push during each contraction.

### Directed pushing

*Directed pushing* is used if you can't feel your contractions and delayed pushing isn't an option or if spontaneous pushing isn't effective. Your caregiver will tell you when, how long, and how hard to push. (See page 233 for more information on directed pushing.)

### Prolonged pushing

Prolonged pushing differs from directed pushing in the length of time you're expected to hold your breath and bear down (ten seconds or more, instead of five to seven seconds).

Not long ago, standard practice in maternity care required that women push for as long and as hard as they could, in order to push out the baby as quickly as possible. Many maternity caregivers are still more comfortable advocating prolonged pushing than spontaneous bearing down. Research shows, however, that prolonged, forceful pushing usually isn't necessary and may sometimes cause problems that are less likely to occur with spontaneous bearing down, including exhaustion of the mother, overstretching of pelvic ligaments and muscles, possible perineal tears, later urinary incontinence (leaking of urine), concerns with the baby's heart rate, and failure of the baby to rotate or descend.[11]

Prolonged pushing, especially in the supine position (on your back), can also decrease the oxygen available to your baby and may cause your blood pressure to drop, both of which can increase the need for a faster delivery with an episiotomy. The second stage may last slightly longer with spontaneous or directed pushing than with prolonged pushing, but babies usually remain in good condition throughout the process.[12]

Prolonged pushing is best reserved for women with inadequate progress in the second stage, even after trying different positions, or for women whose babies are already in distress and may require interventions (such as a forceps delivery, vacuum extraction, or cesarean birth) unless they're pushed out quickly. Well before your due date, discuss prolonged pushing with your caregiver. Include your preferences regarding the practice in your birth plan and discuss them with the staff when you arrive at the hospital or birth center. See pages 232–234 for more discussion on the various pushing techniques.

## Use Different Positions

As long as your labor is progressing well in the second stage and your baby is fine, use whatever positions seem most comfortable to you. If your caregiver is concerned about your progress or your baby's well-being, he or she may recommend that you try a different position. Even if it's uncomfortable, this new position may correct the problem and avoid the need for further interventions.

If your second stage is rapid, try a position that neutralizes the effects of gravity, such as side-lying, to help slow down labor. If progress is prolonged, try positions that take advantage of gravity. Be prepared and willing to change positions every twenty to thirty minutes. (See pages 222–223 for descriptions of positions.)

Some caregivers are comfortable with having a woman give birth in any position she desires. However, most caregivers prefer a position that they're used to (usually semi-sitting or on the back),[13] which might not be the best position for comfort or progress. During pregnancy, discuss your options with your caregiver. If he or she delivers babies in only one position, plan to use several other positions throughout early second stage to aid labor progress. During second stage, if pushing is prolonged, ask whether a change in position might help resolve the situation.

*Note:* If you've received pain medications, your mobility and choice of positions may be limited. (See Chapter 10.)

## PHASES OF THE SECOND STAGE

The second stage has three phases: the resting phase, descent phase, and crowning and birth phase. These three phases share characteristics with the three phases of the first stage. High spirits, little pain, and slow progress characterize the first phases of both stages. Intense contractions, total mental absorption, and steady progress characterize the second phases. Lastly, intense sensations and confusion characterize the third phases.

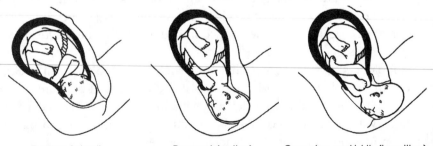

Resting (latent)              Descent (active)              Crowning and birth (transition)

## Resting Phase

After the intensity of transition, your uterus may stop contracting for ten to twenty minutes, allowing you to rest, clear your head, recoup your energy, and grow excited for your baby's imminent arrival. This resting phase is normal and may occur because your baby's head has slipped into your birth canal, causing your uterus, which had been stretched tightly around your baby, to slacken. Your uterus needs a few minutes to adjust to the change, but once it begins to tighten around the rest of your baby's body, strong contractions resume and your urge to push becomes powerful.

The resting phase doesn't occur in all labors. If your baby is low in your pelvis when the second stage begins, or if she's descending rapidly, your body may skip this resting phase or make it brief. Even if this phase doesn't offer you much rest, you probably still become clearheaded and emotionally recharged as you move into the second stage.

If the resting phase lasts longer than fifteen to twenty minutes, your caregiver may ask you to try a position that enhances the effects of gravity to encourage an urge to push. Or he or she may direct your pushing, asking you to hold your breath and bear down even if you don't have an urge to push. Directed pushing may frustrate both you and your caregiver, as labor progress rarely occurs without the urge to push. However, directed pushing may be worth trying before using a medical intervention such as Pitocin (see page 281).

## Descent Phase

During this phase, your baby descends into your birth canal and likely completes rotation to the occiput anterior position (see page 285). At this time, powerful contractions make your urge to push irresistible. You may find bearing down thrilling and rewarding because you can feel progress. Or you may feel alarmed by the full, bulging, stretching feeling in your perineum. You may tense your pelvic floor and "hold back" (see page 262), afraid to let your baby descend. When pushing, it's important to relax your pelvic floor and bulge your perineum (see page 96). Prenatal perineal massage (see page 235) is excellent preparation for the second stage because it teaches you to relax your perineum while it's being stretched. Your partner can help you during this phase by reminding you to relax, open up, bulge your bottom, or ease your baby out. This type of encouragement is usually more helpful than being told to push, push, push!

In this phase, you may need several contractions before you can push effectively. If you have trouble figuring out where to direct your efforts when pushing, ask your caregiver to perform perineal massage or to use a warm compress to give you a location. Using a mirror to watch what happens when you push may also help you figure out how to push more effectively.

Clenching your jaw and clamping your lips together are signs that you're also tensing the muscles in your vagina. By relaxing your face and mouth, you may be able to relax your vagina.

## In Their Own Words

When I was dilated, my midwife told me I was ready to push—but I didn't feel ready! She had me try the squat bar and sitting on the toilet, which just made the pain more intense and didn't give me an urge to push. I remembered reading that there's sometimes a lull between transition and pushing, so I wasn't worried. I asked my doula and my husband to tell the staff that I wanted to push spontaneously when I was ready. My wishes were respected and I slept between contractions until I finally began bearing down.

—Marie

# Holding Back during the Descent Phase

During the second stage, you may tense your pelvic floor (at least briefly) in response to the stretching sensations you feel when your baby's head is in your birth canal. Holding back is normal and usually passes quickly once you feel your baby descending.

To stop yourself from holding back, try telling yourself to let go. If successful, the pain decreases and you won't have a desire to hold back again. However, you may have trouble letting go for one or more of the following reasons:

**The pressure of your baby's head within your vagina alarms you, and you find it difficult to give in to that pressure.**

Remind yourself that holding back tends to increase pain and slow progress. You'll feel so much better after letting go! Listen to your partner, doula, and caregiver when they encourage you to let go and let your baby out.

Try sitting on the toilet for a few contractions. This position may help your perineal muscles release naturally because it's associated with "letting go" of urine or a bowel movement.

Warm compresses on your perineum can help because the moist heat promotes relaxation and relieves the stretching sensation. This simple, inexpensive comfort measure also alleviates perineal pain and reduces the risks of tearing and urinary incontinence (see page 352).[14] In addition, having your caregiver press the cloth on your perineum reassures you that he or she will help guide your baby out. Before your due date, discuss using warm compresses during labor with your caregiver and include the option in your birth plan (see Chapter 8).

*Note:* During this phase, some caregivers use their fingers to stretch a woman's perineum. While this practice may help her push more effectively, research finds that it's often very painful and is no more effective for enlarging the vaginal outlet and preventing a tear than the use of warm compresses or even no treatment.[15]

**You're uncomfortable with having people stare at your perineum.**

Try to recognize that they're watching the progress of your baby, but ask to be covered as much as possible. For example, warm compresses can conceal your perineum as they help relax and stretch it.

**You fear you'll have a bowel movement while pushing.**

Because your baby presses on your rectum while descending, it's normal to pass a small amount of stool when you push. When this happens, your nurse or caregiver interprets it as labor progress. You might not even be aware of it, because your caregiver wipes away and removes the stool discreetly (perhaps with a warm compress, if one is used to help your perineum relax and stretch). Sitting on the toilet for a few contractions may help you dispel this fear and relax.

**If you've been sexually abused, you fear that the sensations of your baby in your vagina will remind you of your abuse.**

It may help to tell yourself that you're pushing your pain out of your body as you push out your baby. Because it's important to separate your abuse from the birth of your child, see page 59 for more information on sexual abuse and childbearing.

If you let yourself release tension and push despite the pain, you'll find that pushing feels better than holding back.

As this phase progresses, the joy and anticipation you feel give you renewed strength. Your perineum begins to bulge, your labia part, and your vagina opens as your baby's head descends each time you bear down. Between pushes, your vagina partially closes and your baby's head retreats. With another contraction, your baby moves farther down, his head becomes clearly visible, and you may be able to see it in a mirror. You may want to reach down and touch his soft, wrinkled head. The normal squeezing of your baby's head by your vagina causes the scalp to wrinkle until his head moves farther down your birth canal.

## Crowning and Birth Phase

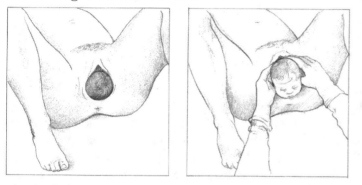

The third phase of the second stage is the *crowning* of your baby's head and her birth. It begins when your baby's head no longer retreats from your vaginal opening between pushes, and it ends when her body completely exits yours. During this phase, your vaginal opening stretches to its maximum, which likely causes a stinging, burning sensation called the "rim of fire." To reduce the risk of a vaginal tear or a rapid birth, you may need to stop pushing to let your vagina and perineum gradually stretch around your baby's head as it emerges. Depending on the speed of the birth, your caregiver may direct you to push only moderately or to push only between contractions. He or she may ask you not to push at all (see page 228 to learn how to resist the urge to push). Your caregiver may support your perineum with warm compresses to prevent your baby's head from coming too rapidly and to help your perineum stretch gradually.

Research finds clear problems with routine episiotomy to enlarge the vaginal opening; nonetheless, some caregivers still commonly perform episiotomies. See pages 289–290 for more information on episiotomy.

### Two Views on Crowning and the Birth

When Grace finally crowned, I knew my wife could push her out, even though she was starting to feel exhausted. Sure enough, she tapped into a source of strength that probably surprised her as much as it did me, and pushed our daughter out. Grace was so slimy! But she was also so gorgeous, I cried when I saw her.
—*Ryan*

When I began pushing, Jacob was holding my left hand and the nurse was murmuring instructions in my right ear. I didn't feel that my contractions were coming close enough together. I could feel a burning sensation as my baby's head slowly moved down. Everything seemed in slow motion. Finally, with a rush of pain and a huge relief, my daughter came out.
—*Paige*

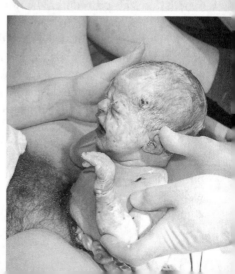

## Protecting Your Perineum from a Large Tear or an Episiotomy

Many women worry that pushing will damage their vaginal tissues, or they fear that an episiotomy will be needed. Here are research-based actions you can take during pregnancy and labor to protect your perineum:

- Choose a caregiver who prefers to avoid episiotomies and has a low rate of doing the procedure (less than 20 percent).
- Good nutrition promotes healthy tissues, so eat well during pregnancy.
- Perform perineal massage regularly for a few weeks before the birth. (See page 235.)
- When you push, use spontaneous bearing down or bear down for only five to seven seconds each time.
- During the birth, use positions that put minimal strain on your perineum, such as side-lying, kneeling, or hands-and-knees. (See page 222.)
- Also during the birth, pant lightly and listen to your caregiver's directions to avoid pushing while your baby's head and shoulders are born.

# Your Baby's Birth

The second stage of labor ends with your baby's birth. If your baby's position is head down (occiput anterior or posterior), first the crown of his head emerges, followed by his brow and face. His head appears bluish-gray and is soaking wet. After his head is out, it rotates to the side to allow his shoulders to slip more easily through your pelvis. One shoulder emerges, followed by the rest of his body, perhaps rather quickly. You or your partner may want to help catch your baby.

Your baby's body may appear bluish at first and may be streaked with blood, mucus, and *vernix caseosa* (a white, creamy substance that protected your baby's skin in your womb). With your baby's first breath, his skin color quickly becomes normal. All babies, regardless of skin color, experience this change in the first minutes of life, as respiration and circulation become stable. See Chapter 17 for more information on your newborn's appearance.

Your caregiver's or birthplace's policy may require that your baby have his nose and mouth suctioned immediately after the birth. However, studies find that healthy vigorous newborns don't benefit from this procedure.[16] During pregnancy, discuss your caregiver's or birthplace's policy on suctioning and include your preferences in your birth plan (see Chapter 8).

While you await the delivery of the placenta, your baby may be dried and immediately placed on your abdomen or in your arms. The umbilical cord is typically clamped and cut around this time; however, there are long-term advantages for your baby if cord clamping is delayed. (See page 267.) The custom in some hospitals is to assess a newborn's well-being while he's in a baby warmer in the birthing room. However, research shows that newborns are warmer and begin breastfeeding earlier when kept skin-to-skin with their mothers; in addition, most women report greater satisfaction when they have their babies with them immediately after the birth than if they're separated from them.[17] Before the birth, find out your hospital's custom on the use of baby warmers; in your birth plan, express your preference to hold your baby immediately after the birth (if he's doing well). Your nurse or caregiver can assess your baby while he's in your arms or at a later time, after he's had at least an hour of skin-to-skin contact with you.

## YOUR REACTIONS AFTER THE BIRTH

After your baby is born, your first response may be, "It's over! No more contractions!" and you may feel grateful and relieved that your baby is finally out of your body. These feelings may initially overtake your interest in your baby, especially if you had a long, tiring labor.

Conversely, you may temporarily forget about your labor and birth the moment you see or hear your newborn. You may be surprised or awed by your baby's appearance. You may hold your breath in suspense until you hear her begin to breathe, smiling with relief and joy when you hear her first hearty cry. If your caregiver needs to inspect your perineum and check for separation of the placenta, you may find the procedures painful and distracting, and you may be unable to focus completely on your baby. After your caregiver has finished these tasks, however, you can return your total attention to your baby.

### In Their Own Words

After my baby was placed on my chest, my body began shaking uncontrollably. The lights were turned back on, and I opened my eyes to stare at this slimy, squirmy thing that had been living inside of me. I always thought I'd need medication, but everything went so fast that I had a natural birth. It was an amazing, scary, and wonderful experience—something I will never forget.

—*Mary Ann*

## A NOTE TO FATHERS AND PARTNERS

The birth of your baby requires great physical effort by your laboring partner, even if she has an epidural. Here are ways you can assist her during this stage:

- Help her change positions and physically support her as needed.
- Encourage her to relax her pelvic floor as she pushes.
- Cheer her on as she pushes, but be sure you don't override her caregiver's directions.

When your baby is born, you may experience happiness, exhaustion, relief, wonder, joy, and love for your partner and your baby—all at the same time. Your baby becomes the focus of your attention.

If your baby can't remain in your partner's arms immediately after the birth (probably because of concerns for his well-being or because the staff want to check him carefully in a baby warmer in the room), stay with him so you can report what you see being done to him to your partner. Talk to your baby; he knows your voice and hearing it calms him.

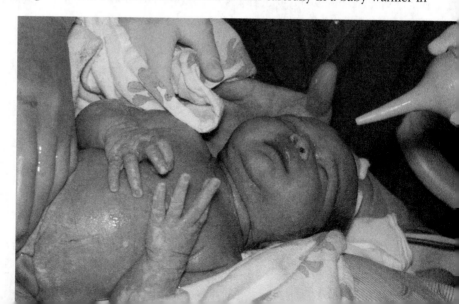

# Third Stage of Labor: Delivery of the Placenta

Typically lasting between ten and thirty minutes, the third stage is shorter and less painful than the earlier stages. It begins with the birth of your baby and ends when the placenta is delivered. The following sections describe what you can expect during this stage and discuss the care your newborn will likely receive immediately after the birth.

## WHAT YOU CAN EXPECT

After your baby is born, contractions stop briefly, then resume with the purpose of separating the placenta from your uterine wall. Although these contractions are typically much less intense than those before your baby's birth, you still may need to use relaxation techniques and rhythmic breathing. Or you may be so engrossed in your baby that you hardly notice these contractions. Your caregiver will probably direct you to give a few small pushes to deliver the placenta. You may appreciate seeing the placenta after it's delivered; after all, it's an amazing organ that allowed your baby to thrive in your womb.

## NEWBORN ASSESSMENT WITH THE APGAR SCORE

Within one minute after the birth and again at five minutes, your caregiver evaluates your baby's well-being by conducting a routine newborn assessment called the *Apgar score*. As soon as your baby is breathing and dried off, your caregiver considers five factors and give a score of zero to two points for each one (see below). A score of seven to ten indicates that your baby is in good condition. A score of six or less means your baby needs additional medical attention and observation.

The Apgar score can be done while you hold your baby. Babies seldom receive a ten on the first score (most babies' hands and feet are bluish for a while after the birth). If your baby's first score is six or less, your caregiver may have her taken to a baby warmer in the birthing room for stimulation or possibly oxygen. The second score is usually higher than the first score, indicating improvement with time or medical assistance.

While Apgar scores help detect babies who need immediate medical attention, they can't predict a baby's overall health or long-term well-being. Your nurse or caregiver performs a thorough newborn exam (within twenty-four hours of the birth) to more accurately assess your baby's condition.

## Apgar Score

| Sign | 0 points | 1 point | 2 points |
|------|----------|---------|----------|
| Heart rate | Absent | Fewer than 100 beats per minute | More than 100 beats per minute |
| Respiratory effort | Absent | Slow, irregular | Good, crying |
| Muscle tone | Limp | Arms and legs flexed | Active movement |
| Reflex irritability (your baby's reaction to something placed in her nose) | No response | Grimace | Sneezing, coughing, pulling away |
| Skin color | Bluish-gray, pale all over | Normal skin color, except for bluish hands and feet | Normal skin color all over |

# CLAMPING AND CUTTING YOUR BABY'S UMBILICAL CORD

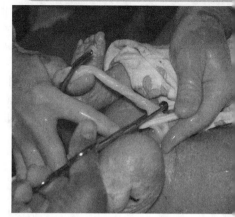

Soon after birth, your baby's umbilical cord is clamped, then cut with scissors. Your partner may cut the cord.

The timing of cord clamping and cutting affects your baby's blood volume. Before birth, your baby's blood circulates via the cord to and from the placenta, allowing the exchange of oxygen, nutrients, and other substances. At birth, one-third or more of your baby's blood is in the placenta,[17] but over the first few minutes, it transfers to your baby. The blood vessels in the cord are gradually compressed by a substance called Wharton's jelly, which expands when the cord is exposed to air. If the cord is clamped immediately, which is still a common practice, your baby doesn't receive a large portion of his blood from the placenta. Delaying clamping until the cord stops pulsating allows your baby to receive as much blood as possible. Some blood remains in the placenta after pulsation stops.

For years, obstetricians and others had been taught that placental blood is "extra" and that if it got to the baby, it could lead to jaundice (see page 389). But this belief has been disproved.[18] In fact, delayed clamping benefits the baby by helping increase blood levels of iron and reduce anemia at ages two months and six months. It may also hasten separation and delivery of the placenta by decreasing its size.[19]

To achieve the optimal blood volume, the baby is placed on the mother's abdomen (level with the placenta) until the cord stops pulsating. Then it is clamped and cut. Holding the baby high above or low below the mother may alter the speed of transfer of blood that passes between the placenta and baby,[20] but placement on the mother's abdomen is the most physiologic and seems appropriate under most circumstances.

In challenging situations, the baby may benefit even more from delayed cord clamping. Some hospitals are waiting a few minutes to clamp and cut the cord after a cesarean.[21] For a baby who needs medical attention or resuscitation, these procedures can often be carried out with the cord intact so the baby, while remaining next to his mother, continues to benefit from oxygenated blood transferring to him.

During pregnancy, discuss delayed cord clamping and cutting with your caregiver and include your preferences in your birth plan.

## COLLECTION AND STORAGE OF UMBILICAL CORD BLOOD

Blood in the umbilical cord is a rich source of stem cells, which generate and continually renew supplies of red cells, platelets, and white cells. Stem cells make it possible for a person to use oxygen, clot blood, and fight infection. Stem cells found in umbilical cord blood are easier to match to another person's tissue than are the more mature stem cells found in bone marrow. As a result, cord blood stem cells can be used to successfully treat people with such diseases as immune deficiencies, severe inherited anemia, and childhood leukemia and other cancers. Stem cells are also used in the search for cures of these diseases.

The value of cord blood in treating diseases has led many expectant parents to consider having their babies' cord blood collected and stored. Cord blood collection is done after the baby's cord is cut, and it's accomplished most successfully within ten minutes after the birth,[19] which means that the baby still benefits from delayed cord cutting (see above). After collection, the stem cells are then separated from the blood in a laboratory and stored either in a blood bank for use by the public or in a private storage facility for later use, if needed, by the child or her family.

The American Academy of Pediatrics (AAP) encourages parents to donate cord blood to public blood banks and cautions against using private cord blood banks.[22] The reason is because most conditions that cord blood stem cells may help treat (such as precancerous changes and genetic abnormalities) already exist in the baby's cord blood, which means that her stored cord blood stem cells won't help treat the condition if she develops it later. (The AAP also points out that private cord blood storage is often expensive.) Publicly donated cord blood is tested for disease and genetic abnormalities before being approved for use.

If you're interested in learning more about cord blood collection, donation, or storage, ask your caregiver, contact your local blood bank, or search the Internet for unbiased sources of information. Do this research well before your due date.

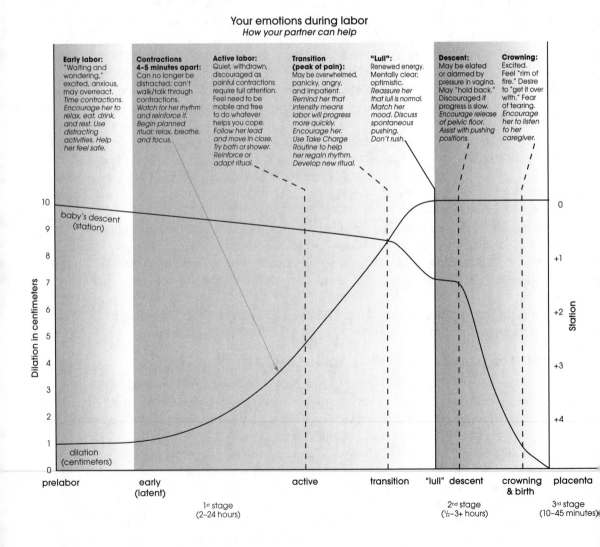

### Your emotions during labor
*How your partner can help*

# Fourth Stage of Labor: Recovery

The fourth stage of labor begins just after the placenta is delivered and lasts until your condition is stable, typically an hour or two after the birth. This stage may last longer if you had anesthesia, if your labor was difficult or prolonged, or if you had a cesarean birth.

After you deliver the placenta, your caregiver checks your perineum and birth canal for bleeding. If you had a vaginal tear or an episiotomy during the birth, your tissues are stitched to speed healing, a procedure that typically lasts less than thirty minutes. Unless you were already given anesthesia in labor, you receive a local anesthetic by injection before your perineum is stitched. Although the stitching should be painless, the injection may sting and you may need to use rhythmic breathing to manage the discomfort.

If your perineum is intact or you have a shallow tear, you don't need stitches, but the area may become swollen or bruised. Whether you have stitches or not, you'll appreciate having an ice pack placed on your perineum to reduce any swelling and relieve discomfort.

After the birth, your uterus begins the process of *involution* (returning to its nonpregnant size). It continues to contract, and by doing so, closes the blood vessels where your placenta was implanted in order to prevent excessive blood loss and to prompt the shedding of the uterine lining that built up during pregnancy. You quickly begin passing *lochia*, the heavy red discharge made of the extra blood and fluid that supported your pregnancy and the uterine lining that sustained your baby. A maternity pad is necessary to absorb the flow.

Once the placenta is delivered, your nurse or caregiver checks your uterus frequently to make sure that it remains firm. If your uterus is relaxed, he or she massages it firmly, causing it to contract and preventing excessive blood loss. Uterine (or fundal) massage can be painful, and you may

want to do it yourself to control the amount of pressure used and perhaps reduce pain to a tolerable level. See page 270 to learn how to do uterine massage or ask your nurse for instructions.

Your contractions during involution may be painful, especially if you've given birth before. Although these *afterpains* are common and aren't nearly as intense as labor contractions, you may need to use slow breathing to help manage them.

After your baby's birth, your legs may tremble for a while, which is normal. A warm blanket may reduce the trembling. You may also realize that you missed some meals during the hard work of labor. Be sure to eat and drink to satisfy your hunger and quench your thirst.

This stage gives you a chance to get to know your baby without disturbances and to let him nuzzle at your breast. Most babies are ready to suckle within twenty to sixty minutes after the birth. See page 405 to learn more information about your baby's first feeding.

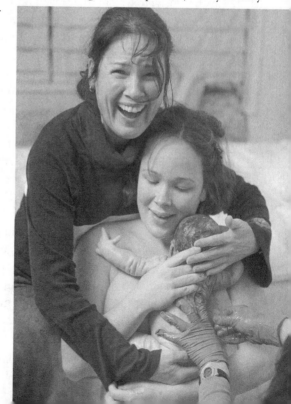

# How to Massage Your Uterus

1. Empty your bladder. Lie on your back and check your uterus by pressing on the area below your navel. If your uterus feels as firm as a grapefruit, you don't need to massage it. If you can't feel your uterus, it has relaxed and softened. Proceed to the next step.
2. With one hand slightly cupped, massage your lower abdomen firmly with small circular movements until you feel your uterus contract and become firm. This action may be painful (but probably less so than if someone else does it). If you can't make your uterus contract, tell your nurse or caregiver. He or she will massage your uterus to make it contract.

Because your uterus can bleed excessively if it's not firm, don't skip this massage on the first couple days after the birth. Afterward, you may periodically check to see if your uterus needs massage to keep it contracted. See page 354 to learn what's done if your uterus doesn't contract or you have excessive bleeding.

## YOUR BABY'S HORMONES IN THE FOURTH STAGE

After the birth, your baby's stress hormones (catecholamines) stimulate her adaptation to life outside your uterus. These hormones absorb fluid in her lungs so she can breathe easily, jump-start her ability to regulate her temperature, and make her alert and heighten her reflexes for the first few hours, during which time she begins feeding, exploring her world, and seeing you for the first time.

During labor, your baby produced beta-endorphins; after the birth, she produces prolactin. She also begins producing oxytocin (the "love hormone") in synchrony with you. These three hormones help strengthen the bond between the two of you, increase her interest in breastfeeding, and stimulate you to care for her. Other people also can produce oxytocin—although to lesser degrees than what you produce—by holding your baby skin-to-skin, keeping eye contact with her, and caring for her.

By snuggling with your baby after the birth, the skin-to-skin contact allows for mutual regulation of hormones as you adjust to your new lives together.

## ENTERING PARENTHOOD

A main characteristic of the fourth stage is that you and your partner are no longer *expectant* parents—you're *parents*! After the birth of your baby, you don't get a chance to regroup before you begin parenting your child. This new role, along with other postpartum changes to your life, may overwhelm or bewilder you. In Chapters 15, 17, and 18, you'll learn about feeding and caring for your baby as well as your emotional and physical adjustment after his birth.

Enjoy your baby's first hours of awake time. He's likely alert, calm, and bright-eyed, as he begins observing and sensing new sounds, smells, sights, touches, and tastes. If the light isn't too bright, he'll stare, particularly at your face. (If the light is too bright, ask someone to dim them or use your hand to shield your baby's eyes.) As your baby cuddles with you, gazes into your face, or suckles at your breast, your curiosity will give way to fascination. These moments are a time for falling in love with each other. Your partner also will want to hold your baby close, perhaps skin-to-skin, and bond with him.

Family-centered and Baby-Friendly hospitals (see page 12) encourage parents and babies to stay together as much as possible after the birth, unless problems develop that require separation.

At these hospitals, the caregiver performs routine observations or procedures on a healthy, normal baby while the newborn is in his mother's or other parent's arms. Before your due date, check your hospital's policy on newborn procedures. If caregivers routinely send healthy newborns to the nursery, ask your caregiver to issue an order to delay or bypass your baby's admission to the nursery. See Chapter 17 for more information on newborn care.

A few hours after the birth, your baby will probably fall deeply asleep. You and your partner may do the same, as exhilaration gives way to fatigue. At that time, someone who's alert should periodically observe your baby's vital signs and yours, including skin color, pulse, respiration, blood pressure, and temperature. Your partner may be as exhausted as you and unable to take on this responsibility until after he or she rests. In the hospital, a nurse does this job. After a home birth, the midwife or a birth assistant makes initial observations before passing the job on to an informed and rested friend or relative.

## PROCESSING YOUR BIRTH EXPERIENCE

Your birth experience isn't really over until you've had a chance to think about and understand it. Giving birth to your child will become one of the most vivid and poignant memories you'll ever have. In order to create a complete story of the experience, you need to compare and contrast your feelings, thoughts, and impressions with those of others who attended the birth, getting answers to any questions, and looking at photos taken during labor and birth. At some point, you may want to tell your story to people who didn't attend the birth but are eager to hear about it. You may even want to write the story or draw or paint a picture of it—each option is a great way to preserve this special memory for you and your child.

Depending on your birth experience, processing it may take weeks, months, or even years. If your birth experience was particularly difficult or disappointing, processing it may take longer than processing an easy and satisfying experience. Dealing with a difficult birth may also bring up strong, disturbing feelings. If this is the case for you, talk about your experience with your caregiver, doula, childbirth educator, or a counselor knowledgeable about childbirth. This person can help you gain perspective and come to terms with your birth experience. See page 352 for further discussion on troublesome or disappointing birth experiences.

## *Key Points to Remember*

- By understanding what happens in each stage of labor, you can anticipate and appreciate the physical accomplishments of each stage, respond well to the accompanying emotional hurdles, and cope with increasingly intense contractions.
- Expect the unexpected in labor. Know that there are steps you can take to respond to any variation in labor, from a rapid labor to a prolonged one.
- Your labor partner's presence and support are vital to your ability to cope with labor.
- Your baby also labors. The two of you labor together and adjust together to your new roles afterward.
- See Appendix B for a quick reference chart that summarizes the stages of labor and briefly explains what you can do during each stage to help labor progress and increase your comfort.

# CHAPTER 13

# When Childbirth Becomes Complicated

Most healthy pregnant women will have normal childbirth experiences, in which labor progresses without significant delay and the baby is healthy, tolerates contractions well, and is in a position that's favorable for birth. For some women, however, complications can arise during labor or birth. In these cases, the well-being of the mother and baby may improve with interventions such as medications, technology, or surgery.

This chapter describes conditions and events that can complicate labor or birth, as well as interventions that may resolve such problems. If your pregnancy is high-risk, you're more likely than not to require some of these interventions. If your pregnancy is low-risk, it's still wise to learn about possible complications and available interventions, just in case an unexpected problem arises during your labor or birth. With this knowledge, you can prepare for how you'll work with your caregiver to have the best birth experience possible.

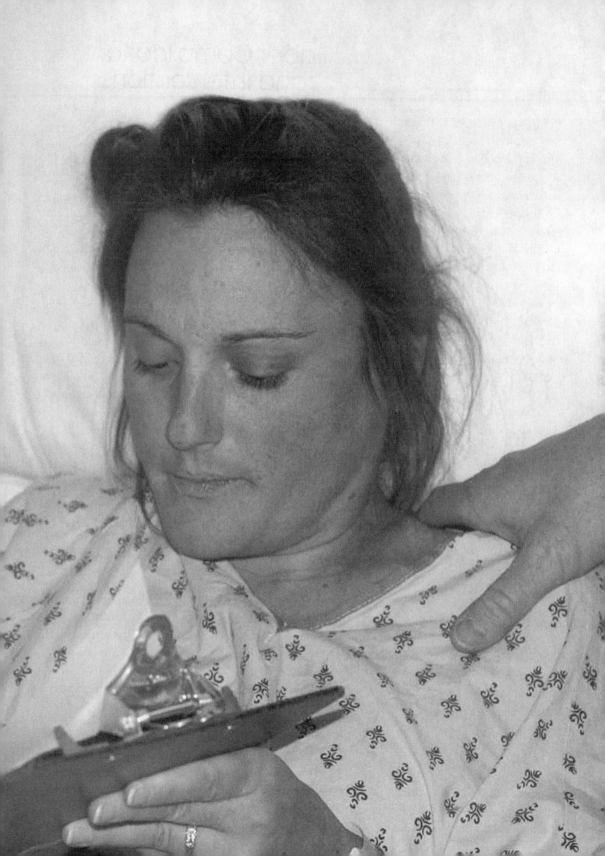

# Labor Complications and Interventions

Although a woman may be having a normal pregnancy, no one can predict whether her labor will be free of complications. Compared to a normal labor, a *complicated labor* is longer, more painful, or more difficult, and may require medical help to ensure the well-being of the mother and baby.

Most labor complications rarely pose immediate problems that require prompt medical attention. If a potential problem arises in labor, such as slow cervical dilation, it may be resolved simply with time, patience, and self-help techniques. The problem becomes a complication only if these approaches don't resolve it. To identify, prevent, or treat a complication, caregivers may use *interventions* such as induction, episiotomy, continuous electronic fetal monitoring, cesarean surgery, and other procedures.

For every complication, there are usually several possible interventions that may resolve it. When deciding which interventions to use, caregivers consider many factors, including:
- The circumstances of the woman's pregnancy and labor
- The woman's preferences for interventions
- Current scientific evidence on the effectiveness of interventions, as well as their benefits and risks
- Hospital policies and customs on interventions
- Legal liability issues
- The caregiver's training and experience
- Professional standards on interventions
- Professional peer pressure to use interventions
- Cost of interventions as well as staff availability to conduct them

The combination of these factors helps explain the wide variation in intervention rates among different caregivers and hospitals across the United States and Canada.

Some labor complications occur more frequently than others. The following are typical problems, numbered in order from most common to least common:

1. The need or wish to start labor
2. Prolonged active labor
3. Concerns about the baby's well-being
4. Prolonged second stage of labor
5. Preterm labor and premature birth
6. Gestational hypertension
7. Multiples (twins, triplets, or more)
8. Breech and other difficult presentations
9. Complications in the third stage of labor
10. Rapid unattended birth
11. Prolapsed cord
12. Seriously ill newborn or infant death

During your prenatal visits, discuss these potential problems with your caregiver and ask the key questions on page 10 to help you make informed decisions about interventions, so you'll know what to expect if a complication arises in your labor.

# The Need or Wish to Start Labor

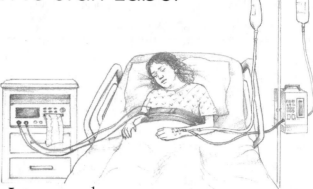

For some women, if the need or wish to start labor at a particular time trumps letting labor start spontaneously, they consent to an intervention called *induction*. The following sections discuss the reasons for induction, describe the medical methods for doing the procedure, and offer alternative non-medical methods to induce labor.

## COMMON MEDICAL REASONS FOR INDUCTION[1]

If a caregiver knows or suspects that any of the following conditions have occurred, he or she closely monitors both the mother and baby for signs of distress. The caregiver also may order tests to assess the baby's maturity and well-being. (See page 144.) If monitoring or test results suggest that the risks of continuing the pregnancy outweigh the risks of induction, the caregiver usually recommends inducing labor.

**Post-date pregnancy**

A *post-date*, or prolonged, pregnancy is one that has lasted to at least forty-two weeks. (Many caregivers shorten that time frame to 40½ weeks or 41½ weeks.) After forty-two weeks gestation, a baby has about a 5 to 10 percent risk of *postmaturity*, a condition in which the placenta stops functioning well, the baby's growth slows or stops, and the risk of stillbirth gradually increases. Tests that assess babies' well-being can help identify those at risk of postmaturity. If postmaturity is suspected, induction is recommended.

**Rupture of membranes**

After a woman's bag of waters breaks, her risk of infection increases. If her labor doesn't start on its own within twenty-four hours (or sooner if she has tested positive for Group B streptococcus—see page 131), her caregiver may recommend induction.

**Lack of growth in the baby**

If a caregiver observes signs that the baby is no longer growing or thriving in the uterus, an induction typically is recommended.

**Genital herpes**

If a woman is having frequent outbreaks of genital herpes in late pregnancy, her caregiver may plan to induce labor between outbreaks to avoid a cesarean birth. (See page 133 for more information on genital herpes.)

**Illness in the mother**

Particular illnesses, such as gestational hypertension or diabetes, can affect the health of the mother or the pregnancy, especially if the illness intensifies over time. (See Chapter 7.) Induction is recommended if the birth will alleviate or cure the illness.

**Fear of macrosomia (big baby)**

In some pregnancies, ultrasound scans suggest that the baby is large for his mother's size and build, or is growing rapidly. Some of these women and their caregivers worry about letting labor begin on its own, because during the wait the baby may grow too big to fit through the pelvis or will experience shoulder dystocia, a rare situation in which the baby's head is born but the shoulders become stuck within the pelvis. To avoid either complication, these women consent to induction in order to give birth to a baby of manageable size.

Studies on the accuracy of ultrasound scan estimates, however, have found a margin of error of at least 10 percent. This finding means that ultrasound scans often overestimate the baby's size. In addition, even if a baby is large, his size won't necessarily cause problems with the birth. In all cases of shoulder dystocia, only 30 percent occur in babies that weigh more than 8½ pounds at birth; this means that 70 percent of cases occur in babies of average or small size. Furthermore, when compared to letting labor begin spontaneously, inducing labor because of a suspected large baby more often causes labor to stop (arrest of labor), increasing the need for a cesarean birth. For these reasons, professional obstetrical and midwifery organizations don't include macrosomia on their lists of medical reasons to induce labor.[2]

## ELECTIVE INDUCTION

The reasons for induction often stem from concerns for the mother's or baby's well-being during labor. Sometimes, however, women request induction—or their caregivers recommend it—for non-medical reasons. This type of induction is called a social or *elective induction.*[3] Opinions vary among maternity care experts on the wisdom of the following reasons for elective induction:

**Convenience for the caregiver's schedule**
If a woman has been seeing a caregiver in a group practice, she may want labor to begin on a day when her caregiver is on call, and avoid having an unknown caregiver attend the birth. Many caregivers prefer inducing their clients' labors because doing so lets them attend the births. Furthermore, in some (but not all) group practices, the caregiver who attends the birth receives the largest share of the maternity care fee.

**Convenience for the family's schedule, support needs, or circumstances**
Many women choose induction so the birth will fit into their family's schedule or into the schedules of those who can help out after the birth. Induction may especially appeal to women who live far from a hospital, those who need to arrange for the care of other children during the birth, or those who have had a previous rapid birth and want to better control the timing of this birth.

**Discomfort in late pregnancy**
Induction often appeals to women who are uncomfortable in the late trimester and are impatient for pregnancy to end.

**Pregnancy reaches term**
A pregnancy reaches term at thirty-seven weeks gestation. Many women request induction at that time, but babies benefit from pregnancies that last closer to forty weeks. Elective induction should not be done before thirty-nine weeks, to allow babies' lungs to mature fully.[3a]

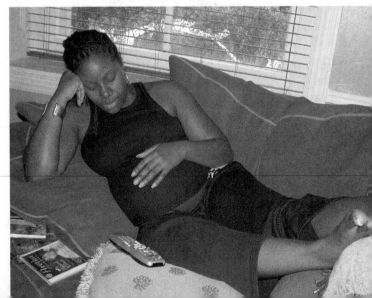

# REASONS TO THINK CAREFULLY BEFORE CONSENTING TO INDUCTION

Medical advances have made induction methods more reliable than they were in the past, when elective inductions were considered unsafe for babies. Today, elective inductions far outnumber medical inductions in many hospitals; in fact, induced labors outnumber spontaneous labors. Although induction may sound tempting when you're anxious to get labor started, consider the following facts before consenting to an elective induction:

- Induction leads to a more medicalized birth, with more interventions, such as intravenous (IV) fluids and continuous electronic fetal monitoring (EFM), and fewer options for natural coping techniques, such as the freedom to move around and the use of the bath or shower for pain relief.
- Depending on the method of induction, the intervention may make contractions more painful than normal, which may increase the need for pain medications.
- Elective induction bypasses the baby's ability to start labor at the optimal time. Babies continue to mature and develop during the last weeks of pregnancy. Even if a pregnancy has reached its due date, the baby may benefit from a few more days in the uterus. (See pages 393–394.) Elective induction can cause a premature birth if done too early, especially for a pregnancy without a clear due date. Elective inductions have contributed significantly to the increasing rate of prematurity in the United States.
- All methods of induction carry possible risks, especially uterine hyperstimulation (contractions that are too strong or too frequent) and the higher likelihood that the baby won't tolerate labor (as indicated by EFM).
- There's no guarantee that induction will get labor started. If induction fails, a cesarean section typically is performed. When compared to first-time mothers whose labors began on their own, those who had elective induction (or whose cervixes weren't ripe before induction) were two to four times more likely to have had a cesarean birth.[4]

If you're considering an elective induction, weigh the risks and benefits of the procedure to you and your baby. If your caregiver suggests an induction, ask the key questions on page 10 to determine whether it's medically indicated or elective. Ask whether there's a desired time frame for an induction to work, and under what circumstances an induction is considered a failure. Also ask if it's possible to wait for labor to begin after a failed induction, or if an immediate cesarean is required. Weigh all these factors so you can make an informed decision.

If you're offered an induction for a non-medical reason and are thoroughly informed of the procedure's risks and benefits, you may decide to wait for labor to begin on its own or postpone induction until later in pregnancy. Or you may consent to induction after concluding its benefits outweigh the potential risks. Whatever you decide, you'll have made an informed decision, which is the best one for you.

## Medical Conditions That Rule Out Induction

In some cases, induction isn't possible because a medical condition compromises the procedure's safety to the mother and baby. Examples of such conditions include a genital herpes outbreak, placenta previa (see page 139), previous surgery to remove uterine fibroids, or a baby with a transverse presentation (lying sideways). If you have any of these conditions, your caregiver won't induce your labor.

# NON-MEDICAL METHODS FOR INDUCTION

If your caregiver recommends induction, you may have time to try non-medical methods to start or speed up labor on your own. Although most of these methods have had little scientific evaluation, they're generally simpler and easier to do than medical induction. They also pose milder risks, although some have unpleasant side effects.

Non-medical methods for induction are less likely to start labor than medical methods; however, if successful, they let you avoid the disadvantages of medical induction (see page 277). Even if only partially effective, they may cause enough cervical changes to allow for a successful medical induction.

The following sections briefly describe self-help techniques and complementary medicine methods for inducing labor. Visit our web site, http://www.PCNGuide.com, to learn more information about them. Before trying any of these methods, *consult your caregiver!* If you think your caregiver might not support your decision to try them, approach the topic carefully in order to avoid receiving an unhelpful response. For example, instead of asking, "Do you think I should try some non-medical induction methods such as walking or acupuncture?" try asking, "Is there any medical reason why I shouldn't try walking or acupuncture to start labor?" That way, if your caregiver disapproves of a technique, he or can give you specific reasons.

*Note:* If you don't have time to try non-medical induction methods, if you don't wish to try them, or if they're unsuccessful, your caregiver can offer you various medical methods of induction. See page 279 for more information.

## Self-help Techniques

The following are activities you can do and actions you can take to try to start labor on your own.

### Walking

Taking long walks can help start labor; however, walking is more effective at keeping active labor going than it is at starting labor, when extensive walking may just exhaust you.

### Intercourse or orgasm

Sexual intercourse and clitoral stimulation (manual or oral) may help start labor. Sexual excitement, particularly orgasm, causes the release of oxytocin and prostaglandins, two hormones that cause uterine contractions and may start labor. Semen also contains prostaglandins. When using this method, frequent sexual activity is more effective than a single act. Try to forget your goal of starting labor and just enjoy the sexual experience.

*Note:* If your bag of waters has broken, don't have intercourse or put anything into your vagina, to minimize the risk of infection.

### Nipple stimulation

Nipple stimulation causes the release of oxytocin, which in turn causes uterine contractions that may start labor.[5] To stimulate your nipples, lightly stroke them, have your partner gently caress or suck on them, or use a breast pump. You may feel contractions within minutes, or you may have to stimulate your nipples for hours (off and on, but perhaps continuously) before experiencing steady contractions.

*Caution:* Occasionally, nipple stimulation causes contractions that last too long (longer than sixty seconds), occur too frequently (more than two in ten minutes), or are too painful. If this happens to you, stop stimulating your nipples.

### Castor oil

Labor may start if the bowels are stimulated to empty. *Castor oil* is a strong laxative that causes powerful bowel cramps and contractions. It's thought to increase prostaglandin production, which may start uterine contractions.[6] Visit our web site for directions on using castor oil to start labor.

Enemas are also used to stimulate bowel movements; however, current studies have found them to be ineffective at starting labor.[7]

### Acupressure

Firm finger or thumb pressure on particular acupressure points may start or speed up contractions. (See page 214.)

## Complementary Medicine Methods

The following non-medical methods are often used along with conventional medicine methods to treat various health-related problems. Because of their potential side effects, these methods require the supervision of a trained professional.

### Herbal tea and tinctures

Various herbal teas and tinctures can induce labor; however, these ingredients may also cause undesired side effects. For example, blue cohosh tea causes uterine contractions, but it can also raise blood pressure to unsafe levels.[8] (Visit our web site for more information.) Use this method only with the guidance of a knowledgeable professional and your caregiver.

### Homeopathic remedies

*Homeopathy* uses diluted derivatives of certain natural substances to stimulate the body to respond in a way that heals or corrects a specific problem, such as a labor that won't start. Although side effects are unlikely, these remedies are best administered by a trained homeopathic practitioner.

### Acupuncture

*Acupuncture* is an ancient Chinese medicine technique that uses needles placed at strategic points along meridians, or energy flow lines, in the body. It has no known risks. There's been little scientific research on the effectiveness of acupuncture to ripen the cervix or start labor, but the few studies on the subject have found acupuncture to be beneficial for induction.[9] (Visit our web site for more information on acupuncture.)

An acupuncturist may also use *moxibustion,* a version of acupuncture that doesn't use needles but instead uses burning herbs placed close to the acupuncture point.

## MEDICAL METHODS OF INDUCTION

Caregivers use a selection of medical methods to start labor. The choice of method depends on the condition of the cervix. Induction is more likely to succeed if the cervix is favorable—that is, it's ripe, anterior, and partially effaced and dilated. The cervix is unfavorable for induction if it's firm, posterior, and not effaced. (See page 168 for further explanation of cervical conditions.)

The philosophy and preferences of the caregiver and hospital also influence the choice of method. If you're scheduled for an induction, ask your caregiver which method will be used so you'll know what to expect.

## Medical Non-drug Methods

The following are brief descriptions of methods for ripening the cervix or inducing labor without the use of medications. Visit our web site to learn more information about them.

### Balloon dilators

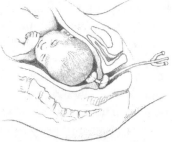

These devices have been found to speed up the onset of labor by ripening the cervix and causing some dilation.[10] A Foley balloon catheter (originally designed to empty the bladder) or a *cervical ripening balloon* is placed within the cervix, where it remains until it falls out when the cervix begins to open or until up to twelve hours have passed and it's removed.

### Stripping (or sweeping) the membranes

This procedure is quick and relatively noninvasive. The caregiver inserts a finger into the cervix to loosen the bag of waters from the uterine wall in order to prompt the release of hormones that start contractions. Your caregiver may suggest this intervention if you've reached or passed your due date and your cervix is very ripe and dilated at least the width of a finger. Although the procedure is painful (it feels like a vigorous vaginal exam) and may cause slight bleeding and cramping, studies have found it to reduce the time until labor begins.[11]

### Artificial rupture of membranes (AROM)

Also called *amniotomy*, AROM is a procedure in which the caregiver breaks the bag of waters with an amniohook, a long plastic device that resembles a crochet needle. It's done either alone or with Pitocin to start labor or to speed up progress in active labor. AROM is rarely successful if the cervix is unfavorable (see page 279), in which case the caregiver uses cervical ripening techniques (see page 281) before trying AROM. See below for more information on using AROM to start or speed up labor.

## Risks and Benefits of Artificial Rupture of Membranes (AROM)

### AROM for Induction

AROM increases the chance of starting labor, especially when used with Pitocin; however, if labor doesn't start after AROM, the chance of a cesarean birth increases. This is because bacteria can enter your uterus after your membranes are ruptured, which increases the risk of infection to you or your baby over time. If labor doesn't progress after AROM, a cesarean section is performed.

If you need an induction for medical reasons, remember that your chance of success increases if AROM is used along with Pitocin. If you consent to an elective induction but want to avoid a cesarean birth, consider trying Pitocin without AROM. If Pitocin doesn't start labor, it can be discontinued and tried again in a day or two. The second attempt may start labor, potentially decreasing the need for a cesarean.

### AROM to Speed Up Active Labor

During contractions in active labor, your bag of waters may bulge through your cervix. Performing AROM at this time may cause your baby's head to press more firmly on your cervix, likely making contractions suddenly more painful and speeding up labor progress. Without AROM, the membranes often remain intact until the second stage of labor, and then break spontaneously.

If your caregiver suggests AROM to speed up labor, ask the key questions on page 10 to help you decide whether to consent to the procedure. If labor is progressing well, you might not need AROM. If labor is progressing slowly, and your caregiver thinks your baby is in a favorable position, then AROM may help speed it up. If labor is progressing slowly because your baby is an unfavorable position such as occiput posterior (facing toward your front) or her head is tilted back or to the side, you may prefer to try other options first to correct your baby's position and speed up labor (see page 286).

The advantage of not rupturing your membranes is that your bag of waters provides your baby some cushioning and room for moving into a more favorable position. In fact, rupturing your membranes may cause your baby's head to stay in an unfavorable position, potentially causing a longer or more painful labor.[12]

## Medications to Induce or Augment Labor

*Pitocin*, commonly referred to as "Pit," is a synthetic version of oxytocin, the hormone that your body releases to start labor. (Syntocinon is another synthetic version of the hormone.) Pitocin is almost always used for medical induction, and it's sometimes used to help *augment* (speed up) a slow labor by increasing the frequency and intensity of contractions. It's administered intravenously, allowing the dosage to be increased, reduced, or stopped, if necessary.

Although Pitocin causes your uterus to contract, it doesn't ripen your cervix. If your cervix is unfavorable for induction (see page 279), cervical ripening methods are necessary before receiving Pitocin (see below). Visit our web site, http://www.PCNGuide.com, for more information on Pitocin.

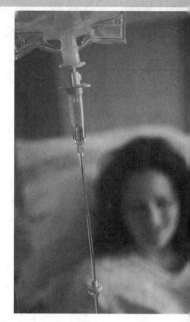

## Medications to Ripen the Cervix

*Synthetic prostaglandins* are medications that mimic prostaglandin, the hormone the body releases to ripen the cervix. They're used especially when the cervix is unfavorable for induction (see page 279).

One type of synthetic prostaglandin is prostaglandin E2 or dinoprostone, which comes in a gel (Prepidil) that's placed next to the cervix to speed up ripening. This medication is also available in a tampon-like device (Cervidil). While both are relatively noninvasive, Cervidil may be the more desirable choice, because the medication can be removed entirely if it becomes necessary to stop ripening.

Another type of synthetic prostaglandin is prostaglandin E1 or *misoprostol (Cytotec)*. The use of this medication is more likely than other synthetic prostaglandins to cause contractions along with cervical ripening. It comes either in a pill that's taken orally or in a gelatin capsule that's placed next to the cervix. See page 282 for more information on misoprostol.

## Two Options If Induction Leads to Slow Labor Progress

Occasionally, labor can take a long time to start with induction. If your labor progress with induction is slow (and your membranes haven't been ruptured), you have two options.

**Option One: Serial Induction**

With *serial induction*, Pitocin is discontinued at night to allow you to eat and sleep. The advantage of this option is that it may improve your chances of a vaginal birth. The disadvantage, however, is that it may take several days for labor to start, which can be emotionally and physically draining for you and your partner. Extra support and patience are essential.

Today, caregivers rely on serial induction less often than they did in the past, mainly because having one family occupy a birthing room for days is costly to both the family and the hospital.

**Option Two: Artificial Ruptures of Membranes (AROM)**

With this option, your membranes are ruptured and your dose of Pitocin may be increased quickly. This more aggressive approach may start labor, but it must do so within a certain time frame (twelve to twenty-four hours). If you don't have steady dilation within this period, the induction is considered a failure and a cesarean section becomes necessary.

# The Strange Story of Misoprostol (Cytotec)[13]

In the mid-1990s, misoprostol was introduced as a quick, inexpensive way to ripen the cervix and induce labor. The use of the drug for this purpose became controversial because the United States Food and Drug Administration (FDA) had approved it for the treatment of stomach ulcers. No careful research had established safe dosages for cervical ripening and labor induction. In fact, the drug company had no legal requirement to scientifically evaluate the safety of misoprostol for these purposes. Using the drug for any purpose other than the treatment of stomach ulcers was (and continues to be) considered "off-label."

At first, the use of misoprostol seemed to be a success, because it helped induce labor quickly. But along with fast labors came severe contractions (uterine hyperstimulation) and distressed babies. Many mothers and babies suffered physical harm, and some died. Many women found labor induced by misoprostol to be traumatic.

Several years passed before sufficient research determined that dosage size and frequency caused the dangerous side effects of misoprostol. Today, it's clear that misoprostol must be given in low doses (typically, 25 micrograms for vaginal use and 50 micrograms for oral use), and dispensed no more frequently than every four to six hours. Sometimes, these low doses are all that's needed to ripen the cervix and start labor; however, misoprostol is usually used along with Pitocin and AROM to increase the likelihood of inducing labor. If labor hasn't progressed with repeated doses of misoprostol or if the baby becomes distressed, the drug is discontinued.

Some researchers believe misoprostol is as safe as other synthetic prostaglandins, all of which have potential undesirable side effects.[14] (Visit our web site, http://www.PCNGuide.com, for more information.) However, misoprostol has special safety considerations. In general, after a woman's membranes have ruptured, giving misoprostol orally is safer than administering it vaginally (to minimize the risk of infection).[15] In addition, the American College of Obstetricians and Gynecologists (ACOG) warns that women with a prior cesarean birth shouldn't use misoprostol, because of the increased risk of uterine rupture.[16]

If you're planning a hospital birth, find out whether its care practices approve the use of misoprostol to ripen the cervix and induce labor, and if so, under what circumstances. Do your own research on the drug and ask your caregiver the key questions on page 10 so you can make an informed decision about whether it's right for you.

## PROCEDURE FOR MEDICAL INDUCTION

If you've consented to a medical method of induction, here's what you can expect to do:

- Call the hospital before leaving home for your scheduled appointment. The hospital staff can't predict the number of women who will be in labor at any one time. If the maternity unit is especially busy at the time of your appointment, you may be told to call back in a few hours to confirm that they have room for you. Be prepared for this possibility so you aren't overly frustrated and disappointed if your appointment is postponed at the last minute.

- Be prepared to wait. An induction may start labor in as little as six to eight hours, or it may take up to three days or longer. Pitocin is the drug most commonly used to stimulate contractions, and it sometimes takes several hours to start labor. Make sure you bring magazines, books, puzzles, needlework, or other projects with you to pass the time.

An induction that begins with an unripe cervix often takes a very long time to work, or it may fail. If your cervix is unripe at the time of your appointment, induction is postponed so you can have prostaglandins or cervical dilators inserted to ripen your cervix. Cervical ripening may require several trips to the hospital.

- Once you're admitted to the hospital for induction, expect to have continuous electronic fetal monitoring (EFM) to keep track of your contractions and record how well your baby tolerates them. Continuous EFM restricts your ability to use self-help comfort measures (see Chapter 11). If available, ask to use wireless (or *telemetry*) monitoring, which allows you to walk and use the shower or bath. If wireless EFM isn't available, try to move around as best as you can.

- Expect to become hungry if hospital policy restricts eating while receiving Pitocin and if contractions take a long time to begin. Pitocin increases the risk of a cesarean section, and the surgery is safest if done on someone with an empty stomach (to prevent food particles from entering the airway). If your hospital restricts eating while receiving Pitocin, you can probably still drink clear liquids.

- Be prepared for contractions that are more intense than normal. Labor is often more painful when it's induced than when it begins spontaneously. It's possible to ease the intensity of contractions by reducing the dose of Pitocin, but this doesn't always work. Furthermore, reducing the dose may make induction less effective.

## Two Views on Medical Induction

The most frustrating thing for me after receiving Pitocin was how it affected my ability to move around. First I got an IV for the Pitocin and fluids. Then I got an epidural, which meant I was hooked up to monitors and stuck in bed. Next I had a blood pressure cuff put on, and then I got a bladder catheter. All those wires and tubes made it really hard to move.

—*Mary*

During labor my contractions repeatedly slowed down whenever I rested, so I walked around to get them going again. Ultimately, my doctor convinced me to use a very low dose of Pitocin so my contractions would become regular. They did, and my baby was at last born after twenty-one hours of labor. Even with the bumps, the experience was remarkable.

—*Melissa*

# Prolonged Active Labor

In the first stage of labor, the early phase is prolonged if it takes longer than usual for the cervix to dilate to 4 to 5 centimeters and enter the active phase. Prolonged early labor usually resolves with time, self-care, and changes to the environment that reduce stress and increase the body's release of oxytocin, the hormone that causes contractions. (See page 245 for more information on prolonged early labor.)

Typically in active labor, cervical dilation speeds up, contractions become more painful, and labor progresses with each contraction. If labor slows or stops in this phase, it may indicate problems with the mother or baby. By taking the same measures that can resolve prolonged early labor or by using the self-help measures described in the next section, a woman may speed up prolonged active labor. However, if these measures don't work, medical interventions may be required.

## First Stage of Labor

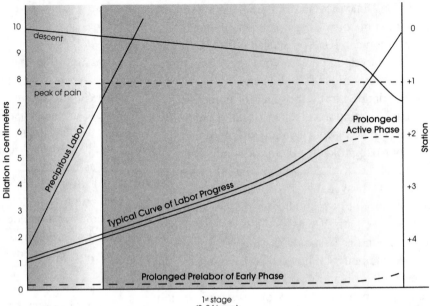

1st stage
(2–24 hours)

Prolonged active labor can result from a number of things affecting the mother, including the following:

- A full bladder
- Medications
- Immobility
- Ineffective contractions
- A baby in an unfavorable presentation or position
- Dehydration and lack of nourishment
- Exhaustion or stress caused by environment, discouragement, anxiety, or fear

The following sections describe these problems and discuss self-help measures and medical approaches for resolving them.

## SELF-HELP MEASURES TO SPEED UP ACTIVE LABOR

When active labor is prolonged, the way to speed it up depends on the cause of the delay. In many cases, you may be able to solve the problem on your own, depending on how rested you are, the amount of pain you have, your state of mind, and whether you have emotional support and encouragement. These factors influence whether you can use the following measures and for how long.

**Full bladder**

A full bladder can delay labor progress and increase pain, so empty your bladder every hour or so.

**Medications**

If you've received pain medications or other drugs that may have slowed your labor, allow time for them to wear off, if it's safe to do so.

**Immobility**

If you've been lying in one position for a long time, walk or stand to let gravity help your baby descend. Or shift from lying on one side to sitting or to the hands-and-knees position. Use these positions even if you're attached to an IV line and an electronic fetal monitor.

**Ineffective contractions**

To enhance the effectiveness of contractions, try acupressure, nipple stimulation, walking, and standing. (See pages 278–279.)

**Unfavorable presentation or position of baby**

To improve the presentation or position of your baby within your pelvis, try the techniques described on page 286.

**Dehydration and lack of nourishment**

To keep hydrated and provide fuel for the hard work of labor, drink plenty of fluids and eat foods that give you energy (if allowed).

**Exhaustion or stress**

If you're discouraged, anxious, fearful, or exhausted, you need reassurance, encouragement, a safe and nurturing environment, and help with comfort measures and relaxation techniques (see Chapter 11). A doula can relieve your emotional stress and uncertainty, and can reassure and guide both you and your partner. (See page 23 for more information about doulas.) You can also reduce stress and build confidence by referring to the information you've learned in this book and in other resources on pregnancy and birth, or in your childbirth preparation classes. Lastly, don't forget your nurses and hospital staff—their help can sustain you.

## MEDICAL CARE FOR PROLONGED ACTIVE LABOR

When active labor slows down or stalls, your caregiver's goal is to assess and maintain your baby's well-being as well as your own. If you're both tolerating the delay, there may be time to let the problem resolve itself or to determine the cause of the delay and intervene as necessary. Additional vaginal exams are likely, to check for progress in cervical dilation and in your baby's descent or rotation. Your baby's heart rate is monitored closely, possibly with continuous electronic fetal monitoring. You may receive IV fluids to prevent or treat dehydration, and you may begin to welcome medications for relaxation and pain relief if your labor is unduly long. To try to speed up labor, your caregiver may rupture your membranes (see page 280), or he or she may administer Pitocin to augment your labor by increasing the frequency and intensity of contractions.

In a planned home birth or birth at a birth center, a transfer to the hospital becomes necessary if you need Pitocin or if your baby isn't tolerating labor well. Prolonged active labor is the most common reason for transfer to the hospital during labor in a planned out-of-hospital birth.

If the monitoring of your baby's heart rate shows that he isn't tolerating labor well, or if your labor continues to lag even after receiving Pitocin, you and your caregiver may decide a cesarean section is necessary.

## SLOW ACTIVE LABOR CAUSED BY YOUR BABY'S POSITION

One of the most common reasons for prolonged active labor is a baby who's in an unfavorable position, or *malposition*, and doesn't fit into the pelvis as well as a baby in a favorable position does. About 25 percent of women begin labor with a baby in the occiput posterior (OP) position, in which the back of the baby's head is toward the mother's back. This malposition can prolong labor because the baby's head must rotate further than usual to face the mother's front, or occiput anterior (OA), the favorable position for birth. In addition, when the baby is OP, cervical dilation and the baby's descent might not progress efficiently.

By the transition stage of labor, most OP babies have turned to the OA position on their own, although some turn after transition. When low in the birth canal, some OP babies are turned by the caregiver, who reaches inside the vagina and rotates the baby's head to the OA position. This

## In Their Own Words

procedure has a significant success rate.[17] Other babies are born in the OP position (sometimes called "sunny side up"), or are born by cesarean section.

If your baby is OP or otherwise malpositioned (such as a brow or face presentation—see page 295), you may have considerable back pain during and sometimes between contractions, possibly because your baby's head is pressing unevenly on your sacrum, straining your sacroiliac joints and causing pain in your lower back. Back pain also may occur when your baby is transverse (lying sideways) or even OA.

Back pain or prolonged active labor is sometimes caused by a subtle malposition called *asynclitism,* in which the baby's head is tilted and the top of it isn't centered on the cervix. With asynclitism, the head doesn't press evenly against the cervix (which makes dilation less efficient) and it doesn't fit through the pelvis as well as when it's centered on the cervix. When the baby's head is tilted, the part of the head that emerges first through the birth canal is larger than when the top of the head emerges first.

Asynclitism is difficult to diagnose during labor, partly because it's not as clearly associated with back pain as the OP position is. Clues that suggest asynclitism include delayed dilation or uneven dilation, in which most of the cervix dilates completely while the remainder doesn't, creating a "cervical lip". Another clue is a swollen cervix that seems to have closed a few centimeters. After the birth of the head, its shape is also a clue to the baby's position. If the head has some off-center elongation, it indicates that the baby's position was asynclitic.

## What You Can Do If Your Baby Is Malpositioned

It can be difficult to identify a baby's position; even seasoned caregivers and nurses often misidentify it.[18] For this reason, assume your baby is malpositioned if your labor progress has slowed, if you have back pain, or if you have irregular or coupling contractions (occur in pairs with a short break between the first and second contractions). At any point in labor, try the positions and comfort measures described on pages 228–232 to help optimize your baby's position and manage back pain. With continued use, these positions should guide your baby into a favorable position. Once your baby's head fits into your pelvis, back pain often subsides and labor progress improves.

## MEDICAL APPROACHES TO RELIEVE BACK PAIN

If you continue to have intense back pain even while using the positions and comfort measures described on pages 228–232, here are a few medical approaches that may help relieve the pain.

### Sterile Water Block

If you have severe back pain but want to minimize use of pain medications, the *sterile water block* is a promising option. To administer a sterile water block, your caregiver or nurse injects tiny amounts of sterile water into four places on your lower back. The procedure provides almost immediate pain relief by rapidly increasing endorphin production in the area around the injection sites. The effects last for an hour or two, and the procedure can be repeated. The first injections may feel like bee stings for up to thirty seconds, but additional injections may be less noticeable. While the sterile water block can relieve back pain, it doesn't relieve abdominal pain.[19]

If you're interested in the sterile water block, discuss it with your caregiver.

## Medications for Pain Relief

If you have severe back pain during a prolonged active labor and want medications for relief, you can ask your caregiver or nurse for an epidural or spinal narcotics. (See Chapter 10.)

# Concerns about the Baby's Well-being

Most healthy full-term babies get a better start in life if they undergo labor. Contractions jump-start many processes that improve a baby's transition to life outside the womb, such as breathing, temperature regulation, alertness, and suckling.

During a contraction, the amount of oxygen that's available to the baby varies. Although most babies compensate for this variation well, a few can't and instead show signs of distress. For these babies, electronic fetal monitoring (EFM) of their heart rate patterns indicates they're not getting the optimal amount of oxygen during contractions. Babies in this situation are described as having *nonreassuring fetal heart rate*, also called *fetal intolerance of labor* or simply "fetal distress." See page 252 for more information.

The presence of *meconium* (a baby's first waste) in the amniotic fluid may also indicate that a baby isn't compensating well for the varying amount of available oxygen during contractions. When a baby's oxygen supply is low, her intestines cramp to send oxygen-rich blood to other areas that need oxygen the most (such as her brain). This cramping causes meconium to pass from the intestines into the amniotic fluid, giving the fluid's normal clear color a brownish or greenish tint. (If there's a lot of meconium, the fluid becomes dark brown or black.) When a woman's bag of waters breaks, the caregiver notes the presence of meconium and assesses the baby's health. See page 253 for more information about this condition.

Although EFM and the presence of meconium don't always identify oxygen-deprived babies (see page 313), caregivers won't hesitate to take measures to improve the baby's well-being if either assessment indicates distress.

## What You Can Do If Your Baby Has a Nonreassuring Heart Rate Pattern

If your baby has a nonreassuring heart rate pattern, you'll need professional help to resolve the problem. Follow your caregiver's or nurse's requests to change positions, and breathe deeply; these measures are often enough to restore your baby's heart rate to normal.

## Medical Care for Babies in Distress during Labor

When a baby shows signs of distress, sometimes the problem resolves itself without intervention. For example, if your baby is pressing on the umbilical cord and constricting the flow of oxygen-rich blood, he may shift his position so he moves off the cord, thereby restoring normal blood flow.

If intervention is necessary, there are several options to restore a baby's heart rate to normal. For example, you may breathe oxygen by mask and change your position to increase your baby's heart rate. If Pitocin is causing contractions that are too intense, your dose can be reduced to slow or stop contractions, increasing the amount of available oxygen to your baby. If you're not receiving Pitocin, you can receive a *tocolytic* (anti-contraction) medication to slow or stop contractions and allow oxygen levels (and thus your baby's heart rate) to improve.

If the volume of amniotic fluid is too low to cushion the umbilical cord, your caregiver may use *amnioinfusion*, a procedure that replaces enough water in your uterus to remove the pressure on the cord caused by your baby's head or trunk. If these interventions don't resolve the problem and your baby's condition worsens, a cesarean section may be necessary. See page 313 for more information.

# Prolonged Second Stage of Labor

The second stage of labor begins when your cervix is fully dilated and ends with the birth of your baby. In this stage, labor progress may slow or stop for reasons that can cause a prolonged active phase (such as exhaustion or a malpositioned baby). In those cases, the same measures that can resolve a prolonged active labor can be tried to resolve a prolonged second stage. (See page 283 for more information.) Sometimes, receiving an epidural prolongs the second stage. (See page 259 for information on delayed pushing with an epidural.)

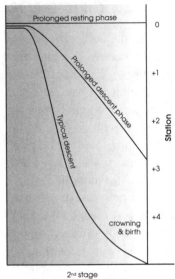

One problem that's unique to the second stage is a baby that doesn't descend through the birth canal, despite hours of pushing by her mother. In this situation, following the measures described on page 289 often can help with the baby's descent.

In rare circumstances, a prolonged second stage is more difficult to resolve than usual. For example, the baby can fit through the upper part of the pelvis (pelvic inlet), but she can't rotate and descend through the lower part (pelvic outlet).

A second rare problem is a short umbilical cord, which can cause the baby's heart rate to slow during contractions or limit her descent because the cord can't stretch enough for her passage through the vaginal opening. Sometimes, a cord that's of sufficient length can pose the same problem as a short cord, if it's wrapped around the baby; however, in most cases the cord remains loose enough to prevent a problem.

In both of these examples, a cesarean section may be required if time and the measures taken to resolve the problem aren't successful.

Shoulder dystocia is a rare but potentially serious complication that occurs when the baby's head has been born, but the birth of her shoulders is delayed because they're too broad to fit through the pelvis. It becomes critical for the baby to finish being born quickly, because her oxygen supply from the cord may be reduced. The caregiver may ask the mother to change position, as this may resolve the issue. The caregiver may also use skilled maneuvers to rotate the baby and deliver the shoulders. Often an episiotomy is necessary (see page 289), and sometimes the baby's collarbone breaks in the effort to get her out quickly. A newborn's collarbone is flexible and usually heals quickly.

# What You Can Do If the Second Stage Is Prolonged

If your baby isn't descending during the second stage, a change in position can help resolve the problem with time, as long as your baby is handling labor well. Try squatting, lap squatting, the supported squat, or the dangle (see pages 221–223). These positions may be the best aids to help your baby descend and rotate because they use gravity and allow for maximum enlargement of the pelvic outlet.[20] You may also try the standing, semi-sitting, and hands-and-knees positions. If you don't have apparent progress after twenty to thirty minutes in one position, change to another one.

If you're unable to use these positions because of your caregiver's preference or because an epidural limits your movements, or if you try them but they don't work, your caregiver may ask you to try the exaggerated lithotomy position, in which you're flat on your back with your knees drawn up toward your shoulders. This position may help your baby move beneath your pubic bone.[21]

If tension in your perineum seems to interfere with your ability to effectively bear down—even after receiving warm compresses and reminders to relax—try sitting on the toilet to encourage the muscles of your perineum to release.

If trying various positions doesn't enhance your labor progress, your caregiver may suggest that you use prolonged pushing (see page 259). In this situation, the advantages of prolonged pushing may outweigh the drawbacks.

# Medical Care for Prolonged Second Stage

With a prolonged second stage, the caregiver carefully monitors the baby's heart rate. If your baby seems to be tolerating labor, expect your caregiver to encourage you to continue your efforts to speed up labor, such as using various positions.

If your attempts are unsuccessful, your caregiver may recommend using a medical procedure to facilitate the birth, such as vacuum extraction, forceps delivery, episiotomy, or cesarean section. Your caregiver also may recommend these interventions if you're exhausted and unable to push effectively, if you've received medications that inhibit your efforts and slow your labor, if Pitocin augmentation isn't helping (see page 281), or if your baby is no longer tolerating labor. The following sections briefly describe episiotomy, vacuum extraction, and forceps delivery; visit our web site, http://www.PCNGuide.com, to learn more information about them.

## Episiotomy

An *episiotomy* is a surgical incision of the perineum that enlarges the vaginal outlet. The procedure is performed just before the baby's head is born, as the perineum is stretching. An episiotomy has been found to shorten the time to birth by five to fifteen minutes, which may be necessary for the baby's well-being if he's in distress. A caregiver also may recommend an episiotomy if forceps are used to deliver the baby, or if shoulder dystocia is suspected (see page 288).

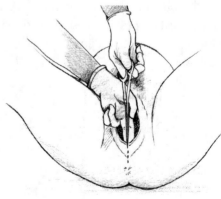

After the birth, an episiotomy is repaired with sutures, and the mother may experience moderate to severe pain during the first few days. See page 336 for more on information on healing and comfort after an episiotomy or a spontaneous tear.

# Routine Episiotomy

The use of episiotomy was once standard practice in maternity care, but well-designed studies performed in the 1990s found no benefit and some risks to routine episiotomy.[22] As a result, the practice has declined in recent years.

Caregivers who continue to perform routine episiotomies (some of whom have rates as high as 80 percent) tend to hold on to two outdated beliefs, despite the studies that have disproved them: One, a spontaneous tear is always worse than an episiotomy; two, an intact perineum has been overstretched and is therefore more damaged than one that has had an episiotomy.

Other caregivers reserve episiotomies for situations in which there are problems with the birth. These caregivers usually have episiotomy rates between 5 and 20 percent. (Many midwives' rates are less than 10 percent.) They point out that most spontaneous tears (which occur in half of all vaginal births) are smaller than the average episiotomy; furthermore, serious large tears are more likely to occur *with* an episiotomy than without one.

If avoiding an episiotomy is important to you, discuss it with your caregiver at a prenatal visit. Rather than asking if your caregiver does routine episiotomies, ask for his or her opinion on the practice and when he or she thinks it's necessary. If you're uncomfortable with the answers, you may want to consider changing caregivers. (See page 20 for more information.) In addition to choosing the right caregiver, follow the measures on page 264 to help safely avoid a tear or an episiotomy.

*Note:* Be aware that if your baby is in distress in the late second stage, your caregiver may decide that an episiotomy is necessary for your baby's well-being.

## Vacuum Extraction and Forceps Delivery

A *vacuum extractor* is a silicone suction cup, and *forceps* are long steel tongs. Either instrument can be applied to the baby's head to help make a vaginal birth possible, although the vacuum extractor is used more often than the forceps. Both instruments, however, are used much more frequently on women who have received epidural pain medication than on women who haven't.

To use either instrument, the caregiver pulls on it as the woman pushes during contractions. When used according to established safety protocols, both instruments are generally safe for babies, although bruising, swelling, and scraping of the baby's head often occur. To protect the baby, the caregiver discontinues use of the instruments if it's obvious the baby isn't descending. At that point, a cesarean section becomes necessary.

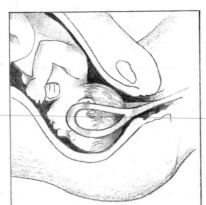 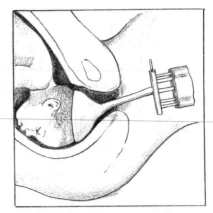

# Preterm Labor and Premature Birth

A labor is preterm if it begins before the thirty-seventh week of pregnancy. If a preterm labor isn't stopped, a premature birth occurs. The younger a premature baby's gestational age is, the more problems she's likely to have.

Certain indicators can identify women at high-risk for preterm labor, if caught early in pregnancy. Risk factors include a previous miscarriage, a prior premature birth, and a cervix that's short, ripe, or dilating early in pregnancy. For women with these risk factors, caregivers may recommend options such as bed rest, medications, and cervical cerclage, to stop preterm labor and prevent a premature birth. See page 136 for more information about the risk factors for preterm labor as well as its prevention and treatment.

Some women have no risk factors for preterm labor and are caught by surprise when they begin showing signs of the complication (see page 137). If you experience any signs of preterm labor, *call your caregiver immediately!* The methods used to prevent a premature birth are more likely to succeed if preterm labor is detected before your cervix has dilated to 2 centimeters. After evaluating your cervix's condition and your baby's well-being as well as your own, your caregiver will decide whether it's in your and your baby's best interest to try to stop labor.

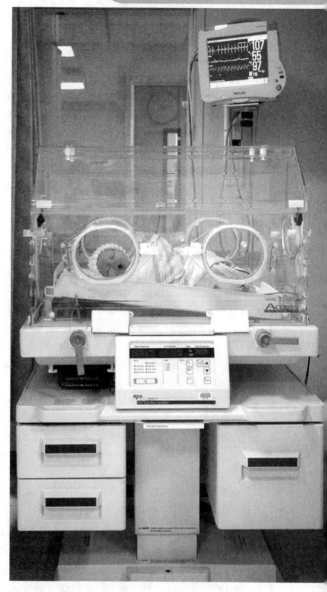

Because the management of preterm labor is a high-risk situation, it usually involves the specialized skills of an obstetrician. If your caregiver isn't an obstetrician and you develop preterm labor, he or she may work closely with one to manage the problem. If a premature birth is unavoidable, a pediatrician or neonatologist (a pediatrician specialized in the medical care of newborns) is typically present at the birth for immediate evaluation and treatment of the baby.

The following sections describe the steps that are commonly taken if preterm labor is suspected or confirmed, as well as the care given to a newborn if a premature birth is unavoidable.

# WHAT TO EXPECT IF YOU HAVE PRETERM LABOR

If you begin showing signs of preterm labor, expect the following:

- When you call your caregiver or birthplace to report preterm contractions, you may be asked to drink one or two large glasses of water and lie down for an hour, then call again if the contractions continue. The rationale for this advice is that mild dehydration sometimes causes contractions.
- If you go to the hospital or clinic for advice, your contractions are then evaluated with an electronic fetal monitor, and you may receive a vaginal exam or ultrasound scan to discover whether your cervix is changing. If it isn't changing, you aren't in preterm labor. Instead, you may have an active or irritable uterus, and may be told to rest more to calm your contractions.
- If your cervix is changing, your caregiver then checks whether your baby's lungs are mature enough so he can breathe on his own after the birth. To make this determination, your caregiver withdraws a small amount of amniotic fluid from your uterus (*amniocentesis*) and analyzes the surfactant levels to determine whether the lungs are mature.
- If your baby is immature and birth seems unavoidable, the focus of care shifts to prevention of *respiratory distress syndrome (RDS)*—the most common complication of premature birth. In this situation, your caregiver may try to delay the birth for a day or two in order to allow time for *corticosteroids* to speed up the maturing of your baby's lungs.[23] The administration of these medications has reduced the incidence of RDS by 40 to 60 percent. Corticosteroids also help decrease intracranial bleeding (brain hemorrhage) in a newborn.
- The drugs used to stop or slow preterm labor are powerful and have strong side effects. Although the highest doses are usually used only for a day or two, lower doses of some of these drugs, combined with bed rest, may be used for a longer period to keep preterm contractions from increasing in frequency and intensity. The following are the classes and examples of drugs used to prevent preterm labor:
  * Beta-mimetic agents (terbutaline and ritodrine)[24]
  * Calcium channel blockers (nifedipine)[25]
  * Prostaglandin inhibitors (naproxen and indomethacin)
  * Oxytocin receptor antagonists (atosiban)[26]

  Magnesium sulfate, a drug frequently used to treat gestational hypertension, also has been used to stop preterm labor; however, this use has proved unsuccessful. Instead, this drug produces extremely uncomfortable side effects for the mother and is dangerous to the baby.[27]
- During preterm labor, giving the mother systemic pain medications (such as narcotics or narcotic-like drugs) usually isn't recommended because these drugs can affect the baby's heart rate and sometimes his breathing after the birth. Therefore, in early labor, plan to use relaxation and breathing patterns for pain relief. In active labor or during the birth, you can continue these techniques or you can request regional anesthesia (epidural), which has less effect on newborns than systemic pain medications have.

# Care of the Premature Baby

If your baby is born prematurely, expect your caregiver and the hospital staff to take the following measures:

- If your baby is born before the corticosteroids have had enough time to mature her lungs, treatment for RDS becomes necessary, which includes administering oxygen and mechanical assistance with breathing. In addition, your baby may need to have *surfactant* instilled into her lungs. This substance allows the lungs to expand during an inhalation and remain partially inflated during an exhalation.[28]
- If your baby is very premature, you may need to transfer to a hospital with an intensive care nursery and highly trained nurses and neonatologists. Because your baby is at high-risk, her heart rate may require continuous monitoring.
- Depending on your baby's condition, you might not be allowed to hold her right after the birth. Most premature infants are taken to either a *special care nursery* or a *neonatal intensive care unit (NICU)*, where they stay until they can breathe on their own, stay warm at room temperature, and breastfeed or take a bottle.
- Your premature baby may require prolonged hospitalization. Most hospitals recognize that having parents participate in their baby's care benefits both the child and the adults. (See page 394.) Expect the hospital staff to encourage you to spend as much time with your baby as you can. They may even provide you with sleeping arrangements.

## *Kangaroo Care*

Kangaroo care is a method of treatment in which newborns are kept in skin-to-skin contact with one of their parents as much as possible. Proponents of Kangaroo care believe it's the most effective way to promote a baby's well-being, especially for a premature or sick baby. It also helps parents show love for their baby by allowing them to participate in his care.[29]

With Kangaroo care, as soon as the newborn's condition is stable after the birth he's placed nude on his mother's bare chest or abdomen (or that of the other parent or loved one, if the mother is unavailable). A blanket covers both of them. The caregiver and staff encourage the parents to give Kangaroo care for extended periods several times a day.

Studies show that a baby's growth and development improve with Kangaroo care.[30] He spends more time in deep sleep, more time in the quiet-alert state (see page 382), and less time crying. He has fewer episodes of apnea (suspension of breathing) and fewer episodes of bradycardia (slow heart rate). His temperature stabilizes, and he gains weight more rapidly, which can lead to a shorter hospital stay if he's ill or was born prematurely. Although all babies benefit from Kangaroo care, a premature baby's health particularly improves when allowed to smell his parents' familiar scent, hear their heartbeats,[31] and absorb their body heat. The skin-to-skin contact often helps ease any anxiety he may have from being connected to the various monitors, IV lines, and tubes for oxygen and food.

If you're at risk for preterm labor and premature birth, contact the newborn nursery to learn about their policies on Kangaroo care and how to arrange for it.

# Gestational Hypertension and Preeclampsia

If you have gestational hypertension, expect your caregiver to monitor your blood pressure and your baby's well-being closely throughout your pregnancy. If the condition is mild and stable—and remains that way—your pregnancy is typically allowed to continue to term. (To learn more information about hypertension and preeclampsia in pregnancy, see page 140.) However, be aware that preeclampsia rarely improves and often worsens as pregnancy continues. In severe cases, or when blood tests indicate HELLP syndrome (see page 142), most caregivers recommend managing a woman's labor in order to keep her blood pressure down and prevent seizures from eclampsia.

Caregivers commonly recommend inducing labor in women with preeclampsia, because ending the pregnancy is often the first step to resolving the problem. Some caregivers also recommend an epidural because of its suspected side effect of lowering blood pressure; however, studies haven't shown this practice to be effective.

# Multiples (Twins, Triplets, or More)

When compared to a pregnancy with only one baby, a pregnancy with multiples is at higher risk of complications, such as preterm rupture of the membranes, preterm labor, preeclampsia, prolonged labor, prolapsed cord, and babies who are malpositioned or who are premature or small in size for their gestational age. In addition, although labor with multiples often progresses normally, the birth is usually more complicated than the birth of a single baby. For example, a woman's overstretched uterus sometimes can't contract efficiently, which slows labor progress and increases the risk of postpartum hemorrhage (see page 299).

The risk of all these difficulties increases as the number of babies increases. If you're pregnant with multiples, expect more medical supervision and more interventions than are usual with a single baby at term.

Timing the birth of multiples is a controversial topic. Some caregivers believe that waiting for labor to begin on its own can affect the babies' well-being; they argue that multiples are born healthier if labor is induced or a cesarean section is scheduled between the thirty-seventh and

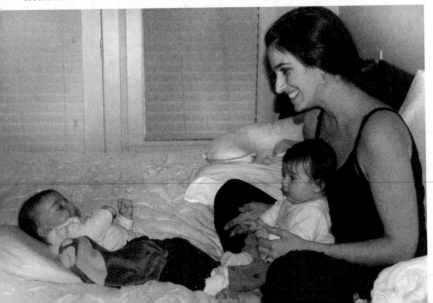

thirty-ninth weeks of pregnancy. Studies of these claims, however, have found inconsistent results. Other caregivers believe that the physiological process of labor and birth best benefits mother and babies; they wait for labor to begin spontaneously while monitoring the pregnancy and the babies' well-being closely.[32]

With vaginal births of multiples, caregivers may recommend epidural anesthesia, in case an intervention that may be painful for the mother is needed to deliver one or more of the babies (such as forceps delivery). Although twins are often born vaginally at term (see below for more information), the rate of cesarean birth for twins is higher than for single babies, and the rate increases with the number of babies. In fact, it's rare for triplets or more to be born vaginally at term. See Chapter 14 for more information on cesarean birth.

## VAGINAL BIRTH OF TWINS

If you're pregnant with twins, expect to receive an ultrasound scan during labor to help identify your babies' presentations (that is, the parts of their bodies that will emerge first from the birth canal). The results help your caregiver determine whether a vaginal birth or cesarean birth is best for your babies' well-being and your own. If a vaginal birth is attempted, it likely occurs in an operating room in case a cesarean section becomes necessary.

For the vaginal birth of twins, the most favorable presentation is vertex (head down), and in most cases both babies are vertex at the time of the birth. However, if both babies are breech (buttocks, legs, or feet over the cervix), a cesarean is usually performed. If the first baby is vertex and the second baby is breech, your caregiver may attempt to turn the second baby after the vaginal birth of the first, or the second baby may be born in the breech presentation. The birth of the second baby usually occurs within five to thirty minutes after the first, and the delivery of the placenta (or placentas) occurs after both babies are born.

# Breech and Other Difficult Presentations

Typically at birth, the baby positions herself so her head is over the cervix; this vertex presentation is the most favorable for a vaginal birth. In about 5 percent of births, however, the baby is in a less favorable presentation.

Face and brow presentations occur in less than half of 1 percent of births, and they usually prolong labor. The very rare shoulder presentation (*transverse lie*) occurs in about 1 in 500 births. Because a baby in this position turns to a vertex presentation only occasionally, a cesarean birth is usually necessary.

The breech presentation (buttocks, legs, or feet over the cervix) occurs in 3 to 4 percent of births, although the incidence rises with multiples or premature births. The three types of breech presentation are:

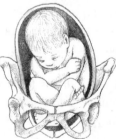

- Frank: the baby's buttocks are over the cervix and her legs are straight up toward her face (the most common breech presentation)
- Complete: the baby appears to be sitting cross-legged over the cervix
- Footling: one or both of the baby's feet are over the cervix

In the United States, breech babies are typically born by cesarean section. To help avoid a cesarean, many women try to turn their breech babies before the birth by using different self-help techniques or complementary medicine methods. Some women consent to a medical method to try to turn their babies. The following sections describe these techniques and methods.

# SELF-HELP TECHNIQUES TO TURN A BREECH BABY

By the thirty-fourth to thirty-sixth week of pregnancy, your baby should assume his birth position and presentation. Your caregiver learns this information during your prenatal visits at that time. If your baby is breech, you may wish to try self-help techniques or complementary medicine methods (see page 297) to encourage him to turn to a vertex presentation.

The effectiveness of some of these self-help techniques to turn babies hasn't been formally studied; however, others have been studied and found to be mostly ineffective.[33] Nonetheless, these techniques help some babies turn and they pose few (if any) risks. Even if their chances of success are low, trying them may decrease your risk of cesarean birth.

*Note:* Although these techniques pose minimal risks, check with your caregiver before attempting any of them.

## Breech Tilt Position

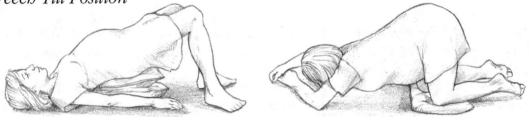

In the breech tilt position, your hips are higher than your head. Before trying it, check with your caregiver to make sure there aren't any medical reasons for avoiding it. (If you're in good health and your baby is thriving, your caregiver probably won't object.) Have your partner nearby to help you.

One way to do the breech tilt position is to lie on your back with knees bent and feet flat on the floor. Raise your pelvis and place enough firm cushions beneath your buttocks so your hips are 10 to 15 inches higher than your head. (Ask your partner to help place the cushions.) Or instead of using pillows to tilt your body, lie head down on a wide flat board (such as an ironing board) that's tilted so one end is on a chair and the other is on the floor. If the board is wobbly, have your partner hold it steady and help you get on and off the board.

Another way to do the breech tilt position is by getting into an exaggerated open knee-chest position. From the hands-and-knees position (see page 222), place a firm cushion or two beneath your knees. Then with your partner's help, carefully lower your chest to the floor or bed so your buttocks are high in the air.

Do the breech tilt position for about ten minutes three times a day, when your baby is active. To ease discomfort, make sure your stomach and bladder are empty. Try to relax your abdominal muscles and visualize your baby somersaulting so her head is in position over your cervix. You may feel your baby squirm as her head presses into the top of your uterus (fundus).

## Use of Sound

During active phases, babies can hear well and often respond to sounds. By playing pleasing or familiar sounds so they seem to come from low in your uterus, your baby may move his head down to hear them better.

You can play music through headphones placed on your belly just above your pubic bone. Or your partner can lay his or her head in your lap and talk to your baby. The sound should be at a comfortable volume. Use this harmless technique for as long as you like.

## Use of Cold on Your Fundus

If your baby's head is near your fundus (the top of your uterus), she may move her head down if the area becomes uncomfortably cold. To do this technique, place an ice pack on your fundus, making sure to have a layer of cloth between the ice pack and your skin. The typical advice is use the ice pack for no longer than twenty minutes at a time, but you may choose to use it for longer periods, if it's comfortable for you. You can also decide how often to use the technique during the day.

## COMPLEMENTARY MEDICINE METHODS

The following methods are used to try to turn a breech baby without the use of medical equipment or intervention.

### Acupuncture

Acupuncture is used for numerous health-related purposes, including turning breech babies (see page 279 for a description of the technique). The acupuncture point associated with this purpose is Urinary Bladder 67, which is located on the outside tip of each little toe. To try to make the baby move out of the breech position, a trained acupuncturist places needles in both locations of this point.

Your acupuncturist may also use moxibustion (see page 279), and you may be taught the technique so you can do it yourself several times each day. Some scientific trials of moxibustion report that its success rate for turning breech babies by the onset of labor is 50 percent.[34]

### Webster Technique

This technique for turning breech babies is based in chiropractics. It involves the analysis of the mother's pelvis, an adjustment of her sacrum, and relief of abdominal muscle tension. The goal is to relieve any uterine constraint that may be preventing the baby from moving into a favorable birth position.[35]

Although this technique hasn't been formally studied, its popularity is growing. To find a chiropractor trained in the Webster Technique, visit the web site for the International Chiropractic Pediatric Association at http://www.icpa4kids.com.

## EXTERNAL VERSION

If self-help techniques or complementary medicine methods don't cause your breech baby to turn, your caregiver may try a medical procedure called *external version* and begin discussing your options for birth. External version is usually done around the thirty-seventh to thirty-eighth week of pregnancy, but some women consent to the procedure earlier in pregnancy on an experimental basis to evaluate success and safety.[36]

---

## Two Views on a Breech Birth

At the thirty-fifth week of pregnancy, when we learned our baby was breech, we went to a chiropractor and an acupuncturist. Fortunately for us, our baby turned head down two weeks later, and we were able to have the birth we'd planned.

—Megan and Peter

We'd planned a natural birth, but found out at thirty-five weeks that our baby was breech. We tried acupuncture, moxibustion, lights, talking, and pelvic tilts; nothing worked. We then tried an external version, which also didn't work. So we scheduled a cesarean section for a day after the due date, to allow for our baby's full development. Our caregiver helped us make a cesarean birth plan that would let us have the best possible birth experience.

—Jamie and Jonathan

Studies of external version indicate that it's a safe procedure with a roughly 65 percent success rate.[37] For unsuccessful external versions, the baby either didn't turn or had turned but resumed a breech presentation. In these cases, the babies usually were born by cesarean section.

Here's what to expect if you consent to an external version:

1.  Your baby receives a non-stress test before and after the version, to determine his well-being. (See page 144.)

2.  Using ultrasound scans, your caregiver confirms that your baby is breech; estimates the volume of amniotic fluid; visualizes the uterus, cord, and the site of the placenta; and plans the direction in which to move your baby. External version isn't done if the volume of amniotic fluid is low or if you have uterine abnormalities. The procedure may be avoided if the placenta is implanted in the front wall of your uterus.

3.  You receive an injection of a tocolytic drug (such as terbutaline), which relaxes your uterus. The drug may make you feel nervous and a little shaky, but try to remember that a relaxed uterus makes the procedure easier to do.

4.  Using ultrasound scans for guidance and to monitor your baby's heart rate, your caregiver presses and pushes on your baby through your abdominal wall, encouraging him to turn to a vertex presentation.

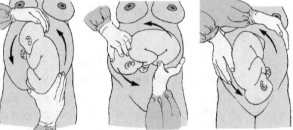

External version takes five to ten minutes. If your baby's heart rate shows that he's in distress, the procedure is stopped. If the placenta begins to separate from your uterine wall during the procedure (a rare event) or if your baby remains in distress after it's stopped, a cesarean section may be necessary.

It may take only a nudge or two to get your baby to turn. Or it may take constant, intensifying pressure on your abdomen to encourage movement. Try to relax your abdominal muscles and use light breathing (see page 225) to help you tolerate the procedure and give your caregiver the time needed to turn your baby. Your partner or doula can help you by maintaining eye contact and encouraging you to maintain rhythmic breathing. If you need a break, say so. Your caregiver can hold your baby in place until you've caught your breath and are ready for the procedure to be resumed.

Your caregiver may offer you an epidural or spinal block to reduce discomfort. Although anesthesia may make external version more comfortable for you and it may increase the procedure's chances of success (because you can better tolerate the pressure for as long as is necessary to turn your baby), it's unclear whether using anesthesia presents more risks than not using it. Anesthesia prolongs both the procedure and its recovery time; furthermore, it's expensive. With support from your partner or doula, it's likely that you can handle the discomfort of external version without medication.

*Note to partners or doulas:* Your help can make the difference in whether an external version succeeds in turning the baby. To encourage relaxation and help maintain rhythmic breathing, use the Take Charge Routine (see page 256).

## BIRTH OPTIONS FOR A BREECH BABY

Although vaginal breech births usually result in healthy babies, they carry potential risks that don't exist for vaginal births with vertex presentations. For example, a breech birth increases the risk of prolapsed cord (see page 302) or even spinal cord injury, a rare problem that can occur if the baby's head is tilted back (hyperextended) when it passes through the birth canal.

Another potential risk is a compressed cord. During a vaginal breech birth, the baby's feet and body are born before her head. As the baby's head comes through the cervix and birth canal, it can compress the cord and reduce the amount of oxygen in the blood coming from the placenta.

Also, because the baby's feet and buttocks are smaller than her head, they may be born before the cervix dilates enough for her head to pass through. In this event, the birth of her head may be delayed, which may cause the baby distress.

Because of the potential complications of vaginal breech births, cesarean sections have become routine for delivering breech babies in the United States. The trend toward cesarean surgery for breech babies began in the 1970s, as safety improvements led to its increased use. As the number of vaginal breech births declined, fewer caregivers learned the skills to conduct them, which led to a further decline. Then in 2000, a large influential study found that breech babies born by cesarean had better outcomes than those born vaginally.[38] Consequently, vaginal births of breech babies in the United States plummeted. (Recent criticisms of this study, however, have charged that it has many faults that affect the reliability of its conclusions.)

In other parts of the world, vaginal breech births are common. For many major hospitals in Europe and Australia, for example, they're routine. The Society of Obstetricians and Gynaecologists, which is based in Canada, recently published a practice guideline that supports vaginal breech births in selected cases.[39] It advocates screening for breech babies with high chances of having a safe vaginal birth, then planning vaginal births for those babies. The association also uses protocols that allow for an immediate cesarean, if necessary. When caregivers follow this practice guideline, about half of breech babies are born vaginally, the number of complications associated with vaginal breech birth decrease markedly, and both mother and baby fare well.

One day, maternity care in the United States may support vaginal births for breech babies. In the meantime, if your attempts to turn your breech baby are unsuccessful by the thirty-seventh to thirty-eighth week of pregnancy, it's time to consider a planned cesarean birth. See page 327 to learn how to prepare for the best possible cesarean birth.

# Complications in the Third Stage of Labor

The third stage of labor begins with the birth of your baby and ends with the delivery of the placenta. The following sections describe complications that may arise during this stage.

## POSTPARTUM HEMORRHAGE

*Postpartum hemorrhage* is the excessive loss of blood (more than 500 milliliters or 2 cups) during the first twenty-four hours after the birth. It occurs in 20 percent of women, making it the most common problem during the third stage.

The treatment of postpartum hemorrhage depends on its cause. The three main causes of postpartum hemorrhage are uterine atony; vaginal, cervical, or perineal lacerations; and retained placenta or placental fragments. The following sections describe these conditions and their treatments.

*Note*: For any of the causes of postpartum hemorrhage, treatment may require IV fluids or a blood transfusion if the bleeding is severe. Also, the excessive loss of blood may lead to symptoms of shock, such as rapid pulse, pale skin, trembling, faintness, feeling cold, and sweating.

## Uterine Atony

Uterine atony is poor uterine muscle tone, and it's the most frequent cause of postpartum hemorrhage. If your uterus doesn't contract after the birth, your caregiver will massage it to encourage contractions. Nursing your baby or lightly stroking your nipples also helps contract your uterus by stimulating the release of oxytocin. If these measures don't control bleeding, your caregiver may give you medications, such as Pitocin, to promote contractions. Visit our web site, http://www.PCNGuide.com, to learn more information about these medications.

## Lacerations

Lacerations (or tears) of the cervix, vagina, or perineum may occur, regardless of whether you have an episiotomy. If you have lacerations, they'll be sutured to control bleeding. Your vagina also may be packed with sterile gauze to further stop blood flow. (See page 336 for comfort measures that you can take to ease the pain of a laceration.)

## Retained Placenta or Placental Fragments

If the placenta or fragments of it aren't expelled from your uterus, they interfere with postpartum contractions and allow blood to flow freely through vessels at the site where the placenta attached to your uterine wall. When this happens, the placenta or fragments are removed, you receive Pitocin or another medication to contract your uterus, and your uterus is massaged to promote further contractions. You can continue treatment by massaging your uterus yourself and by breastfeeding your baby (which stimulates the release of oxytocin, a hormone that causes contractions).

In rare cases, the placenta can't be separated from the uterine wall (placenta accreta). The only safe treatment for this serious complication may be a hysterectomy (removal of the uterus).

# Rapid Unattended Birth

Some women's labors are much faster than usual. They begin with intense contractions that are less than four minutes apart and progress rapidly. If your labor is this fast, head for the birthplace immediately, or if planning a home birth, call your midwife. To travel to the birthplace, do *not* drive yourself. Instead, have your partner or someone else drive you there.

If your labor progresses so quickly that you push and strain involuntarily and can see your baby's head at your vaginal opening or feel him coming down the birth canal, stay at home—don't travel. It's better to have shelter and essential supplies to help with an unattended birth than it is to rush to the birthplace and risk having an unattended birth along the way. If, however, you decide to travel to the birthplace and you begin to give birth en route, have the driver pull over to the side of the road, help you deliver your baby (see page 301), and then drive you both to the hospital.

## POSSIBLE PROBLEMS AFTER A RAPID UNATTENDED BIRTH

Usually after a rapid unattended birth, both the mother and baby are fine; however, complications may develop, which is why medical professionals should assess both the mother and baby as soon as possible after the birth. If you have a rapid birth, medical help is most likely only minutes away. In the meantime, you may be able to help resolve the following potential problems or prevent them from worsening:

# Quick Checklist for a Rapid Unattended Birth

Do as many of the following tasks as possible if you expect a rapid birth without the attendance of your caregiver or a medical professional. A rapid birth can be hectic, but try to remember to use what you've learned about the birth process, as well as relaxation and breathing techniques.

1. Get help, if possible. Call your partner, your caregiver, the hospital, or 911. If your partner can't physically be with you, try to enlist the help of another person—even a child—to assist you.
2. Gather clean sheets, towels or paper towels, tissues, and extra clothing to be used during the birth and for your baby.
3. Wash your hands.
4. Remove all clothing from your bottom and vaginal area.
5. Lie on your side or sit leaning back. Make sure you're in a clean place with enough room for your baby to rest as she slips out of your body.
6. Put a sheet, towel, or some clothing under your bottom.
7. Try not to hold your breath if your body is pushing. Keep panting through each contraction until your baby is born.
8. After your baby is born:
   - Wipe away any mucus from her nose and mouth. Remove any membranes covering her face.
   - Wipe her head and body to dry her.
   - Place her on your bare abdomen or chest to keep her warm.
   - Cover your baby and yourself using cloths, towels, or clothing.
9. Don't cut the cord.
10. Put your baby to your breast, and let her breastfeed, if possible.
11. If you're at home, await the birth of the placenta. (If the placenta isn't expelled in fifteen to twenty minutes, try kneeling to see if gravity can help it come out. If unsuccessful, then go to the hospital.) If you're in a car, have your partner or another person drive you and your baby to the hospital.
12. Place the placenta nearby in a bowl, newspaper, or cloth. (It'll still be attached to the cord and your baby.)
13. Place towels or a pad between your legs to absorb the blood flow.
14. Go to the hospital or get medical help as soon as possible to check both you and your baby. A medical professional will also cut the umbilical cord and check your placenta.
    *Note:* The medical emergency team may arrive in time to help you with some of the these tasks.

**If your baby doesn't breathe spontaneously**

Have someone call 911, if possible. Place your baby on his stomach with his head lower than his trunk, then rub his back briskly but gently. If he doesn't respond within thirty seconds, hold his ankles together and smack the soles of his feet sharply. If your baby still doesn't breathe, check for mucus in his mouth with your finger. If you know how to give infant CPR, do so. If you don't, call 911 for help.

## In Their Own Words

I went into labor with my second child two weeks early. My husband and I headed to the hospital, but I was ready to push before we arrived. We'd called 911, then called my doula, who told my husband what to do and coached me to breathe and tell my two-year-old that I was okay. The ambulance arrived just as the baby was born. We were all fine, but continued on to the hospital for observation and rest. Labor and birth took just an hour from beginning to end. What an adventure!

—*Kirsti*

### If you have excessive bleeding from your vagina

Some bleeding normally occurs after labor and birth, both before and after the placenta is expelled. However, excessive bleeding (more than 500 milliliters or 2 cups) may indicate a postpartum hemorrhage, especially if you begin to have symptoms of shock such as rapid pulse, pale skin, trembling, faintness, feeling cold, and sweating. If you or your partner suspect that you have a postpartum hemorrhage, call 911. Firmly massage your fundus (the top of your uterus) in a circle until the uterus contracts, and encourage your baby to nurse (or you or your partner can stroke your nipples) to stimulate the release of oxytocin, a hormone that causes contractions. To avoid shock, lie down and elevate your hips so they're higher than your head. Get to the hospital or call for an ambulance if you haven't already done so.

# Prolapsed Cord

During a normal vaginal birth, the umbilical cord stays high in the uterus as the baby descends through the birth canal and out the vaginal opening. With a *prolapsed cord*, however, the cord slips below the baby so it's either in the vagina or lying between the baby and the cervix. Although a prolapsed cord is rare (about 1 in 400 pregnancies), it's a potentially serious complication because the baby's body can compress the cord, especially during contractions, and reduce the amount of oxygen available to her.

A prolapsed cord can occur when your membranes rupture with a gush of amniotic fluid and the cord is allowed to slip toward the vaginal opening because your baby's body doesn't block its passage. This can happen if your baby is premature or in a breech or transverse (lying sideways) presentation, or if her head isn't yet engaged in your pelvis and is still "floating high." If you're pregnant with multiples, the risks of prematurity and malposition increase, which further raise the risk of prolapsed cord.

At your prenatal visits in late pregnancy, ask your caregiver to check your baby's position by using ultrasound scans or feeling your abdomen by hand. If your membranes rupture with a gush and you know that your baby is in a breech or transverse position, take the following steps to help ensure her well-being:

1.  Get into an open knee-chest position (see page 229) so gravity can help move your baby away from your cervix and possibly off the cord. You might or might not be able to feel the cord in your vagina.
2.  Arrange for immediate transportation to the hospital.
3.  Remain in the knee-chest position in the vehicle or ambulance.
4.  When you arrive at the hospital, tell the staff that you may have a prolapsed cord. If a prolapsed cord is confirmed, a nurse will insert a hand into your vagina keep your baby off the cord. Expect to have a cesarean section as soon as possible. If the cord isn't prolapsed, you can resume your plans for coping with a normal labor.

If your baby's head is still unengaged but low in your pelvis, you probably can follow your caregiver's advice for managing ruptured membranes (see page 174).

If you don't know whether your baby's head is low or high in your pelvis, the risk of a prolapsed cord is less if the position of the head is unknown than if the head is known to be high. Regardless, you may wish to take the above steps as a precaution.

# Seriously Ill Newborn or Infant Death

Although most babies are born healthy and normal, others regrettably aren't. Some babies are born with health problems (congenital problems) or birth defects. Other babies are born dead (stillbirth) or die around the time of birth from genetic abnormalities, birth trauma, or infection. These tragic events are uncommon, but they do occasionally occur.

If your baby dies or has a serious health problem, you'll experience deep, long-lasting grief, sadness, anxiety, and despair. To help you cope should either of these possibilities happen, during pregnancy decide your preferences for care. The following sections describe what to expect if your baby dies or has a health problem, as well as care options you may want to think about. By making these decisions in advance, you can have peace of mind that you won't have to make them when grief or worry is affecting your ability to think clearly.

## SERIOUSLY ILL NEWBORN

If your baby has a serious health problem, you can help by contributing to his care whenever possible. It's likely that you or your partner can spend time with your baby, even if he's in a special care nursery. If your baby is transferred to a hospital that specializes in the care of seriously ill babies, you may be able to arrange for an early discharge from your hospital so you can visit your baby. (If an early discharge isn't possible, your partner may need to divide his or her time between visiting you and being with your baby.) Because of the special nutritive qualities of colostrum and breast milk (see Chapterr 18), you may want to nourish your baby by breastfeeding him or by bottle-feeding him your expressed milk.

The number of people and machines involved in your baby's care may worry and exhaust you. You may become impatient with staff if you feel that they're not fully answering your questions about your baby's condition, treatment, and prognosis. To help you feel more in control of the situation, consider keeping a notebook with you so you can jot down your questions as they arise and record the answers as you receive them. You can also keep track of your baby's treatment and progress.

## INFANT DEATH

If you have a stillbirth or your baby dies soon after birth, you'll have to make several tough decisions. The emotional grief and sadness that follows an infant death will consume you, making it difficult to think clearly. To ensure that everyone knows your preferences for care in the event of stillbirth or infant death, it's helpful to think about them in advance and note them in a special birth plan (see page 155).

To help you begin thinking about your options, ask your caregiver or childbirth educator how families are typically cared for after a stillbirth or infant death. Then begin thinking about your specific preferences. For example, if your baby dies before labor begins, do you want your labor induced?

If so, when? Do you want to be awake and participate in the birth? Do you want the support of a doula or someone other than your partner (who will also need support during this difficult time)?

After the birth, do you want to recover in an area that's separate from other mothers and babies on the postpartum floor, or somewhere else in the hospital? Do you want to have an early discharge from the hospital? Do you want to have an autopsy done to help find the cause of death?

What may make your memories of your baby more meaningful? You may want to hold your baby so you can physically acknowledge her existence. You may want to name your baby or have a religious ceremony for her, such as a baptism. You may want to photograph her, have her footprints taken, or obtain a lock of her hair. You may want to have a funeral or memorial service to provide an opportunity for family and friends to grieve together, say good-bye to your baby, and express their love and concern for you.

## COPING WITH A SERIOUSLY ILL NEWBORN OR AN INFANT DEATH

If your baby has a health problem, you and your partner will need to support each other and rely on supportive family, friends, and community resources to help you with the care of other children, transportation, food preparation, housecleaning, and notification of events to extended family, coworkers, and others. You may want to join a support group for parents in a similar situation.

If your baby is stillborn or dies after the birth, you and your partner will need the opportunity to grieve. The grieving process is necessary for coming to terms with your loss, but it's a painful and exhausting experience, as you feel often overwhelming numbness, sadness, shock, disbelief, fear, anger, blame, and guilt. Make sure you and your partner frequently discuss what each of you is feeling; your reactions during the grieving process may differ at times. Rely on any emotional and practical help that family, friends, and community resources can provide. Also consider joining a group for parents who have experienced an infant death. While nothing can take away the pain of losing a baby, this group can offer support at an extremely difficult time. (See Appendix C for a list of resources.)

To help you accept the death of your baby, at some point in the grieving process you'll need to review the birth experience and reflect on it. Recall the events with your partner, caregiver, doula, attending nurse, or childbirth educator. Use their recollections to help you write a record of your birth experience. Because remembering these events can be overwhelming, consider asking a counselor, therapist, hospital chaplain, or spiritual leader to help you work through your emotions.

Take plenty of time (months to years) to heal emotionally and physically. Eventually, you and your partner will reach a level of acceptance, although the sorrow may always remain. Allow yourselves to acknowledge your baby's life and savor the good memories from pregnancy, the birth, and the special time you had with him.

# Key Points to Remember

- Although most labors are normal, complications sometimes arise. Many problems are anticipated due to conditions such as a pregnancy with multiples, a preexisting illness in the mother, malposition, or developmental problems in the baby. Other problems are unexpected, such as a premature birth, post-date pregnancy, prolonged labor, distress in the baby, or postpartum hemorrhage.

- When a complication in childbirth arises, numerous medical and non-medical interventions are available to increase the chances of resolving the problem and improving the well-being of both you and your baby. By becoming fully informed about these interventions, you can decide whether they're right for you and can participate meaningfully in your care.

- Although rare and often unexpected, tragedies in childbirth—such as injury to the mother, serious health problems for the baby, or even death of the baby—can occur. To help you cope should such a misfortune happen to you, it's wise to think about your care preferences and make any practical decisions during pregnancy, when you can think about them clearly.

# All about Cesarean Birth

A *cesarean birth* (also called a "cesarean section," "C-section," "cesarean delivery," or simply "cesarean") is a surgical procedure used to deliver a baby through incisions in the mother's abdomen and uterus. It's the most common surgery performed in the United States. In high-risk situations, a cesarean can be a lifesaving procedure, vital for preserving the health of mothers and babies. While a cesarean is a relatively safe and routine procedure, it's still major surgery and should be used only when its potential benefits outweigh its possible risks.

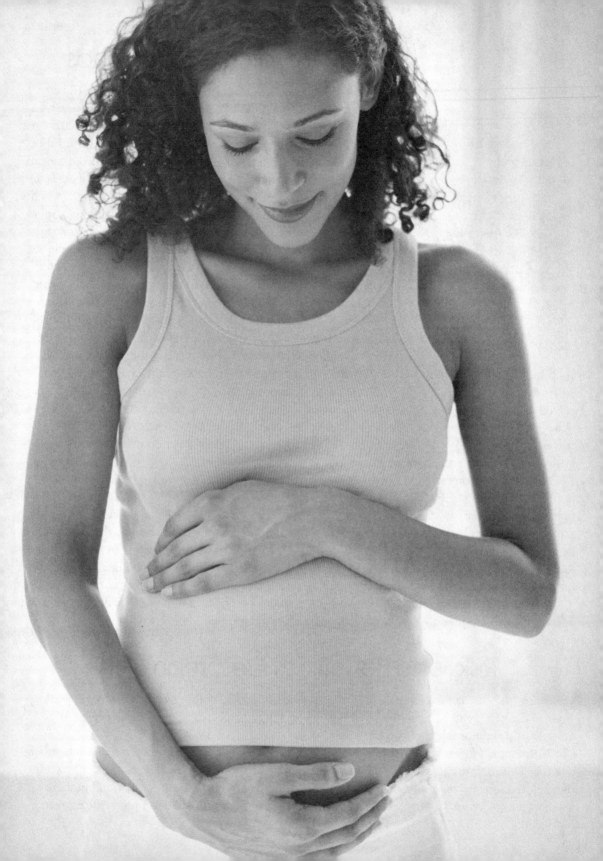

# Cesarean Birth Trends

In 1970, about 5 percent of birthing women in the United States had a cesarean birth. From 1985 to 2001, the cesarean birth rate ranged from 20 percent to 22 percent. In 2002, rates began increasing dramatically. In 2008, nearly one-third of birthing women in the United States (32.3 percent) had cesareans.

Pregnant women, their caregivers, and cultural beliefs all contribute to the rising cesarean birth rate. For example, when compared to pregnant women of just a generation ago, more of today's pregnant women are older, obese, or carrying multiples. These factors can lead to situations that may make vaginal birth risky. As cesarean surgery has become safer, medical schools have stopped teaching physicians the skills that can make vaginal birth in certain situations (such as a breech presentation of the baby) possible. In addition, caregivers often overuse medical practices known to increase the chance of cesarean birth (such as labor induction and continuous fetal monitoring) and underutilize practices known to increase the chance of vaginal birth (such as continuous labor support). Finally, Western culture embraces technology and the perceived safety it provides. As a result, women and their caregivers may prefer to deliver by cesarean, believing that the technology lets them better control the birth process. Some caregivers practice "defensive medicine," which arises from a fear of legal action if they don't do everything technologically possible to control the birth process.

Many people worry that too many babies are born by cesarean. Two leading health organizations, the U.S. Department of Health and Human Services and the World Health Organization, have recommended a primary cesarean (a woman's first cesarean) rate of 15 percent, a percentage that's roughly half that of the current U.S. rate. These organizations observed that rates higher than 15 percent seem to harm mothers' health without improving their babies' well-being. In fact, despite the sharp increase in cesarean births over the past decade, the number of babies' deaths hasn't fallen and the number of mothers' deaths may be rising.

Maternity care experts suggest that pregnant women can do several things to reduce the chance of having a cesarean birth without jeopardizing their health or their babies' well-being.

# Risks and Benefits of Cesarean Birth

Cesareans may be planned, unplanned, or emergency surgeries. With a *planned cesarean*, you may have weeks or months to learn the procedure's benefits and risks, explore whether vaginal birth is an option, and prepare a cesarean birth plan.

With an *unplanned cesarean*, you begin labor expecting a vaginal birth, then a problem arises (such as failure to progress in labor) and you must make an unexpected decision. It may seem difficult to ask questions and make choices while coping with the challenges of labor, but there's usually time to discuss your options. Some women believe it's worthwhile to prepare a cesarean birth plan in anticipation of an unplanned cesarean.

## Reducing Your Chances of Having a Cesarean Birth

Read "Ten Steps to Improve Your Chances of Having a Safe and Satisfying Birth" on page 30. After reviewing those recommendations, follow these guidelines:

1. If your baby is breech at thirty-five weeks, attempt to turn her using positions, sound, acupuncture, or chiropractic techniques. Ask your caregiver about external version. (See page 297.)
2. Avoid induction for non-medical reasons or for debatable medical issues. (See pages 275–276.) Research shows induction increases the risk of cesarean.[1]
3. If labor progress is slow, try a variety of positions and movement to speed it up. Or try self-help techniques, including nipple stimulation, relaxation techniques, eating or drinking, and emotional support to reduce fear and anxiety. (See Chapter 11.)
4. If your caregiver recommends a cesarean for failure to progress or fetal distress, ask the following questions: How much time do we have to decide? Can I labor for another hour before having a cesarean? What other options can I try? Can I change positions? Start or stop Pitocin? Start or stop pain medication? Have oxygen or IV fluids? Use tests to check my baby's well-being? Use vacuum extraction or forceps delivery? If you're uncomfortable with your caregiver's response, ask for a second opinion. Continue to ask questions until you feel that you understand your caregiver's answers. Once you do, you can make an informed decision.

Be prepared for the possibility that a cesarean may still be necessary for a safe birth.

See page 327 for information on how to have the best possible cesarean birth.

Despite the prevalent use of the term *emergency cesarean*, this surgery is fairly rare. It occurs when a life-threatening situation arises and a physician must deliver a baby within minutes. Time for questions may be limited, and the mother must emotionally process events later.

When considering a cesarean birth, you should weigh the surgery's possible risks against its potential benefits and against the risks and benefits of a vaginal birth. In general, if a vaginal birth presents greater risks to you or your baby than a cesarean birth, then the risks of a cesarean are worth taking.

## RISKS OF CESAREAN BIRTH[2]

Why does a high cesarean rate concern maternity care experts? At first glance, cesarean birth seems to be a quick, safe, and easy way to deliver a baby without the pain and uncertainty of labor. A closer look at the procedure, however, reveals major risks, leading experts to recommend limiting cesareans to only those cases in which vaginal birth is unsafe or impossible.

The following effects are more likely to happen with a cesarean birth than a vaginal birth. They're listed in order of most common side effects to rare complications.

## Fact or Fiction?

*Because a planned cesarean is more predictable and controllable, it's safer for mothers and babies.*

**Fiction.** While cesarean surgery is a vital tool for coping with high-risk situations, it's not safer than a vaginal birth and shouldn't be used without a clear medical reason. Studies show that low-risk mothers who had planned cesareans are nearly three times more likely to suffer from severe complications or die than those who had vaginal births.[3] Likewise, babies born by planned cesareans are more likely to be admitted to the neonatal intensive care unit (NICU). In one study, the chance of infant death was 1.77 per 1,000 for babies born by cesarean. By comparison, the chance of death was 0.62 per 1,000 for babies born vaginally.[4]

### Effects on the mother

- Longer hospital stay
- Pain from the incision
- Increased blood loss
- Infection
- Rehospitalization and/or admission to the intensive care unit (ICU)
- Injury to the bowel, bladder, or ureter (a muscular tube which connects the kidney to the bladder)
- Hysterectomy
- Blood clots
- Complications from anesthesia
- Death (very rare)

### Effects on the baby

- Less immediate contact with his mother
- More likely to have trouble breastfeeding
- Breathing problems at birth
- Admission to the neonatal intensive care unit (NICU)
- Asthma
- Scalpel injury during the surgery
- Death (rare)

### Effects on future pregnancy and birth

- Adhesions (excess scar tissue that binds together tissues in the abdomen)
- Higher probability of cesarean birth
- Higher rates of the potentially life-threatening conditions of placenta previa, placenta accreta, placental abruption, and ectopic pregnancy
- Infertility or reduced fertility
- Increased risk of uterine rupture
- Doubled risk of stillbirth

## BENEFITS OF CESAREAN BIRTH

The benefits of a cesarean depend on why your caregiver has recommended the surgery. Below are reasons caregivers recommend a planned, unplanned, or emergency cesarean.

### Cesareans planned for clear medical reasons[5]

- Placenta previa (see page 139) or a uterine tumor that blocks the cervix
- Malformed or injured pelvis
- Severe preeclampsia, in which case induction is ruled out (See page 140.)
- Genital herpes, if the infection occurs in late pregnancy
- Human immunodeficiency virus (HIV), if the viral load is over 1,000 copies per milliliter[6]
- Transverse lie, in which the baby lies horizontally in the uterus
- Twins if the first baby is breech; triplets or more
- Certain birth defects, problems with the baby, or medical problems with the mother

## Cesareans planned for less clear medical reasons

- Prior cesarean (See page 323.)
- Recurrent genital herpes with active lesions at the beginning of labor
- Breech presentation (See page 295.)
- Twins if the first baby is presenting head down
- Large baby (See page 275.)

Under these conditions, some caregivers recommend a cesarean; others don't.

## Cesareans planned without medical reason

- Fear, convenience, and so on (See below.)

## Unplanned cesareans for situations that arise in labor

- Failure to progress/cephalo-pelvic disproportion (See page 312.)
- Variations in the baby's heart rate that indicate possible distress (See also page 313.)

## Emergency cesarean

- Placental abruption (See page 140.)
- Prolapsed cord (See page 302.)
- Uterine rupture (See page 323.)
- Urgent health problems with mother or baby

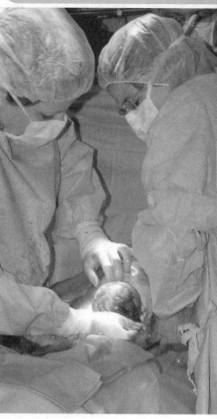

## *Cesareans without Medical Reason*

Some women request a cesarean birth because they fear vaginal birth, want to avoid labor pain, believe the surgery will preserve their pelvic floor (avoid perineal laceration and sexual function problems, and prevent urinary incontinence), want to schedule the birth for convenience, want to feel more in control of the birth process, or have some other non-medical reason. These planned cesareans are considered "maternal request cesareans" " or "elective cesareans."

In 2003, the American College of Obstetricians and Gynecologists issued a statement that affirms physicians are ethically justified to perform a cesarean at a mother's request. But a statement from the Society of Obstetricians and Gynaecologists of Canada argues that physicians should perform a cesarean only when medically necessary. Statements from other organizations of maternity care professionals also warn that no evidence suggests cesarean births are as safe as vaginal births for the mother or baby. For example, recent studies show that low-risk healthy women planning to deliver by cesarean have a nearly 3 percent chance of developing severe complications during birth, while those planning a vaginal birth have a less than 1 percent chance.[7] A statement from the National Institutes of Health declares that, due to specific complications that can result in the mother or baby, maternal request cesareans aren't recommended for women who plan to have more babies, and shouldn't be performed before the thirty-ninth week of pregnancy.[8]

If you're considering requesting a cesarean, it's important to learn about both vaginal and cesarean birth so you can make an informed decision. If your goal is to avoid labor pain, remember that while a planned cesarean may eliminate labor pain, it may result in weeks of painful recovery.

## Advice from the Authors

If your caregiver recommends a cesarean during labor, here are a few ways to ask for alternatives. Thinking ahead of time helps prepare you in case you're not able to think on the spot.

- How much time do I have to make the decision? Is the situation urgent?
- What will happen if we wait another hour? What can I do during that hour to help move labor along? Are there any other procedures or medications that may help my labor progress?
- What are the problems you worry may arise, and what other alternatives do we have for preventing or treating those problems?

If preserving your pelvic floor is your reason for a planned cesarean, know that within a few months after the birth, there's no difference in occurrences of incontinence or sexual dysfunction between women who birthed vaginally and those who had a cesarean. To limit your chances of developing perineal pain, tears, and incontinence in a vaginal birth, use side-lying or hands-and-knees position during the second stage of labor (pushing phase), don't hold your breath or strain for prolonged times, and avoid an episiotomy and forceps delivery. To limit your chances of incontinence throughout life, do Kegel exercises, don't smoke, and maintain a healthy weight.

If fear of pain, fear of vaginal birth, or a need to feel in control is driving your desire for a cesarean, there are steps you can take to make vaginal birth seem more manageable. Take childbirth preparation classes to better understand the reality of labor and learn pain-coping techniques, hire a doula for support, talk with women who have had positive birth experiences, and consider seeking counseling to address your fears.

In rare circumstances, these measures aren't enough and a cesarean may be appropriate for preserving your psychological well-being.

## HOW COMMON IS EACH REASON FOR A CESAREAN?

The following is a rank-order list of the most common reasons caregivers give for recommending a cesarean:

1. Failure to progress in labor (See below.)
2. Concerns about the baby's heart rate (See page 313.)
3. The mother has had a previous cesarean (See page 323.)
4. Concerns about the mother's health
5. Concerns about the baby's health
6. Baby that's breech or in another unfavorable position

About 40 percent of cesareans are planned, and about 60 percent are unplanned and occur because of problems or concerns that arise during labor, such as those listed above.[9] The factors that lead to planned and emergency cesareans are typically beyond your control. For an unplanned cesarean, there was a time when you and your caregiver might have made different choices that could have prevented the need for a cesarean (see "Ten Steps to Improve Your Chances of Having a Vaginal Birth" on page 30), but that time has passed. Consequently, when your caregiver recommends a cesarean, surgery often is the safest option.

## *Understanding Failure to Progress*

*Failure to progress* is the most common reason caregivers recommend a cesarean for first-time mothers. The term can mean two things:

- Labor is taking longer than expected for the cervix to dilate to ten centimeters.
- The pushing stage is taking longer than expected.

A long labor or delivery isn't necessarily harmful, and if both mother and baby are doing fine, it's not automatically a reason for a cesarean. Some people call failure to progress "failure to wait long enough."

Sometimes caregivers diagnose failure to progress as *cephalo-pelvic disproportion (CPD)*, which means the caregiver believes the baby's head is too large to fit through the mother's pelvis. Even if you had ultrasound scans to check the size of your pelvis and your baby, they aren't always accurate. CPD is impossible to predict, often because the position or angle of the baby's head—and not the baby's size—causes a poor fit in the mother's pelvis. To help avoid this problem, mothers should move and change positions in labor so their babies can get in the best possible position for birth. (See page 220.)

A caregiver can't reliably diagnose failure to progress during the early phase (before your cervix is 5 centimeters dilated), because this phase can progress very slowly and still be normal. (See pages 242–247.) If you become exhausted during the early phase, medications may help you rest. (See page 191.)

If your caregiver diagnoses failure to progress in active labor (after your cervix is 5 centimeters dilated), ask what alternatives to a cesarean are available to help get labor moving. These may include changing positions or other coping techniques (see pages 228–231), augmenting your labor (see page 281), or taking pain medication to help you relax.

If progress is very slow during the pushing stage, ask your caregiver about using different positions, warm compresses, manual rotation of your baby's head, vacuum extraction, or forceps delivery to help birth your baby vaginally. (See page 289.)

Although trying these options may help labor progress, if they don't work—or if there are compounding factors, such as concerns about your baby's heart rate or your ability to continue pushing—your caregiver may recommend a cesarean.

## Understanding Concern about a Baby's Heart Rate

Concern about the baby's heart rate is the second most common reason for a cesarean for first-time mothers. The clinical term for this concern is *nonreassuring fetal heart rate*, sometimes also called *fetal intolerance of labor* or "fetal distress."

Monitoring the baby's heart rate is how caregivers monitor his well-being (see page 252), but interpreting this heart rate is challenging. A change in fetal heart rate patterns may indicate that the baby is having problems. But a decreased heart rate may also mean that there was a short-term decrease in oxygen, and the baby is compensating well by conserving it. Monitoring the baby's heart rate electronically gives caregivers clues about the baby's *current* well-being, but it can't accurately predict the baby's *long-term* well-being. The following are reasons why electronic fetal heart rate monitoring isn't a reliable tool for determining a baby's long-term well-being.

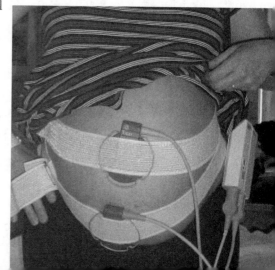

- How different caregivers interpret the same heart rate pattern varies widely. When analyzing the same heart rate pattern, one caregiver may determine the baby is fine, while another may diagnose fetal distress.

- Heart rate monitoring has a high rate of *false positives*, in which the heart rate pattern indicates distress but the baby is fine.
- While nonreassuring fetal heart rate patterns have led to an increased rate of cesareans, the surgery hasn't reduced the number of birth injuries or infant deaths.[10]

In addition to electronic fetal heart rate monitoring, fetal scalp stimulation is a simple, quick, and accurate way to learn more about how the baby is handling labor. (See page 254.) During a vaginal exam, a caregiver presses on the baby's scalp. If the baby's heart rate rises, she's likely handling labor just fine; if it doesn't change, she might not be doing well.

When there are significant concerns about the baby's heart rate, some caregivers recommend a cesarean quite quickly. Others are willing to wait and see whether the baby's heart rate pattern improves or at least doesn't worsen, while trying to hasten labor progress. These caregivers have lower cesarean rates for nonreassuring fetal heart rate patterns, and the babies are born just as healthy as babies born by immediate cesarean.

If your caregiver recommends a cesarean because of concern about your baby's heart rate, ask questions to learn how worrisome it is and whether waiting for an improved heart rate pattern is possible. Also ask whether another caregiver may recommend against a cesarean because of your baby's heart rate pattern. With these answers, you can better understand your options.

# The Cesarean Procedure

Whether a cesarean is planned, unplanned, or an emergency, knowing the procedure demystifies the surgery and helps you prepare for having a cesarean birth, especially if you weren't expecting one.

## PREPARATION FOR A PLANNED CESAREAN

At your final prenatal visit, you're instructed not to eat anything for the eight hours before the surgery (in case you need general anesthesia) and to arrive at the hospital two hours before the procedure.

## PREPARING FOR THE SURGERY

First, a hospital staff member asks you to sign a consent form stating that you understand the reasons for the cesarean and its risks and benefits. A nurse shaves your abdomen and the upper portion of your pubic hair, and then you're given a liquid antacid medication. The nurse starts an intravenous (IV) drip for fluids and medications, then inserts a catheter to drain urine from your bladder (to reduce the risk of bladder injury). You can request that the nurse insert the catheter after you've received anesthesia.

## ANESTHESIA

For a planned cesarean, most women have spinal blocks because of their ease of administration, rapid onset, and degree of anesthesia. Twenty percent of women have epidural anesthesia, and a small percentage have general anesthesia.

For an unplanned cesarean, caregivers prefer giving women regional anesthesia (epidural or spinal). If you already have an epidural catheter in place, the anesthesiologist increases the dosage of medication to numb you completely from chest to toes. If you don't, the anesthesiologist administers a spinal block. Epidurals and spinal blocks let you stay awake and alert, but prevent you from feeling pain during the surgery. If you have regional anesthesia, your partner may be with you in the operating room.

General anesthesia, which makes a woman unconscious for surgery, is used only for these rare situations:

- Emergency cesareans, when the baby must be delivered within minutes
- Unplanned cesareans in small hospitals with limited anesthesia services
- Instances in which an anesthesiologist can't successfully place an epidural or spinal, or a woman can't tolerate a regional anesthetic

If you have general anesthesia, hospital policy might not allow your partner to be in the operating room. For more information on pain medications, see Chapter 10.

## THE OPERATING ROOM

In the operating room (OR), the staff includes the primary obstetrician, an assisting physician or midwife, an anesthesiologist, a surgical nurse who handles sterile instruments, a nurse for your baby, and an assisting nurse. There may be others present if there are concerns about your baby's health. The anesthesiologist is next to your head throughout the surgery. Let him or her know if you feel any pain, nausea, or other discomfort. To remain calm and relaxed, use the visualizations, slow breathing, and relaxation techniques that you learned in childbirth preparation class or on pages 216–220.

During surgery, you're on your back, usually with a foam wedge under your left hip to reduce supine hypotension. (See page 89.) The nurse washes your abdomen with an antiseptic, drapes a sterile sheet over your body, and places a surgical screen at your chest to prevent you from viewing the surgery or touching the surgical area.

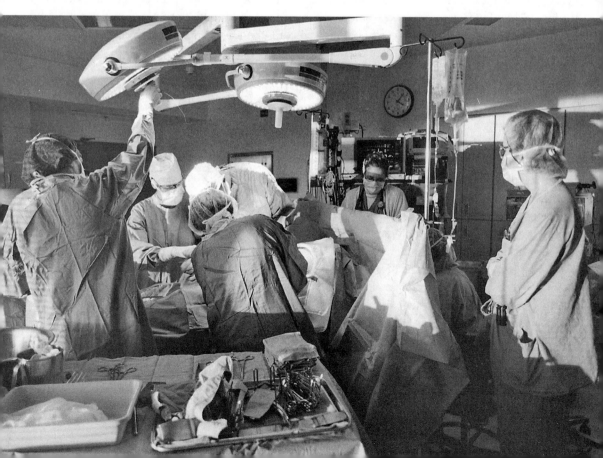

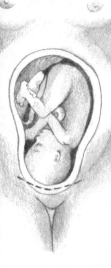

## THE SURGERY

First, the obstetrician cuts through your abdominal wall (skin, fat layer, and a fibrous layer of connective tissue called "fascia"). This cut is typically a *transverse incision*, or horizontal cut, 4 to 6 inches across and 1 inch above your pubic bone (a bikini cut). In unfavorable conditions (such as placenta previa or a transverse baby), for obese women, or in an emergency, this cut may be a vertical incision between the navel and pubic bone (a classical cut).

The obstetrician then manually separates your abdominal muscles and cuts through a fibrous tissue (the peritoneum) that encases your abdominal cavity. He or she then makes a low transverse incision in your uterus. In some cases, it's a low vertical incision. In very few cases, it's a classical incision, a vertical cut in the upper uterus.

After making a small incision, the obstetrician stretches the opening wide enough for your baby's head to fit through. To control bleeding, he or she cauterizes the ends of cut blood vessels, and you may smell a burning odor. If needed, he or she breaks your membranes, and you soon hear the suctioning of amniotic fluid.

Then the obstetrician reaches in to extract your baby as the assisting physician presses on the top of your uterus to help push out your baby. You may feel intense pulling and tugging while they work on you, but you shouldn't feel pain. The obstetrician first lifts out your baby's head (or, if breech, his buttocks). He or she may cup a hand around your baby or apply a vacuum extractor to his head. Then fluids are suctioned from your baby's nose and mouth before the obstetrician lifts him completely out, clamps and cuts the umbilical cord, then holds him up for you to see.

## Immediate Baby Care

The operating room staff may care for your baby at a warming table or they may take your baby to the nursery. During a vaginal birth, contractions squeeze fluids out the baby's airway, but a baby born by cesarean doesn't have that advantage. For this reason, your baby's mouth and nose may need additional suctioning.

The staff evaluates your baby with Apgar scores and a newborn assessment and may do other procedures, including administering eye ointment, injecting vitamin K, and measuring height and weight. (See pages 370–371.)

If your baby is having trouble breathing (which is more likely after a cesarean than a vaginal birth), she may need assistance, supplemental oxygen, and extra observation in the nursery. If she's premature, she may be given surfactant medication, which makes breathing easier.

A cesarean surgery takes about one hour, but your baby is born just ten to fifteen minutes after surgery begins. As soon as possible after the birth, a nurse or your partner should bring your baby close to you. He or

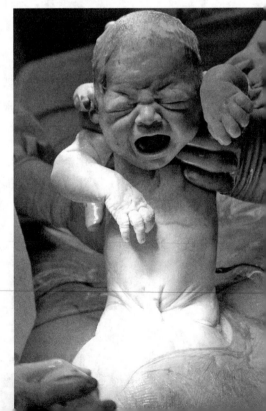

she can hold your baby so you can get to know her while the obstetrician repairs the incisions.

## During the Repair

At the beginning of the repair, Pitocin is added to your IV to make your uterus contract and prevent excessive bleeding. Then the obstetrician manually removes the placenta through the incision site and inspects it.

The obstetrician may lift out your uterus completely for repair, or he or she may do the repair internally. Some physicians feel they can do a better repair if the uterus is outside the abdomen; however, external repair can cause nausea and vomiting.[11] To close the incision in your uterus, the obstetrician uses stitches that will dissolve. Most experts recommend obstetricians use the double-layer suturing method,[12] which requires suturing both the inner and outer layers of the uterus, thereby creating a stronger scar that's less likely to reopen in future labors. The obstetrician then repairs your abdominal muscles, closes your skin with staples or stitches, and bandages the area.

During the repair, some women develop pain in their shoulder area, which is caused by air that has entered the surgical area. This "referred pain" soon subsides on its own.

During or after the surgery, you may feel nauseated, anxious, or panicky. You may tremble all over. Medications can help ease these discomforts, but may make you so drowsy that you sleep through your baby's first hours. Instead, try slow, deep breathing and ask for a cool cloth on your forehead to help ease nausea. Warm IV fluids or blankets over your shoulders can help reduce trembling. If you decide you need medications, ask for those that let you stay awake and alert.

After the surgery, you may return to the room where you labored, or you may go to a surgical recovery room. Then staff will transfer you to a postpartum room a few hours after the surgery.

## In Their Own Words

While they were finishing the surgery, I started shaking. I wanted to hold my baby, but I was worried the trembling would disturb her. They gave me medication for the shaking, but then I fell asleep for the next hour. I wish I had just put up with it, and snuggled my baby. Instead, I slept for her first hour—and no one even thought to take a photo of her during that time, so I feel as though that part of her life was lost to me.

*—Maria*

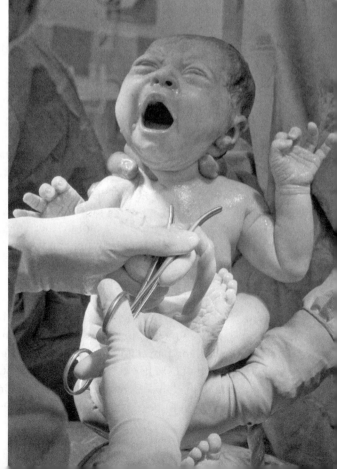

## Common Q & A

**Q:** My wife and I just found out she'll need a cesarean. I want to support her in the OR, but I'm worried I'll pass out when I see blood. What can I do?

**A:** Ask ahead of time if you can bring an extra support person (doula, friend, or family member) into the OR in case you need to leave. Be sure to let the anesthesiologist know about your concerns. He or she will have good ideas for what you should do. Plan to stay close to your wife's head, where the surgical screen will prevent you from seeing the surgery, and focus on her face, giving encouragement and reassurance.

## A NOTE TO FATHERS, PARTNERS, AND OTHER SUPPORT PARTNERS

When the surgery begins, you may feel pushed to the side as the experts do their work. But you have an important role to play. Your job is to support your partner and be the primary caretaker of your baby while the surgery is completed.

During the surgery, you'll sit by your partner's head, behind the sterile area. If you're interested, you may stand and watch the surgery, but you must stay behind the screen and out of the staff's way.

Whether you sit or stand, hold your partner's hand, talk to her, stroke her hair, and rub her shoulders. Help her with relaxation techniques and visualization. The medication may make her feel as though she can't take a deep breath. She may panic and say, "I can't breathe." Rest assured, she can breathe—otherwise, she couldn't talk! Coach her through slow breathing, reminding her that she's breathing well, even though she can't feel it.

After your baby is born, go where your partner directs you. Most likely, she'll want you to stay with your baby, but she may want you close by her side. If hospital policy allows for two support people in the OR, one of you can stay with your baby and the other can remain with your partner.

If you're with your baby in the OR, tell your partner everything you notice about your baby and describe all the details of what's happening to him. As you talk, your familiar voice will soothe your baby. Usually, you can touch and hold your baby shortly after birth. In that case, your main goal is to bring him to your partner as quickly as is safely possible so they can begin to bond.

If you go with your baby to the nursery, or if medication and the stress of the surgery makes your partner fall asleep, pay attention to all the events so you can tell her about them later. Take lots of photos. Think of other ways you can capture these moments for her. For example, you may ask visitors (even grandparents) to refrain from holding your baby until after your partner has had a chance.

Remember that it's important for your partner and baby to begin breastfeeding as soon as possible after the birth. Babies often become sleepy an hour or two after birth, so it's best if the first feeding happens before then. Some mothers can begin breastfeeding in the OR while their surgeries are completed, but others begin nursing in the recovery or postpartum room. If your partner is groggy from medication, she may need your help holding your baby as he nurses. If she has trouble latching him onto her breast, ask a nurse, doula, or lactation consultant for help. You may be tempted to help her rest by feeding your baby by bottle, but resist that urge. Introducing a bottle at this time may make breastfeeding challenging. Get the contact information of a local lactation consultant or breastfeeding hot line you can call if you and your partner have breastfeeding questions when you're back home.

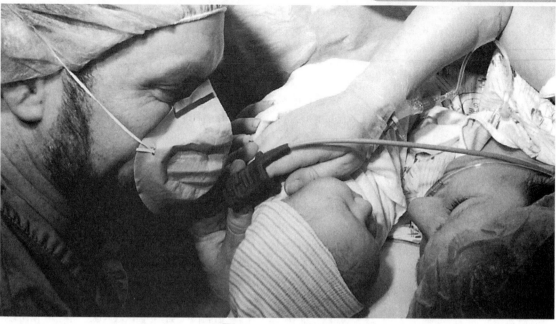

# Recovery

After you've had a cesarean birth, you experience all the normal parts of postpartum physical recovery (see Chapter 15) and learn to care for your newborn. But there's one additional factor—you're recovering from major surgery!

Here's an overview of what to expect when recovering from a cesarean: For the first twenty-four hours, you need help doing everything—holding your baby, rolling over, sitting up, walking, and using the toilet. For the first two weeks, you're sore, move slowly, and need help with baby care and household tasks. At six weeks, your body should feel back to normal.

The following sections provide more detail on the recovery process.

## YOUR HOSPITAL STAY

A cesarean birth requires a hospital stay of two to four days. During that time, your nurses regularly monitor your vital signs, check vaginal bleeding (lochia), ask if you're urinating and moving your bowels, and check your incision to ensure it's healing well. Nurses are a wellspring of information, advice, and breastfeeding assistance. Take advantage of this valuable resource!

## PAIN MEDICATION

During the surgery, you may be given epidural or spinal narcotics that provide many hours of pain relief. Alternatively, after the surgery you may be given patient-controlled analgesia (PCA). PCA lets you push a button to release a narcotic into your IV when you need more pain relief. (The amount of the narcotic is controlled so overdose isn't possible.)

Take enough medication to be comfortable. When you're in pain, it's hard to move around, bond with your baby, learn parenting skills, and relax for breastfeeding. (Only low concentrations of the medication reach your baby through your breast milk, so the effects on your baby are slight.)

## Supporting Your Belly (Splinting)

When you first get up after a cesarean, it may feel as though your belly is sagging and needs support. It may even feel as though your insides are shifting around. Your belly may hurt whenever you change positions, cough, or laugh. To support the area during these times or whenever you need comfort, try using your hand, a pillow, or a rolled-up towel to press gently against your incision area.

Don't let medications wear off completely. Take your next dose when it's due, even if you're not hurting yet.

Although the medication options provide effective pain relief and let you move around, itching and nausea are frequent side effects. Other medications counteract these side effects, but they may cause drowsiness or diminish pain relief. If your medications make you groggy, ask to have the dosage decreased or medication changed.

After about twenty-four hours, you're given oral pain medications, which you may need for several days to a week. As the pain subsides, reduce the dosage or switch to regular acetaminophen or ibuprofen. If you don't need pain relief, you may stop using pain medications, even if you haven't taken all of them.

### PHYSICAL ACTIVITY

Moving as soon as possible after the surgery boosts blood circulation, which lowers the risk of blood clots, and improves digestion and lung function. But don't overdo it. For the first two weeks, minimize lifting heavy objects and climbing stairs. These activities strain your abdominal muscles.

### Rolling Over, Sitting, Standing, and Walking

Within a few hours after a cesarean birth, you're encouraged to sit on the side of the bed. If you're on your back, roll onto your side by "bridging": Bend your knees, press your feet into the bed, and lift your hips. With your hips elevated, rotate them to one side so one hip is directly above the other. Rest your bottom hip on the bed, then use your arms to push yourself to a sitting position with your legs dangling over the side of the bed. Rest for a moment; this move may make you dizzy, especially the first few times you do it.

With the nurse's help, stand by pushing down with your hands. Stand as tall as you can—you won't harm your incision even though it may hurt and feel as though it's pulling apart.

Within eight hours of the surgery, you should be able to walk to the bathroom with help. Within twelve hours, you should be able to walk short distances independently; within twenty-four hours, you should be able to walk the hospital hallways.

### Exercises and Physical Activity

The following exercises are recommended to help your body recover from a cesarean.

**First day after surgery**

*Deep Breathing:* Take a few deep breaths, bringing air all the way down to your belly. This movement gently exercises your abdominal muscles.

*Coughs:* Hold your hands over your incision, inhale deeply and exhale with either a gentle huffing cough or a forceful short puff. This movement dislodges any accumulated mucus from your respiratory system.

*Ankle Pumps:* Flex and point your feet and rotate your ankles to help circulation and prevent blood clots in your legs.

### Days two to four

*Knee Bends:* While lying on your back in bed, flex your feet, bend one leg while sliding your heel toward your bottom, then straighten the leg. Repeat with your other leg. This motion helps prevent blood clots in your legs.

*Tension Relievers:* While sitting, roll your shoulders and rotate your ankles.

*Abdominal Pull-ins:* Pull in your belly as if making yourself look thin, then relax.

### For the first two to four weeks

- Rest and take it easy. Don't lift anything heavier than your baby and don't drive. Limit climbing stairs, reaching into high cabinets, doing laundry, vacuuming, entertaining visitors, and so on.
- Don't have sex.
- Check with your caregiver about when to begin the postpartum exercises described in Chapter 15.

## DIGESTION, ELIMINATION, AND GAS

Abdominal surgery can slow digestion and lead to problems with gas, gas pains, constipation, and urination. As soon as you can walk to the bathroom, your bladder catheter is removed.

Some hospitals' policies require that women consume nothing by mouth for twenty-four hours after a cesarean, then only clear liquids until day two or three. Research has shown, however, that women who are allowed to eat when desired (within four to eight hours after surgery) have more satisfactory recoveries. They experience less gas, resume moving their bowels sooner, require less IV fluid, and can expect an earlier discharge from the hospital.[13] Ask your caregiver about your hospital's policy and note in your cesarean birth plan that you want to resume eating shortly after the surgery.

During the first few days after the surgery, take the stool softeners that your nurses give you, drink lots of water, and gradually add high-fiber foods to your meals. To minimize gas, avoid consuming iced drinks, carbonated beverages, and very hot or cold foods. To help digestion, walk, change positions often, and rock back and forth in a chair.

## INCISION CARE

After the surgery, you're shown how to clean the incision area and check for swelling and infection. (It's normal for the area to itch and ooze a watery yellow or pink discharge.) Gently clean and dry the wound daily. Avoid touching the incision without first washing your hands. Twenty-four hours after the surgery, you can shower or bathe as usual. Dry thoroughly, then wear loose, comfortable clothes. If you're overweight, make sure air can circulate around the incision area so it stays clean and dry.

If tape was used to close your incision, it eventually comes off on its own. If staples or clips were used, your caregiver removes them and applies tape to the incision before you leave the hospital. He or she can tell you further what to expect.

After six weeks, your scar shouldn't cause you discomfort, although it may still feel stretched or pulled. It may also feel numb for three months or more. When the feeling returns, you may experience some "zinging" or prickly sensations, due to the healing of damaged nerve pathways. After the incision has healed, you may notice a hard ridge along it. This is scar tissue, which tends to shrink and attach to the soft tissue underneath. Massage the scar tissue in different directions (along and across the scar) and roll it between your thumb and index finger. These motions ensure the different layers of skin, tissue, and muscles can move freely underneath. If the massage is painful, do it more gently. Massage your scar a few times every day (five minutes each time).

See page 337 for postpartum warning signs of an infected incision.

## BREASTFEEDING

Breastfeeding can be more challenging after a cesarean birth, but successful breastfeeding is possible if you know how to manage potential challenges. Some research suggests that, when compared to women who had vaginal births, fewer women who had cesarean births start breastfeeding, or they quit breastfeeding sooner. With education and support, however, initial breastfeeding rates and breastfeeding duration are similar for both mothers who had cesareans and those who didn't.[14]

After your surgery, finding a comfortable position to breastfeed may be problematic. To protect your incision from your baby's weight and wiggling, lie on your side or use the football (or clutch) hold. If using the cradle hold or cross-cradle hold, first place a pillow on your incision. (See page 406 for information on breastfeeding positions.) Your partner or a nurse can help adjust the number and position of pillows to support your baby and protect your incision. They can also help check your baby's latch onto your breast.

Your baby may be quite sleepy, depending on what medications you had during the surgery. Have patience as she figures out how to latch onto your breast and feed. Also, if your baby needed extensive suctioning of her nose and throat after birth, she may have trouble latching onto your breast during the first days. Skin-to-skin contact between you and your baby helps calm her and promotes a good latch.

The surgery may delay when your milk comes in. Frequent feedings is the best way to increase your milk supply. The sooner you initiate breastfeeding after the birth and the more often you breastfeed your baby, the more milk she takes, and the more milk you make.

After the surgery, you may have a higher chance of acquiring a bacterial or yeast infection, which can cause sore nipples. (See page 422.)

## EMOTIONAL REACTIONS TO HAVING A CESAREAN BIRTH

Women have all sorts of feelings about having a cesarean birth. Reactions often depend on prior hopes and expectations. If you learn you need a planned cesarean, you may feel relieved that you don't have to go through labor. Or you may feel disappointed that you don't get to experience childbirth. You may worry about your medical condition or the surgery and its risks. Or knowing exactly what to prepare for may reduce your anxiety.

If the need for an unplanned cesarean arises during labor, you may be disappointed or you may be relieved that labor is about to end. You may feel frustrated that you worked so hard for all those hours only to have your baby delivered surgically. Or you may be frightened about facing something you never expected to happen. If concerns about your baby's heart rate led to the cesarean, you may worry about your baby's well-being.

### Coming to Terms with Your Feelings about the Cesarean

When the surgery is over and you know your baby is fine, you may feel acceptance (if you felt the surgery was necessary), anger (if you didn't feel part of the decision-making), disappointment, guilt, resentment, or relief. Sometimes women don't feel any particular emotions about the cesarean right away, but do eventually.

For some women, a cesarean leads to low self-esteem. They don't feel confident about their mothering skills because of their failure to birth "normally." They have trouble connecting emotionally to their babies because the birth wasn't what they'd wanted. They may feel emptiness or sadness when recalling the birth, instead of feeling fulfillment and joy.

If your cesarean birth depresses you, you may feel guilty and upset. You may feel as though you should "just be happy" to have a healthy baby. Know that it takes time to let go of the birth you envisioned and it's perfectly normal to grieve for one thing as you celebrate another. If possible, talk honestly and openly about the birth with people who understand your feelings.

Sometimes, understanding the reason for the surgery can help you better accept the birth. Your recollection of the experience might not be complete, especially if labor was exhausting or the cesarean was an emergency. Ask your caregiver to discuss with you the events that led to the cesarean, or review your hospital chart together.

Also consider talking with your childbirth educator, doula, or a counselor about your birth experience. Look into joining a support group, such as the International Cesarean Awareness Network (ICAN), or search online for discussion groups that may help you find others who had similar experiences. Continue using these resources until you come to terms with your birth experience and can move forward with your life as a new mother.

# Vaginal Birth after Cesarean (VBAC)

If you've had a cesarean and are pregnant again, you need to decide between planning another cesarean birth or planning a *trial of labor after cesarean (TOLAC)*, in which labor is allowed to begin and progress with the hope of having a *vaginal birth after cesarean (VBAC)*.

## MAKING THE CHOICE BETWEEN VBAC AND REPEAT CESAREAN

It's your right and responsibility to decide whether to have a repeat cesarean or try for a VBAC. After reading this section on VBAC, discuss with your caregiver the medical benefits and risks specific to your situation. Because caregivers' views on VBAC vary widely, you may want to consult with multiple providers. Also consider the emotional and practical issues unique to your situation that may affect your decision. For example, you might have lingering fears of labor that may stall a TOLAC, or there might not be a caregiver or hospital near you that permits VBAC.

## MEDICAL BENEFITS AND RISKS OF VBAC VERSUS REPEAT CESAREAN

In March 2010, the National Institutes of Health held a consensus development conference to conduct a professional assessment of the currently available data on VBAC. The panel concluded that the benefits of TOLAC to the mother might be balanced by the increased risks to the baby; however, the benefits of a repeat cesarean to the baby might be balanced by the increased risks to the mother. Consequently, when TOLAC and repeat cesarean are medically equivalent options, women and their caregivers should work together to make a decision, and the woman's preference should be respected.[15] In July 2010, the American College of Obstetricians and Gynecologists (ACOG) agreed that attempting VBAC is a safe and appropriate choice for most women.[15a]

When analyzing the benefits and risks of TOLAC and repeat cesarean, you need to examine the relatively rare but real risk of *uterine rupture*, the separation or opening of the scar from the uterine

# What Influences My Chance of Uterine Rupture?

Although the thought of uterine rupture is scary, the chance of its occurrence is relatively small (one-third of 1 percent for TOLAC).[16] Here are some general guidelines of the risk:

- The chance of rupture is **lowest** for a woman who has had only one prior cesarean with a low transverse scar and who hasn't been induced.
- The chance of rupture is **higher** if the woman has had more than one prior cesarean, had an infection after a prior cesarean, had a cesarean less than eighteen months ago, or has had labor induced.
- The chance of rupture is **highest** (and VBAC is too risky) for a woman who has had a vertical incision or an inverted T- or J-shaped incision for a prior cesarean, had a rupture from a previous labor that caused problems, or has had an ultrasound scan that found the uterine scar to be less than 2½ millimeters thick.[17]

incision. If rupture occurs, it often results in a hysterectomy for the mother (14 to 33 percent risk) and can lead to the death of the baby (6 percent risk).[18]

However, the vast majority of women considering TOLAC or repeat cesarean won't experience uterine rupture with either option. With TOLAC, the risk of rupture is 325 in 100,000, or about one-third of 1 percent; with a planned repeat cesarean, the risk of rupture drops to 26 in 100,000.[19]

After balancing the rare chance of rupture against all other factors, the overall risk of the baby's death is 130 in 100,000 for TOLAC and 50 in 100,000 for repeat cesarean.[20] Although this risk may seem alarming, it's similar to the risk of the baby's death for a first-time mother laboring with an unscarred uterus (about 100 in 100,000).

Even with the increased chance of rupture, vaginal birth carries fewer overall risks than surgical birth. For example, when compared to repeat cesarean, TOLAC carries a lower risk of hysterectomy, blood transfusion, and deep vein thrombosis; it also involves a shorter hospital stay. The overall risk of maternal death is less than 4 in 100,000 for TOLAC and more than 13 in 100,000 for repeat cesarean.[21]

Weighing the benefits and risks of a VBAC against those of a repeat cesarean can be challenging, and it's best to closely consult with your caregiver to better understand your options. If your risk of uterine rupture is high (see above) or your chances of having other complications in labor are high, a planned cesarean may be best for you. A planned cesarean has fewer risks than an unplanned cesarean that occurs after a failed TOLAC. If your risk of uterine rupture is low and your chances of VBAC success are favorable (see page 325), your best option may be to attempt a VBAC.

## Monitoring for and Managing Uterine Rupture

During a VBAC labor, the caregiver closely monitors both mother and baby for uterine rupture, which he or she can diagnose by carefully observing the baby's heart rate, the shape of the mother's abdomen, and the mother's blood pressure. If a caregiver suspects a rupture, the mother has an emergency cesarean to prevent excessive bleeding and distress to the baby. With careful monitoring and quick intervention, the majority of babies are fine at birth after a rupture.

## Improving Your Chances of Having a Successful VBAC

1. Choose a caregiver who proves his or her support of VBAC by having a high VBAC attempt rate and a success rate of 70 percent or more. You may have to interview several providers. Discuss your goals and preferences and ask questions about how you can work together toward a successful VBAC experience. If your current caregiver doesn't support your goals, consider finding a new one.
2. Consider hiring a doula who has had a VBAC herself or has worked with women who have had VBACs.
3. Take a childbirth refresher class or a VBAC class.
4. If your cesarean birth was traumatic or you feel anger, mistrust, or fear about your next birth, talk with a birth counselor, childbirth educator, or doula to help you deal with these feelings. You may also want to contact your local branch of the International Cesarean Awareness Network (ICAN). This organization's mission is to prevent unnecessary cesareans through education, provide support for cesarean recovery, and promote VBAC. They're a good source of local information and emotional support. You can also find abundant information on their web site, http://www.ican-online.org, including the paper "Your Right to Refuse: What to do if your hospital has banned VBAC."[22]
5. Avoid induction with Pitocin or prostaglandins. One study showed the risk of uterine rupture was less than one-half of 1 percent for spontaneous labor, just over 1 percent if labor was induced with Pitocin, and just under 1½ percent with prostaglandins.[23] If induction is necessary, non-drug methods, balloon catheters, and rupture of membranes may be safer for a VBAC. (See pages 278–280.)
6. Try to minimize medications for pain relief and use other interventions only if necessary.
7. Review "Ten Steps to Improve Your Chances of Having a Safe and Satisfying Birth" on page 30 and "Reducing Your Chances of Having a Cesarean Birth" on page 309.

By following these suggestions, you'll have done all you can to ensure a vaginal birth. But always remember that there's no guarantee a cesarean won't become the wise option if serious problems arise during labor. Consider writing a VBAC birth plan as well as a "best possible cesarean" plan to use if a repeat cesarean becomes the safest option. (See page 329.)

### Likelihood of VBAC Success

Most women who plan a TOLAC achieve a vaginal birth (60 to 94 percent).[24] VBAC is more likely if a woman is younger than forty and has had a prior vaginal birth, and if the reason for her previous cesarean hasn't recurred and her labor is progressing well. VBAC is less likely in the following situations:

- The mother has had multiple prior cesareans, has complicating medical conditions, or is obese.
- Gestation is over forty weeks and the baby is estimated to weigh over 9 pounds.
- Labor is induced or augmented.

## AVAILABILITY OF VBAC

Before 1980, common thought was "once a cesarean, always a cesarean." From the 1980s to 1999, experts recommended VBAC because they believed it was safer than repeat cesarean. However, in 1999 and again in 2008, the American College of Obstetricians and Gynecologists (ACOG) recommended that hospitals permit VBAC only when a physician, staff, and anesthesia were immediately available to provide an emergency cesarean.[25] As a result, due to staffing and liability concerns, hospital policies turned against VBAC. By early 2010, one-third of hospitals no longer permitted VBAC and one-half of physicians stopped offering it as an option.[26]

Many maternity care experts disagreed with the ACOG recommendation. The American Academy of Family Physicians as well as the 2010 National Institutes of Health panel questioned the rationale behind it.[27] In July 2010, ACOG changed their stance, stating that if a laboring woman arrived at a hospital that didn't support TOLAC, she should not be forced to have a repeat cesarean against her will. However, during prenatal care, a physician who is uncomfortable with VBAC may refer the patient to another physician. If you prefer to try for a VBAC but can't find a caregiver that supports your decision, consider relocating for the end of your pregnancy to a friend's or relative's home near a hospital and caregiver that support VBAC.

## EMOTIONAL REACTIONS WHEN DECIDING BETWEEN A REPEAT CESAREAN AND A VBAC

Some women who have had a prior cesarean may have emotional challenges choosing between a VBAC and a repeat cesarean. Emotional challenges also can arise during labor for women who choose VBAC. Because fear and anxiety can slow or complicate labor, it's best to address these emotional issues during pregnancy. See Chapters 10 and 11 to learn ways to help labor progress smoothly.

### Fear

The thought of laboring again may seem more frightening than the risks of major surgery. You

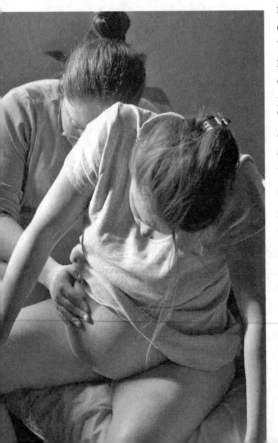

may fear labor pain, a long labor, uterine rupture, complications, another cesarean, failure to deliver "normally," or simply the unknown. Discuss your fears with your caregiver, childbirth educator, doula, or cesarean support group that supports VBAC. These people can reassure you and support your decision. They can help you identify the most distressing parts of your previous birth and help you plan how to avoid or address them. For example, you may plan not to wait for hours before having a cesarean if you have another long labor that doesn't progress.

### Shame or guilt

You may feel ashamed that you might have done things that led to a prior cesarean birth, or you may feel guilty for having agreed to a cesarean. Talk with others who understand your feelings so you can forgive yourself and approach this birth from a fresh perspective.

### Lack of confidence

You may doubt your ability to give birth vaginally and hesitate to invest time and effort in a VBAC because you don't want to be disappointed. Remember that each pregnancy and birth is different. Get to know women who have had successful VBACs. You may find they also lacked confidence and hope before giving birth. Ask what helped them become confident enough to birth vaginally. For example, perhaps they visualized the birth experience they'd hoped for.

### Feeling pressured

You may feel pressured by caregivers, friends, or family to make one decision or another. Always remember that you have the right to make an informed decision. Others can provide information and opinions, but only you can make the choice that's best for you and your family.

### Stress in labor

In addition to the emotional hurdles that arise in most labors (see graph on page 268), specific events in a VBAC labor may raise your stress level.

- When early labor is underway, you may suddenly second-guess whether a VBAC is such a good idea. Be prepared for this "moment of truth" beforehand by thinking of ways to deal with it.
- Particular events in labor may trigger flashbacks of your previous labor that ended in a cesarean. Don't suppress them, even if they're unpleasant. Acknowledge them openly and note how things are different this time.
- A big hurdle may be reaching the point in labor that led to a previous cesarean. Until you pass that point, you may continue to question your ability to birth vaginally. After you've passed it, you can breathe a sigh of relief and enjoy a boost of optimism.

# Having the Best Possible Cesarean Birth

## Two Views on VBAC

I gave birth to my daughter by unplanned cesarean. I was disappointed for quite a while afterward, because I'd had my heart set on delivering vaginally. When I got pregnant again, I didn't waste any time learning all I could about VBAC. I know there's no guarantee I'll deliver vaginally this time, but I want to do all I can to better my odds.

—*Jana*

When my first labor failed to progress, I ended up needing a cesarean. I remember thinking at the time, "Thank goodness! I'm sick of this pain!" Now I'm pregnant again, and I'm not keen to repeat that labor experience. Part of me wants to skip it all together, but another part realizes that recovering from a C-section is no piece of cake, either. I think I need to learn how to better handle the labor pain so I can avoid the pain of cesarean recovery.

—*Samantha*

Whether or not a cesarean birth is what you want, you can have a satisfying experience. The following steps will help you make your cesarean birth the best it can be.

### Educate yourself.

- Learn about the cesarean procedure from books, classes, and discussions with your caregiver.
- Find out your birthplace's policies and regulations for cesareans.

### If a planned cesarean is necessary, prepare in advance.

- Take care of yourself in pregnancy. Eat well and exercise regularly if possible. The more physically fit you are before the surgery, the quicker you recover afterward.

## Common Q & A

**Q:** I've heard of "natural cesareans" or "slow cesareans." What are they?

**A:** Historically, cesareans were emergency procedures that emphasized rapid delivery and immediate access to the baby for resuscitation. As cesareans have become more commonplace and oftentimes less urgent, some obstetricians have begun doing the surgery more slowly and encouraging immediate skin-to-skin contact between the mother and baby after the delivery. This woman-centered, baby-friendly way of doing cesareans is new, and your caregiver might not be aware of it. Learn more about natural cesareans and find a journal article to share with your caregiver by visiting http://tinyurl.com/la83t2.

- Tour the hospital, including the special care nursery. Ask to have any lab work, tests, and paperwork done before the day of surgery. Meet with an anesthesiologist to discuss options and learn what medications he or she will use.
- If hospital policy allows for two support people in the OR, ask a friend or family member to join you with your partner for the surgery. Or consider hiring a doula. Her calm, familiar presence and knowledge of cesareans can reassure you. Plus, after your baby is born, she can remain by your side while your partner stays with your baby.
- Take a breastfeeding class with your partner so you both know ways to help make nursing after a cesarean easier.

### Wait for labor to begin (or at least until week thirty-nine of pregnancy).

If your caregiver recommends a cesarean before your labor begins, be certain that there are clear medical reasons for the recommendation. There are definite advantages to waiting until labor begins on its own. Ask that your caregiver schedule the surgery as close to your due date as possible, and also ask about amniocentesis to verify your baby's lung maturity before surgery.

- Labor benefits babies. Babies born by scheduled cesarean without experiencing labor are four times more likely to develop persistent pulmonary hypertension, a potentially life-threatening situation.
- Severe complications, including breathing difficulties, infection, and other problems that require admission to the neonatal intensive care unit (NICU), are twice as likely for babies born at thirty-seven weeks than are babies born at thirty-nine weeks.[28]
- Not waiting for labor to begin for a planned cesarean can lead to accidental prematurity if the estimated gestational age is wrong. Knowing the exact date of conception, having an ultrasound scan early in pregnancy that documents a gestational age, or having the baby's lung maturity verified are ways to better estimate an accurate gestational age.

### Prepare a cesarean birth plan.

Even if you're planning a vaginal birth, consider writing a cesarean birth plan. (See Chapter 8 for more information on birth plans.) Here are questions to consider asking at a prenatal appointment to learn about your options:

- Can I have two support people in the OR with me?
- What will be the atmosphere in the OR? Can I choose music to play? Will the staff narrate what's happening? Will they chat with me to keep me relaxed during the procedure? Will they stop chatting if I request it?
- Will staff lower the screen or use a mirror so I can see my baby's birth? Are there restrictions on photographing and video-recording the birth?

- Can my partner announce our baby's sex? Will you do minimal suctioning of my baby's nose and mouth? Can I have skin-to-skin contact with my baby after birth? Will newborn exams be done where my partner and I can see our baby? If possible, can my baby stay in the OR during my repair? Will breastfeeding be initiated as soon after the birth as possible?
- Will you do internal repair and double-layer suturing? (See page 317.)
- If I experience anxiety, trembling, or nausea, will I be offered non-drug options for coping or medications that will keep me alert?
- Can I start eating whenever I wish after the surgery?

If the options and answers don't satisfy you, consider switching to a different caregiver or birthplace.

## Understand the reasons for a cesarean.

If you're having a planned or unplanned (but nonurgent) cesarean, ask your caregiver as many questions as you need to fully understand the benefits, risks, and alternatives before consenting to surgery. If you have an emergency cesarean, talk with your caregiver after the birth about why it was needed. This information may help you feel that the decisions made during the birth were necessary at the time, which can help you accept the events of birth.

## Insist on early, frequent contact with your baby.

Cesarean delivery, narcotic pain medications, and high levels of stress at birth may delay breast-feeding and affect breast milk production. The more time you spend nestling with your baby and the more frequently you nurse, the sooner your milk supply increases. Skin-to-skin contact also enhances the emotional bond between you and your baby.

## Develop a postpartum plan.

The postpartum period is more challenging when you're recovering from major surgery, so plan ahead for the extra support you'll need. See page 158 for more information.

## *Key Points to Remember*

- More than 30 percent of women giving birth in the United States have cesareans. Although a cesarean is a relatively safe surgery, vaginal birth has fewer overall risks. For this reason, birthing women and their caregivers should consider a cesarean only when the potential medical benefits clearly outweigh the possible risks.
- There are steps you can take to increase your chances of a vaginal birth, and important questions you can ask if your caregiver recommends a cesarean.
- VBAC is a viable option for many women with prior cesareans; however, policies at your local hospital may limit access to a VBAC.
- Preparing a cesarean birth plan helps ensure that if you need a cesarean, you'll have a positive birth experience that lets you feel nurtured and cared for.

# CHAPTER 15

# What Life Is Like
# for a New Mother

The days, weeks, and months that follow your baby's birth are a time of major physical, emotional, and social readjustment and recovery.

After the birth, your reproductive organs return to their prepregnant state (usually within six weeks). You begin to lose the extra weight you gained during pregnancy. Your breasts begin to produce milk. These physical changes are normal, but they can seem more difficult than you expected.

During the first weeks, most new parents experience sudden mood changes. You may feel joyous and energetic one moment, then exhausted, let down, or even disappointed the next. Caring for your baby may also upset the equilibrium within your family until you can adjust your roles and schedules.

This chapter describes the typical changes that can affect the lives of a new mother and her family, and offers ways to help smooth your adjustment to parenthood.

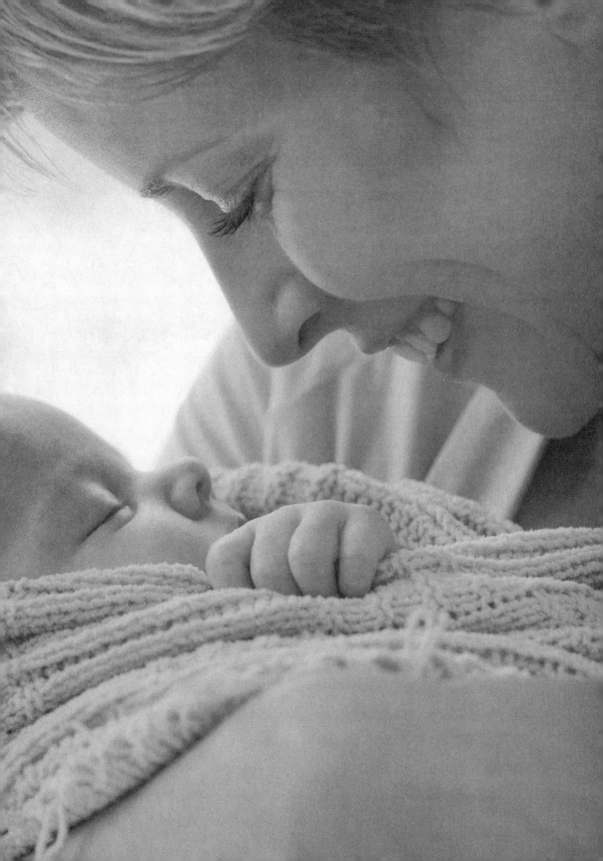

# Factors That Influence Your Adjustment to Postpartum Life

Every woman adjusts to life with a new baby differently. Some women seem to find a comfortable balance in their lives within weeks. Others take months to adjust, and some never do.

Why do some women adjust to postpartum life more easily than others do? Numerous factors can influence the adjustment process. Some factors are internal, such as the health of the pregnancy. Others are external, such as the strength of a new mother's support network.

The following are favorable or positive factors that can help ease your adjustment to parenthood. The more of these factors you have, the more likely your adjustment to postpartum life will be smooth. The fewer of these factors you have, the more likely your adjustment will take longer than the typical eight to twelve weeks. You might not be able to control some of these factors, but developing a postpartum plan can help improve others. (See Chapter 8.)

**Before pregnancy**
- Positive experience with how you were raised
- Good mental and physical health (you and your family)
- Minimal exposure to trauma
- Positive experience with previous pregnancies, births, and baby care

**During pregnancy**
- Planned pregnancy
- No pregnancy complications
- Pregnant with only one baby
- No need for prolonged bed rest or treatment for a high-risk pregnancy
- Minimal financial worries
- Physically undemanding job
- Adequate sleep
- Good relationship with the baby's father or your partner
- Presence of other supportive people

**During labor and birth**
- Normal, uncomplicated birth
- Presence of continuous, competent care and support from staff, your partner, and other support people

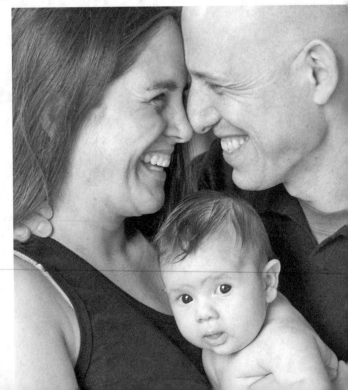

**Early postpartum period**
- Immediate contact with your baby (including breastfeeding)
- Minimal postpartum pain
- Good health (you and your baby)

**Later postpartum period**
- Delaying the return to employment until you feel ready
- Your baby's easy temperament and continuing health
- No feeding problems
- Adequate sleep for the whole family
- Positive emotional state
- Continuing supportive relationships with your partner, family, and friends

# Your Care in the Days Following the Birth

If you have a vaginal birth in a hospital, your postpartum stay is typically one to two days (unless a medical reason necessitates a longer stay). If you have a cesarean birth, your stay is usually two to four days. At a freestanding (unaffiliated with a hospital) birth center, your stay is typically three to six hours. At a home birth, your midwife leaves about three to four hours after the birth.

Before leaving the hospital or birth center (or your midwife leaves your home), ask your caregiver for information on newborn care and postpartum recovery. If you're birthing at a hospital, attend classes offered on these topics during your stay.

Ideally, your caregiver and your baby's caregiver (or a mother/infant nurse) should examine you and your baby on the third or fourth day after the birth, to detect jaundice, dehydration, or excessive weight loss in your baby and to check your physical recovery, help you with any feeding challenges, assess and treat pain, and answer your questions about baby care. If you develop pain or a fever before this scheduled visit—or if your baby looks yellow (see page 389), has trouble feeding, or seems sleepy or listless—request an appointment for as soon as possible.

Learn about possible warning signs that indicate problems with your health or your baby's health (see pages 337 and 393). Contact your caregiver and your baby's caregiver with any health concerns. For non-medical concerns, your childbirth educator, a breastfeeding counselor, doula, or experienced parents may provide helpful advice and information.

# Your Physical Recovery: Early Postpartum Period

Immediately after the birth, your caregivers will closely observe your physical condition. They'll frequently check your temperature, pulse, respiratory rate, and blood pressure. They'll monitor vaginal bleeding; your uterus's size, firmness, and position; and the functioning of your bladder and bowels. If you had anesthesia, they'll monitor the return of feeling and movement in your legs.

## UTERUS

Your uterus returns to its prepregnant size—a process called *involution*—about six weeks after the birth. Immediately after the birth of your placenta, you can feel the top of your uterus (fundus) at your navel. Your uterus involutes (drops) the width of one finger each day and is firm and tight to prevent heavy blood loss from the site where the placenta attached to your uterus. Soon after the birth, you or your nurse massages your uterus, stimulating it to contract. (See page 270 for instructions.) Nursing your baby also helps stimulate the uterus to contract.

As your uterus contracts, you may experience discomfort or pain. These *afterpains* often occur during breastfeeding and are more common if you've given birth before. To ease the pain, relax and use slow breathing patterns (see page 224). Ibuprofen or prescribed medications may also help. Afterpains typically disappear after the first week.

*Lochia* is the bloody, fleshy-smelling discharge that flows from your uterus and out your vagina for up to six to eight weeks after the birth. For the first few days, the flow looks like heavy menstrual flow. Passing jellylike clots is normal, especially in the first days. The flow amount may change with your activity or body position. Lochia is heavier when you change positions, are overactive, breastfeed, or have a bowel movement. If flow increases, remind yourself to slow down and rest. Within ten days, lochia diminishes and becomes pale pink or rust in color. Over the next several weeks, it becomes white, yellowish white, or tan. (See page 337 for warning signs.)

If you're not breastfeeding, you'll probably resume menstruation four to eight weeks after the birth. If you're breastfeeding, you might not menstruate for several months or until you wean; however, you can become pregnant, because you may ovulate before your period returns. Your first few periods may be heavier and longer than usual or they may be lighter than usual, but they'll eventually return to normal.

## CERVIX AND VAGINA

As your uterus approaches its prepregnant size, so does your cervix. After the birth, your vagina gradually regains its tone, and your labia remain somewhat looser, larger, and darker than before pregnancy.

## BREASTS

For the first twenty-four to seventy-two hours after the birth, your breasts secrete colostrum (highly nutritious fluid that's your baby's first milk). Mature breast milk appears between the second and fifth day. At that time, your breasts may become engorged, which may present feeding challenges. (See page 419.)

### If You're Not Breastfeeding

If you decide not to breastfeed (or can't), your breasts typically undergo the same initial changes as breastfeeding mothers. To reduce milk production and increase comfort, apply ice packs and avoid breast stimulation. On the second or third day after the birth, wear a snugly fitting sports bra or wrap an extra wide elastic bandage across your breasts and around your chest to compress your breasts and decrease the swelling that occurs as your milk comes in. Rewrap the elastic bandage every few hours. Keep your breasts bound for twenty-four to forty-eight hours.

Once your milk comes in, apply ice to your breasts for twenty minutes every four hours or so to decrease the pain from inflammation and swelling. Use ice packs or an elastic bandage to hold several bags of frozen peas or corn in place over your bra or shirt. Consider taking ibuprofen or acetaminophen (Tylenol) for pain relief.

If you're not breastfeeding because your baby has died, suppressing your milk may cause you to experience a "second grieving" for your baby who can't have the milk. Know that you don't have to immediately suppress lactation if you don't want to. Some mothers express and donate their milk in honor of their babies. (See page 303 for more information on newborn death.)

## HORMONAL CHANGES

When you deliver the placenta, your estrogen and progesterone levels drop rapidly and remain low until your ovaries begin producing these hormones again. If you breastfeed, your production of prolactin and oxytocin increases, while estrogen and progesterone levels remain low until you wean your baby.

# CIRCULATORY CHANGES

During pregnancy, you accumulate extra blood and fluid. When giving birth, bleeding naturally occurs as the uterus contracts to compress the blood vessels that flowed to the placenta. During an uncomplicated vaginal birth, the average blood loss is about 1 cup. If you had an episiotomy or a sizable perineal tear, you may lose more blood. You continue to lose blood in your lochia for a few weeks. See page 299 for signs of excessive blood loss.

In the early postpartum period, you urinate often and sweat heavily (especially at night) to lose the extra fluid accumulated during pregnancy. You may lose as much as 5 pounds of fluid during the first week after the birth.

# ABDOMINAL AND SKIN CHANGES

After giving birth, your abdominal muscles are loose, and take several months to regain firmness. Exercise speeds up the process. Your stretch marks fade from red to silver but don't completely disappear. If your skin darkened during pregnancy, the pigmentation will fade. Any increased hair growth also disappears gradually.

If you pushed hard for a long time during the birth, the rapid changes in blood pressure during and between pushes may have caused broken blood vessels in your eyes and on your face and neck. They typically disappear within a week or two of the birth.

# HEMORRHOIDS

*Hemorrhoids* are swollen varicose veins in the rectal area that may be as small as a pea or as large as a grape. They may itch, bleed, sting, or ache, especially during a bowel movement. Many women develop hemorrhoids during pregnancy; some develop them after a vaginal birth. Most hemorrhoids disappear in the first postpartum month. To prevent hemorrhoids or to reduce discomfort and promote healing, follow these suggestions:

- Take steps to prevent constipation. (See page 120.)
- Do your Kegel exercises (see page 95), with emphasis on the anal muscles.
- Use witch hazel on the area.
- Take sitz baths. (See page 336.)
- Avoid heavy lifting. If you must pick up a heavy object (such as an older child), do a Super Kegel (see page 96) and hold it as you lift.

If these measures don't help prevent hemorrhoids or reduce their discomfort, see page 353.

# BOWEL AND BLADDER FUNCTION

After the birth, you may have trouble urinating because of a tear near your urethra or swelling around it (from the birth or a bladder catheter). To help start the flow, try to relax your perineum, drink lots of liquids, or pour warm water over your perineum (or try urinating in the shower or bathtub). If you still can't urinate, call your caregiver.

The birth may cause you to become constipated because of loose abdominal muscles, episiotomy, hemorrhoids, or a sore perineum. Iron supplements and narcotic pain medications may also cause constipation. Prevent constipation by eating lots of fresh and dried fruits, vegetables, and whole-grain cereals (to increase your fiber intake) and by drinking plenty of water. Adding a tablespoon of flax meal to your food also may help. When you're able, walking and exercising your abdominal muscles help restore normal bowel function, as does moving your bowels when you have the urge (instead of waiting until later). If your caregiver prescribes a stool softener, follow the instructions for use.

When moving your bowels, support your perineum by gently pressing toilet paper against your stitches to prevent the tissue from bulging and stretching.

If these suggestions don't help and you remain uncomfortable, your caregiver may prescribe a laxative, suppositories, or an enema.

## PERINEAL CARE

Your perineum needs special care after the birth, especially if you're bruised or swollen, or had stitches for an episiotomy or a tear. (See below to learn how to care for your perineum.) Stitches dissolve in two to four weeks, and the tissue usually heals within four to six weeks, although you may feel discomfort for some time. Discomfort during intercourse may persist for months. See your caregiver if the discomfort worsens or continues beyond several months.

## Steps for Perineal Care

Follow these steps to relieve perineal pain, promote healing, and prevent infection.

- Apply ice to your perineum to reduce swelling. Soon after the birth, your nurse or midwife will apply an ice pack to your perineum. For the next several days, continue to use ice intermittently to soothe pain from a tear, episiotomy, or hemorrhoids. To make an ice pack, put crushed ice or a frozen wet washcloth in a zip-close plastic bag and wrap it in several layers of paper towel. Hold it in place with your perineal pad. Or dampen a maxi pad with witch hazel and freeze it before use.
- Begin doing Kegel exercises immediately after the birth (see page 95). Frequent pelvic floor exercises increase circulation, promote healing, and reduce swelling. They also help restore strength and muscle tone. Don't be discouraged if you can't do Kegels as well as you could before the birth. Your strength should improve quickly.
- After urinating, clean yourself by pouring warm water over your perineum from front to back (to prevent infection from organisms in the rectal area). If you birth in a hospital, you may be given a "peri bottle" (squirt bottle filled with warm water) to wash yourself. Use toilet paper to gently pat yourself dry from front to back.
- Don't use tampons before your postpartum checkup.
- Don't douche.
- Take a sitz bath to help relieve perineal soreness: Sit in a clean tub of warm water for ten to twenty minutes. After the bath, lie down for fifteen minutes to decrease swelling caused by the warm water. If you like, use cold water. It can be as soothing as a warm bath and doesn't increase swelling.
- Sit on a plastic donut pillow to lift your perineum off the surface you're sitting on. If you don't have a donut pillow, make your own by rolling a bath towel lengthwise and shaping it into a horseshoe shape. Sit on the pillow with both buttocks supported.
- Sit on a firm surface if your stitches are causing pain. You may find sitting on a firm surface more comfortable than sitting on a soft one or on a donut, either of which can separate the edges of your incision. To help keep your incision pressed together and avoid pain, sit down on one buttock first, then ease onto the other buttock.
- Lie down and rest as often as you can in the first weeks after the birth. When sitting or standing, gravity can increase swelling and cause the pelvic floor to ache.

## Warning Signs after the Birth That Require Medical Attention

Report any of the following warning signs to your caregiver.

| Warning Signs | Possible Problems |
|---|---|
| Fever (oral or temporal artery temperature of 100.4°F/38°C or higher) | • Uterine infection<br>• Bladder or kidney infection<br>• Breast infection (mastitis)<br>• Infection of episiotomy or tear<br>• Infection of cesarean incision<br>• Other illness |
| Burning with urination; blood in urine | • Bladder or kidney infection |
| Inability to urinate | • Swelling or trauma of the urethral sphincter |
| Swollen, red, painful area on the leg (especially the calf) that's hot and tender to the touch | • Thrombophlebitis or deep vein thrombosis (blood clot in the blood vessel); do **not** rub or massage the area. |
| Sore, reddened, hot, painful area on breast(s), along with fever and flu-like symptoms | • Breast infection (mastitis) |
| Passage of blood clot larger than a lemon followed by heavy bleeding, or any bleeding heavy enough to soak a maxi pad in an hour or less | • Passage of some (but not all) of a retained placenta<br>• Uterine infection |
| Vaginal discharge that has an extremely foul odor (like spoiled fish); vaginal soreness or itching | • Uterine infection<br>• Vaginal infection |
| Increased pain at site of episiotomy or tear; may be accompanied by foul-smelling or pus-like discharge | • Infection of episiotomy or tear<br>• Reopening of incision or tear |
| Opening of cesarean incision; may be accompanied by pus-like discharge or blood | • Infection of cesarean incision |
| Appearance of rash or hives; may be accompanied by itching | • Allergic reaction to medication |
| Severe headache that begins after the birth and is worse when upright and less painful when lying down | • Spinal headache following regional anesthesia |
| Any sudden onset of pain that's new, such as abdominal tenderness or burning near perineal stitches when urinating | • Uterine infection<br>• Reopening of perineal tear or incision |
| Pain and tenderness in front or back of pelvis, accompanied by difficulty walking and a "grating" sensation in pubic joint | • Separation of pubic symphysis (cartilage between the pubic bones in the front of your pelvis) |
| Feeling extremely anxious, panicky, or depressed; accompanied by rapid heart rate, difficulty breathing, uncontrollable crying, feelings of anger, or inability to sleep or eat | • Postpartum mood disorders, including anxiety and panic attacks, obsessive thinking or worrying, or depression |
| Frightening relationship with your partner; being verbally or physically abused | • Domestic violence increases during pregnancy and after the birth. If you need to talk or get help, call the National Domestic Violence Hotline, 800-799-SAFE (7233) or 800-787-3224 (TTY). |

# Your Physical Recovery: Later Postpartum Period

Within three to eight weeks after the birth, your caregiver will give you a general physical examination (including a pelvic exam) to assess your recovery and to discuss any physical or emotional problems you may have. You also may discuss your family-planning preferences. After the checkup, your caregiver will recommend that you have regular Pap smears.

If you notice any of the warning signs listed on page 337 before your checkup, call your caregiver immediately for an appointment.

## BREAST SELF-EXAMINATION

Your caregiver may recommend that you examine your breasts every month. To learn how to examine your breasts, visit the Susan G. Komen for the Cure web site at http://www.komen.org/bse. It's best to check your breasts right after your menstrual period, when they're softest. If you're breastfeeding, check your breasts on the first day of each month, after a feeding.

Although only a small percentage of breast changes indicate cancer, tell your caregiver about any thickening breast tissue, lumps that don't disappear within a day or two, or nonmilk discharge. A medical examination can determine whether the changes are benign (harmless) or suggest a problem. Early detection and treatment of cancerous tissue can help prevent the growth and spread of the disease.

# Caring for Yourself after the Birth

After giving birth, you can help your recovery by eating well, getting adequate rest, and asking others for help with household chores, meal preparation, and other tasks that you may find difficult to accomplish while caring for your baby.

## NUTRITION

In the postpartum period, continue eating healthful foods, as you did during pregnancy. (See Chapter 6.) If you're breastfeeding, see page 417 for nutrition suggestions.

Don't drastically change or restrict your diet to lose weight. The maximum amount of weight you should lose per week is 1 to 2 pounds. Most new mothers lose pregnancy weight gradually over several months without special effort.

If you're anemic, your caregiver may recommend that you continue taking prenatal vitamins and iron supplements. To prevent constipation, ensure your diet contains plenty of fiber.

## REST AND SLEEP

When you first begin caring for your baby, finding time to sleep may seem impossible. If you're not tending to your baby's needs, you're trying to finish household chores or attempting to take a shower.

However, fatigue and sleep deprivation can greatly challenge your physical and emotional recovery, so make sleep a top priority and take every opportunity to nap. Even if you can't sleep, simply resting gives you the energy to meet your baby's often unpredictable needs.

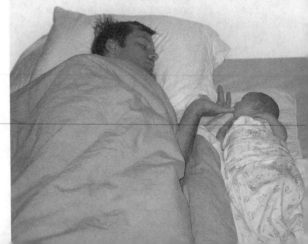

You may notice that your baby sleeps as much during the day as she does at night. This sleep pattern is common and temporary for newborns. As you baby grows, she'll begin to sleep longer at night when you and your family do. (See page 380.) If you're used to sleeping only at night, or if your baby naps for short periods and wakes up frequently, the advice to "sleep when your baby sleeps" may frustrate you. In addition, constantly listening for your baby's cries may make you feel wired and unable to sleep.

You'll eventually adjust to being awake at night and learn how to rest and sleep when you can. But what can you do in the meantime? Try the following suggestions to help you relax and fall asleep:

- First, commit to making sleep a priority, right after meeting your baby's needs. Someone else can do household tasks, or they can wait until you're rested.
- Give yourself permission to do whatever it takes to be able to rest, such as turning off the phone, sitting outside, taking short walks, having a bath, eating and drinking particular food and beverages, having a massage, or taking pain medication.
- Limit visitors; don't worry about being a gracious host. If a visit lasts too long, ask the guests to leave, or excuse yourself with your baby and retire to your bedroom.
- Try relaxation techniques such as the relaxation countdown (see page 218).
- Keep your baby close to you so you don't strain to listen for her (which can interfere with your ability to rest).
- Conversely, you may find that your baby's sounds increase your anxiety and restlessness, especially if you're extremely tired. In that case, let someone else tend to your baby in another room while you rest. Once you're rested, anxiety usually decreases.
- If your partner is available, take turns caring for your baby throughout the night. Or try scheduling parenting shifts: One parent goes to bed early, while the other is responsible for caring for your baby during the night. The parent who went to bed first takes over care early the next morning, allowing the other parent to sleep in. If you're breastfeeding, you may need to adapt this schedule to accommodate feeding patterns.

## Recipe for Sleep in the First Weeks after the Birth

Many first-time parents use the following approach to get an adequate amount of sleep until their babies begin to sleep for longer stretches.

1. Ask yourself how much sleep you needed before pregnancy to function well. Six hours? Eight hours? That's the amount of sleep you now require every day.
2. Because feedings and baby care prevent you from getting this amount of sleep in one stretch, you'll need more time in bed to meet your sleep requirement. Stay in bed until you've slept enough (meals and trips to the bathroom are obvious exceptions). Each time you wake up, keep a mental note of how long you slept.
3. Don't brush your teeth, shower, or dress until you've met your sleep requirement. If you require eight hours of sleep, it may take from 10 PM until noon (or later) the next day to get out of your pajamas!

*Notes:* You may find that having your baby sleep with you (or in the same room) makes it easier to get enough sleep, because you can care for your baby quickly. Also, if you have other children, this approach may require the help of another adult who can care for them while you sleep.

## ASKING FOR HELP

After the birth, you may be upset to realize that you can't do things (such as manage your household) as well as you could before the birth. You may find it difficult to ask for help, but having support will speed your postpartum recovery.

Accept any offer that will make it easier for you to rest, shower, or otherwise care for yourself. Someone may offer to do the dishes and laundry, shop for groceries, vacuum and dust, or simply watch your baby. If you're concerned about meals, someone can cook and freeze meals in advance, or bring a meal every day for the first few weeks.

If you're unable or unwilling to ask friends and family for help, consider hiring part-time household help or a postpartum doula (see page 27) for a few weeks after the birth. Many communities have agencies that specialize in postpartum home care.

# Postpartum Fitness

Immediately after giving birth, your body begins recovering from the event as your mind begins reordering your priorities to emphasize rest, healing, and caring for your baby. In the early postpartum period, there's little time or need to resume or begin a vigorous exercise regimen. However, moderate activity (such as walking) and gentle conditioning exercises (see below) can help speed your recovery. If your labor and birth were normal, you can begin doing these exercises when you feel ready, whether that's a few days or a few weeks after the birth. Follow your caregiver's guidelines about exercise and other activities such as driving, stair climbing, and lifting.

After several weeks to months, you may want to resume more vigorous exercise. Listen to your body and increase your intensity gradually. You're over-exercising if you become exhausted, experience any pain, or have increased vaginal bleeding. (See page 337 for postpartum warning signs.) In that case, consult with your caregiver before resuming the exercise.

As you increase your fitness level, your energy, motivation, and endurance will improve.

## EXERCISES TO CONDITION YOUR MUSCLES AND RELIEVE TENSION

In the postpartum period, your abdominal muscles require exercise to recover their former shape and strength while avoiding further separation or diastasis (see page 341). Your pelvic floor muscles need exercise to increase circulation, reduce swelling and promote healing in the perineum, and restore vaginal and rectal muscle tone. When these muscle groups are in good condition, they provide core muscle support for your entire body.

You can do conditioning exercises, as well as exercises that relieve tension, with your baby near you. For example, each time you change a diaper, contract your pelvic floor muscles or do pelvic tilts. Before or after feeding your baby, do head tilts and shoulder circles. During a feeding, try doing transverse abdominal contractions.

The following sections describe these and other exercises.

### Core and Postural Exercises

Every day or so, try doing the following conditioning exercises, especially the pelvic floor contraction. Whenever exercising your abdominal muscles, first contract the pelvic floor muscles to support them.

# Reducing the Separation of Your Rectus Abdominis Muscles

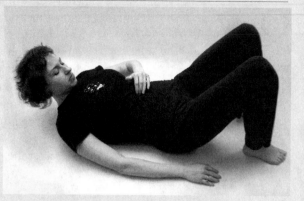

Before you begin doing any abdominal muscle exercise other than transverse abdominal contractions and pelvic tilts (see pages 96–97), check your rectus abdominis muscles for separation. These are the muscles from your chest to your pubic bone. As your abdomen grew and stretched during pregnancy, the connective tissue between these muscles may have begun separating painlessly and without bleeding to prevent the muscles from overstretching. Separation is normal, but your help is required to close the gap.

To check for separation, lie on your back with your knees bent. Press the fingers of one hand into your abdomen just above your navel. Slowly raise your head and shoulders. The rectus muscles will tense, letting you detect any gap. A slight gap (1 inch or less) indicates normal muscle separation after pregnancy; it doesn't need to be closed. A larger gap between the muscles (2 to 3 inches) indicates that you need to close the gap before doing crunches and other conventional abdominal exercises. If you don't close a wide separation, strenuous exercise that requires abdominal stabilization will only increase the separation and defeat the purpose of the exercise.

To help narrow a large gap, do transverse abdominal contractions and head lifts (see below). Progress to more advanced abdominal exercises after the gap has narrowed to the width of one or two fingers and when your abdominals can keep your rectus muscles closely aligned without your support.[1]

### Pelvic Floor Contraction (Kegel or Super Kegel Exercise)
See page 95 for instructions. Immediately after the birth (vaginal or cesarean), do two to three short Kegels whenever you can, then progress to five full Kegels each hour. Gradually work toward holding the contraction for up to twenty seconds (the Super Kegel).

### Pelvic Tilts I, II, and III
See page 97 for instructions. Remember to contract the pelvic floor when performing these exercises.

### Transverse Abdominal Contractions
See page 96 for instructions. This exercise helps close a separation of the rectus muscles while toning your abdominals and flattening your stomach. It becomes progressively easier to do over time. Begin with three sets of contractions per day and increase the number of sets as you like.[2]

### Head Lifts
*Aim:* To help close a separation of your rectus muscles while toning your abdominals and flattening your stomach.

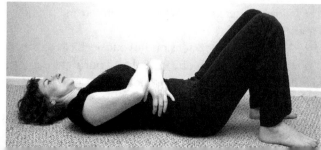

## Common Q & A

**Q:** I know I should exercise to help my recovery, but I just can't find the time. What can I do?

**A:** As your baby grows and begins to need your care and attention less frequently, you'll have more time for exercise. In the beginning, exercising outside the home might not appeal to you. If you'd rather avoid the hassle of having to look presentable and getting to class on time, exercise at home with your baby by dancing with him or doing postpartum exercises with him next to you. No matter how long it's been between showers, you're the best thing your baby has seen!

When you feel ready, schedule walks with other new mothers or take a postpartum exercise class to motivate you to get moving and reconnect with the outside world.

*Exercise:* Lie on your back with your knees bent. Cross your hands over your abdomen, placing them on either side of your waist. Inhale; as you exhale, raise your head. At the same time, pull your bellybutton toward your spine and use your hands to pull the side abdominal muscles toward each other (see photo on page 341). Hold for a slow count of five. Slowly lower your head and rest.

*Repetition:* To close any separation, repeat twenty times each day and increase repetitions as you're able. The separation should regain its normal ½-inch (or smaller) width within several weeks. Progress to more advanced abdominal work only after the separation is within this normal range.[3]

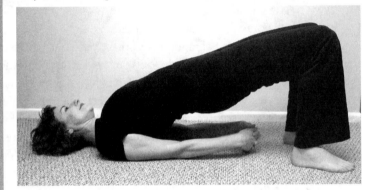

**Bridge Pose**

*Aim:* To tone your hamstrings and buttocks.

*Exercise:* Lie on your back with your knees bent and your arms resting on the floor along your sides. Inhale; as you exhale, lift your tailbone off the floor, then each vertebra, until your weight is resting on your shoulders. Push your feet into the floor and keep your thighs parallel to each other (not rolled outward). To protect your neck, avoid turning your head. If you like, clasp your hands together under your back and press your arms into the floor to lift your chest.

*Repetition:* Hold the position for several breaths, then roll back into the starting position. Repeat the exercise five to ten times each day.

**Pectoral Stretch, Hip Flexor Stretch, and Posture Check**

See pages 99–100 for instructions.

## Tension Relievers

The following exercises relieve muscle tension and promote overall relaxation.

**Head Tilts**

*Aim:* To relieve muscle tension in your neck caused by holding your baby.

*Exercise:* Look straight ahead and tilt your right ear toward your right shoulder and hold for ten seconds. Don't let your left shoulder rise. Repeat on your left side.

*Repetition:* Do this exercise once a day or as often as feels good.

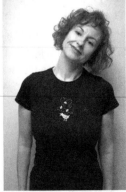

## Peek-a-boo Yoga

Here's a fun way to stretch your body and bond with your baby. Start on your hands and knees. Place your baby on his back underneath you so your eyes are level with his. Then follow this sequence of poses, which are described on pages 100–103):

- Cat pose
- Child's pose (Stretch your arms above your head with your forearms cradling your baby.)
- Opposite-limb extensions
- Child's pose
- Downward-facing dog
- Child's pose
- Downward-facing dog
- Child's pose
- Half-dog pose
- Bridge pose (While you do this exercise, move your baby to the side, perhaps on his tummy. Or hold him on your abdomen)
- Corpse pose with five-minute meditation (Your baby can be either on your abdomen or next to you.)

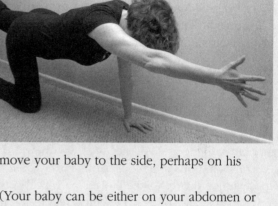

**Shoulder Circles**

See the instructions on page 99. This exercise relieves tension in your shoulders and upper back caused by holding your baby.

**Relaxation and Slow Breathing**

*Aim:* To relax and rejuvenate your body and to release mental stress that accompanies baby care.

*Exercise:* Use the same relaxation techniques you found helpful during pregnancy and birth. For example, try five minutes of slow breathing (see page 224), passive relaxation (see page 216), relaxation countdown (see page 218), or the five-minute meditation (see page 102).

*Repetition:* Do this exercise whenever you have a moment to recognize what a phenomenal job you're doing as a new parent!

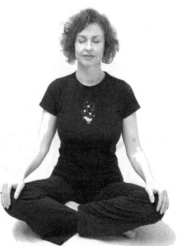

# POSTPARTUM FITNESS AFTER A CESAREAN BIRTH

If you've had a cesarean birth, see Chapter 14 for activities that are appropriate for the first few days after surgery, such as deep breathing, knee bends, and abdominal pull-ins, and rolling from back to side while bridging. Pelvic floor exercises are also fine to do.

Your caregiver will probably recommend that you wait six weeks before doing any strenuous activities, including the postpartum exercises described on pages 340–343. Consult with your caregiver before starting an exercise regimen.

## POSTPARTUM FITNESS AFTER A CHALLENGING PREGNANCY OR BIRTH

If you were pregnant with multiples, were on bed rest, or had a difficult pregnancy or birth, your recovery may be more challenging than other women's. Conserve your energy initially, until you can do things more normally. As you resume your daily activities, your strength will return. When you're able to exercise, expect to tire quickly. Set reasonable expectations and try not to compare your progress with other women's. Be patient with yourself and celebrate every accomplishment.

## A NOTE TO FATHERS AND PARTNERS

When your partner is ready, gently encourage her to exercise, but don't pressure her. Help her make time for exercise, and consider exercising with her so you can spend some time together while improving your health.

# Adapting to Postpartum Life

As a new parent, you may sometimes yearn for the simpler, more predictable life you had before you began tending to your baby's seemingly never-ending needs. You may wonder how long it'll take you to physically recover from the birth and to balance the interests and demands of your former life with the joys and needs of your new life with your baby.

At some point after your baby's birth, you'll experience postpartum adaptation (also called "postpartum recovery"), the process by which your life generally returns to more predictable patterns. You can take care of daily demands, feel rested most of the time, and begin to enjoy previous interests again. Your body is healing, and you can meet your baby's needs with growing confidence. (See page 332 for factors that influence your adjustment to postpartum life.)

The following sections describe areas of your life that will be affected by your baby's arrival and may require special attention as you adapt to your new role. Visit our web site, http://www.PCNGuide.com, to download a work sheet to help you prepare.

## Parenting Groups and New-parent Classes

Connecting with other new parents is one of the most helpful ways to ease the transition to parenthood. (See Appendix C for information on specialized support groups for complicated circumstances.) By attending a parenting group or new-parent class, you can learn about other parenting styles, hear new solutions to common parenting problems, see other babies' development, and discover that you're 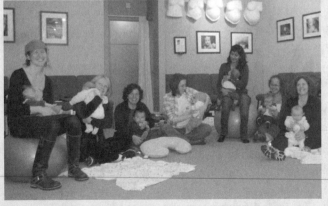 not the only one overwhelmed by postpartum life.

Hospitals, churches, community colleges, and community organizations may offer parenting groups and classes. Many of these target mothers, but most welcome fathers and partners. Plan ahead by learning about local groups and classes before your baby's birth.

# YOUR SEX LIFE AFTER THE BIRTH

Many caregivers recommend that new mothers don't have intercourse for the first six weeks, but this time frame is arbitrary. If you and your partner want to resume intercourse as soon as possible after the birth, it's probably safe to do so after any stitches have healed and the amount of lochia has decreased. But be gentle; you may be sore at first. In addition, after giving birth (and for as long as you breastfeed), hormonal changes reduce vaginal lubrication. A water-soluble lubricant can help.

If you'd rather wait until well after the birth to resume your sex life, that's perfectly normal. Having a sore perineum, a demanding baby, little help, and extreme fatigue can affect your ability to enjoy sex. You may even fear it. Cuddling with your partner and gently enjoying each other's bodies (with or without orgasm) can help you both relax and show your love.

If you find even touching undesirable, express those feelings honestly but respectfully, especially if your partner has an interest in sex. Discuss other ways you can show your love for each other until you're ready to resume a physical relationship.

Whenever you choose to have intercourse, remember that you can become pregnant whether or not you've begun to menstruate. Your caregiver can help you choose a family-planning method. For example, using a condom in combination with spermicidal foam, cream, or jelly is safe and effective contraception soon after the birth. To learn more options, visit http://www.4woman.gov/faq/birth -control-methods.pdf and http://www.plannedparenthood.org/health-topics/birth-control-4211.htm.

If you're breastfeeding, you may leak breast milk during intercourse, especially when you have an orgasm. The hormone oxytocin plays a strong role in both orgasm and milk ejection (let-down). Some women wear a bra and nursing pads when having sex. Others choose to ignore the leaking or find humor in the situation. As one woman said, "When the milk starts flowing, my partner and I know I'm having a good time!"

# ADJUSTING TO PARENTHOOD

Parenting is learned skill; it's not instinctive. Your ability to parent depends on several factors, including how your parents raised you, parenting styles you've seen, experiences you've had with young children; knowledge of the physical, emotional, and intellectual abilities and needs of children; and the temperament and needs of your baby.

Even if you haven't had much experience with babies, your baby is your best teacher. You can learn about her abilities, needs, and development by observing her behavior and responses to your care, reading baby-care books, or attending parenting classes.

The early weeks of parenting aren't always easy, but if you (and your partner) are nurtured and receive help, you'll have the time and energy to care for your baby and build strong family bonds.

# PARENTING WITH A PARTNER

If you're parenting with a partner, you both don't need to do things the same way to appreciate each other as parents. If you have different approaches, discuss your views and arrive at a comfortable solution together so you both feel respected, supported, and involved. Consult with your baby's caregiver, a parent educator, a postpartum doula, or a baby-care book for ideas. Let the small problems go (such as a diaper put on backward) so you can work out the large issues together (such as how to respond to crying). Try not to interfere with each other's parenting or protect each other from the realities of baby care.

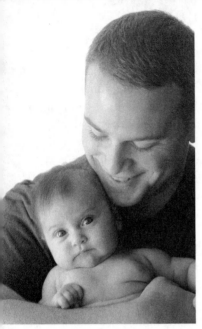

## A NOTE TO FATHERS AND PARTNERS

Once the excitement of having a new baby has faded, your baby's constant demands and frequent crying may begin to tax everyone's endurance. You may feel frustrated that your partner can soothe your baby and meet his needs better than you, especially if she's breastfeeding.

Despite your feelings, your baby and his mother need your continued support and care. By acknowledging that both parents are under a lot of stress and by sharing the parenting duties, you'll strengthen your relationship with your partner and your family.

To learn more about baby care and soothing skills, read Chapters 17 and 18.

## CHANGES IN FAMILY RELATIONSHIPS

The birth of a baby can bring many emotional and social changes to immediate and extended family. Relatives, especially grandparents, are usually eager to be a part of your baby's life. Think about what role they want to play—and the role you want them to play. Then try to discuss ideas and expectations with them before the birth. The sample letter on page 347 may help you express your thoughts.

If you have other children, a new sibling might or might not be a welcome addition. See Chapter 19 for information on preparing an older child for a new baby.

Some new parents find that the demands of baby care challenge their relationship, especially if it was strained before the birth. If your relationship with your partner is troubled after the birth, see page 361 for help.

If you're a single parent, you may want (or need) the help of your family. See page 362 for a discussion on single parenthood.

## RETURNING TO WORK

For some new mothers, returning to work after the birth is necessary because they're the only ones in their families able or available to work. Many other new mothers return to work to contribute to their families' financial well-being or to advance their careers, or because they simply love their jobs. Whatever the reason, if you decide to return to work after the birth, see pages 28 and 362 to learn more information about your options.

# Postpartum Emotional Challenges

After giving birth, your emotions will fluctuate, partly from extreme changes in your hormone levels and partly from fatigue, inexperience or uncertainty with baby care, loneliness or isolation, changes to your normal routine, and your baby's around-the-clock demands. Mood swings may also be caused by a disappointing or difficult birth, an unexpected illness or condition in your baby, a personally stressful situation (social, financial, or physical), or a personal or family history of mood disorders.

For most women, these emotional fluctuations are mild and decrease within a few weeks (see page 348). For others, the mood swings are overwhelming, long-lasting, and may require treatment.

# A Letter to Grandparents

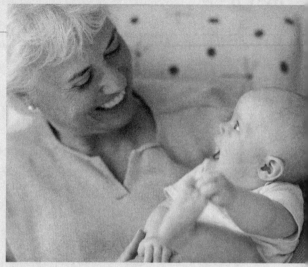

*Although grandparents are the focus of this letter, you can adapt it to suit another family member or friend and to reflect your circumstances.*

Dear Grandparents,

Congratulations on the birth of your new grandchild! This arrival continues your family for another generation. If you're wondering how you can best help the new parents' transition to parenthood, we have some suggestions.

The new parents need to know that you think they're the best parents your grandchild can have. They need to hear that parenthood is challenging, tiring, and one of the most important and rewarding experiences they'll ever have.

You'll find that some things have changed since you raised children, and some have remained the same. You need to honor the new parents' decisions and parenting style, even if their ways differ from your own. Please offer advice only when asked and help the new parents find up-to-date answers to their questions. Reading the same books they're reading about newborn care and feeding may help.

The new parents need to have hands-on experience to learn the skills that all parents need to develop. While it may be tempting to tell them how to do things, or to do things for them, don't interfere. If you're invited to help, recognize the request as an honor. Ask how you can help, and be willing to cook meals, do laundry, shop, and clean the house so the new parents can master caring for their baby. You'll work hard, sleep little, and leave tired—but you'll be appreciated.

If you can't be with the new family or if your relationship with them is strained, think of another way to support them. For example, you can help pay for a postpartum doula, diaper service, meals, or travel expenses for another family member to help them. The new parents will appreciate your gesture, and it can help reconcile a troubled relationship.

Remember your first weeks as new parents and try to have realistic expectations. For example, forgive the new parents if they forget to thank you for your help and gifts. Your care and concern will enhance not only your relationship with your grandchild, but also your relationship with her parents.

With best wishes for joyful grandparenting,

*Penny,* *Janet,* *Ann*

Grandmothers and coauthors of *Pregnancy, Childbirth, and the Newborn*

## BABY BLUES

About 80 percent of new mothers experience *baby blues* (or the "blues"), usually within the first week after the birth. Symptoms of baby blues include the following:

- Crying easily
- Feeling overwhelmed or out of control
- Feeling exhausted, anxious, or sad
- Lacking confidence as a parent

Baby blues are normal and rarely last longer than two weeks. You can diminish the condition by getting more rest, reducing any pain you're experiencing, and surrounding yourself with supportive family and friends. If you're feeling sad or upset, get support immediately. A few encouraging words may be all you need to feel better. Without support, you may have a tougher time shaking baby blues.

## POSTPARTUM MOOD DISORDERS

About 20 percent of new mothers develop postpartum mood disorders (PPMD), which are more serious than baby blues. See Chapter 16 for a complete discussion of PPMD.

# Putting Parenthood into Perspective

Parenting a baby upsets the equilibrium in one's life, and you may wonder how much time you'll spend caring for your child. The following chart illustrates predictable life phases.

You live roughly the first third of your life before becoming a parent. During this time, you develop as an individual and may begin a relationship with someone and consider starting a family with him or her.

You spend the next third of your life having and caring for your children. During this time, many couples are caught up with child care and careers, and they neglect to nurture their relationship. Make time with your partner for conversation and shared activities. Also make time for your own interests so you keep growing as an individual, as well as a parent and partner.

You spend the last third of your life with an "empty nest." Your children are grown and living elsewhere, and you and your partner are once again just a couple. This phase may come with reduced responsibilities or different duties such as caring for your aging parents. You may have time to pursue interests—perhaps grandparenting! One of you will outlive the other at some point, and that person must draw on the support of family and friends, as well as on interests and passions, to find a new way in life.

From the moment your child is born, you'll be a parent for the rest of your life. However, your time spent as a parent of a baby is brief. Enjoy it!

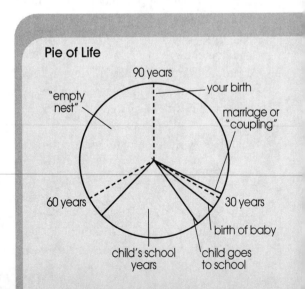

**Pie of Life**

# Key Points to Remember

- The postpartum period is a time of physical and emotional readjustment and recovery. Everyone's adjustment is unique. Factors that arise before, during, and after pregnancy and birth all affect your recovery.

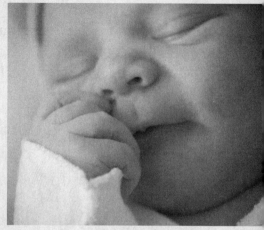

- Your body undergoes many normal changes in the postpartum period. You can help your recovery by eating well, exercising when ready, asking for help when needed, and getting adequate sleep. Be aware of any warning signs that may indicate a problem with your physical or emotional recovery. (See page 337.)

- Transitioning to parenthood can be frustrating and overwhelming at times, but most parents adjust well with help and support.

- Although you'll be a parent for a lifetime, the time you'll spend on baby care is brief.

# CHAPTER 16

# When Post Partum Becomes Complicated

Our culture embraces a joyous picture of new motherhood: A stylish, slender mother tending to her beautiful, chubby baby with minimal signs of stress or fatigue. But this depiction doesn't represent reality. After the birth, many mothers just try to get through the days and nights with a newborn as best as they can. They may need months to become confident, comfortable, and happy with baby care and their new roles as mothers.

For some women and their families, postpartum recovery is more challenging than usual because of a traumatic birth experience, a physical condition that makes recuperation difficult, an emotional complication such as postpartum depression, or a strained relationship. This chapter addresses some of these unexpected and uncommon complications and troubling situations that can challenge the postpartum period. It also offers empathetic advice and solutions so you can learn how to manage these complications and focus on enjoying life with your baby.

# Traumatic Birth Experience

If birth was much worse than you'd expected, you may feel traumatized, sad, angry, and confused. In the weeks and months afterward, as your baby needs less immediate care and you have time to think about your experience, these feelings may intensify.

Ignoring feelings of extreme sadness, fear, loss, or anger won't make them go away. An event such as a new preg-nancy or the birth of a friend's baby can unexpectedly bring up unresolved feelings you may have about your labor, birth, and postpartum experience.

To deal with these feelings, talk with your caregiver (or someone knowledgeable about birth) about your experience to help you understand how events unfolded. You may want to work with a therapist or counselor who can help you acknowledge the unusual difficulty of your experience and find healthy ways to express your feelings and be an advo-cate for yourself, your baby, and your family. For example, if you choose to have another baby, you can work with your caregiver on a plan for having a better birth experience.

# Physical Challenges after the Birth

Physical challenges can prolong postpartum recovery and make it more painful than usual. After giving birth, you may find it difficult to sit, walk, or carry your baby. You may be in constant pain and require frequent medical appointments or even hospitalization. If you're in this condition, you'll need extra help and support from family members, friends, or professionals such as lactation consultants or postpartum doulas. These people can help take care of you, your baby, your family, and your household.

The following sections discuss common physical challenges after birth and comfort measures to help manage them.

## LARGE EPISIOTOMY OR SEVERE PERINEAL TEARING

To reduce the pain from a large episiotomy or severe perineal tearing (laceration), use the comfort measures discussed on page 336 and take any prescribed pain medication. Because constipation is a common side effect of narcotics such as Vicodin, see page 120 for tips to treat constipation. To reduce swelling, lie down as often as possible. If the pain worsens, contact your caregiver to detect problems that need further treatment.

## URINARY INCONTINENCE

For a short time after giving birth, you may have urinary *incontinence*, a condition that causes you to leak urine when you have a full bladder, exercise, cough, or sneeze. Leaking usually stops on its own within weeks of the birth.[1] To treat urinary incontinence, practice your Kegel exercises (see page 95) frequently each day. Use maxi pads or incontinence pads to protect clothing.

Sometimes, leaking happens even without a full bladder or exercise, and it can persist for more than a month or two. This condition is more serious—and often embarrassing and depressing. Talk with your caregiver about treatment options. If necessary, consider asking your caregiver to recommend a physical therapist to evaluate the effectiveness of your Kegels and suggest other exercises and therapies.[2] In rare cases, caregivers recommend surgery if the condition persists for more than a year.

## FECAL INCONTINENCE

After giving birth, you may have fecal incontinence, an embarrassing and upsetting condition that causes you to uncontrollably pass gas or leak stool.[3] The condition may persist for the first few weeks after the birth. (If it persists for more than a month, contact your caregiver.)

To treat fecal incontinence, practice your Kegel exercises. Research shows that Kegels can help a woman regain bowel control.[4] Use incontinence pads to protect clothing. Consult with your caregiver about medications or changes to your diet that can help stop fecal incontinence. On rare occasions, caregivers recommend surgery to correct the problem.

### Advice from the Authors

**Asking for Help**

When asking family members and friends for help during your postpartum recovery, you may find that people are more eager to help if given specific tasks such as cooking meals, shopping, housecleaning, or holding your baby. This way, your loved ones don't have to worry their help is misdirected, unwanted, or duplicated by someone else. Plus, by letting people know what you'd like them to do, you ensure you get the kind of help you need when you need it.

## PERSISTENT HEMORRHOIDS

Pregnancy often causes hemorrhoids (dilated veins in the anus and rectum that can cause pain or itchiness). Most hemorrhoids disappear in the first month following the birth; however, some persist for months.

To help prevent and treat hemorrhoids, follow the recommendations in on page 335. If these measures don't provide adequate relief, consult with your caregiver about any outpatient procedures that may help. In rare circumstances, a caregiver may recommend surgery to correct the problem.

## SEVERE ANEMIA

*Anemia* is a condition in which the number of red blood cells is lower than normal. Many women are mildly anemic during pregnancy and after the birth, but 2 to 4 percent of women become severely anemic from postpartum hemorrhage. Anemia is also a risk factor for developing postpartum depression (see page 357).[5]

Symptoms of anemia include weakness, lightheadedness, shortness of breath, and overwhelming fatigue. A caregiver can diagnose anemia by analyzing a blood sample.

To treat anemia, caregivers advise women to take an iron supplement and eat iron-rich foods. (Visit our web site, http://www.PCNGuide.com, for more information on iron-rich foods.). Caregivers rarely order a blood transfusion to treat anemia unless the blood loss is life threatening.

If you have severe anemia, you'll need extra help with baby care and housework. When getting up from sitting or lying down, move slowly. Have someone accompany you to the bathtub or shower to prevent falling if you become lightheaded.

## LATE POSTPARTUM HEMORRHAGE

Late postpartum hemorrhage is a large loss of blood occurring between twenty-four hours to six weeks after the birth. Infection or retained fragments of the placenta usually cause the bleeding, which occurs in 1 percent of women. If a woman loses a significantly large amount of blood, she may develop anemia (see page 353).

To treat late postpartum hemorrhage, a caregiver removes the fragments of placenta using medications or a D&C (see page 128), or treats a uterine infection with antibiotics.

## BACK AND HIP PAIN

After giving birth, many women experience pain in the lower back or pelvic region. Sometimes, the pain results after a woman twists or overstretches her lower back or pelvic and hip joints while she's numb from epidural or spinal anesthesia. This pain may last for the first few days or weeks after the birth, and many caregivers recommend ibuprofen for relief. If you develop this pain and it interferes with your ability to walk or roll over, ask your caregiver to refer you to a physical therapist.

If you injured or broke your tailbone (coccyx) before the birth, your baby's passage through your pelvis may flex or even re-break your tailbone, causing pain and bruising. Even if you didn't injure or break your tailbone before birth, it may break or become injured during birth if your baby is large. The tailbone will reset itself, but it may take weeks to months. Taking ibuprofen, applying heat or cold packs, and sitting on a firm surface can help relieve pain.

Sometimes in pregnancy or during birth, the pubic joint in the front of the pelvis (pubic symphysis) widens or separates, causing some women to experience mild to debilitating pain in the pubic region after giving birth. Because pubic pain isn't well documented, caregivers may underestimate the severity of the condition or even dismiss it as normal pain that will disappear with time.

To treat pubic pain, avoid lifting objects and making movements that cause pain, such as stair climbing, vacuuming, and spreading your legs or knees wide apart. Use a walker or a sturdy baby stroller if walking is especially painful. Working with a physical therapist can speed recovery.

## NUMBNESS AND PAIN IN YOUR HANDS

After birth, you may experience numbness, tingling, weakness, or pain in your hands and wrists. These symptoms may stem from the swelling around the nerves in your wrists (for example, carpal tunnel syndrome), caused by extra fluid your body retained in pregnancy. After the birth, the swelling diminishes as the fluid level naturally decreases over time; however, until it does, repetitive activities—such as holding, lifting, and carrying your baby—can exacerbate these symptoms.

To treat numbness and pain, try to keep your wrists in a neutral position (not bent or curled) when handling or feeding your baby. Consider buying wrist splints if keeping your wrists in a neutral position is difficult. If symptoms don't improve, ask your caregiver to refer you to a physical therapist or hand specialist for ultrasonic therapy, custom splinting, exercises, or corticosteroid treatments.

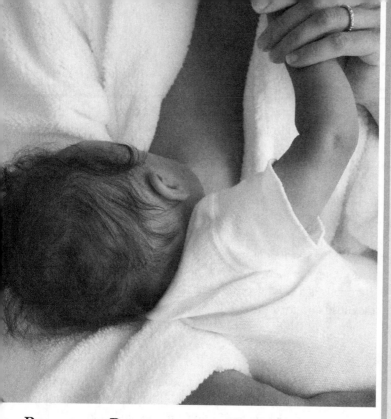

## PERSISTENT BREASTFEEDING PROBLEMS

In the first weeks after the birth, most breastfeeding women experience sore nipples and breast fullness. But some women have intense breastfeeding challenges that continue for weeks or months. If you find breastfeeding to be an ongoing painful, time-consuming challenge and you dread the next feeding, you may feel angry, sad, or even depressed because your breastfeeding experience isn't what you expected.

If breastfeeding problems make you think about quitting breastfeeding, contact a lactation consultant or other breastfeeding expert for support, information, suggestions, and tips. These professionals can tell you whether and how soon the problem can be fixed, and they can help you adjust your approach to nursing if necessary. If the problem requires medical attention, they can refer you to a physician who specializes in breastfeeding medicine, dermatology, or infectious disease. Some communities offer support groups for women with breastfeeding challenges.

Despite having excellent support and a commitment to breastfeeding, some women have problems that don't improve, causing exhaustion and despair. These women realize that stopping breastfeeding is the only solution—one that may cause great sadness or great relief. If you're in this position, a lactation consultant or your caregiver can help you sort out your feelings with the decision, acknowledge the hard work you put into breastfeeding, and show you how to feed your baby with formula. If you have strong negative feelings about your breastfeeding experience, consider talking to a counselor to help you come to terms with your decision.

For more information on breastfeeding challenges, see pages 419–424 and pages 428–434.

# THYROID PROBLEMS

Three to eight months after giving birth, 5 to 7 percent of women develop postpartum thyroiditis, a two-phase condition in which the thyroid gland first becomes inflamed and overactive (hyperthyroidism) and then returns to normal function or becomes underactive (hypothyroidism).

Symptoms of hyperthyroidism typically last a short time and include feeling overheated, muscle weakness, shakiness, anxiety, rapid heart rate, inability to concentrate, and weight loss. The thyroid may recover completely from hyperthyroidism, but if the inflammation damaged the gland, it may then become underactive.

Symptoms of hypothyroidism include tiredness, constipation, memory loss, intolerance of cold, muscle cramps, weakness, weight gain, and inadequate breast milk production. Hypothyroidism may disappear and the thyroid function may return to normal. If the gland remains underactive, caregivers typically prescribe thyroid hormone replacement medication.

If you experience these symptoms, don't ignore them or blame them on sleep deprivation. Instead, call your caregiver. Because thyroiditis is a risk factor for developing postpartum depression (see page 357), it's important to diagnose and treat the condition or rule it out as the cause of your symptoms.

# GALLBLADDER PROBLEMS

The gallbladder is a small organ that receives bile from the liver and concentrates it before sending it to the digestive tract to aid with fat digestion. Pregnancy hormones slightly increase the risk of developing gallstones, caused by a slowdown in the passage of bile from the gallbladder. When the stones leave the gallbladder, they may clog the bile duct and cause sharp and extreme pain.

Symptoms of gallstones include nausea, vomiting, abdominal bloating, burping, gas, indigestion, and steady, increasing pain in the upper abdomen, under the right shoulder, or between the shoulder blades. The pain often occurs after eating fatty foods or at night and lasts thirty minutes to several hours. If you experience sweating, chills, fever, yellow skin, or clay-colored bowel movements, see your caregiver immediately. The treatment for gallbladder problems is laparoscopic surgery.

# POSTPARTUM HIGH BLOOD PRESSURE (HYPERTENSION)

Hypertensive disorders (high blood pressure) affect 6 to 8 percent pregnancies in the United States.[6] For most women with gestational hypertension (see page 140), blood pressure returns to normal after the birth. Some women, however, continue to have high blood pressure, and a few women develop the condition after the birth.

Little information exists on preventing or treating postpartum hypertension,[7] but complementary medical approaches (such as acupuncture, meditation, and yoga) may help augment traditional medical therapies.

If you develop postpartum hypertension, your blood pressure will most likely return to normal, but it may remain a continuing health concern. To monitor your blood pressure and find an effective medication for treatment, you'll need to see your caregiver frequently. While these appointments can complicate postpartum life, they're necessary to ensure your health. If breastfeeding, ask your caregiver or a lactation consultant if a blood pressure medication is safe for nursing.

# Emotional and Mental Health Challenges

*Postpartum mood disorders (PPMD)* include the emotional conditions that can develop in the first year after giving birth, such as anxiety and panic disorder, obsessive-compulsive disorder, postpartum depression, bipolar disorder, and post-traumatic stress disorder. About 20 percent of women will develop one of these conditions or a combination of them after giving birth.

PPMD are more serious than "baby blues" (see page 348) and can complicate the postpartum period significantly. They can be emotionally paralyzing and cause feelings of hopelessness and isolation. In addition, our culture finds PPMD shameful, which may lead affected new mothers to hide their symptoms and not seek the help they need and deserve.

The following sections describe PPMD and their risk factors. As you read about the conditions, know that the severity of the symptoms varies among women.

## POSTPARTUM ANXIETY AND PANIC DISORDER

About 10 percent of women have postpartum anxiety and panic attacks; however, those women with a history of anxiety and panic disorder have an increased risk of developing the condition after giving birth. Symptoms include shortness of breath, sensations of choking, lightheadedness, faintness, rapid heart rate, chest pain, nausea, and diarrhea. If you develop this disorder, an overwhelming fear of being alone, dying (you or your baby), or leaving your home may immobilize you.

## POSTPARTUM OBSESSIVE-COMPULSIVE DISORDER (OCD)

About 3 to 5 percent of women develop postpartum OCD, a condition characterized by obsessive (uncontrollable) thoughts and compulsive rituals to protect the baby. All mothers typically have instincts to protect their babies, but these instincts are extreme in women with postpartum OCD. Examples of obsessive thoughts include a fear of being a "bad" mother, of hurting the baby, or of germs. Compulsive rituals can include constant hand washing (hundreds of times each day), frequent housecleaning, excessively checking on the baby, or constantly ensuring that doors are locked. Not surprisingly, these rituals interfere with normal daily living.

## POSTPARTUM DEPRESSION

*Postpartum depression* occurs in 10 to 20 percent of new mothers. For a woman with a history of depression, the risk of developing the condition increases to 30 percent. For a woman with past postpartum depression, the risk increases to 70 percent.[8]

Postpartum depression generally occurs between two weeks to one year after the birth, although the onset typically begins between the sixth week and the sixth month. Symptoms vary in severity among women and include the following:

- Feelings of hopelessness, despair, and exhaustion
- Feelings of extreme inadequacy and low self-esteem
- Lack of energy
- Loss of interest in everything
- Inability to sleep, even when an opportunity arises
- Overeating or forgetting to eat
- Constant crying
- Surprising and frightening outbursts of anger at loved ones
- Recurring thoughts about hurting oneself (even committing suicide) or the baby

## BIPOLAR DISORDER OR MANIC DEPRESSION

Bipolar disorder (BD) occurs in 2 percent of the population. A woman diagnosed with BD before pregnancy will likely relapse if not treated during pregnancy and the postpartum period.

BD usually begins with extreme mood elevation, energy, and grandiose thoughts within a few days to weeks after the birth. A long-term period of depression may follow. Suicide is a risk during both mania and depression. A woman with BD needs the care of a psychiatrist or therapist with expertise in treating the condition.

## POSTPARTUM POST-TRAUMATIC STRESS DISORDER

After the birth, post-traumatic stress disorder (PTSD) may result from a difficult or frightening birth or from traumatic situations such as an unexpected illness, sudden problems for the baby, or insensitive or hurtful care. PTSD can also occur when birth triggers memories of a traumatic event such as a frightening hospital experience, physical or sexual abuse, or rape.

Common symptoms of PTSD include preoccupation with the trauma, flashbacks to the event or recurrent nightmares (both possibly accompanied by anxiety and panic attacks), anger or rage, and extreme protectiveness of oneself or the baby.

## RISK FACTORS FOR PPMD

While no one can predict who will have PPMD, the following factors increase your risk of developing one of the conditions:

**History of mental health challenges**

- Panic disorder, OCD, depression, or BD (or history of these challenges in an immediate family member)
- Physical, emotional, or sexual abuse
- Eating disorders
- Substance abuse (or living with someone who's abusing drugs or alcohol)

**Challenges with menstruation, pregnancy, birth, or your baby**

- History of severe premenstrual symptoms
- History of infertility or miscarriages
- Unplanned and unwanted pregnancy
- Traumatic pregnancy or birth
- High-needs baby or a baby with a chronic medical condition
- Feeding problems with your baby

**Temperament**

- Low self-esteem
- High expectations to be perfect and in control

## Myths and Facts about PPMD

**Myth:** All women feel sad, anxious, or angry after giving birth. The feelings will go away if I just "tough it out" or ignore or deny them.

**Fact:** Acknowledging how you feel and getting help will speed your recovery.

**Myth:** Having PPMD means I'm a weak person.

**Fact:** Strong, intelligent women have PPMD. You didn't cause the condition by anything you did.

**Myth:** Having PPMD means I'm a "bad" mother.

**Fact:** Many women with PPMD think only "bad" mothers ever get angry or have thoughts about hurting themselves or their babies. It may help you to know that these thoughts don't make a mother "bad." All mothers do the best they can, and women with PPMD who recognize that these thoughts are harmful don't act on them.

**Myth:** If I take medication for PPMD, I can't breastfeed.

**Fact:** Medications that are compatible with breastfeeding exist. Check with your caregiver or therapist.

### Recent stressful life events

- Death in the family
- Moving to a new home
- Changing jobs or losing a job
- Getting married, separating, or divorcing
- Financial pressures
- Excessive sleep deprivation

### Lack of support

- Unsupportive partner or no partner
- Unsupportive friends or family
- Poor or absent relationship with your mother

### Health issues

- Thyroid disease
- Anemia[9]

### Inflammation

Research shows that inflammation and a lack of omega-3 fatty acids in a woman's diet are major risk factors for PPMD (as well as for depression in the general population).

Consuming too many omega-6 fatty acids (found in vegetable oils and many processed foods) can cause inflammation. Late pregnancy and postpartum stressors (such as sleep deprivation, major life stress, and pain) also raise inflammation levels.

Consuming omega-3 fatty acids (found in fish, flax meal, and other foods and supplements) can lower high levels of inflammation and prevent or treat postpartum depression and possibly other PPMD.[10] For more information on omega-3 fatty acids, see page 114.

# TREATING PPMD

If you have any of the risk factors for PPMD (see page 358), arrange for professional help before the birth so you can report any symptoms quickly and begin treatment. Early treatment can shorten the duration of PPMD.

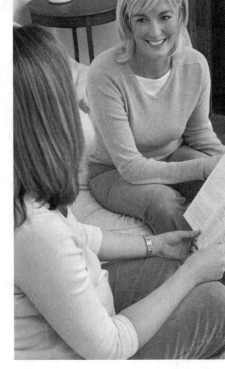

Appropriate treatment for PPMD depends on the severity of the symptoms and may include therapy, medications, and lifestyle changes such as the following suggestions:

- Eat well.
- Avoid alcohol, caffeine, and over-the-counter sleep medications.
- Exercise regularly.
- Get information about PPMD and their treatments.
- Get enough sunlight or use a light box to decrease the risk of developing seasonal affective disorder (SAD).
- Take time for yourself each day—even if it's just for five minutes.
- Get adequate rest and sleep.
- Get enough omega-3 fatty acids to reduce inflammation. (See page 359.)

Other treatment options include the following:

- Attend a PPMD support group, which helps women and their families understand the conditions, recognize the causes, and learn about resources for support. Your caregiver, childbirth educator, local hospital, or health department can refer you to a support group in your area. You can also contact Postpartum Support International by phone (800-944-4773) or by visiting their web site at http://postpartum.net.
- Get counseling or therapy. Choose a therapist or psychiatrist who specializes in PPMD.
- Take prescribed medication for anxiety, OCD, depression, and bipolar disorder.
- Get counseling along with taking medication (which can help with a more rapid recovery than taking medication without counseling).

## A Note to Fathers, Partners, and Relatives

PPMD can affect the whole family. Women with PPMD often worry about their ability to be physically and emotionally available to their babies. You may worry, too.

To help a mother with PPMD, encourage her to get treatment, provide support and care, gather information on interacting with a newborn, help with housework, and find ways to ensure she gets rest and sleep.

Getting enough sleep may be the most important step to recovery, but it can also be the most challenging. Help with nighttime feeding and parenting so the mother gets two or more three- to four-hour stretches of sleep each night. Consider getting support from other family members, a postpartum doula (see page 27), or mother/baby support groups.

## POSTPARTUM PSYCHOSIS

*Postpartum psychosis* is a rare condition that's more serious than PPMD. It occurs soon after birth in about .01 percent of women. Symptoms include severe agitation, mood swings, depression, and delusions. Women with postpartum psychosis need immediate care and psychiatric treatment. Hospitalization is often necessary at the onset of the condition, at which time women take medications to treat symptoms. Once home, women continue taking medications (monitored by a psychiatrist) and receive ongoing psychotherapy.

# Social and Relationship Challenges

The postpartum period can become more challenging than usual if there are problems in your relationship with your partner or if the relationship is abusive. You may also feel stress if you feel your partner isn't taking on a fair share of the parenting and housekeeping tasks.

If you're a single parent, or if you need to return to work early or to a hostile or unsupportive workplace, you may have additional stress.

The following sections discuss these challenges and suggest ways to manage them.

## YOUR RELATIONSHIP WITH YOUR PARTNER

Research finds that many spouses (especially women) become less satisfied with their marriages after the birth of their first babies.[11] Caring for a newborn disrupts family life and can cause chaos and confusion until the family establishes new comfortable patterns.

New parenthood can leave little time to nurture a couple's relationship. If a new mother believes her partner isn't as supportive as she expected, or if the couple's lifestyles and activities grow apart after becoming parents, the relationship can become strained.[12] Relationship problems may also arise if relatives are intrusive or unsupportive, or if the baby is high-needs or has serious medical needs.

How can relationships survive the strain of new parenthood? Having a good relationship before the birth best predicts that a couple will have continued satisfaction with the relationship after the birth. Also, if both parents wanted to have the baby, they're more likely to be happy with their relationship than if one of them had reservations about adding to the family.[13]

## Two Views on Relationships after the Birth

I had an unexpected, frightening, and very premature birth. My son spent a month in the neonatal intensive care unit and another month in the special care nursery. Because my marriage was strong, my husband and I together faced the fears and challenges of having a baby born so early. It did take months for us to feel safe taking our son out in public, but now he's almost a year old, and we see he's a strong and hearty boy. I'm grateful my husband and I had each other to lean on during that first tough year.
—*Morgan*

The birth of our son was a frightening time. I worried that I might lose both my wife and my child. Over the next months, I came to be in awe of both my wife's and son's resilience. Yes, there were some tough days and weeks, but we just took one day at a time. Now we have a sturdy one-year-old, and we are talking about having another baby.
—*James*

If your relationship with your partner becomes strained after the birth, improving matters will usually require a joint effort. First, you and your partner need to agree that a problem exists. Second, you need to agree to get the counseling that's critical to the relationship's survival and to your baby's healthy development. (If one of you refuses to get help, the other will still benefit from counseling.)

Professionals and resources that can help your relationship include marriage or couples counselors, religious counselors with professional expertise in helping families, or courses designed to provide practical, researched-based strategies for building strong relationships between couples, such as Becoming Parents Program, Inc. (http://www.becomingparents.com) and Bringing Baby Home (http://www.bbhonline.org).

## ABUSE AND DOMESTIC VIOLENCE

Abuse and domestic violence (any combination of verbal, psychological, emotional, sexual, economic, or physical abuse) affect rural and urban women of all ages, physical abilities, and lifestyles and of all religious, ethnic, socioeconomic, and educational backgrounds. The only risk factor for abuse and domestic violence is being a woman,[14] and the risk increases during pregnancy and especially after the birth.[15]

If you're in an abusive relationship, you are *not* at fault. The goal of abuse is to leave you feeling confused, ashamed, powerless, hopeless, and out of control. National and local agencies can help you and your children. Memorize the phone number for the National Domestic Violence Hotline, 800-799-SAFE (7233), and call if you need to talk to someone or need resources, including help making an escape plan for you and your children.

## SINGLE PARENTHOOD

About 30 percent of new mothers are single parents, some by choice and others by circumstance. For some single mothers, money is tight, and they need to find affordable child care and return to work soon after the birth. Others have jobs that pay well and provide excellent maternity leave benefits. For still others, the father may provide financial support or family members may provide a home and help with child care.

If you're a single mother, you'll need support as you recover from the birth and gain confidence as a parent. New parenthood can be socially isolating, especially if there aren't adults to talk to in the days following the birth. Organizations and networks exist that provide single mothers with opportunities to talk with one another. Visit http://www.singlemothers.org or http://www.singlemothersbychoice.com to learn more information.

## RETURNING TO WORK

By three months after giving birth, 60 percent of employed, first-time mothers in the United States return to work.[16] During pregnancy, a three-month leave from work after the birth may seem reasonable; however, by the third postpartum month, new mothers are just getting to know their babies and establishing a relationship with them. Many women dread having to leave their babies in someone else's care, especially when no other options are available.

In addition to finding suitable and affordable child care, mothers need to figure out how to get their babies to and from the care location. Breastfeeding mothers must also determine how much milk to pump and store. If either the mother or baby has health complications or feeding difficulties, or if the mother has PPMD (see page 357) or a stressful or unsupportive job, returning to work can be even more challenging. Once back at work, many mothers worry how sleep deprivation will affect their ability to function.

If your child-care options are unacceptable or your work situation is unbearable, try to negotiate with your employer for a delayed return to work, work shorter or flexible hours, or work part-time or from home. If these options aren't possible, you and your family will need to ask yourselves some tough questions: Should you quit your job? Should you try to find another job? Can your family's budget function without your income? How much energy do you want to devote to improving your workplace's attitude toward new parents and families? See page 28 for information to help you answer these questions.

If you want to help improve maternity and family benefits in the United States, support political action groups such as MomsRising (http://www.momsrising.org), whose efforts seek to change public policy on maternity and family leave and other benefits for mothers and families.

## Key Points to Remember

- For some women and families, physical, emotional, or social challenges can complicate the postpartum period and prolong recovery and adjustment to life with a newborn.
- Acknowledging the difficult circumstances of your postpartum period and seeking help are essential for recovery.
- If your pregnancy has been complicated or if you anticipate problems during birth or afterward, find supportive resources and explore options before the birth to reduce further postpartum complications and provide help if necessary.

# CHAPTER 17

# Caring for Your Baby

After months of waiting, meeting your newborn can be an overwhelmingly emotional experience. You rejoice at finally being able to hold your baby in your arms, but you may begin to worry how best to keep her happy and healthy. You realize there's so much to learn about your baby and how to care for her.

This chapter describes general baby care (such as diapering, bathing, and calming your baby, and where and how to put her to sleep) as well as your baby's abilities and communication skills. It also covers medical care, including newborn warning signs that indicate when you need to seek medical help, and discusses care for babies with special needs. With this information—along with time, practice, and guidance—your ability to care for your baby will soon become second nature.

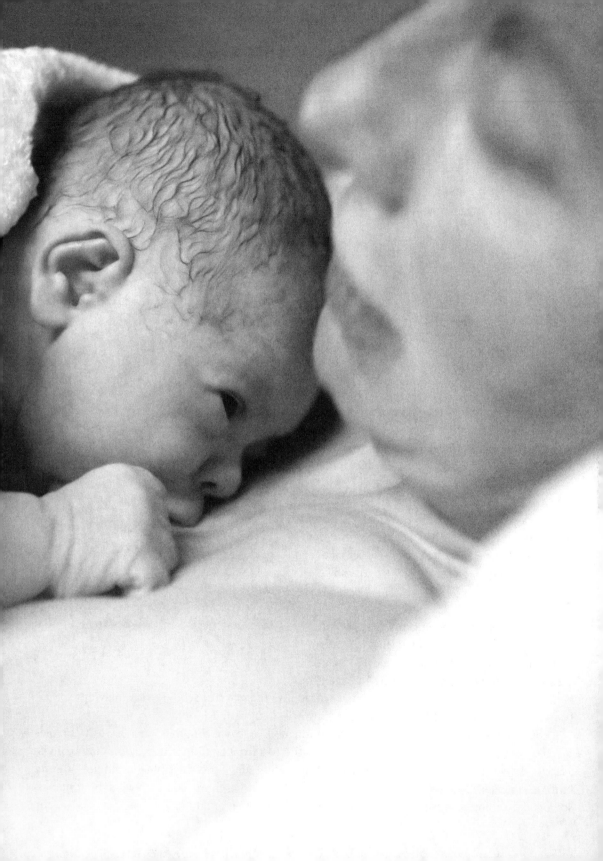

# Meeting Your Baby

If you and your baby are doing well immediately after the birth, the best place for him is on your bare chest, with just a blanket covering you both. This skin-to-skin contact allows the two of you to bond and gives you a chance to discover all the things that make your baby unique. These first few moments together also provide you with some wonderful memories. The following sections describe what you can expect as you get to know your newborn.

*Note:* In some circumstances, additional time is necessary for mothers and babies to get acquainted. If you had a long and tiring labor, your recovery may delay the enjoyment of meeting your newborn. If your baby has trouble adjusting to life outside your womb, he may need to be separated from you so medical staff can care for him.

## YOUR NEWBORN'S APPEARANCE

When you first meet your newborn, her appearance may surprise you, especially upon seeing the large size and unexpected shape of her head, her tiny hands and feet, her enlarged reddened genitals, her initial dusky blue coloring, and her little body streaked with blood and vernix caseosa (creamy white substance that protected her skin). These features can make a strong first impression, but they're completely normal. You'll probably find that you can't take your eyes off your new baby.

### Body

The average full-term baby weighs 7 to 7½ pounds and measures about 20 inches in length. A newborn's shoulders and hips are narrow, his belly is round, and his arms and legs are relatively short, thin, and flexed.

### Head

Your baby's head is large in proportion to her body. Her head may be molded (that is, appear cone-shaped or longer than expected) from pressures within your pelvis during birth. Her

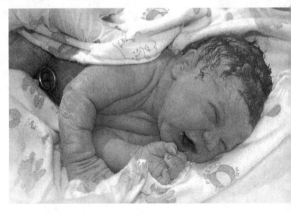

head will return to a normal round shape within a few days. Her scalp or face may appear bruised and swollen, but bruising and swelling will disappear with time.

Your baby's skull has two soft spots called fontanels (areas where the bones haven't completely fused). A large, diamond-shaped fontanel is on the top front portion of her skull, and a smaller, triangle-shaped one is at the back. The larger fontanel usually closes by eighteen months after the birth; the smaller one closes by two to six months. A thick, tough membrane covers the fontanels, so gently brushing or washing your baby's hair and scalp won't hurt her.

## Hair

At birth, your baby may have a full head of hair or be nearly bald. You may also notice lanugo (fine, downy body hair) on your baby's back, shoulders, forehead, ears, and face—especially if he's premature. Lanugo usually disappears during the first few weeks after the birth.

## Eyes

Fair-skinned babies usually have gray-blue eyes at birth; dark-skinned babies have brown or dark gray eyes. If your baby's eye color is going to change, it usually does so by the time she's six months old. Her tear glands won't produce many tears until she's about a month old.

## Sucking Callus (Blister)

Intense sucking often causes a painless white callus on the center of a baby's upper lip. Sometimes the callus peels. It doesn't need treatment and gradually disappears as the lip toughens.

## Skin

At birth, your baby's skin is dusky blue, wet, and streaked with blood and varying amounts of *vernix caseosa*, the white creamy substance that protected your baby's skin before birth. Within a minute or two after your newborn begins breathing well, his skin color changes to normal tones, beginning with his face and trunk and soon reaching his fingers and toes. The vernix often remains in skin creases even after bathing. Gently rub it into your baby's skin; there's no need to remove it.

A fair-skinned newborn baby often looks blotchy. After a few weeks, his skin has a more even color, although it may appear blotchy when he's cold.

Also common on a fair-skinned baby's skin are stork bites and angel kisses, red areas formed by a collection of tiny blood vessels near the skin's surface. They often appear on the baby's eyelids, nose, forehead, or back of the neck. Most aren't caused by injury and usually fade or disappear within six to nine months; however, some (especially those on the neck) may be permanent.

Mongolian spots (areas of dark pigmentation) commonly appear on the lower back and buttocks and occasionally on the thighs or arms of some babies, usually of Native American, Asian, African, or southern European descent. Although the spots are black and blue, they're not bruises. They gradually fade and usually disappear by the time the child is four years old. If your baby has Mongolian spots, make sure those who care for him know that the marks aren't bruises.

Many babies have peeling skin, particularly at the wrists, hands, ankles, and feet. Babies born after their due dates peel more than babies born at term. The peeling is normal and doesn't usually require treatment. If cracks on the wrists or ankles bleed, apply skin ointment such as A&D ointment (available at pharmacies).

## Breasts

During pregnancy, your hormones may have caused your baby's breasts to swell. Some babies (male and female) leak milk from their nipples. Both swelling and leaking is normal and doesn't require treatment. Don't try to express milk from your baby's nipples; doing so may cause infection. The condition typically disappears within a week or two after the birth.

## Genitals

Your hormones during pregnancy also may have caused your baby's genitals to swell. If your baby is a boy, he may have an unusually large, red scrotum. If your baby is a girl, she may have milky or bloody vaginal discharge called a "pseudo menstrual period." This discharge indicates that her uterus has had a healthy response to your hormones and is now shedding its first lining. The conditions for both sexes are normal, temporary, and don't require treatment.

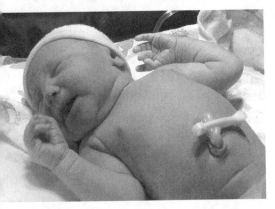

## Umbilical Cord

Immediately after your newborn's umbilical cord is cut, it's bluish-white and 1 to 2 inches long. To stop the bleeding, your caregiver applies a plastic cord clamp or tie umbilical tape around the cord. The cord clamp is removed when the cord is dry, usually before your discharge from the hospital or within twenty-four to forty-eight hours after the birth. The tape doesn't have to be removed. Usually within one to two weeks after the birth, your baby's umbilical cord will fall off.

## YOUR NEWBORN'S REFLEXES

When you observe your newborn, you may notice that loud noises, bright lights, or quick movements startle her or make her fling her arms and legs out and straighten her body, especially when she's on her back. This physical response (called the "Moro reflex") is one of the normal early reflexes that indicate good neurological health.

Another early reflex is when your newborn firmly grasps your finger when you place it on her palm. (Reflex or not, this action is simply wonderful!) The stepping (or automatic walking) reflex occurs when your baby alternately moves each foot when she's held upright and her feet bear weight. Your baby's sucking and swallowing reflexes let her eagerly suckle milk from your breast or a bottle nipple. She also may suckle your breast or suck on her fingers or yours to soothe herself. Your newborn responds to a touch on her cheek or lips by turning toward it and opening her mouth wide. This rooting reflex is especially pronounced when she's hungry.

Your baby's caregiver checks these reflexes in the newborn exam (see page 369). As your baby matures, many of these early reflexes will disappear.

Whether awake or asleep, your baby may yawn, quiver, hiccup, stretch, or cry without apparent reason. Many of these behaviors are reflexive and beyond your baby's control. Hiccups are especially common soon after feeding and don't require treatment.

Some reflexes are protective. Your baby coughs to help move mucus or fluid from her airway. She sneezes when she needs to clear her nose or when it's irritated, or when a bright light shines in her eyes. She blinks if something touches her eyelashes, and she pulls away from a painful stimulus such as a blood draw from her heel. If lying on her stomach, she lifts her head and turns it to the side to avoid being smothered. If something is placed over her nose and mouth, she twists away from it, mouths it vigorously, or attempts to knock it away with her arms.

## YOUR NEWBORN'S BREATHING PATTERN

You may notice that your baby breathes more rapidly than you do (between thirty and sixty times per minute). You also may notice that he has periods of irregular breathing, which can be worrisome but is normal. When your baby sleeps, he may snort, squeak, pant, groan, and even occasionally pause his breathing. These irregularities usually disappear a month or two after the birth, when you'll notice that his breathing is more regular.

If you're worried whether your baby's breathing patterns are normal, observe him as he sleeps. If you see the irregularities described in the previous paragraph, don't be concerned. However, if you observe signs of respiratory distress (such as blue lips, a struggle to breathe, flared nostrils, or a deep indentation of the chest with each breath), call your baby's caregiver immediately.

## YOUR NEWBORN'S BOWEL MOVEMENTS

Your baby's first bowel movements (*meconium*) will be a sticky, green-black substance that was in her intestines before birth. By two to three days after the birth, she'll produce brown, brown-green, or brown-yellow stools that are the consistency of cake batter. After your milk has come in (by three to four days after the birth), your baby will produce yellow, green, or brown stools that are mostly watery but may be curd-like.

The frequency and consistency of bowel movements depend on the baby and on the food she eats. Breastfed newborns typically poop after each feeding, or produce at least two large runny stools each day after their mothers' milk has come in. Formula-fed babies poop frequently in the first several days after the birth. When they're a week old, they may produce one to two putty-like stools each day.

# What Happens after the Birth

If you give birth at a hospital, your baby will typically stay in your room ("room-in"), and you and your family will provide basic baby care, including diaper changes. This arrangement allows you to get acquainted with your baby and discover questions you may have about his care. Your nurses, caregiver, and other hospital staff can help you find answers.

If you give birth at a birth center, you'll probably go home three to six hours after the birth. If you give birth at home, your caregiver will likely leave three to six hours after the birth. At either birthplace, your caregiver can answer any questions you may have about newborn care. You may also consult with a doula, lactation consultant, or your childbirth educator.

Regardless of where you give birth, your caregiver will likely evaluate your newborn soon after the birth. The following sections describe common tests and procedures including circumcision, a procedure to consider if you have a baby boy (see page 372).

## NEWBORN TESTS AND PROCEDURES

The table on pages 370–371 describes common tests and procedures that evaluate your baby's health and ensure she remains healthy. They're part of routine newborn care, and many are required by state or province government. Find out which tests and procedures your state or province mandates by contacting its public health department. You also may ask whether you can request further tests or procedures, or can decline some routine ones.

If you give birth at a birth center or at home, talk with your midwife about when and where she'll offer these tests and procedures.

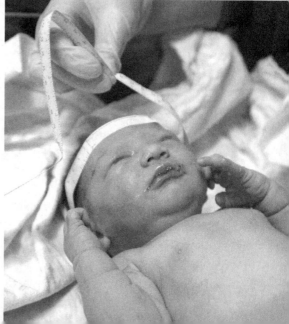

## Newborn Tests and Procedures

Protocols for tests and procedures vary somewhat among caregivers. Ask your caregiver which tests are routinely performed at your birthplace and which are used only if medically indicated. You can find further information about these procedures on our web site, http://www.PCNGuide.com.

| Test or Procedure | What It Is | Comments |
|---|---|---|
| Apgar score | Immediately after the birth, your caregiver will evaluate your baby's well-being by a quick assessment of key factors. | See page 266 for a full discussion on this routine assessment. |
| Infant vital signs | Your caregiver or nurse assesses your baby's temperature, heart rate, and respiration to ensure she's adjusting well, to detect any problems with her heart or lungs, or to determine whether she needs to be warmed. | A normal heart rate for infants is 90 to 160 beats per minute; normal respiration is 30 to 60 breaths per minute. Your baby should appear pink and breathe easily (that is, without grunting, flared nostrils, or a deep indentation of her chest with each breath). If there's a concern, your baby's caregiver will assess her or admit her to the hospital nursery. Normal axillary (underarm) temperature of newborns is between 97.4°F (36.3°C) and 99.5°F (37.5°C). If your baby has a fever, she'll be admitted to the nursery and may have a septic workup and antibiotics. If she's too cool, she'll be placed on your bare chest and covered with warmed blankets, or placed under a special warming light in your room or in the nursery. |
| Vitamin K | Vitamin K is injected into your baby's thigh soon after the birth to enhance blood clotting and possibly prevent a bleeding disorder.[1, 2] | Breastfed babies are slower to produce adequate amounts of vitamin K than formula-fed babies. Formula contains small amounts of vitamin K.[3-5] |
| Newborn eye care or prophylaxis | Erythromycin or tetracycline ointment (or, rarely, silver nitrate drops) is placed in your baby's eyes within an hour after the birth to prevent infection and possible blindness if she was exposed to gonorrhea or chlamydia in the birth canal.[6] | All treatments can cause temporary blurring of vision. In the first hour after the birth, your baby is very alert and wants to gaze at you. Wait until after that hour before giving treatment. Eye prophylaxis can't prevent all possible eye infections caused by viruses or bacteria other than chlamydia and gonorrhea. |
| Septic workup (only when medically indicated) | Your baby's blood is drawn and cerebrospinal fluid may be obtained by spinal tap; samples are sent to a laboratory to be tested for bacteria. Results are available in 48 hours. | If infection is suspected, your baby will be admitted to the nursery for intravenous (IV) antibiotics. If tests results are normal, antibiotics will be discontinued. If tests show the presence of bacteria, your baby will stay in the nursery for a full course of antibiotics. |
| Test for jaundice (used only when there are concerns) | Your baby's blood is drawn from her heel and is sent to a laboratory, where the bilirubin level is determined. Sometimes, a jaundice meter is used to estimate bilirubin levels by flashing a light onto your baby's forehead. | If your baby's skin and the whites of her eyes are yellowish, an elevated bilirubin level is suspected. Most jaundice is mild and disappears with little or no treatment. (See page 389 for more information on jaundice.) |

| Test or Procedure | What It Is | Comments |
|---|---|---|
| Hepatitis B vaccination | Your baby is given an injection (shot) to immunize her against hepatitis B, a blood-borne viral infection that can lead to liver infection, cirrhosis, or liver cancer. | Side effects are rare, other than localized pain and tenderness at the injection site. Some parents choose to delay vaccination to avoid stressing the newborn. Others question the need for a baby to receive this vaccine unless the mother is carrying the virus, since a baby is highly unlikely to get hepatitis B from the usual modes of transmission (IV drug use or sexual encounters). See pages 386–388 for more information on vaccinations. |
| Test for hypoglycemia (low blood sugar) | Your baby's blood is drawn from her heel to test for hypoglycemia. | Hypoglycemia is most common in babies that weigh more than 8 pounds 13 ounces or less than 5 pounds at birth, or in babies who had preterm or postterm births. It also can occur in babies who are cold or whose mothers are diabetic or received large amounts of IV fluids with dextrose during labor. Hypoglycemia can lead to respiratory distress, lethargy, slow heart rate, seizures, and (rarely) death. Treatment includes frequent breastfeeding or formula feeding. In more serious cases, the baby may be given IV dextrose. |
| Infant security | All hospitals should have policies to prevent kidnapping and to ensure all babies are properly identified, which can safeguard against accidentally switching infants. | All babies should be given wrist and ankle bands at birth that match their mothers'. All staff caring for babies should wear easy-to-read identification badges, and the hospital should have a written plan that details how it'll respond if an infant is missing (a very rare situation). Having your baby in your room and never leaving her unattended are the best ways to keep your baby safe. |
| Newborn hearing screening | Your baby's caregiver will assess her hearing in the first days after the birth using a device for about 10 minutes while she's sleeping. | Caregivers typically test the hearing of newborns who are born prematurely, who have a family history of hearing deficits or deafness, or who have been exposed to pathogens or medications that put them at risk for hearing loss. However, health care professionals are considering universal screening because 50 percent of babies with hearing deficits have no known risk factors. |
| Newborn screening[7] | Your baby's blood is drawn from her heel before she's a week old. (If the first sample was collected within the first 24 hours of birth, a second specimen is collected before she's 2 weeks old.)[9] The blood is then screened for various rare conditions. | Although screening detects rare conditions that most babies don't have, affected babies greatly benefit from early diagnosis and treatment. These conditions include sickle cell anemia, beta thalassemia, phenylketonuria (PKU), hypothyroidism,[8] and galactosemia. The American College of Medical Genetics recommends that caregivers screen newborns for twenty-nine conditions; however, states and provinces vary widely in the number of conditions that they screen. Visit http://www.marchofdimes.com for more information about these conditions and tests. |

# CIRCUMCISION

*Circumcision* is the surgical removal of the foreskin covering the glans (tip) of the penis. It may be the oldest-known surgery (dating back around six thousand years) and is done worldwide for social, cultural, religious, and medical reasons. It's performed in hospitals and clinics, and at ceremonial sites.

Some communities practice circumcision more often than others. For example, the Jewish and Islamic communities use circumcision as a religious ritual. It's a common procedure in North America, Africa, and the Middle East; however, it's uncommon in Latin America, South America, Europe, Australia, and the Far East.

The benefits and risks of circumcision are debatable among health care professionals. Parents of baby boys will need to gather information on the subject (preferably during pregnancy) so they can make an informed decision about whether to give their written consent to have their sons circumcised.

The following sections provide facts about circumcision, as well as information about the procedure and aftercare.

## Facts about Circumcision

Think about the following facts carefully as you consider circumcision. Consult with your baby's caregiver to learn more about the benefits and risks of the procedure.

- There are few medical reasons for circumcision. Social or religious factors may guide your choice.
- The American Academy of Pediatrics (AAP) says circumcision has potential medical benefits as well as risks, and parents should be well informed before making the decision.[10]
- The procedure usually takes less than thirty minutes. Healing takes seven to ten days.
- A newborn will feel the pain caused by the procedure.
- Health care providers recommend an injection of local anesthesia to reduce the pain of circumcision.[11] Complications from anesthesia are rare and include bruising at the injection site. Applying local anesthetic creams to the penis an hour or so before the procedure may decrease pain, although less effectively than an injection of anesthesia.[12] Sucking on a special pacifier that delivers a small amount of sugar water during the procedure also may reduce pain.
- Out of 1,000 newborn circumcisions, 2 to 6 will develop minor to serious complications, including irritation of the glans from rubbing against wet diapers, painful urination, bleeding, infection, and scarring of the urinary outlet (where urine exits the penis).
- Health insurance might not cover the caregiver's fee for doing the procedure or the hospital's or clinic's fee for using its equipment.
- Some studies find a connection between an intact (uncircumcised) penis and urinary tract infection (UTI) in the first year of life; however, the risk of infection is low (about 1 percent).[13] Exclusive breastfeeding can significantly reduce the risk of UTIs (by 300 percent).[14]
- Contrary to previous reports, no evidence suggests that circumcision prevents cancer of the prostate gland or certain sexually transmitted infections (STIs). International studies do link circumcision with a reduced risk of human immunodeficiency virus (HIV) infection; however, the U.S. Centers for Disease Control and Prevention (CDC) doesn't recommend circumcision to prevent HIV, citing that circumcision itself carries risks and provides only partial protection. They recommend other proven prevention measures such as correct condom use.[15]
- Opinions differ about whether newborn circumcision affects adult sexual performance. Some experts say it does, while others argue it doesn't.
- In 2003, 56 percent of boys in the United States were circumcised. (In some regions, rates were as low as 31 percent.) By 2009, the rate dropped to 32.5 percent nationwide.[16]

## The Circumcision Procedure

If you decide to have your baby boy circumcised, talk with his caregiver about the potential risks and benefits of the procedure, including the use of anesthesia.

Before the procedure, you need to sign a consent form. Then your baby is placed on his back in a special plastic bed, with Velcro straps holding his body and limbs firmly in place. He then receives anesthesia. After it has taken effect, his penis is washed with an antiseptic. A sterile sheet with a hole in the center (to reveal the penis) is placed over his trunk. The foreskin is separated from the glans and removed by one of three instruments: Gomco clamp, Plastibell device, or Mogen clamp. Circumcision takes about five minutes, and you may be allowed to stay with your son during the procedure.

## Care of the Circumcised Penis

After the circumcision, ask your baby's caregiver or the medical staff how to care for your son's penis. If a Mogen clamp or Gomco clamp was used to remove your baby's foreskin, he'll usually have Vaseline-covered gauze applied to the circumcision site for twenty-four hours, at which time the gauze typically falls off. Watch for bleeding, inability to urinate, or swelling; if you observe any of these signs, call your baby's caregiver. If the gauze doesn't fall off after twenty-four hours, wrap the area in a warm, moist washcloth or give your baby a bath. Once the gauze is soaked, gently remove it. (If you can't, call your baby's caregiver.) Once the gauze is removed, apply an ointment, such as A&D ointment, or diaper cream on your baby's diaper where it touches his penis to prevent irritation at the circumcision site.

If a Plastibell device was used to remove your baby's foreskin, a small plastic ring will remain on his penis, with a suture thread tying the foreskin tightly to the device. The device and foreskin usually fall off seven to ten days after the circumcision. Do not pull the ring off; let it fall off on its own. At the circumcision site, you may see small yellow or white patches of normal, healing tissue. Report any swelling, bleeding, inability to urinate, or pus-like discharge to your baby's caregiver.

## Care of the Intact (Uncircumcised) Penis

If you decide against circumcision, know that a newborn's intact foreskin doesn't usually retract (pull back) but instead adheres to the glans. Don't force back your baby's foreskin to clean the glans. Regular bathing will keep the area sufficiently clean. The foreskin will gradually loosen as your son matures. Most boys' foreskins are fully retractable when they're between four and eight years old. Once your son's foreskin can be easily retracted, the glans can be cleaned with just soap and water.

# Caring for Your Baby at Home

If you give birth in a hospital or birth center, you may feel both excitement and anxiety when heading home with your newborn. If you give birth at home, your caregiver's departure after the birth may cause the same feelings. Once the anticipation of the birth is over, many new parents suddenly realize that they're responsible for this tiny person, and they wonder whether they're up to the challenge.

Caring for a baby becomes easier with practice. During the first days and weeks after the birth, you'll begin to master diapering, bathing, dressing, and comforting your baby. To learn about these tasks, try to take a newborn care class before the birth. If that's not possible, ask whether the hospital

## Two Views about Leaving the Hospital

The hospital stay was very pleasant. I didn't want to leave! I enjoyed getting spoiled with attention, and I was nervous to be on my own with a newborn.
—*Michelle*

Leaving the hospital felt like such a big, momentous event. Then we arrived home, and that was really exciting for the first few minutes. Then we sat down, looked at each other, and said, "Okay, now what?" We realized that we had to figure out what this parenting thing was all about.
—*Alice*

or birth center offers a "crash course" that you can take before you're discharged. If you give birth at home, ask your caregiver about baby care during your last prenatal appointments or before she leaves after the birth. You may also consider hiring a postpartum doula to help you with baby care (see page 27).

The following sections are an introduction to the basics of baby care.

## CAR SAFETY

It's the law in the United States and Canada that every baby traveling in a vehicle must be restrained in a car seat that meets current federal safety standards. If you give birth in a hospital or birth center, before you're discharged you'll need to have a car seat that's the right size for your newborn correctly installed in your vehicle, according to the manufacturer's instructions. For the latest information on car seats, visit the American Academy of Pediatrics' web site, http://www.aap.org/family/carseatguide.htm, or visit http://www.saferchild.org/carseat.htm.

If your baby is premature or weighs 5½ pounds or less before discharge, the hospital or birth center staff will place your baby in the car seat for an hour to assess her ability to breathe adequately. If your baby can't breathe well at any point during the hour, the staff will remove her from the car seat and provide a special car bed to ensure safe transport.

## DIAPERING YOUR BABY

Today's parents have several options to manage their babies' waste, from cloth diapers to disposable diapers to no diapers at all.

**Cloth diapers** have come a long way since diaper pins were used to fasten them. The design of most cloth diapers is similar to that of disposable brands, with Velcro tabs and elastic around the leg holes. Cloth diapers are usually used with a diaper wrap or plastic pants to prevent leaks. You can use a baby diaper service (if available in your area) to provide clean diapers and take away used ones. Or you can buy cloth diapers and launder them at home.

**Pocket diapers** have a diaper wrap on the outside and a fleece liner on the inside, which can keep your baby dry and reduce diaper rash. You can fill the pocket between the inner and outer layers with a cloth diaper, hemp, or other material that can be more absorbent than a cloth diaper. Launder pocket diapers at home according to the manufacturer's directions.

**Disposable diapers** come in various sizes and styles. Although they may be more convenient than other diapering options, they also may be more expensive. You'll need to properly dispose used diapers according to the directions on the package.

**Ecologically friendly disposable diapers and biodegradable diapers** can be composted if wet with only urine. With some brands, a portion of the diaper can be flushed if it's poopy (check manufacturer's instructions).

To learn how to diaper your baby and figure out the size and quantity of diapers you'll need, ask your childbirth educator, nurse, or parent educator. You can also ask the staff at a specialty baby store or diaper service, or any experienced parent. You may also find helpful information online by using the search terms *diaper choices* to find web sites that review cloth diapers and disposable diapers.

Some parents use a diaper-free method called **elimination communication (EC)** and avoid using diapers entirely or part of the time. EC is a common practice worldwide, where access to diapers and the ability to launder them is limited or unavailable. This method requires paying close attention to a baby's cues to urinate or have a bowel movement, but it eliminates or reduces the cost of diapers and is ecologically friendly. Parents practicing EC dress their babies with the diaper area open and unrestricted. When they observe their babies' cues to urinate or have a bowel movement, they hold their babies over a sink or special potty. Some parents begin practicing EC soon after birth; others wait until their babies are older. Some use this method around the clock; others only during the day or while at home.

## Common Q & A

**Q:** My son's diapers are always leaking. Is the kind of diaper I'm using to blame? Or is there another reason?

**A:** The cause for the leaking may well be a matter of positioning. Try pointing your baby's penis down as you diaper him. That way, the urine will be directed toward the most absorbent part of the diaper.

## Diaper Rash

If the skin on your baby's diaper area becomes irritated, he may have diaper rash. Many substances can cause diaper rash, including urine and stool, some laundry detergents, or chemicals used in some disposable diapers. Diaper rash also can appear if you inadequately launder your baby's cloth diapers.

To prevent or treat diaper rash, change your baby's diapers frequently and rinse his skin with water at each change. Before putting on a new diaper, wait a few minutes to allow your baby's clean bare skin to air-dry (or blow-dry the diaper area with a hair dryer set on low or no heat).

If using cloth diapers, run them through an extra rinse cycle to reduce irritation from detergents, or use a milder detergent. To reduce the amount of ammonia (from urine) that stays in cloth diapers even after laundering, add a ½ cup of vinegar to the diaper pail or to the rinse cycle. Because plastic pants can trap moisture and cause irritation, you may need to switch to a different type of diaper cover.

If these treatments don't work, you also may consider applying a diaper rash cream to the irritated area after you clean and dry it. To choose a cream that's safe and effective, visit http://www.cosmeticsdatabase.com. If the diaper rash persists, consult your baby's caregiver.

## Constipation

Constipation is the production of small, hard, dry stools that can be painful to pass. The condition is more common in formula-fed babies than in breastfed babies, because formula is harder to digest than breast milk.

If you're breastfeeding your baby, about a month after the birth you may notice that she has begun pooping only once a day or even once a week. This change doesn't indicate constipation. Instead, it shows that her digestive system has begun to efficiently use more of your milk. If you're still concerned, call her caregiver.

## *Diarrhea and Vomiting*

Diarrhea (frequent, watery bowel movements) and vomiting are serious conditions for babies because they can cause dehydration quickly. Formula-fed babies experience diarrhea and vomiting much more often than exclusively breastfed babies, probably because formula is harder to digest than breast milk and also may be exposed to more contaminants.

Symptoms of diarrhea include more frequent stools that may smell foul, look bloody, or contain mucus. An affected baby may appear ill, weak, or listless. If you see any of these signs, call your baby's caregiver for advice.

## BABY CLOTHES AND EQUIPMENT

As you prepare for your baby's arrival, you may wonder if you need all the items available in baby stores and departments. See page 160 for a list of typical baby clothing and equipment. After reviewing your options, choose the items that appeal to you and are appropriate for your family.

## BATHING YOUR BABY

Newborns need bathing only once or twice a week.[17] You can bathe your newborn with a wet soft cloth, but a tub bath may be a more enjoyable experience for you both. Babies stay warmer and calmer when immersed in warm water than when given a sponge bath. The warm water also may soothe fussy babies, and it won't increase the risk of infection in the cord or a newly circumcised penis.

To give your baby a tub bath, fill a sink or baby bathtub with comfortably warm water. Hold your baby securely with his head resting in the crook of your arm or the bend of your wrist, with your hand gently grasping his arm. Lower him into the water so it covers his body, but not his head and neck. With your free hand, use only water to clean his eyes and face. Next, wash his hair with mild soap, massaging his head with your fingers or a soft brush. Wash his body with water or with a mild baby soap. Let your baby enjoy the warmth of the water. When the bath is done, make sure his skin and hair are completely dry before dressing him.

Many parents enjoy bathing with their babies as a way to relax together. To bathe with your baby, fill the bathtub with comfortably warm water. Get into the tub first and have someone hand you your baby. If no one is available, line your baby's car seat with a towel (to keep him warm and the car seat dry if you return him there after the bath), set him in it next to the tub, then pick him up once you're in the water. Lay him on his back on your thighs so the water covers his body but not his neck and head. Enjoy relaxing in the water together. Wash his body with water or with a mild baby soap. When you're done bathing your baby, hand him to someone who can wrap him in a warm towel or place him back in his towel-lined car seat.

# CORD CARE

Many different rituals and treatments have been used to promote the separation of the umbilical cord from a baby's abdomen while preventing infection. However, researchers have studied only a few for their effectiveness.

One such study compares two treatments: cleaning the cord with rubbing alcohol at each diaper change or letting the cord dry naturally. While the results show that infection didn't develop from either treatment, the cord that dried naturally separated a day earlier than the cord treated with rubbing alcohol.[18] These findings suggest that the best cord care requires minimal intervention.

To care for your baby's cord, follow these recommendations:

- Wash your hands before touching the cord.
- Use baby soap (or no soap) to bathe your baby, to maintain the acid pH of her skin that helps reduce bacteria growth.
- To keep the cord dry and clean, fasten your baby's diaper, diaper wrap, and plastic pants below the cord.
- If the cord is soiled, gently clean it with warm water and let it dry thoroughly.
- If the cord area is red, emits a foul odor, oozes pus, or bleeds bright red blood in a spot larger than a quarter, call your baby's caregiver. (*Note:* When the cord falls off, some dark brownish-red blood or clear yellow sticky fluid at the separation site is normal.)
- If your baby leaves the hospital with a cord clamp attached, have her caregiver or the hospital staff remove it at a later date. (Or you can remove it if given clear instructions from a medical professional.) Do not cut off the cord clamp.

# Your Baby's Communication

Although your baby can't talk, he can communicate his needs, likes, and dislikes through *infant cues*. Your baby may let you know he's hungry by rooting, sticking out his tongue, being wakeful, or sucking on his hand. He may yawn and half-close his eyes to tell you he's sleepy.

If you don't respond to your baby's early cues, he may begin to fuss and cry to let you know he's hungry, lonely, uncomfortable, or overstimulated. By the time you see this late cue, it may take longer to satisfy his needs because you must first calm him. For example, feeding your baby is harder if you wait until he cries than if you respond to his early feeding cues. (See Chapter 18.)

As you get to know your baby, you'll be better able to interpret the cues described in the following sections.

## ENGAGEMENT CUES

When your baby is calm, quiet, and alert, she has subtle ways to get your attention and keep it. Her body relaxes, her eyes brighten and open wide, and she stares at you intently. If you ignore these engagement cues or look away, she may vocalize or move her arms to catch your attention. When you return her gaze, a quiet exchange begins as she explores your face. When she needs a brief rest to process what she has seen, she may turn or look away until she's ready to return her gaze to you.

During these exchanges with your baby, be sensitive to her needs by returning her gaze when she wants your attention and by letting her rest without coaxing her to look at you.

From birth your baby can imitate some of your facial expressions. For example, shape your mouth into an O and hold the expression for ten seconds where your baby can clearly see you; repeat this action several times. If your baby is quiet and alert, she'll shape her mouth into an O.

You can also do this exercise when sticking out your tongue or lower lip; your baby will mimic these expressions as well.

When your baby is around six weeks old, she'll begin to smile and coo to initiate an exchange and in response to your smile. (These endearing interactions make many parents fall deeper in love with their babies!)

Your baby can best teach you what calms or agitates her. When your responses to soothe your baby are effective, she becomes calmer and less fussy, and she relaxes into your body as you hold her. If your responses overstimulate her, she may stiffen, arch her back, or spread her fingers wide as if trying to push something away. If you miss these disengagement cues, she may cry loudly.

To help you learn more about your baby's cues and abilities, consider taking a parent-infant class or consulting with your baby's caregiver or nurse, your childbirth educator, or other experienced parents.

# CRYING

Contrary to traditional thought, you won't "spoil" your baby by responding whenever he cries. When your baby cries, he's not manipulating you for your attention; he simply has no other way to tell you he needs something. Crying is often your baby's last attempt to communicate that he's hungry, overstimulated, tired, or uncomfortable. He may cry because he has gas and needs to be burped. He may cry because he has a wet or dirty diaper (especially if he's feeling cold), a diaper rash, or sore circumcision site. He may cry if he's ill or simply because he wants to be held and rocked.

Responding to your baby's crying helps develop his trust in your ability to meet his needs. Try to respond before he becomes so upset that he can't calm himself easily. Your baby will become more agitated if you are upset, so try to stay as calm as possible by talking quietly to him and moving slowly and calmly around him.

Soothing your baby is easier if you know why he's crying. But occasionally, you might not immediately know the reason for his distress, which can naturally be frustrating. In those cases, try comforting him with any of the following calming techniques. Give each one several minutes to work before trying another, and be careful not to overstimulate your baby.

- Try feeding your baby first. Some babies need to nurse frequently before taking a longer (more than one hour) rest between feedings.
- Take a bath with your baby. The warm water may calm him, and he may even breastfeed.
- Give your baby a gentle massage.
- Take your baby for a walk in a baby carrier or stroller.
- Try the Five S's (see page 379).

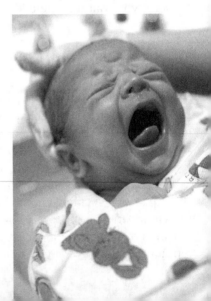

If nothing seems to calm your baby and you find yourself losing your temper, put him safely in his bed or car seat and take a short break. If after five to ten minutes your baby is still agitated and you still feel angry and frustrated, never shake or roughly handle him, no matter how upset you are. Instead, call your partner, a relative, a friend, or a neighbor to help you.

Although at first you may have trouble figuring out exactly why your baby is crying, let your instincts and feelings guide you. You'll become more comfortable in your ability to calm your baby with time, practice, and advice from your baby's caregiver, a supportive relative or friend, or a new-parent group.

# The Five S's

Dr. Harvey Karp suggests calming babies using a five-step method called the Five S's. This method provides babies with a familiar and comforting womb-like environment. Some babies need all five steps, while others are calmed by just a few.[19]

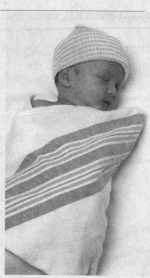

**Swaddling**

Swaddling increases how long your baby sleeps by preventing her from startling herself awake.[20] You can swaddle your baby in a large, lightweight blanket; a commercial swaddling blanket; or sleep sack with her arms tucked inside. Your nurse, midwife, or doula can show you how to swaddle your baby, or there are many commercial swaddling products on the market. (For example, Dr. Karp offers an instructional DVD.) You can also provide a swaddle-like environment by tucking your baby snugly inside a baby carrier, sling, swing, or bouncy seat. Visit our web site, http://www.PCNGuide.com, to learn an effective double swaddle technique.

**Side or stomach position**

Hold your baby in your arms on her side (which may aid digestion) or on her stomach with gentle pressure against her abdomen. Being held on her back may cause her to startle easily.

**Shushing**

Make a shushing sound near your baby's ear or use white noise (continuous noise such as a fan or radio static) loudly enough so she can hear it over her crying.

**Swinging**

Repetitive motion such as swinging helps soothe babies. Swing your baby by swaying, rocking, jiggling, or gently bouncing with her on an exercise ball. You also can gently swing her from side to side in a hammock made by holding two corners of a blanket while someone else holds the other two corners. To give yourself a chance to eat or rest, consider using a baby swing.

**Sucking**

Let your baby suck on a pacifier or your finger. Feeding her can also calm her; however, you'll have likely already tried this as a calming technique, because hunger is a typical reason for crying.

## Colic or Fussy Periods

When babies are between three and twelve weeks old, most have predictable fussiness in the evening and early night (a time some parents call "fuss and feed"). In the past, this fussy period was called *colic*, defined as three or more crying episodes each week for three or more weeks, with each episode lasting three hours or longer.[21]

Dr. T. Berry Brazelton, an expert in infant development, states that this fussy period is a normal "touchpoint" or parenting challenge.[22] His research reveals that an overload of stimuli (such as bright lights, loud noises, and feelings of hunger) throughout the day causes the predictable fussiness. As the day progresses, the baby's immature nervous system begins to cycle into shorter sleep periods, more frequent feeding, and more fussiness.[23] At the end of the fussy period, babies usually settle into their longest stretch of sleep that may last three hours or longer.

If your baby is fussy or colicky, use the suggestions on page 378 to calm him. Because overstimulation often causes excessive crying, use a calming technique consistently for several minutes before trying something new. Remember that the calmer you are, the easier it is for your baby to settle down.

Although all babies have gas, if your fussy baby seems especially gassy, use comfort holds that provide pressure against his abdomen, such as those illustrated at right, to help alleviate the pressure. You may have heard the suggestion to

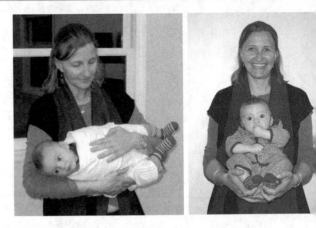

give your baby simethicone (Mylicon) drops; however, research hasn't found them to treat gas any more effectively than a placebo.[24] Some parents give their babies "gripe water" to alleviate gas. This supplement generally contains potentially gas-reducing ingredients such as fennel, spearmint, and ginger.

Parents sometimes mistake colicky symptoms for those of gastroesophageal reflux (GER or reflux). With this condition, some of the acidic stomach contents flow up into the esophagus, making the tissue inflamed and painful. Babies with GER often arch and stiffen during feedings, may spit up or cough, may have sour breath, and are especially uncomfortable when placed on their backs. The difference between colic and GER is that reflux symptoms are constant during the day and night. Also, GER can be treated with medication and by positioning the baby upright after feedings and for sleep.

If your baby is constantly crying in addition to vomiting, spitting up, or having a cold, a fever, or constipation, consult with his caregiver.

Fussy periods can be stressful to new parents, and you may want to ask your baby's caregiver, other parents of colicky babies, or members of a parent-baby support group for advice on soothing your baby and coping with the stress. If you're spending several hours each day soothing your baby, take a break now and then. Let a trusted person relieve you so you can take a walk. Or take your baby on a walk with another new parent and baby. As with most parenting challenges, these fussy periods will end with time, your growing confidence as a parent, and your baby's increasing maturity.

# Your Baby's Sleeping and Waking Patterns

After a period of wakefulness after the birth, many babies sleep for much of the first day. They rouse only briefly and might not be interested in feeding. Other babies, however, are awake, fussy, and feed frequently during the first day.

After babies have adjusted to their new environment, they sleep twelve to eighteen hours in a 24-hour period, typically in short but frequent intervals. As long as a baby feeds well and is growing well, how long she sleeps at any one time isn't a concern.

When your baby is older, she may awaken at night to feed and then fall back to sleep. If your baby awakens because she's hungry, she'll root, suck on anything close by, and wave her arms and legs vigorously. If you don't respond to these early feeding cues, she'll cry. For more information on feeding your baby, see Chapter 18.

# SLEEP LOCATION

Upon first learning they're pregnant, many expectant parents plan on creating a separate nursery filled with adorable decorations and a lovely crib. However, experts recommend that babies sleep in the same room as their parents in the early months to reduce the risk of sudden infant death syndrome or SIDS (see page 391).

Some parents choose to have their baby sleep in a cosleeper or in a basket, bassinet, or crib near their bed. This placement allows parents to quickly respond to the baby's needs and to comfort him with the sounds of their breathing.

Other parents find they get more sleep if they tuck their baby in bed with them. Because a newborn has long wakeful periods at night just as he did while in the womb, where he was snug and warm, he may sleep better with his parents in their bed than by himself in another location. Many families put their babies in a crib, bassinet, or cosleeper at the beginning of the night, and then move them into their bed as morning approaches to get a few more hours of sleep.

As your baby grows older and needs you less at night, you can move him to a crib or his own bed in your room or another room. Or he can continue sleeping in your bed with you. It's your decision.

Wherever your baby sleeps, you need to place him in a safe space and position him on his back on a firm surface to reduce the risk of SIDS. See page 392 for more information on safe sleeping spaces.

# YOUR BABY'S SLEEP-ACTIVITY STATES

Experts have identified six sleep-activity states that babies experience: deep sleep, light sleep, drowsiness, quiet alert, active alert, and crying. While each state has specific characteristics, the way that babies change from state to state varies. Some babies move gradually from one state to another, while others make abrupt transitions. Some spend more time asleep or in a quiet-alert state than others; some spend more time crying. Your baby's temperament affects his states; you can't control them.

Identifying the following states in your baby will help you give him appropriate care.

## Sleep States

In **deep sleep** your baby is still and relaxed; her breathing is rhythmic. She occasionally jerks or makes sucking movements, but rarely awakens. She doesn't need anything from you at this time, so use it as an opportunity to rest and take care of yourself.

**Light sleep** is the most common sleep state in newborns. Your baby's eyes are closed, but they may move behind her eyelids. She moves, makes momentary mewing or crying sounds, sucks, grimaces, or smiles. She breathes irregularly. She responds to noises and efforts to arouse or stimulate her. When your baby moves and makes sounds, wait a few moments to see if she's awakening to a drowsy state and needs care, or if she's falling back to deep sleep.

## Awake States

When your baby is **drowsy,** he appears sleepy, his activity level varies, and he may yawn or startle occasionally. His heavy-lidded eyes, which open and close for brief periods, lose focus or appear cross-eyed. He breathes irregularly and slowly reacts to sensory stimuli. If you hope he'll fall asleep, try shushing or patting him to help him settle down. If you hope he'll awaken, try picking him up, singing to him, or dancing with him.

## Tummy Time

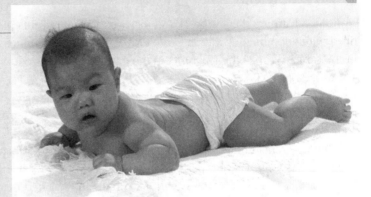

Because babies need to sleep on their backs and spend time in car seats and swings, the back of their heads can become flattened from contact with a firm surface. To prevent your baby from developing a misshapen head and to give her an opportunity to lift her head and strengthen her neck muscles, frequently place her on her tummy when she's awake for as long as she's happy in that position. Also limit the amount of time your baby spends in car seats and other baby equipment that put pressure on the back of her head. Many babies fuss when they're first learning to lie on their tummies. Over time, they'll tolerate tummy time and eventually will begin to enjoy longer sessions. Here are ways to provide supervised tummy time:

- Lay your baby across your lap.
- Lay your baby on the floor with a nursing pillow supporting her chest.
- Lay your baby on an exercise ball, hold her steady, and roll the ball gently forward and back.
- Hold your baby tummy-side-down while practicing postpartum exercises. (See page 343.)

In addition, holding your baby upright in your arms or in a baby carrier (such as a Moby Wrap or ERGObaby carrier) will provide tummy-time benefits.[25]

**Quiet alert** is the most pleasing and rewarding state for parents. Your baby lies still and looks at you calmly with bright, wide eyes. He breathes with regularity and focuses attentively on what he sees and hears. By providing him something to look at, listen to, or suck on, you encourage him to spend longer times in this state. (See pages 385–386 for information on playing with your baby.)

**Active alert** is the state that indicates your baby is starting to need something, although he might not know what it is yet. He can't lie still; he may be fussy. His eyes are open but not as bright and attentive as when he's in a quiet-alert state. He breathes irregularly and makes faces. Hunger, fatigue, noises, and too much stimulation readily affect your baby and may lead to fussing or crying.

When your baby reaches this state, try to determine what he needs. If he shows feeding cues, feed him. If he looks away, he probably needs less stimulation. If you act immediately, you may bring him to a calmer state before he begins to cry.

**Crying** is your baby's last attempt to tell you he can't cope any longer. If he's hungry, overstimulated, tired, sick, gassy, frustrated, wet, cold, hot, or lonely, he may have first tried communicating with subtle cues. If his needs continue to go unmet, he communicates his distress by crying. In this state, he also moves his body actively, opens or closes his eyes, makes unhappy faces, and breathes irregularly. Sometimes, crying is a way to let himself enter another state. More often, however, he needs you to feed or comfort him.

## RECORDING YOUR BABY'S SLEEPING AND ACTIVITY PATTERNS

At times, your baby's apparently inconsistent sleeping and activity patterns may puzzle you. However, by charting your baby's feeding, sleeping, quiet-alert, and crying or fussing periods for a week, you can see when and how long your baby typically sleeps, is awake and content, or cries. You may notice that she has a fussy period at a certain time. Or you may learn that she takes a long nap at roughly the same time every day.

After charting for a week, you may discover that your baby's sleeping and activity patterns are somewhat consistent. As your baby matures, the patterns will continue to change. Visit our web site, http://www.PCNGuide.com, for a sample chart that you can use to record your baby's patterns.

# Your Baby's Growth and Development

Your baby has a unique appearance, temperament, and personality. His activity level and sleeping and eating patterns differ from those of all other babies, as do his responses to pain, hunger, or boredom.

Some babies are easy to care for; others are more difficult. For example, you may need additional patience and flexibility if your baby reacts to stimuli intensely, adapts to changes in his environment slowly, has a high activity level, and has mostly unpredictable feeding, sleeping, and activity patterns. As you get to know your baby's temperament, you'll learn to care for him in an effective and satisfying way.

Although your baby's temperament will probably change little over time, his abilities will quickly change. Because normal development patterns vary widely from one baby to the next, don't worry if your baby develops later or earlier than another baby. If, however, you notice that your baby misses some developmental milestones (see below) or is consistently older than the approximate age when he reaches a milestone, consult with his caregiver. Early detection and treatment may improve your baby's long-term development.

## Developmental Milestones

Here's a list of developmental behaviors or characteristics and the age when your baby is most likely to begin showing them. If your baby was premature, these milestones may occur somewhat later.

| Behavior or Characteristic | Approximate Age |
| --- | --- |
| Looks or stares at your face for short periods | Birth to 4 weeks |
| Holds up his head for a few moments while lying on his stomach | Birth to 4 weeks |
| Pays attention to sound by becoming alert or by turning toward it | Birth to 6 weeks |
| Smiles or coos when you smile, talk, or play with him | 3 weeks to 2 months |
| Lifts head and shoulders while lying on his stomach | 2 to 3 months |
| Holds his head steady when upright | 2 to 3 months |
| Brings his hands to his mouth | 3 months |
| Laughs and squeals | 6 weeks to 4½ months |
| Rolls over from front to back or back to front | 2 months to 6 months |
| Grasps a rattle placed in his hand | 3 to 4½ months |

# YOUR NEWBORN'S SENSES

While getting to know your baby over the first weeks after the birth, you may wonder what she can see, hear, and taste. For years, experts underestimated a newborn's abilities. At one time, it was believed that a newborn responded only to a wet diaper, hunger, or gas. It also was thought that a newborn couldn't see at birth; when she finally could see, she could do so only in black and white. These beliefs, however, are incorrect.

After years of study, experts now know that newborns have amazing capabilities, some of which are described in the following sections.[26]

## Vision

When your newborn is quiet and alert, he can focus on objects 7 to 18 inches away. His vision at birth is about 20/200 and will be about 20/20 by six months.[27] He prefers to look at human faces (especially eyes), round shapes, high contrast of dark and light colors, complex patterns, and slowly moving objects—especially shiny ones. He may be sensitive to bright lights and will open his eyes wider when the lights are dimmed. His eyes might cross or might not seem to focus. As his eye muscles strengthen and mature, his eyes will track together.

## Hearing

Your baby heard your heartbeat, your voice, your partner's voice, and other internal and external noises while inside you. After she's born, she responds to voices, especially higher pitched voices (this is why people unconsciously raise their voices' pitch when talking to babies). She may become calm or alert when she hears familiar voices or sounds, or when she hears white noise (such as a dishwasher or a washing machine) or familiar music. She also startles at sudden, loud noises.

## Smell

Your baby has a refined sense of smell. Within the first week after the birth, he recognizes differences in smells and can even tell the difference between the smell of your milk and another mother's milk. In fact, the smell of your milk when you hold him may excite him to root and suckle.

## Taste

Your baby can taste things that are sweet, sour, salty, or bitter; however, she prefers sweet tastes. When offered something that's bitter, salty, or sour, she turns away.

## Touch

Your baby enjoys being stroked, rocked, caressed, gently jiggled or bounced, and allowed to nestle into your body while being held. He also likes warmth. Infant massage is a great way to touch your baby (see page 385).

# INFANT MASSAGE

Infant massage is an excellent way to calm and soothe your baby and to communicate your love and care. Many communities offer infant massage classes, or you can follow these instructions to give your baby a massage:

1.  Give your baby a bath. Then, after making sure the room is comfortably warm, remove the towel or receiving blanket and lay your baby on her back on the floor and kneel in front of her, or lay her on her back on your lap.
2.  Put a little vegetable oil or olive oil on your palm, then rub your hands together to warm them. (Don't use baby lotion or oil. Baby lotion will soak into her skin too quickly, and baby oil and other petroleum products aren't healthy for babies.)
3.  When you begin touching your baby, keep at least one hand on her until the massage is over. Massage her arms, legs, and other areas that she enjoys having touched. Use as much pressure as she finds pleasurable. Tell your baby what you're doing, or sing a song. Don't massage your baby's belly if her stomach is full, and stop the massage if she's not enjoying herself.
4.  If she's enjoying the massage (and she probably is), here are some motions to try:
    *   Stroking with open palms
    *   Stroking with thumbs or fingers
    *   "Raking" with fingertips
    *   Tapping lightly with fingertips
    *   Massaging your baby's arms or legs with a gentle wringing motion
    *   Doing whatever makes your baby happy

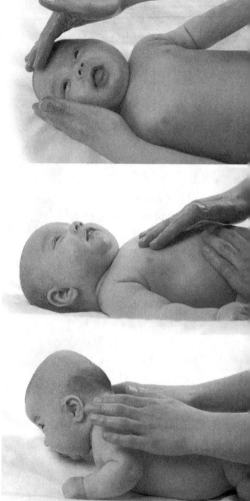

# PLAYING WITH YOUR BABY

For you, play is a way to have fun and perhaps get some exercise. For your baby, play is a way to exercise and learn about himself and the world around him. When your baby grabs and shakes a rattle or plays peek-a-boo with you, he's discovering that he can make things happen. When you talk, coo, laugh, hug, and kiss your baby, he's learning that his responses affect you.

There are many ways to play with your baby every day, such as:

*   Singing and talking to him, or dancing with him
*   Caressing, touching, and cuddling when changing or feeding him
*   Massaging him (See above.)
*   Playing games such as peek-a-boo or playing with age-appropriate toys
*   Having him do exercises with you (See page 343.)

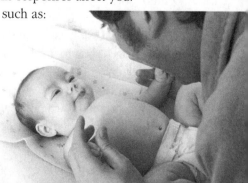

## Advice from the Authors

To learn more information about wearing your baby in a sling or carrier, try these tips:

- Read "Ten Reasons to Wear Your Baby," a great article by Laura Simeon. You can find it online by using the article title as a search term.
- Read *Babywearing* by Maria Blois.
- Learn about different types of slings and carriers at http://www.birthandbeyond.com/howtochbaca.html and http://www.wearyourbaby.com.
- Visit http://www.youtube.com and use "wear your baby" as a search term to find videos that show how to use various slings and carriers.

Play doesn't always need to focus on your baby. He absorbs information from you no matter what you do together. For example, your baby will enjoy hearing you read aloud from a novel or even a newspaper's business section. If you're meeting friends for coffee, your baby will enjoy experiencing new sights, sounds, and smells. Even when you're putting away silverware, your baby can begin to hear numbers if you count each fork out loud as you place it in the drawer.

Use a baby wrap, sling, or carrier to keep your hands free while keeping your baby close as he experiences your everyday activities.

# Medical Care for Your Baby

Making sure your baby is healthy during the weeks and months after her birth will help her become a physically and emotionally healthy child and adult. The following sections describe ways to monitor your baby's health, reduce her risk of catching diseases, and treat illnesses or conditions that she may have, including when to call for medical help.

## WELL-BABY CARE

To make sure your baby is growing well and developing normally, he should have periodic routine well-baby exams by his caregiver. Three to four days after the birth, the caregiver will assess your baby's feeding, check for jaundice, and discuss any concerns you may have. Your baby may have another checkup when he's a week or two old to assess his weight and feeding, give you a chance to ask questions, and possibly repeat newborn screening tests. (See page 371.) Going forward, your baby's caregiver will let you know when to schedule additional appointments.

## VACCINATIONS

Vaccines are biological agents, prepared in a laboratory, that can protect babies and children from specific diseases and their common complications—including death. An administration of a vaccine is called a *vaccination* (or *immunization*). Vaccinations have been one of the most significant health contributions in the last century. The success of some vaccinations has nearly or completely eradicated serious diseases such as polio and diphtheria.

Health care professionals recommend that babies and children receive vaccinations against several diseases according to a schedule that's updated every year by the U.S. Centers for Disease Control and Prevention (CDC). Visit http://www.cdc.gov/vaccines/recs/schedules to see the current vaccination schedule.

Because vaccines introduce a foreign substance to the body, each one has potential side effects after injection. Although the risk of side effects is extremely low, some parents decide not to have their children vaccinated. To these parents, the risks of suffering the possible side effects of a vaccine

## Tips to Protect Your Baby's Health

- Before picking up your baby, before feeding her, and after diaper changes, wash your hands well with soap and water. If you can't wash your hands, use an alcohol-based hand sanitizer.
- Keep anyone with a cold, cough, sore throat, rash, fever, or other signs of illness away from your baby. If you're ill, wash your hands thoroughly before feeding and caring for your baby.
- If you participate in group activities such as parent-baby groups, be sure all participants understand and respect that they should attend only if they and their babies are healthy.
- If your baby is premature or has a chronic health condition, ask her caregiver for additional wellness guidelines.

outweigh the risks of getting the illness. Other parents decide against vaccination because they might not understand the importance of vaccinating their children against diseases that are rarely seen today, such as polio, diphtheria, or even measles. Other parents decide not to vaccinate because of religious or cultural beliefs.

Choosing against vaccination is a decision not to be made lightly. Parents need to make sure their reasons reflect current information. For example, thimerosal (mercury) was once used as a preservative in vaccines and is thought by some to increase the risk of autism. However, manufacturers haven't used thimerosal in childhood vaccines since 2001.[28] The only exception is the influenza vaccine in a multidose vial, which babies shouldn't receive. (After they're six months old, babies should receive the influenza vaccine from a single-dose vial that doesn't contain thimerosal.)

When deciding whether to vaccinate your baby, gather as much reliable information as possible. Some illnesses are more common than others; some vaccines have more side effects than others. To make an informed decision about vaccines, get the current facts from reliable resources such as your baby's caregiver, the CDC hotline at 800-232-SHOT (7468), the National Vaccine Information Center (http://www.nvic.org/), or *The Vaccine Book: Making the Right Decision for Your Child* by Dr. Robert Sears. Visit our web site, http://www.PCNGuide.com, for information about individual vaccines and the diseases they protect against. Many public health departments publish local data about infectious diseases, which can tell you how many cases of diseases such as pertussis, measles, and meningitis have occurred in the past month and year where you live. This information can tell you what illnesses pose the most risk to your baby, which may influence your decision about certain vaccinations.

If you still have trouble making a decision about vaccinations, talk with your baby's caregiver. Most caregivers are willing to discuss your concerns and can help you individualize your approach to vaccination. For example, you may find making the decision more manageable if you consider each vaccine separately. You may decide not to follow the recommended schedule and instead choose to avoid multiple vaccinations at one time by spreading them out over a longer period. (If you're charged a copay for each visit, you may factor this increased cost into your decision.)

If you choose to vaccinate your baby, his caregiver will give you a form that shows completed vaccinations. Many child-care centers, preschools, and schools require proof of certain vaccinations before admitting a child. To find out what vaccinations are required where you live, ask your baby's caregiver. This form is also a reminder of upcoming vaccinations.

If your baby has a reaction to a vaccine, make sure to inform his caregiver so he or she can record it on your baby's vaccination form. You may also want to contact the National Vaccine Injury Compensation Program (VICP), which provides compensation to people who may have been injured by vaccines. For information about VICP, call 800-338-2382 or visit http://www.hrsa.gov/vaccinecompensation.

## TAKING YOUR BABY'S TEMPERATURE

Take your baby's temperature anytime she seems sick (listless, weak, unusually fussy, loss of appetite, runny nose, and so on). To quickly assess whether your baby has a fever, compare the warmth of her chest, abdomen, or back to the warmth of the back of your neck. Both areas should feel about the same temperature. Don't assess your baby's temperature by feeling her hands or feet; a newborn's hands and feet are often cold even though her body is warm.

If your baby feels too warm, take her temperature under her arm (axillary temperature), on her skin (temporal artery temperature), or in her rectum (rectal temperature). Don't use ear probe thermometers, temperature strips placed on the forehead, or pacifier thermometers; they aren't accurate.

Determining whether your baby has a fever depends on which method you use to take her temperature. Your baby's caregiver will tell you when to call for further advice—typically, when your baby's temperature is below 97.4°F (36.3°C) by any method or when her axillary temperature is over 99.5°F (37.5°C) or her temporal artery or rectal temperature is over 100.4°F (38°C).

To take an axillary temperature, place a digital thermometer under your baby's arm. Center the bulb in her armpit, making sure her clothing doesn't touch the bulb. Lower your baby's arm and hold it firmly against her body for five minutes or until the thermometer beeps. Remove it and read the temperature.

A temporal artery thermometer (TemporalScanner) is accurate, noninvasive, and quick when used correctly (moving the probe on the thermometer across your baby's forehead starting above her nose and moving toward her hairline). Several studies of this thermometer have shown it's more accurate than rectal thermometers and ear thermometers (which aren't accurate in babies younger than six months).[29] However, it's also more expensive than a digital or rectal thermometer.

To take a rectal temperature, lubricate the bulb end of a rectal thermometer with nonpetroleum jelly or an ointment such as A&D ointment. Position your baby on her back and hold her ankles in one hand and the thermometer in the other. Gently insert the bulb end into the rectum until you can no longer see the tip (about ½ inch). Hold the thermometer in place for about three minutes. Remove it and read the temperature. After use, clean the thermometer with cold water and soap or with alcohol.

## WHEN TO CALL FOR MEDICAL HELP

If you're worried about your baby's health, write down his temperature and any symptoms that worry you, then call his caregiver. Here's other information your baby's caregiver may wish to know:

• Physical symptoms, such as abnormal temperature, breathing difficulties, coughing, vomiting, diarrhea, constipation, fewer wet diapers than usual, or rash
• Behavioral symptoms, such as listlessness, weakness, loss of appetite, unusual fussiness or irritability, change in typical behavior and activity level (for example, loss of interest in surroundings or in feeding)

- Any newborn warning signs (See page 393.)
- Home treatment you've provided and your baby's response to it, including any medications (What and when?)
- General considerations, such as any recent exposure to illness or someone at home or at day care who's ill

Visit our web site, http://www.PCNGuide.com, to download a work sheet to help you organize your thoughts. Keep a pad and pen handy to write down any advice and suggestions your baby's caregiver may have.

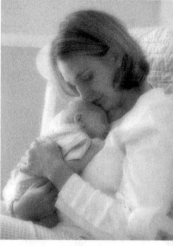

## COMMON HEALTH CONCERNS

The following sections discuss common conditions in newborns that can cause new parents concern but often clear up with minimal treatment.

### Newborn Jaundice

After the birth, your baby has a normal excess of red blood cells that break down into a substance called bilirubin, which she excretes in her bowel movements. If your baby develops *jaundice*, she has an excess of bilirubin that causes her skin or the whites of her eyes to become yellow by the third or fourth day after the birth. About half of all newborns have some mild yellowness in their faces by this time, which disappears without treatment.

Occasionally, the yellowness in your baby is more pronounced on the third or fourth day after the birth and may require treatment. To confirm that your baby's chest is yellow, press your fingers on her breastbone. If the skin looks yellow when you remove your fingers, jaundice may be a concern; call your baby's caregiver to schedule an evaluation.

To diagnose jaundice, your baby's caregiver may take a blood sample from your baby's heel, then use a blood test to measure the bilirubin level. If the level is high enough to warrant treatment, your baby's caregiver will help you make sure your baby is getting enough milk. Inadequate feeding may cause jaundice because a baby who feeds poorly has fewer stools and can't rid her body of bilirubin.

If necessary, your baby will receive *phototherapy*, a procedure that shines a special type of cool light on your baby's skin, causing the bilirubin level to drop. Phototherapy usually continues for two to four days, until further blood tests show that the bilirubin has fallen to a safe level. Your baby can receive phototherapy in three ways.

1. In the hospital, special overhead lights (called "bili lights") are shined on your baby's naked chest or back. Soft pads protect her eyes from the light.
2. At your home or in the hospital, your baby is wrapped in a special blanket to receive phototherapy. You can hold and feed your baby without removing her from the light source.
3. At your home or in the hospital, your baby lies on her back in a net hammock over a phototherapy source.

Jaundice that appears on the first or second day after the birth (early jaundice) is more serious than when it appears on the third or fourth day. It may require intensive treatment, such as phototherapy or, on the rare occasion when the bilirubin level becomes very high, a blood exchange transfusion to lower the bilirubin to a safe level and prevent possible hearing loss or severe neurological damage. If your baby develops jaundice after the first two weeks, have her caregiver evaluate her.

In addition to inadequate feeding, causes of jaundice include prematurity, bruising during labor or birth, exposure to certain drugs given to the mother in labor, liver or intestinal problems, sepsis (infection), and blood incompatibilities such as Rh (see page 135) or ABO incompatibility (when the mother's blood type is O and the baby's is A, B, or AB). Sepsis and blood incompatibilities are typical causes of early jaundice.

## Rashes

In the first week after the birth, some newborns develop red blotches with waxy yellow or white pimples in the middle (erythema toxicum). This characteristic newborn rash appears on the trunk, arms, and legs; doesn't cause itching; and disappears without treatment.

For the first few months, it's common for your baby to periodically have mild facial rashes (smooth pimples, small red spots, or rough red spots). These rashes rarely require treatment. Small white spots (milia) on your baby's nose, cheeks, and chin occur when tiny skin flakes are trapped in small pockets on the skin surface. Milia disappear within a month or two of their appearance. Red bumps (baby acne) may appear on your baby's face in the first several weeks, due to increased oil production that began when some of your hormones transferred to him before the birth. Applying breast milk as a "lotion" may help reduce the rash.

Prickly heat is a common warm-weather rash that appears on overdressed babies. Found most often on the shoulders, trunk, and neck, prickly heat looks like clusters of tiny pink pimples surrounded by pink skin. As it dries, the rash becomes slightly tan. Prickly heat may look worse than it feels to your baby. To avoid this rash, don't let your baby become overheated.

A yellowish, scaly, patchy condition called cradle cap may appear on your baby's scalp and behind his ears. Daily washing or brushing of the scalp may help treat or even prevent cradle cap. Gently comb or brush out the scales using a baby comb, fingernail brush, or soft toothbrush; then wash your baby's scalp with mild soap. Repeat this process every day or every other day until the scales are gone. Massaging your baby's scalp with breast milk or vegetable oil before washing also may help treat or prevent cradle cap.

## Colds

Although it's normal for your baby to have a slightly stuffy nose or make a rattle-like noise when she breathes through her nose, she may have a cold if she has a very runny nose and goopy eyes, is fussier than usual, has trouble eating and sleeping, and perhaps has a slight fever.

To reduce your baby's risk of catching a cold, minimize the number of people she comes into contact with, especially when she's younger than three months. People with colds and other illnesses should stay away from your baby. Make sure all those who want to handle your baby wash their hands thoroughly first.

When your baby has a cold, consult with her caregiver. He or she may suggest using a cool-mist vaporizer near your baby and putting her in a semi-reclined position (such as in a car seat) to sleep. You can clear your baby's nostrils by dripping saline or breast milk into each one, then gently "milking" her nose to clear the mucus. (Breast milk soothes the mucous membranes and contains antiviral and antibacterial properties.) You also can run a hot shower or bath, then take your baby into the bathroom (but not into the tub or shower) to breathe the steam to ease congestion.

Don't give your baby cold medications such as decongestants and cough medicine; they aren't safe for infants.

# MEDICATIONS

Use the following guidelines if your baby's caregiver prescribes medications or vitamins.

- To dispense liquid medication, use a medicine dropper placed between your baby's cheek and gum; don't squirt it on his tongue. Hold your baby in a semi-upright position and let him suck the medicine as you gently squeeze the dropper.
- Another way to give your baby liquid medication is to pour it into an empty bottle nipple, then have him drink it all. When the nipple is empty, fill it with water and have your baby drink it all as well. This ensures that your baby receives a full dose because he'll drink any remaining medicine that was coating the nipple.
- Don't mix medication in with pumped breast milk, formula, juice, or water. If your baby refuses to finish the whole bottle, you won't know how much medication he's received.
- Give only the medication your baby's caregiver specifies. Aspirin—even baby aspirin—is no longer recommended for babies and children because of its association with Reye's syndrome, a serious disease.

# SUDDEN INFANT DEATH SYNDROME (SIDS)

*Sudden infant death syndrome (SIDS)* is the sudden death of a baby younger than one year that remains unexplained after a thorough investigation. The cause of SIDS isn't fully understood.

Almost every parent worries about SIDS at some time. You may have read about the condition or even know someone whose baby died of SIDS. Although there's no way to minimize the loss and grief caused by SIDS, the following facts may help put your fears and worries into perspective:

- SIDS is rare, occurring in about 1 in 2,000 babies in the United States.[30]
- SIDS deaths most commonly occur in babies who are between two and four months old.[31]
- No one—including parents—is to blame for SIDS. It can't be predicted or prevented.
- Death occurs quickly and painlessly; it isn't the result of suffocation, asphyxiation, or regurgitation.
- SIDS isn't caused by vaccinations. In fact, SIDS deaths are statistically more common in babies who haven't been vaccinated.
- SIDS isn't contagious.

For parents faced with a loss by SIDS, support groups can help. The baby's caregiver, a public health nurse, or a childbirth educator can help locate a group. Other resources include First Candle (800-221-7437 or http://www.firstcandle.com) and the American SIDS Institute (800-232-7437 or http://www.sids.org).

You can take steps before and after your baby's birth to help prevent her risk of SIDS.[32] During pregnancy, eat a healthful diet, don't use cocaine or heroin, don't smoke and avoid exposure to secondhand smoke, and have regular prenatal care to help reduce your baby's risk of prematurity.

After your baby is born, breastfeed her. Breastfeeding can lower the risk of SIDS.[33] Also avoid overdressing your baby. To keep her warm, swaddle her or use a blanket or sleep sack. Don't expose her to secondhand smoke, and place her in a safe position in a safe location to sleep (see page 392).

## Safe Sleeping to Reduce the Risk of SIDS

Make sure that everyone who cares for your baby places him on his back to sleep. Placing him on his tummy or side to sleep increases his risk of SIDS. If your baby is unhappy on his back or wakens easily, try swaddling him.

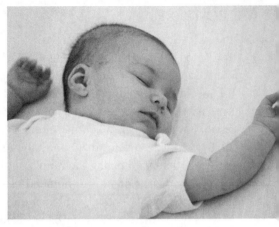

Also make sure your baby's sleep space is safe. Use a firm, flat surface and avoid waterbeds, couches, sofas, pillows, duvets, quilts, comforters, soft materials, loose bedding, soft toys, lambskins, and bumper pads in cribs. Make sure there isn't space between the mattress and headboard or walls, or between the crib mattress and the crib slats. These spaces may entrap your baby and lead to suffocation.

The American Academy of Pediatrics (AAP) recommends that to reduce the risk of SIDS, babies should sleep in the same room as their mothers, but not in the same bed (bed-sharing).[34] This recommendation is controversial,[35] because other experts recommend bed-sharing for such benefits as frequent and convenient breastfeeding, reduced crying, and better sleep for both parents and babies. For more information on bed-sharing and other cosleeping arrangements, read *Sleeping with Your Baby: A Parent's Guide to Cosleeping* by James J. McKenna, an international authority on cosleeping and its impact on the reduction of SIDS.

Parents who choose to bed-share need to follow safety guidelines. A baby shouldn't share a bed with a parent who has consumed sedatives, medication, alcohol, or any substance that causes extreme drowsiness or unawareness, which increases the risk of rolling onto the baby and smothering him. A baby also shouldn't share a bed if a parent is a smoker. If a parent is markedly obese, he or she shouldn't sleep next to the baby to avoid causing a depression in the mattress that baby could roll into on his stomach.

Some parents use pacifiers to help their babies fall asleep. Analyses of several small studies show a small decrease in SIDS with pacifier use, leading the AAP to recommend pacifiers to help babies fall asleep after they're a month old. This recommendation is controversial, because breastfeeding may just as effectively help babies fall asleep. (However, no studies have analyzed this effect of breastfeeding.) In addition, despite parents' efforts to have their baby take a pacifier, only he can decide whether he'll do so.

# Babies with Special Circumstances

Babies who are born early or small for their gestational age may have needs that require special care.

## PREMATURE BABIES

A baby is *premature* if she's born before the thirty-seventh week of pregnancy and weighs less than 5½ pounds. Thankfully, advances in care have increased the survival rates of even very premature babies and have greatly reduced the long-term respiratory and neurological problems experienced by premature babies born just a decade ago. Today, babies born as early as twenty-four weeks gestation can thrive.

# Newborn Warning Signs

If any of the following signs appear in the first month after the birth, report them to your baby's caregiver.

| Warning Signs | Possible Problems |
|---|---|
| Fever (axillary temperature above 99.5°F/37.5°C) | Infection |
| Temperature below 97.4°F/36.3°C (whether taken axillary, by temporal artery, or rectally) | May indicate infection caused by Group B streptococcus (GBS) or other bacteria. |
| Your baby's face, chest, and the whites of his eyes are yellow. | Jaundice (See page 389.) |
| Changes in your baby's behavior, such as listlessness or unusual fussiness or irritability | Illness such as a cold, viral illness, or diarrhea |
| Problems with the umbilical cord, including bright red bleeding, redness around the cord, or a foul odor or pus-like discharge | Infection or other problems with the cord (See page 377 for more information on cord care.) |
| Problems with a circumcision, including continuous bright red oozing or bleeding, swelling, foul discharge, or an inability to urinate | Infection or bleeding from the circumcision site |
| Problems with feeding, including a breastfed baby who feeds fewer than 7 or 8 times in 24 hours, or any baby who feeds poorly | Difficulty with breastfeeding, jaundice, illness, or prematurity (See Chapter 18 to learn about feeding problems.) |
| Fewer wet diapers than expected: In the first week, expect the number of wet diapers to at least equal the day of life (for example, at least 3 wet diapers on day 3). After day 7, expect 6 or more wet diapers in 24 hours. | Inadequate feeding or illness (See page 413 for signs that your baby is getting enough milk.) |
| Problems with bowel movements, including no bowel movement in any 24-hour period in the first month after the birth. After your breastfed baby is a month old, it's normal from him not to have a bowel movement for a day or longer. | Inadequate feeding (See page 369 for a description of normal bowel movements in newborns.) |
| Problems with breathing, including blue lips, a struggle to breathe, flared nostrils, or deep indentations of the chest when breathing | Prematurity, illness, or heart or lung problems |

**Call 911 if your baby can't breathe easily.**

Every day in the womb before term improves a baby's chances of survival and normal development. If a baby's born before term, she looks different than a full-term baby does. She's small, limp, and frail. Her skin is reddish and appears tissue-paper thin, and she has little to no fat or muscle. Her head appears disproportionately large. Vernix caseosa and lanugo (fine, downy hair on her body) are abundant, her fingernails and toenails haven't grown out, and her tiny ears are soft and hug her head. Her cry is feeble, and she may be more difficult to soothe than a full-term baby.

A premature baby is physically vulnerable until she grows older. She sucks weakly, and her swallow and gag reflexes are unreliable. She may need to be fed by a tube into her stomach.

Because her body temperature is unstable (often below normal), she usually stays in a temperature-controlled isolette. Because her lungs are immature, her breaths are irregular, rapid, and often shallow; she may need oxygen to help with breathing. Her ability to absorb food is less efficient than a full-term baby's, although her need for nutrients—especially calories, protein, iron, calcium, zinc, and vitamin E—may be greater.

If you give birth to a premature baby, the experience can be upsetting and frightening. Your baby will need special medical attention that may separate her from you, but she also needs to feel your touch and hear your voice, even when inside an isolette.

Your baby's nurse may encourage Kangaroo care, in which you hold your baby so her bare skin lies against your bare chest (see page 293). Your closeness, breathing movements, and warmth will help regulate her breathing, keep her warm, and comfort her (and thus you). With regular Kangaroo care, premature babies typically grow faster. If you're at risk for preterm labor, contact the newborn nursery to learn about their policies on Kangaroo care and how to arrange for it. (For more information on preterm labor, see page 136.)

If your baby is too immature to breastfeed, you can express milk and have it fed to her through a tube that passes from her mouth to her stomach. Your milk differs from the milk of a mother whose baby is full-term; its composition is designed to meet your premature baby's nutritional needs. It also contains antibodies and immune boosters that help protect her from infection and disease.

Feeding, touching, and caring for your premature baby will help you both cope as she grows stronger. For additional support, you may want to contact a group that provides information, assistance, and emotional support to parents of premature babies. The group may have a library of helpful books and also may supply you with clothing small enough for your baby. For more information about premature babies, check with your childbirth educator, caregiver, or local hospital.

## Babies Who Are Small for Gestational Age

Babies who are small for gestational age (SGA) are smaller in size and weight than expected at birth, given the length of time they were in the womb. This condition has several possible causes, including an inadequate transfer of nutrients across the placenta to the baby; the effects of some drugs (such as tobacco) taken during pregnancy; some congenital and genetic malformations; and certain infections, such as toxoplasmosis. Sometimes the cause is unknown.

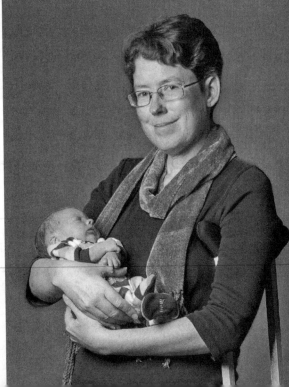

SGA babies present challenges to parents that are similar to those of premature babies. SGA babies don't move easily from state to state (for example, from active to quiet alert or from drowsy to deep sleep—see pages 381–382). They're often fussy and more difficult to soothe than newborns of normal size and weight. Parents spend lots of time calming and quieting SGA babies; successful soothing techniques include frequent feeding, gentle rocking, quiet talking, and maintaining a calm environment.

Parents soon learn that SGA babies can handle only one source of stimulation at a time. Too much stimulation—such as talking to the baby while jiggling or feeding him—overwhelms and agitates him, typically making him cry.

If your baby is SGA, he'll become less intense and fussy as he matures. In the meantime, your sensitivity to his special needs will help you both cope.

## Key Points to Remember

- Every newborn has a unique appearance and temperament. Babies teach their parents what they need by giving cues.
- Crying is often your baby's last attempt to communicate that she's hungry, overstimulated, tired, or uncomfortable. Try to respond to your baby's early cues so you meet her needs before she cries.
- Creating a womb-like environment will help calm your crying baby. The Five S's method (see page 379) can be an especially effective tool.
- Swaddling and cosleeping may increase how long your baby sleeps.
- Be aware of newborn warning signs (see page 393) to know when to seek medical help.
- Learn about vaccinations so you can make an informed decision about vaccinating your baby.
- You can significantly reduce the risk of SIDS by always placing your baby on her back to sleep.

# CHAPTER 18

# Feeding Your Baby

During pregnancy, your body nourishes your baby as he grows from an amazingly tiny fertilized egg to a fully developed newborn who weighs several pounds. After the birth, you continue to nourish him with breast milk, formula, or both. Although either type of nourishment helps your baby triple his birth weight and grow 10 to 12 inches during his first year, only breast milk provides nutrients that encourage the rapid, healthy growth of his brain, nervous and digestive systems, and the development of his immune system.

Whether you feed your baby breast milk or formula, *how* you feed him is also important to his growth. The way your baby gets nourishment influences his physical, social, and emotional well-being,[1] and feeding him with care and love whenever he shows he's hungry helps foster his emotional development, encourage bonding, and strengthen family ties.

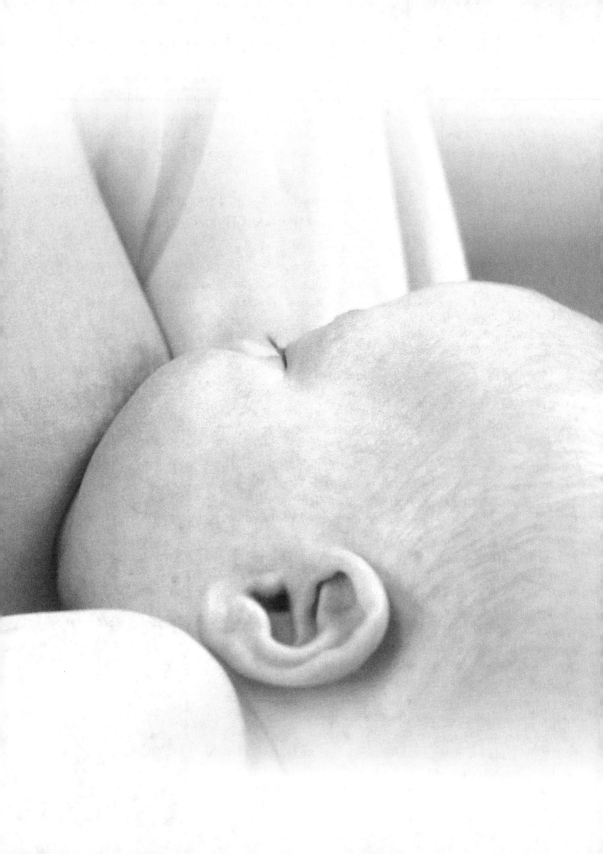

# Breast Milk or Formula?

Whether to feed your baby breast milk or formula (or both) is a personal choice. Before making a decision, it's important to become well informed about breastfeeding, feeding expressed breast milk by a bottle, and formula feeding. Each method of feeding may have advantages and drawbacks, depending on your unique circumstances.

## WHY HEALTH CARE PROVIDERS RECOMMEND BREAST MILK AND BREASTFEEDING

Except in certain rare instances (see page 400), almost all health care providers recommend breastfeeding because of its health benefits for both babies and mothers.

Breast milk's nutritional composition is ideal for babies. Unlike cow milk and formula, breast milk adapts to meet your baby's changing nutritional needs. It's also more easily digestible than the alternatives. Breast milk enhances the development of your baby's brain and may contribute to a higher IQ and better cognitive test scores.[2,3]

Babies who are exclusively breastfed for at least three months have fewer and less severe allergies than formula-fed babies.[4,5] Breastfed babies are much less likely than formula-fed

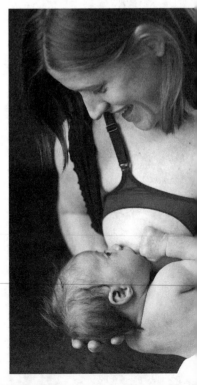

babies to be hospitalized for infections;[6,7] overall, they have fewer ear infections, respiratory infections, urinary tract infections (UTIs), and infections from bacterial meningitis. Breastfed babies also have fewer occurrences of diarrhea and vomiting. In addition, studies show that breast milk can lower a baby's risk of dying from sudden infant death syndrome (SIDS).[8,9]

Looking ahead to your baby's future, breastfeeding can reduce the incidence of some diseases that occur later in life, such as insulin-dependent diabetes mellitus, asthma, obesity, leukemia, lymphoma, and multiple sclerosis.[10]

For you, breastfeeding reduces postpartum bleeding and helps your uterus shrink to its normal size faster. Breastfeeding reduces your risk of some diseases, including premenopausal breast cancer, ovarian cancer, and osteoporosis.[11] Studies show that mothers who breastfed have fewer hip fractures after menopause than do women who never breastfed.[12]

Your family will likely find breastfeeding to be both economical and convenient. (It's virtually cost free and always available.) It also promotes a close, nurturing relationship between you and your baby.

# IF YOU HAVE CONCERNS ABOUT BREASTFEEDING

Despite health care providers' endorsement of breastfeeding, you may doubt breastfeeding's advantages. Maybe you had previous trouble breastfeeding or question its convenience. Perhaps you're concerned about your ability to breastfeed when you return to work. You may worry that a medical condition will make breastfeeding difficult or harm your breast milk, or you may be pregnant with more than one baby. Your partner may worry that breastfeeding will reduce his or her opportunity to parent.

These concerns may lead you to decide that breastfeeding won't work for you, but talk to your caregiver, a lactation consultant, your baby's caregiver, or a childbirth educator about your circumstances before making a decision. You may discover that your concerns about breastfeeding are unfounded or can be addressed.

For example, if you had previous trouble breastfeeding, talk with a lactation consultant during pregnancy to discuss how it can be different this time. If you remain unsure, give breastfeeding a try, knowing that you can stop if it's unsuccessful.

If you doubt that breastfeeding can be more convenient than formula feeding, talk with families who breastfeed and those who formula feed to get an idea of just how more or less convenient one method is than the other.

Returning to work can present challenges to breastfeeding, but they can be overcome or minimized. See page 431 for further information.

A medical condition can affect breastfeeding. For example, breastfeeding is more difficult for a premature baby or one with a congenital condition such as Down syndrome or cleft palate. A lactation consultant can show you special techniques for feeding a baby with physical challenges. Breastfeeding or providing pumped breast milk can be an excellent way to help your premature or special needs baby grow and stay healthy.

A breast reduction might or might not affect your ability to breastfeed. If you've had this surgery, get the support of a lactation consultant before giving birth.

If you're pregnant with twins, triplets, or more, breastfeeding may be challenging, but even if you can't always nurse your babies, you can still provide them breast milk by expressing it. See pages 424 and 429 for more information.

If your partner or others worry that breastfeeding will eliminate an opportunity to care for your baby, point out there are many other ways they can actively parent. They can cuddle and soothe your baby; they can bathe her and change her diapers. As your baby grows, her need for social interaction increases dramatically, giving others many occasions to interact with her. For you, a partner or others can provide support and encouragement if difficulties with breastfeeding arise.

After considering your circumstances and concerns, if you decide not to breastfeed, see pages 435–437 to learn about formula feeding. If you want to breastfeed but discover that you can't, seek the support of your caregiver or a lactation consultant to help you adjust to a different method of feeding.

## How to Find a Qualified Lactation Consultant

*Lactation consultants* are breastfeeding experts who recognize the value of breastfeeding and dedicate their work to its promotion, support, and protection. An International Board Certified Lactation Consultant (IBCLC) is someone who has successfully passed an exam administered by the International Board of Lactation Consultant Examiners (IBLCE). Look for a lactation consultant who has earned these internationally recognized credentials. Here are ways to begin your search:

- Ask your childbirth educator or your local La Leche League group to refer you to an IBCLC.
- If you're birthing in a hospital, ask your caregiver or nurse whether the hospital has a breastfeeding service that employs lactation consultants.
- Visit http://www.ilca.org, the web site for the International Lactation Consultant Association (ILCA), to find referrals.

If you can't find an IBCLC, find a nurse trained in breastfeeding support, a doula, midwife, La Leche League Leader, childbirth educator, experienced breastfeeding mom, or another breastfeeding expert in your area to help you.

## WHEN HEALTH CARE EXPERTS RECOMMEND FORMULA FEEDING

There are a few cases in which health care providers recommend formula feeding over breastfeeding or breast milk. For example, if a baby has galactosemia (a rare condition in which the baby can't digest the sugar in breast milk), formula becomes necessary. In most cases, however, the mother's health is the reason for the recommendation. Formula feeding is best if the mother is HIV positive (and lives in a developed country),[13,14] has untreated tuberculosis, takes certain medications that may harm the baby (such as lithium or radioactive medications), uses street drugs (such as heroin, cocaine, or methamphetamines), is receiving high doses of methadone, or has had extensive breast surgery.

Some women's concerns about breastfeeding are psychological. For example, some are overly anxious about nursing in public; others chronically worry that they might not produce enough milk or that breastfeeding may damage their breasts' appearance. For most women, these concerns are mild and talking with a lactation consultant, obstetrician, or midwife may sufficiently address them. For other women, however, these concerns are overwhelming anxieties, especially if a woman is a survivor of sexual abuse. If you have serious concerns, talking with a lactation consultant or a caregiver can help you decide whether formula feeding is appropriate. If formula feeding is recommended, see page 435 for further information.

## CONCERNS ABOUT FORMULA

In the 1980s, the United States Congress enacted and amended the Infant Formula Act, mandating that manufacturers include in their formula at least minimum levels of twenty-nine nutrients and maximum levels of nine nutrients. Despite these regulations, formula doesn't contain most of the more than two hundred nutrients and components that are present in breast milk. This deficiency may explain why formula can't (and breast milk can) enhance the development of a baby's immune system.

Some kinds of formula are less healthful than others. For example, babies fed low-iron formula are more likely to have anemia (which results in lower cognitive test scores) than breastfed babies or babies fed iron-fortified formula.[15]

Occasionally, manufacturing errors put formula at risk for contamination. When this happens, the formula is recalled, worrying parents whose babies have consumed the recalled formula.

# How Breastfeeding Works

Simply explained, breastfeeding is the interaction between you and your baby as he suckles at your breast. Your body began preparing for breastfeeding long before you became pregnant. When you were in your early teens, increasing amounts of the hormone estrogen stimulated the growth of the ductal system within your breasts. The ductal system provides the pathways for milk to flow out of the nipple.

During pregnancy, your breasts prepare for lactation (milk production and secretion) through a complex interplay of hormones that causes rapid growth of the ductal system and the lobular system, which is responsible for milk production. Blood supply to your breasts supports this growth and delivers the nutrients in breast milk.

During the second trimester and as early as the sixteenth week of pregnancy, the hormone *prolactin* stimulates the production of *colostrum* (the first milk); the hormone human placental lactogen (HPL) stimulates your breasts to secrete colostrum. After you give birth, progesterone levels fall and prolactin levels increase, triggering breast milk production. These amazing changes occur naturally during pregnancy and the postpartum period.

## ANATOMY OF YOUR BREASTS

Your breasts are well designed to make milk. Each breast contains seven to ten milk-producing units called lobes. Each lobe contains branches of *alveoli* (cells that make milk) and milk ducts. Milk flows from the alveoli through the ducts and leaves your breast through five to ten nipple openings.[16] As your baby compresses the *areola* (the darker skin around each nipple) with her lips and gums and massages it with her tongue, she draws milk into her mouth. *Montgomery glands* are the small bumps on the areola that secrete a lubricating substance, which keeps the nipple supple and helps prevent infection. (Use only water to clean your breasts; soap removes this special lubrication.)

Your breasts likely look different during pregnancy. They're probably larger with more visible veins and stretch marks. Your areolae may appear larger and darker; these changes help your newborn see your nipples. Your Montgomery glands also appear larger. Colostrum may leak from your breasts or dry into a crust on your nipples. These physical changes show that your breasts are responding to pregnancy hormones and preparing to make milk.

Of all women, 2 to 6 percent have accessory mammary tissue, extra breast tissue under the arm or below the breast that may have a nipple.[17] This tissue may swell during pregnancy and as milk comes in. If left alone, the tissue diminishes, but placing cold packs on the area may decrease discomfort.

Contrary to popular belief, your breast size doesn't determine the quality or quantity of the milk you produce. Bigger breasts simply have more fatty tissue surrounding the milk-producing structures than smaller breasts have. Breasts, areolae, and nipples of all sizes and shapes are usually perfect for breastfeeding.

## How Your Body Makes Breast Milk

Prolactin and oxytocin are two hormones that play a significant role in milk production and milk ejection (flow). When your baby suckles at your breast, the action stimulates the anterior pituitary gland in your brain to release prolactin into your bloodstream. Prolactin causes the cells in the alveoli to draw water and nutrients from your blood to make milk. Your baby's suckling (or even when you hear him cry) also prompts the posterior pituitary gland to release oxytocin. Oxytocin makes the muscles around milk-producing cells contract and expel milk. It also makes the ducts widen and shorten, helping with milk flow. This process is called the *let-down reflex* or *let-down*.

You have two or more let-downs from each breast during each feeding.[18] During the first weeks after the birth, let-down might not occur until several minutes after your baby has begun suckling. After you and your baby have established a good breastfeeding relationship, let-down occurs within seconds.

Let-down sensations vary widely. During the first few days of breastfeeding, you might not feel your milk let down. Afterward, you still might not feel it, or you might feel a tingling, itching, or flowing sensation. If you don't feel your milk let-down, you'll know it has occurred when you hear your baby swallow, see milk in his mouth, or feel uterine cramping.

The frequency and duration of feedings strongly affect your milk supply. The more your baby suckles and drains your breast, the more milk you produce.

Conversely, you may make less milk if you delay or limit feedings, use a pacifier, offer supplements (formula, water, or other liquids), or schedule your baby's feedings to every three to four hours. The reason is because of a protein in breast milk called feedback inhibitor of lactation (FIL). When your breast is full of milk, FIL slows milk production. When your baby frequently drains your breast, there is less FIL and milk production increases.[19]

To help develop a good milk supply, feed your baby frequently (that is, in response to his feeding cues—see page 410) and let him feed for as long as he wants.

## Composition of Breast Milk

The first milk your breasts produce is colostrum, a yellowish or clear syrupy fluid that's ideally suited to your newborn's needs. Colostrum helps speed the passage of meconium (first bowel movement) and establish the proper balance of healthy bacteria in your baby's digestive tract. Because colostrum is rich in antibodies, it protects your baby from infection. It's also higher in protein than mature milk. On average, you make just over 1 ounce in the first twenty-four hours after giving birth, which is exactly what your baby needs. The volume of colostrum produced increases over the next few days.[20]

After making colostrum, your breasts produce transitional milk, which has a yellowish tint and is higher in fat, calories, and volume than colostrum but lower in protein.

Usually by the end of the first week after the birth, you produce mature milk. This bluish white liquid looks like skim milk and contains more calories than colostrum or transitional milk. By the time your mature milk comes is, the volume of milk production has increased substantially. On average, by the fifth day postpartum, you make about 16½ ounces of milk a day. By three to five months, you make 25 ounces a day; by six months, 27 ounces.[21]

The composition of mature breast milk varies from the beginning of each feeding to its end. The small amount of milk produced early in the feeding is called *foremilk*. The larger portion of milk released with let-down is called *hindmilk*, which provides most of the calories and contains more fat and protein. As your baby grows, the composition of your breast milk changes to meet her nutritional needs.

## Components of Breast Milk

Vitamins, minerals, enzymes, hormones, and other components make up breast milk. Here are the main ones:

**Nonnutritive qualities**

These components protect against disease and promote healthy development. They include anti-infective properties, anti-inflammatory factors, enzymes, hormones, and growth factors.[22]

**Water**

About 87 percent of breast milk is water, which helps newborns maintain their body temperature. Even in very warm climates, breast milk contains all the water a baby needs.

**Fats**

Cholesterol, essential fatty acids, docosahexaenoic acid (DHA), and other fats account for half the calories in breast milk and are necessary for normal development of a baby's nervous system and brain. Fats also aid visual development and enhance the growth of a special coating on nerves as they grow (myelinization).[23]

**Carbohydrates**

Lactose (milk sugar), the primary carbohydrate, helps a baby absorb calcium. It's metabolized into two simple sugars (galactose and glucose) necessary for rapid brain growth.

**Proteins**

Whey, the primary protein in breast milk, becomes a soft curd when a baby digests it, letting her bloodstream readily absorb the nutrients. (Casein, the primary protein in cow milk and cow milk formula, forms a rubbery curd that babies digest less easily than whey, sometimes contributing to constipation.)

**Vitamins and minerals**

Breast milk provides almost all the vitamins and minerals your baby needs. All breastfed babies and some formula-fed babies need to receive vitamin D supplements. A few babies may need iron supplements, and babies at risk of tooth decay may need fluoride.

*Iron*

A full-term, healthy, breastfed baby rarely needs iron supplementation before six months for two reasons.[24] First, iron in breast milk is in a highly absorbable form, despite its small amount. Second, during late pregnancy, a baby stores up iron.

*Vitamin D*

Vitamin D is essential for your body to absorb calcium. Adequate calcium is necessary for bone growth, the maintenance of bone density, and the normal functioning of your nervous system. A severe deficiency of calcium can lead to rickets, a disease that causes bone deformities. You make vitamin D when you expose your skin to sunlight, or you can obtain it by eating foods supplemented with the vitamin. Because safe levels of sun exposure are difficult to determine and hard to obtain in northern climates, your caregiver may recommend vitamin D supplementation for you or your baby.

A blood test can determine if your levels are adequate. If they are, you don't need supplements and the amount of vitamin D in your milk meets your baby's needs. If not, you can take a supplement with 1,000 to 4,000 international units (IU) of vitamin D.[25] If you don't know your level of vitamin D or if it's inadequate, give your baby liquid vitamin D supplements beginning right after birth. The American Academy of Pediatrics (AAP) recommends that a breastfed baby consume 400 IU of vitamin D daily;[26] the Canadian Paediatric Society (CPS) also recommends this amount except for during the winter months, when 800 IU is advised. Choose a supplement that contains only vitamin D; your breastfed baby doesn't need other vitamins and minerals. (Carlson Baby D Drops and Biotics Bio-D Mulsion are two brands that contain 400 IU of vitamin D in just one drop.)

*Fluoride*

Fluoride is a mineral that protects against tooth decay. Only small amounts are present in breast milk. The natural water resources in some regions contain fluoride. Some communities add fluoride to their water supply; others don't. The American Academy of Pediatric Dentistry recommends that parents have a dentist assess their babies' (or children's) teeth before giving them supplemental fluoride.[27]

# Prenatal Preparation for Breastfeeding

To prepare for breastfeeding, learn as much as you can about it before the birth. Read books on the subject, attend a breastfeeding class, and seek the support of groups such as La Leche League, Nursing Mothers Counsel (NMC), new mothers' groups, or WIC (the U.S. government program for low-income women, infants, and children). Spend time around women who breastfeed so you can see how they nurse their babies and learn how they make breastfeeding part of their busy lives.

Choose caregivers who are committed to supporting breastfeeding. While pregnant, ask your caregiver to assess the changes to your breasts, evaluate your nipples, and look for the presence of scar tissue from biopsies or breast surgeries. Many caregivers haven't had training to assess breasts for breastfeeding, so you may need a referral to a lactation consultant.

Even if your caregiver is trained in breast assessment, a prenatal visit with a lactation consultant is recommended if you've had breast surgeries, are expecting more than one baby, have had a previous unpleasant breastfeeding experience, or have specific concerns about your health, nipples, or breast anatomy. Together, you can determine what steps to take during pregnancy and the postpartum period to create a positive breastfeeding experience.

Arrange for help during the first weeks after the birth. This time is generally the most challenging. Enlist family, friends, or a postpartum doula (see page 27) to help with meals and household tasks so you can focus on feeding and caring for your baby and yourself. Keep the contact information of a lactation consultant and breastfeeding support groups readily available. Lastly, know that with time and experience, breastfeeding becomes much easier, more convenient, and enjoyable.

# Nipple Types and Treatment for Flat or Inverted Nipples

There are three main types of nipples.[28] Knowing your nipple type lets you know what (if anything) you can do to help make breastfeeding go more smoothly. To determine your nipple type, place your thumb and index finger above and below your areola at its edge and gently squeeze them together under your areola.

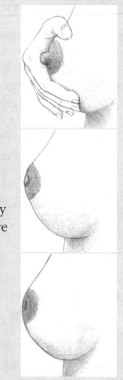

1. **Typical nipples** elongate or protrude (stick out) when squeezed. They're the most common type.
2. **Flat nipples** flatten or move inward (retract) when squeezed.
3. **Inverted nipples** are tucked into the areola. When squeezed, some protrude while others remain inverted, probably because tiny bands (adhesions) bind the tissue.

If you have flat or inverted nipples, some correction often occurs naturally during pregnancy,[29] as hormonal changes enlarge the nipples and improve their ability to protrude. If your nipples remain flat or inverted, you may have trouble starting breastfeeding. In that case, here are a few suggestions:

- Contact a lactation consultant to help with early breastfeeding.
- Consider using a nipple shield, an ultrathin silicone device that you place over your nipple. When your baby sucks on it, he pulls your nipple and milk into his mouth. Don't use a nipple shield without a lactation consultant's help; you may need her expert advice to transition to breastfeeding without it.
- Your baby's sucking also helps *evert* (draw out) your nipple. But if your baby has difficulty latching on, consider using a breast pump before each feeding to draw out your nipples. A lactation consultant or the maternity nurses can show you how to work the breast pump and may suggest other ideas, such as using commercial "nipple enhancers" designed to draw out nipples. (Evert-it or Avent Niplette are two brands.)

# Breastfeeding Basics

If you've never breastfed before, the techniques of breastfeeding may seem awkward and difficult at first. With experience, time, guidance, and support, your skills should improve. This section discusses the basics of breastfeeding that can help you create a beautiful relationship between you and your baby.

## FIRST FEEDINGS

The first feedings are a special time for you and your baby to get to know each other. Most newborns are alert and interested in feeding or nuzzling in the first hour after birth. Take advantage of this time to establish your milk supply and avoid early breastfeeding problems. Research shows that frequent and unrestricted feedings help prevent engorgement (painful swelling of the breasts) and promote an abundant milk supply.[30,31]

## Two Views on First Feedings

It amazed me that my daughter seemed to know what to do at my breast. It was almost as though she'd practiced for feeding while in the womb. I was surprised by how vigorous her suck was. After the first feeding, we all seemed to relax and rest.

*—Kim*

My daughter was born by cesarean. Medications from the surgery had made me sleepy for the first feeding, so my husband had to hold her and help her latch on. (At that point, we really wished he'd come to the breastfeeding class with me!) Although we had some problems with bad latch and sore nipples in the beginning, we got the hang of breastfeeding by three weeks.

*—Peggy*

Here are some tips to make the first feedings a positive experience:

- Breastfeed as soon as possible after the birth.
- Keep your baby with you (preferably skin-to-skin) and let her suckle frequently.
- Try to nurse in a calm, peaceful environment so you and your baby can relax and focus on feeding. If you give birth in a hospital, there may be a lot of distracting activity during the first hour after the birth. (See pages 266–269.) Make sure your caregiver and nurses know (by telling them directly or noting it in your birth plan) that you want to breastfeed your baby as soon after the birth as possible.

If you have a cesarean birth, the completion of the surgery and your recovery may delay the first feeding beyond one hour postpartum. In this case, you need extra help establishing breastfeeding. (See page 428.)

- Don't hesitate to ask some or all visitors to leave the room. If this idea makes you uncomfortable, have your partner or a nurse ask them to leave.
- Take advantage of the breastfeeding knowledge of experienced staff or your doula. They can offer you invaluable reassurance, encouragement, and support.

## BREASTFEEDING POSITIONS

There are several positions for breastfeeding, and each one has special advantages. Whichever position you choose, try to get comfortable and use the basic guidelines in the next paragraph to allow for your baby's participation in getting a good latch and taking plenty of milk.

Bring your baby to your breast with his nose near your nipple and his ears, shoulders, and hips in a straight line. Nestle him close to your body and support his body from his neck to his hips. When you stabilize his body, he can easily move his head and help with the latch. You can use a pillow to support your arm while feeding.

### Cradle Hold

Cradle your baby's head in the crook of one arm and have her facing your breast. Use your forearm to support her body and your hand to support her buttocks.

The advantages of this hold are:

- It's usually the easiest and most comfortable position for you once your baby is nursing well.
- Many mothers use it after learning to breastfeed, because it's convenient for a bigger baby.

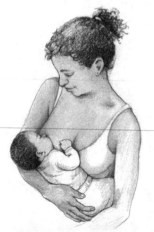

## Cross-cradle or Alternate Cradle Hold

Hold your baby with the arm opposite of the breast from which you're feeding, with his tummy against your chest. For example, if your baby is feeding from your right breast, use your left arm to support his trunk. Support his head with your fingers and thumb on the nape of his neck behind his ears. (Don't press on his head; this may cause him to pull away from your breast.)

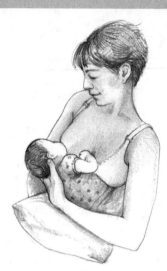

The advantages of this hold are:

- Supporting your baby's neck and shoulders with your hand instead of your forearm allows you and your baby to have more control of his head.
- It's usually the easiest position to learn how to latch him onto your breast.
- It's especially helpful for a premature baby or a baby who's having difficulty latching onto your breast.

## Football or Clutch Hold

Tuck your baby beside your body. Support her body with your arm and cradle the nape of her neck with your fingers and thumb. Bring her up toward your breast as needed so she can easily latch on—she may be lying on her back or side or be sitting up against your chest.

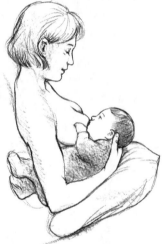

The advantages of this position are:

- It's easy to see that your baby has latched on effectively.
- It may be the most comfortable if you had a cesarean, because your baby isn't pressing on your incision.
- It's helpful if you have large breasts, because your baby's chest helps support your breast.

## Lying Down

Lie on your side with your lower arm tucked around your baby. (Or you can lie on your side with your lower arm placed under your head.) Lay your baby on his side, tucked alongside your body facing your lower breast. Use pillows for your comfort. To feed from the top breast, lean over slightly to bring your nipple toward your baby's mouth.

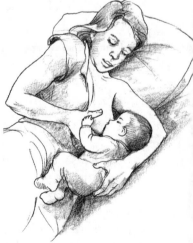

The advantages of this position are:

- It's easy to rest during feedings.
- It's comfortable if you have hemorrhoids or are recovering from an episiotomy or tear.

The disadvantages of this position are:

- It often takes practice to learn.
- It may be difficult to see if your baby has latched on well. Have someone check the latch.

# Helping Your Baby Latch onto Your Breast

1. **Use a comfortable breastfeeding position.** The cross-cradle hold is used in the following example.
2. **Hold your baby close to you.**
   - Have his body touch your chest and his arms near your breast instead of tucked between the two of you. (You may need to lay your other breast over his diaper.)
   - Support his head with your fingers and thumb behind his ears—this allows him to move his head, which will help him latch on more easily. (Avoid pressing on the back of his head with your hand.)
   - If you lean back with your feet up on a footstool, it's easy to keep him near you.
3. **Bring your baby to your breast.** If you hold your breast with your hand, keep your fingers and thumb away from the areola. Allow your breast to remain where it naturally falls and avoid moving it.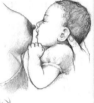
4. **Help your baby have a good, deep latch.**
   - Have his nose and upper lip near your nipple.
   - Press on his upper back so his head tilts back slightly.
   - Place his chin on your breast and his lower lip on the outer edge of areola. This encourages him to open his mouth and grasp the areola and nipple.
   - Wait for him to open his mouth WIDE (as if yawning), then bring his upper lip over the nipple.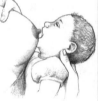
5. **Indicators that your baby has a deep latch on the breast include:**
   - His chin indents your breast and his nose is near or barely touching your breast.
   - He has more areola in his mouth near his lower jaw, and you see more areola above his lips.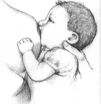
   - You hear and see him swallowing—that is, you hear an "ugh" sound and see a pause in suckling.
   - After feeding, your nipple should be evenly rounded or the same shape as before feeding. It should not looked compressed or have a ridge in the middle or on one side.
6. **Keep your baby close during the feeding.** Press on his upper back with your palm, tuck his bottom in close to you, or lean back. Use pillows to support your arm.

If you have trouble getting a good latch when your breasts are very full, use hand expression to make the areola more graspable. Breast pressure or compression can increase the milk flow, to encourage sucking and swallowing. (See pages 420–421.)

## *Baby Sitting Upright*

Seat your baby on your lap (or on a pillow on your lap) so she faces you and her legs straddle your leg or body. Support her back with your forearm, and support her shoulders and neck with your hand.

The advantages of this position are: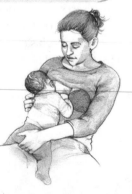
- It's easy to see if your baby has a good latch.
- It's helpful if your baby has gastroesophageal reflux or if you have a very active let-down and a large volume of milk. Sitting upright helps your baby swallow the rapidly flowing milk without difficulty.

# CHALLENGES WITH THE LATCH DURING THE FIRST DAYS

Some babies seem to know how to nurse right from birth, while others seem sleepy or uninterested or have difficulty latching on. (See below.)

During the early feedings, your baby may immediately *latch* onto your breast, tugging and sucking energetically. She may grasp and pull on the nipple so firmly, it surprises you with some discomfort. Or she may tentatively lick and mouth your breast, struggling to get a good latch. Try not to worry if your baby doesn't nurse on the first try or if every feeding seems to take a lot of work before she latches well. If your baby's nose was suctioned at birth, she may need time for the stuffiness to clear before latching onto your breast successfully. A long labor can tire babies, and some medications can make them drowsy or uncoordinated. If your baby is drowsy, try the suggestions on page 415 to rouse her.

You, too, may need rest and nourishment to combat the fatigue of a long, difficult labor. In addition, you may have painful uterine contractions (afterpains) when nursing, especially if this baby isn't your first. Afterpains gradually subside over the first week postpartum, and slow breathing and other relaxation techniques should help you cope in the meantime (see Chapter 11).

Whether your baby nurses well or not, the stimulation of her nuzzling, licking, and closeness to your body encourages milk production. With patience, perseverance, and the help of a knowledgeable lactation consultant or other breastfeeding expert, you and your baby can learn to nurse well.

# WHEN YOUR BABY LATCHES WELL[32]

When your baby latches effectively onto your breast, she can get the milk she needs easily. Signs of a good latch are usually easy to spot. Just before your baby latches on, she opens her mouth as wide as a yawn, with her tongue down and forward. She then draws your nipple and much of the areola into her mouth, giving her a deep latch. Her chin indents your breast and her nose is close to your breast. Her lips (especially the lower lip) are flanged outward and her tongue is extended over her lower gum.

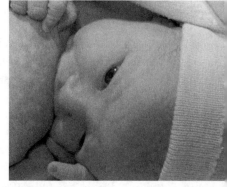

Your baby begins feeding with short, rapid sucks, her jaw moving rhythmically as she suckles. After the milk has let down, she settles into a slower pattern, with bursts of sucking and short pauses. You can hear her swallow. In the first few days, she may need to suckle five to ten times before she has enough milk to swallow. Once the milk has come in, you can hear her swallow each time she suckles. A swallow may sound like a "huh" rather than a loud gulp.

## When Your Baby Doesn't Latch Well

When your baby doesn't latch effectively onto your breast, he might not get enough milk and breastfeeding may become difficult. Like the signs of an effective latch, signs of an ineffective latch are easy to spot:

- Your baby's lips are pursed as though sucking on a straw.
- His cheeks appear sunken, because there's not enough breast tissue to fill his mouth.
- You hear clicking noises during a feeding.
- You don't hear him swallow.
- He slips off your breast and roots frantically.
- You feel nipple pain that continues after the first minute of feeding.

To correct an ineffective latch, contact a lactation consultant or other breastfeeding expert for help.

## WHEN TO FEED YOUR BABY

Your baby shows she's hungry by giving *feeding cues*. Typical feeding cues include the following:

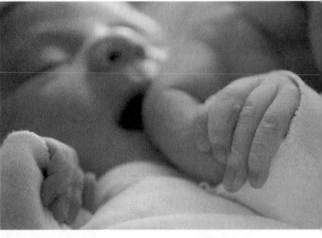

- Your baby roots toward anything that touches her cheeks or lips.
- She brings her hand toward her mouth.
- She thrusts out her tongue often or makes lots of mouth movements.
- She makes lots of body movements.
- She awakens from a drowsy state.

Most babies show these cues to signal hunger long before beginning to fuss or cry, which are last-ditch attempts to communicate their needs. Trying to feed a crying baby is difficult, so watch for your baby's feeding cues and promptly feed her whenever she's hungry.

## BURPING YOUR BABY

When your baby feeds (or cries), he may swallow air that travels to his stomach, causing fullness and possible discomfort. Burping releases the swallowed air, and until he can burp on his own (around two weeks old), he needs help doing so. Even after your baby can burp on his own, he still may need help burping if he gulps air.

If breastfeeding, try burping your baby after he's done nursing at each breast. If bottle-feeding, burp him after he takes two ounces. First, place him in one of the following positions:

- *Over-the-shoulder*: Place your baby high on your chest with his head peeking over your shoulder. Support him well across his back and buttocks.
- *Over-the-lap*: Lay your baby on his tummy across your lap.
- *Sitting and rocking*: Sit your baby on your lap so he faces your side. Place your thumb and index finger under his chin with your palm supporting his chest and your other hand supporting his back. Gently rock him from his front to his back.

Next, gently pat or rub your baby's back. If after a minute or two he hasn't burped, stop trying. He doesn't need to burp.

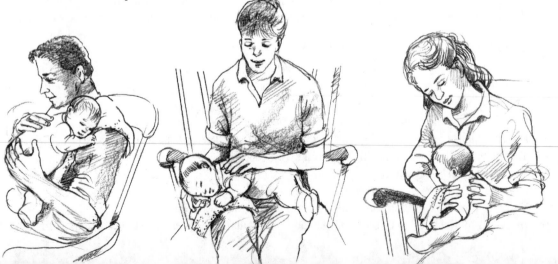

# WHEN YOUR BABY SPITS UP

During or after feedings, many babies *spit up* a dribble or more of milk (up to 2 to 3 tablespoons is common). A newborn has an immature sphincter muscle at the top of the stomach, which lets milk and swallowed air back up the esophagus. Spitting up usually isn't harmful if it occurs only occasionally and the baby is otherwise healthy and growing well. Babies typically outgrow the tendency to spit up around six months old, when they've begun to eat solids.

Your baby is more likely to spit up if you have a strong let-down reflex and an abundant milk supply, causing her to eat too much too quickly or swallow air. Try leaning back when nursing or sitting your baby up during feedings, to help her manage the rapid milk flow. (See page 408.) Your baby may also spit up if she cries hard before a feeding.

You can reduce spitting up by burping your baby when she's done nursing from each breast. (If feeding your baby formula, burp her after every 2 ounces she consumes, and don't overfeed her.) To keep milk in your baby's stomach after a feeding, gently position her upright in your arms, on her side if she's awake, or sitting in a car seat or swing with her head elevated.

If your baby continuously spits up or frequently vomits with force (projectile vomiting), she may have a more serious condition. Call your baby's caregiver when you see the following signs:

- Your baby seems in pain when spitting up (may be gastroesophageal reflux—see page 380).
- Your baby vomits after every feeding and doesn't poop frequently.
- Your baby vomits after each of two to three consecutive feedings and seems weak, limp, or lethargic.

# Your Baby's Feeding Patterns

During the first days, weeks, and months of your baby's life, the frequency and duration of his feedings change to facilitate his growth. A nursing mother's breasts adapt to these changes to meet baby's changing needs. This section describes typical feeding patterns of babies.

## THE FIRST DAYS AFTER THE BIRTH

After feeding vigorously during the first few hours postpartum, many healthy newborns show little interest in eating until they're twenty to twenty-four hours old. By that time, most babies perk up and are eager to feed again.[33] However, mothers should keep trying to feed their babies throughout the first day.

As your newborn becomes more awake after the birth, she may want to feed more frequently,[34] perhaps in clusters (feeding five or more times in three hours followed by a period of deep sleep) or constantly until your milk comes in. To help ensure your milk comes in soon and in an ample volume, watch for your baby's feeding cues (see page 410) and feed her as soon as you see these signs. Newborns need to feed at least eight times every twenty-four hours (that is, about once every three hours), but some may feed fifteen to eighteen times during the first days.

### Increasing Breastfeeding Success during the First Days

If your baby nurses well soon after the birth, breastfeeding has gotten off to a good start. Watch for your baby's feeding cues and feed him when he's hungry, or at least once every three hours.

Babies nurse most vigorously at the first breast offered. Let your baby nurse from the first breast for as long as he likes (ten to thirty minutes on average in the early days). When he detaches from the breast on his own, offer the other breast. (He might or might not take it.) Begin the next feeding with the breast you offered second at the previous feeding. By alternating the breast you offer first, you make sure your baby's suckling stimulates both breasts to make milk. If you forget which breast to offer first at the next feeding, press your fingertips against your breasts and offer the one that feels most full.

If your baby remains with you after the birth, you can watch for his feeding cues and feed him when he wants. If your baby spends time in the hospital nursery, you must rely on the nursing staff to let you know when he's hungry. Request that the staff bring your baby to you for feeding, day or night.

Also make sure to ask the staff not to give your baby any bottles. When full-term, healthy babies breastfeed frequently in response to their feeding cues, they don't need supplemental bottles of formula, sugar water, or plain water. In fact, the routine use of supplemental bottles can increase problems with breastfeeding by diminishing your baby's hunger and interfering with his desire to nurse. When your baby spends less time at your breast, your milk supply might not increase enough to meet his needs.

Additionally, sucking on a bottle nipple is entirely different from suckling at a breast. A newborn who feeds from both a bottle and a breast may develop *nipple confusion* (difficulty adapting to different sucking patterns and differences in flow). If a baby has trouble breastfeeding, he may find feeding from a bottle easier and begin to refuse the breast.[35]

Pacifiers can also cause problems with breastfeeding in the first days and weeks after the birth. Using pacifiers to delay feedings or to distract your newborn interferes with your development of an adequate milk supply. Pacifiers also may diminish your baby's interest in feeding by satisfying his need to suck, which may lead to poor weight gain. (See page 414.) Avoid offering your baby a pacifier until after breastfeeding is well established.

If your baby hasn't nursed well before you're both discharged from the hospital (or after the first day following a home birth or birth-center birth), get help from a lactation consultant or other breastfeeding expert right away to prevent your baby from becoming dehydrated or losing too much weight.

## THE FIRST WEEKS AFTER THE BIRTH

If your baby is nursing frequently, you can expect your milk to come in on the second to fifth day after the birth. When this happens, your body gradually stops making only colostrum and begins to make milk. When your milk comes in, your breasts become heavy, full, and tender. Your nipples may appear flattened because of the swelling. You may begin to seek ways to relieve breast fullness (see page 419).

As your baby gets older, she begins to eat every one to three hours. As the weeks pass, she consumes more milk at each feeding, which may reduce the number of feedings. She also begins to feed less at night and more during the day and evening. Because babies don't always eat on a regular schedule, your baby may cluster her feedings, eating four to five times in five to six hours and then sleeping for several hours.

## THE FIRST MONTHS AFTER THE BIRTH

When your baby is two to three weeks old and has recovered from the birth, he begins to fuss and fret for about an hour (or longer) every evening as a way to cope with new stimulation. During this time, your baby cries, feeds frequently (as often as every thirty to forty minutes), takes brief rests, then cries and feeds again. The frequent nursing stimulates your breasts to make more milk to meet your baby's greater needs. See page 379 for ways to soothe a fussy baby.

Your baby also may experience similar fussy and challenging stages at ages six weeks, three months, and six months. At these times, babies are acquiring new skills. At three weeks old, your baby awakens to his world. (See page 383.) At about six weeks old, he starts to interact with others by smiling. At three months old, he's very alert to his surroundings, recognizes one parent from another, and can become easily overstimulated. At about six months old, he masters sitting unaided.

The acquisition of new skills can affect feeding and sleep patterns until your baby masters them. For example, when he's around three months old, his environment may so distract him that he eats less frequently during the day, only to wake more at night to feed. Don't let these changes trouble you. Feeding your baby in a quiet, dimly lit (even dark) place can help him feed more during the day. Usually within a few days to a week, your baby returns to a more predictable feeding pattern.

# Making Sure Your Baby Is Getting Enough Breast Milk

By the third or fourth day after the birth, most babies lose from 5 to 8 percent of their birth weight. Once their mothers' milk is in, babies steadily gain weight. Full-term babies usually regain the weight they lost and return to their birth weight by the tenth to fourteenth day postpartum.

After your milk comes in (around the third to fifth day postpartum), you can watch for the following six signs to ensure that your baby is getting enough of your milk.

**Suckles frequently**

Your baby feeds vigorously at least eight to twelve times in twenty-four hours.

**Swallowing**

You hear your baby swallow often. Sometimes during a feeding, he swallows after every suck. Sometimes he sucks a few times before swallowing. He fully extends his jaw when swallowing.

**Satisfaction**

Your baby seems satisfied after most feedings. Your breast feels softer.

**Soaking**

For the first week after the birth, expect the number of wet diapers to at least equal the day of your baby's life (for example, he should wet three or more diapers on day three). After your milk comes in, expect at least six to eight wet cloth diapers in twenty-four hours. Because disposable diapers wick away moisture from your baby's skin, it's difficult to tell how often he's urinating. If using disposables, place a tissue or small piece of paper towel in your baby's diaper where his urine will wet it.

**Stools**

After your milk comes in, your baby produces at least three poopy diapers in twenty-four hours. The stools usually are yellow and seedy. For the first month or so after the birth, many babies poop after almost every feeding, or up to twelve times per day. Later on, they usually poop less often.

# Signs That Your Baby Isn't Getting Enough

When your baby doesn't get enough of your milk, her risk of dehydration or problems with weight gain increase. If you observe any of these signs, schedule an appointment with your baby's caregiver to have your baby assessed and weighed:

- Your baby feeds fewer than eight times in twenty-four hours.
- She doesn't produce at least one poopy diaper in twenty-four hours.
- She has few wet diapers or produces urine that appears to have reddish "brick dust" in it.
- Your baby seems constantly hungry and is seldom content after feedings.
- Your baby's feedings worry or concern you.

Some signs are more serious than others. If you notice any of the following signs, call your baby's caregiver immediately:

- Your baby is lethargic and has no interest in nursing.
- The inside of her mouth doesn't glisten with moisture. (A baby's lips can appear dry normally).
- When you gently pinch the skin on her arm, leg, or abdomen and then let go, her skin stays "tented."
- Her eyes, face, chest, and abdomen are yellow. (See page 416 for more on jaundice symptoms.)

**Scales**

Your baby should gain ½ to 1½ ounces per day. When he isn't getting enough milk, other signs besides poor weight gain present themselves. (See above.)

If your baby's weight doesn't return to his birth weight ten to fourteen days postpartum, there are two possible explanations:

- Your baby has trouble getting enough milk.
- You might not be producing enough milk and need to take measures to increase your milk supply. (See page 416.)

## WHEN YOUR BABY DOESN'T GET ENOUGH MILK

Following are several possible reasons why a baby can't get enough milk. In some cases, babies are the cause; in others, parents or other caregivers introduce the problem. In still other cases, a medical condition prevents babies from nursing effectively.

**Ineffective latch**

If a baby can't latch well onto the breast, she can't get enough milk. (See page 409.) If you can't help your baby latch well, get help from a lactation consultant. Most latch problems can be corrected; the sooner you get help, the sooner you can resolve the problem.

**Scheduled feedings**

Breastfed newborns, especially ones who gain weight slowly, need to feed more frequently than once every three hours. All newborns need to feed at night; feeding shouldn't be postponed until the morning. Feed your baby whenever she shows an interest in nursing, day or night. (See page 410 for feeding cues.) Let her nurse for as long as she wants.

## Feeding from only one breast

If you offer your baby only one breast, you risk inadequate milk production and may limit the amount of milk she gets. Always offer your baby the second breast. For the first week, she may nurse very little from the second breast, but she may want to nurse from both breasts as she grows over the next month or so. When your baby is a month or two old, she may nurse from only one breast at most feedings if you have a good milk supply.

## Pacifiers

Giving babies pacifiers can lead to faulty sucking patterns and may shorten the overall duration of breastfeeding.[36] If you try to soothe your baby or delay a feeding by giving her a pacifier, she may develop an inability to suckle effectively at the breast, which may slow her weight gain. For breast-feeding success, avoid using pacifiers, especially in the early weeks of breastfeeding.

## Sleepy baby

Most parents appreciate a baby who sleeps a lot, but long periods between feedings may prevent your baby from getting enough milk. For the first month after the birth, especially if your baby isn't gaining weight well, try waking her every two to three hours during the day and every three to four hours at night. If she sleeps so soundly that you simply can't wake her, wait thirty minutes and try again. Your baby might not get much milk if she's very drowsy during feedings, pauses for long intervals, or falls asleep even though she spends a long time at the breast. See below for suggestions on how to wake a sleepy baby. If she remains sleepy or lethargic and you can't get her to nurse, call her caregiver.

*Note:* After a baby has returned to her birth weight (usually ten to fourteen days postpartum) and is growing well, you don't need to wake her for feedings.

## How to Wake a Sleepy Baby

Once newborn babies are twenty-four hours old, they need to feed at least eight times in a 24-hour period. If your baby doesn't awaken from a light sleep to feed, try these suggestions to wake him:

- If he's swaddled, unwrap him. Remove his clothes (leaving just a diaper).
- Dim the lights so he can open his eyes. Talk to him.
- Hold him in a supported standing or sitting position.
- Massage his arms, legs, and chest.
- Rub expressed colostrum or milk onto his lips. Be patient; if he only nuzzles at first, that's a good start.
- Press on your breast to enhance milk flow and entice him to suckle more vigorously. (See page 421.)
- Burp him (see page 410) or change his diaper.
- Change to another feeding position or switch to your other breast.

After you've tried for ten to fifteen minutes to wake your baby, let him sleep in your arms and try again when he starts to waken.

If you continue to have trouble feeding a sleepy baby, get the help of a nurse, lactation consultant, or breastfeeding expert. If your baby isn't breastfeeding well by twenty-four hours after the birth, ask about using a breast pump to express your milk. Pumping stimulates your breasts to make more milk and ensures that your baby gets your colostrum.

**Jaundice**

High levels of bilirubin in the blood cause jaundice (see page 389), which causes a yellowish tint on the face, chest, abdomen, and the whites of eyes. If your baby exhibits these signs, call her caregiver. Getting an inadequate amount of milk increases the incidence of jaundice, which sometimes appears in the first two weeks after the birth. Jaundiced babies are often sleepy and uninterested in feeding; this disinterest can further diminish milk intake. Frequent breastfeeding helps relieve jaundice. Avoid giving your baby bottles of water; bilirubin isn't excreted in urine, and water supplements may reduce the amount of milk your baby consumes. Once jaundice is treated, your baby becomes more interested in feeding.

# INADEQUATE MILK SUPPLY

Sometimes, a baby doesn't get enough milk because his mother isn't producing enough to meet his current needs. If your milk supply can't meet your baby's needs, try the following suggestions:

- Feed frequently, at least eight to twelve times in twenty-four hours.
- Never limit feedings. Let your baby feed for as long as he likes. (Usually ten to thirty minutes at each breast.)
- Make sure that your baby latches well onto your breast and that you can hear him swallow as he suckles. If you don't, detach him from your breast and have him latch on again.
- To reduce your stress and increase breast stimulation, have a "babymoon." That is, spend a full twenty-four hours in bed with your baby. Pick a time when you can enlist a postpartum doula (see page 27), family, or friends to help with meals, household chores, and other children so you don't have to leave the bed except to use the bathroom. Spend the day nursing as often as possible, snuggling skin-to-skin with your baby, eating and drinking well, sleeping, nurturing yourself, and letting others nurture you. Besides helping restore your milk supply and letting you catch up on needed rest, this time of unrestricted nursing can help improve your baby's weight gain and provide a wonderful opportunity to learn about him.
- Get help from a lactation consultant, who may suggest the following:
  * Rent a commercial-grade electric double breast pump. Pump after each feeding for ten to fifteen minutes. (If your baby can't nurse, you can still build your milk supply by pumping whenever he takes a bottle.)
  * If you need to supplement your baby's feedings, use a syringe or feeding device to feed your expressed breast milk (or prescribed formula) to him through a tube attached to your breast. (See page 426.) This way, your baby receives all his milk from your breast and stimulates it to make more milk.
- Take an herbal medication such as fenugreek, by itself or with blessed thistle, to possibly increase your milk supply. Your lactation consultant or caregiver can tell you how much to take and let you know when you shouldn't take an herbal medication (for example, if you're diabetic).
- Take a prescribed medication such as Reglan or Domperidone. The latter isn't available in U.S. pharmacies, but your lactation consultant can help you obtain it when appropriate. Domperidone has fewer side effects than Reglan, and the American Academy of Pediatrics (AAP) has approved it for nursing mothers.[37] Because of the potential risks of Reglan, try using the other measures listed above before taking it.

## When Your Milk Supply Dwindles

You've had an adequate milk supply and your baby has gained weight well, but lately you've noticed your milk supply has decreased. What's the problem? Consider the following possibilities, all of which can reduce your milk supply:

- You've begun to take birth control pills containing estrogen.
- You've begun using a prescribed estrogen cream to treat vaginal dryness.
- You've recently returned to work or another time-consuming activity, which has made you nurse less frequently.
- You're offering your baby more supplemental bottles and not breastfeeding as often.
- You're possibly pregnant.

If you can determine the reason for your dwindling milk supply, take the steps on page 416 to increase it. If you don't produce more milk, seek a lactation consultant for help.

## When You Have a Problem with Let-down

Extreme stress, inadequate nipple stimulation, and excessive amounts of alcohol, caffeine, and tobacco may delay or inhibit the let-down reflex.[38] To help resolve this problem, try to reduce your stress, give your baby full access to your nipples as she latches onto the breast, and eliminate or limit your intake of alcohol, caffeine, and tobacco. If the let-down reflex continues to give you trouble, contact a lactation consultant for help.

## Common Q & A

**Q:** My wife is exclusively breastfeeding our son. Is there anything I can do to help?

**A:** A father, partner, or other person provides a breastfeeding mom with extra pairs of eyes, ears, and hands. Sometimes a mom has trouble seeing if the baby is latching onto the breast well. You can help check the latch. As your baby latches onto the breast, you can hold his hands out of the way until he has latched on.

You can also help evaluate how much milk your baby consumes by watching for rhythmic jaw movements and periodic pauses, and listening for swallowing noises that sound like "huh."

# Your Nutrition While Breastfeeding

During pregnancy, your body prepares for lactation by storing 5 to 7 pounds of extra fat to provide some of the extra calories necessary for milk production in the early months. In the first month after the birth, you lose a large amount of the weight you gained during pregnancy, but you may maintain some (or all) of this extra fat for the entire time you breastfeed.

In addition to the stored fat, your body draws on your vitamin and mineral reserves to make milk. Although your body can produce plenty of healthy breast milk regardless of what you eat, eating a poor diet may deplete your nutritional stores over time. Eating poorly also affects your health and your overall well-being.

To maintain your nutritional stores, make sure your diet consists of a variety of healthy foods and includes additional protein (which helps produce milk) and calcium. Many women's diets don't include enough calcium, as well as vitamin B, thiamine, folic acid, vitamin D, zinc, and magnesium.[39] A diet that's deficient of these vitamins and minerals reduces a mother's nutritional stores and poses health risks for both her and her baby.[40,41] If your diet doesn't contain adequate amounts of these vitamins and minerals for breastfeeding (see page 403), your caregiver may recommend that you take a vitamin and mineral supplement.

During pregnancy, you may have avoided eating certain foods that might have posed a health risk to your baby, such as soft cheeses, raw fish, and luncheon meats. Happily for you, eating these foods—and generally all foods—doesn't harm your breast milk and doesn't harm your baby when he consumes it. An old wives' tale warns that nursing women should avoid eating cabbage, broccoli, and spicy foods to prevent their babies from developing colic, but there's no evidence to support this theory. (See page 419 for information on food sensitivity.)

Instead, the foods you eat flavor your breast milk, which benefits your baby by introducing the flavors of foods he'll eventually eat at the family table. For example, researchers found that babies drank more breast milk when their mothers took garlic capsules.[42] Researchers also found that breastfed babies ate peas and beans more readily than did formula-fed babies,[43] likely because they recognized the flavors of these vegetables in their mothers' milk.

Contrary to myth, increasing the volume of fluids you drink doesn't increase your milk production. Having a well-hydrated body simply keeps you from feeling thirsty and maintains your overall well-being. You know you're drinking enough fluids when your urine is pale yellow.

What about caffeine? Will a cup or two of coffee affect breast milk? How about a little chocolate (which contains a chemical that's similar to caffeine)? If you drink caffeinated beverages or eat foods with caffeine, know that less than 1 percent of the caffeine you consume appears in your breast milk. Consuming a serving or two a day doesn't affect your baby. If, however, you limited caffeine consumption during pregnancy, you may find you're sensitive to it postpartum.

What about alcohol? When you drink an alcoholic beverage, the concentration of alcohol in your blood approximately equals the alcohol content in your breast milk. This means that the effects of the alcohol on your baby when he consumes your milk corresponds to the amount of alcohol you drank. Although research hasn't shown that consuming the occasional drink is harmful, it's generally best to avoid drinking alcohol or drink only occasionally until after your baby is weaned. Researchers found that babies consumed less breast milk after their mothers drank alcohol than did babies whose mothers didn't drink before nursing.[44]

If you drink alcohol, consume it in moderation. Don't drink more than 8 ounces of wine, two beers, or 2 ounces of liquor per day.[45] In addition, breastfeed your baby before having a drink. That way, you satisfy his needs and allow time for the reduction or elimination of the alcohol in your bloodstream (and breast milk) before he needs to nurse again.

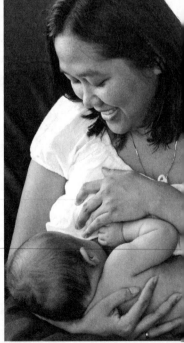

What about dieting? By three months after the birth, many women have burned the 5 to 7 pounds of fat they acquired during pregnancy for milk production. After you've reached your prepregnancy or desired weight, consume enough calories to maintain your weight. Compared to the number of calories you required before pregnancy, you may need only about 300 more calories per day while breastfeeding. (If you're breastfeeding multiples or a newborn and a toddler, you need more calories.)

If, however, you haven't shed the extra weight and find those extra pounds frustrating, limit your weight loss to 1 pound per week. Be sure to consume at least 1,500 calories a day and avoid liquid diets and diet medications. Severely restricting calories compromises your nutritional health and may make you produce less breast milk.[46]

# FOOD SENSITIVITY

In rare cases, a mother eats a food that adversely affects her baby. For example, the baby may become excessively fussy or develop eczema (patches of dry skin), a rash, or diarrhea after consuming breast milk containing protein from certain foods. A baby born into a family with a history of food allergies may react to some of the foods her mother eats. The most common food allergens include cow milk, soy, wheat, eggs, fish, shellfish, and nuts.

If you think a certain food bothers your baby, eliminate it from your diet for a week or so and see if your baby improves. (If you eliminate milk, be sure to get enough calcium from other foods or a supplement.) Discuss your concerns with a lactation consultant or your baby's caregiver. He or she can help you identify the food causing your baby's problem and provide you with nutritional guidelines.

Some babies react negatively when their mothers eat large quantities of certain foods. For instance, if you eat an entire bowl of cherries, drink a pitcher of juice, or consume an enormous amount of chocolate, your baby may become fussy or otherwise bothered after nursing. The solution is prevention: Eat all foods in moderation.

Some foods (such as kelp, seaweed, or those containing artificial colors) and vitamin and mineral supplements can tint the color of breast milk, but they don't pose problems for babies.

# Early Breastfeeding Challenges and Solutions

Almost every woman has questions or challenges with breastfeeding in the first months. Some are serious and require more information and assistance, but others are common, predictable, and can be handled easily.

## BREAST FULLNESS AND TENDERNESS

When your breasts are full, the best way to relieve the normal discomfort and swelling you experience is to nurse frequently. Full breasts can lead to swollen, flattened nipples and areolae, which your baby may have trouble latching onto. You can soften your nipple and areola by hand-expressing a few drops of milk. (See page 420.) Applying warm packs or standing in a warm shower may also start milk flow, making the areola softer and easier for your baby to latch onto. Once your baby is feeding, press on your breasts (see page 421) to enhance milk flow. Let your baby feed for as long as she wants on the first breast. If she doesn't feed from the other breast, hand-express or use a pump to reduce fullness in that breast. If your baby can't nurse even after you've expressed milk from your breast, seek a lactation consultant for help and support.

If your breasts are tender after feeding, apply a cool, moist pack or an ice pack to your breasts. If you use an ice pack, first wrap it in a dishtowel or apply it over light clothing. Some women find applying cool cabbage leaves to their swollen breasts reduces tenderness and swelling. Although science hasn't confirmed the leaves' effectiveness, they do no harm and may be soothing.[47] You may take ibuprofen to reduce discomfort and relieve inflammation.

The fullness and tenderness you experience when your milk comes in is sometimes called engorgement, but these feelings aren't symptoms of true engorgement, which is a more serious condition caused by unrelieved breast fullness. True engorgement may produce a fever higher than 101°F (38°C), acute continuing breast pain, tingling and numbness in the arm and fingers,[48] and difficulty removing milk from the breasts even with a pump. Although the breast fullness and

## Softening Your Areola by Hand Expression

To soften your nipples to make them easier for your baby to grasp, follow these steps before he latches on.

1. Place your thumb at the top edge of your areola (where it meets your skin) and your fingers on the bottom edge.
2. Lift your breast with your fingers and thumb. (To keep them from slipping to the end of your nipple, gently press your breast toward your chest with your hand.)
3. Gently squeeze your breast for five to ten seconds. Then move your fingers and thumb to other locations at the edge of your areola. Continue squeezing and pressing your breast against your body until milk releases.
4. Stop when you see a few drops of milk or when the areola is smaller in diameter.

tenderness when milk comes in usually don't last longer than a day or two and can be relieved by the mother, treating true engorgement may require the help of a lactation consultant.

## SORE NIPPLES

Your nipples may become sore any time you breastfeed, but sore nipples are most common during the first weeks. You may have sore nipples only when your baby first latches on, or the soreness may last throughout the entire feeding and between feedings. Sore nipples may cause discomfort or intense pain, but treatment almost always resolves the problem.

For example, a common cause of nipple soreness is overly vigorous or incorrect pumping. To fix this problem, carefully read the information on page 425 about correct pumping. Other common causes for sore nipples include the following.

### Early Tenderness

Research shows that most women's nipples are tender at the beginning of feedings, but the tenderness usually lasts only a few weeks.[49] As your baby learns to nurse, his mouth tugs, compresses, and rubs your nipple and areola. The resulting discomfort can make you stiffen in pain and breathe rapidly. As the feeding progresses for thirty seconds or so, the pain lessens or ends. After the feeding, your nipples may appear slightly reddened, bruised, or swollen. To help reduce or prevent early tenderness, hand-express a few drops of milk to soften the areola before feeding, then help your baby latch on well.

### Poor Latch

If your nipples remain sore throughout the feeding (and possibly afterward) or they begin to crack and even bleed, a poor latch is likely the cause. A baby might not latch on well if her mothers' breasts are too full or are engorged, or they have flat or inverted nipples. A baby also may have trouble latching on if she bites instead of suckles, if she tucks her lower lip inward during feedings, or if her mouth is only slightly open (not wide open) and she latches onto only the nipple.

# Enhancing Milk Flow with Breast Pressure and Compression

When your breasts are very full, pressing on your breast helps the milk flow toward your nipple. Sometimes called breast massage, this method doesn't call for you to rub your breast in circles. Instead, you apply breast pressure or compression. With these techniques, you press milk toward the nipple openings and into your baby's mouth, which prompts a burst of suckling.

**Breast pressure**

1. When your baby takes long pauses at the breast or stops suckling, put your palm on your chest near the outer edge of your breast.
2. Slide your palm on your breast until you feel the firm milk glands.
3. Press gently from the outer breast toward the nipple. Stop before you get close to the areola. Pressing near the areola can affect your baby's latch.
4. When your baby begins to suckle less, move your hand to another part of your breast and repeat these steps.

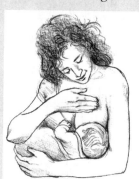

This technique helps relieve breast fullness, helps empty plugged ducts, and provides more high-calorie hindmilk for your baby.[50]

**Breast compression**

1. Cup your breast with your hand, placing your thumb and one to two fingers near the outer part of your breast.
2. Squeeze your finger(s) and thumb together and slightly press into your breast, then out toward your nipple.
3. When your baby begins to suckle less, cup your breast in another position on the breast and compress it again.

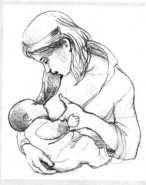

This technique helps babies eat more, especially those who are gaining weight slowly, and entices sleepy babies to continue feeding.

Premature or ill babies may latch on poorly. A neurological or anatomical condition may prevent otherwise healthy babies from latching on and sucking well. For example, a tight frenulum ("tongue tie") describes a condition in which the thin membrane that extends from the bottom of the tongue is too short to let the tongue protrude from the mouth.

Having sore nipples because of a poor latch can make you dread breastfeeding. Here are suggestions for prevention and treatment:

- Correct the latch. (See page 409.) Correcting a poor latch relieves most of the soreness instantly, even if your nipple is cracked and bleeding.
- Nurse frequently. If you delay feeding, your breasts become fuller, making it more difficult for your baby to latch on.
- Start on the least sore breast, because babies feed vigorously at the beginning of a feeding.
- To soften the areola and make latching on easier, hand-express some milk before feeding. (See page 420.)
- If you're sore where your baby's bottom lip rests on your breast, she may be tucking that lip inward over her gum. Gently pull her lip out when she feeds.
- Before pulling your baby from the breast to reposition her, first slip your finger into her

## Advice from the Authors

When you have breastfeeding questions, concerns, or need extra encouragement, consider these sources of support:

- Your caregiver or your baby's caregiver
- Hospital staff (Ask if they have a breastfeeding hotline or if it's okay to call the labor and delivery unit with questions.)
- Lactation consultant
- Physician specializing in breastfeeding medicine
- La Leche League group or any new moms' support group
- Someone who has successfully breastfed her baby
- National Women's Health Center: http://www.women shealth.gov/
- Web sites on breastfeeding support, including http:// www.womenshealth.gov/ breastfeeding, http://www.llli .org, http://www.breastfeeding .com, and http://www.breast feedingonline.com
- Online forums on breastfeed ing, including http://forums .llli.org/, http://www.mother ing.com/discussions/, and http://www.kellymom.com

mouth and break the suction so your nipple comes out easily.

- If you use nursing pads, change them whenever they become wet.
- Take a pain relief medication, such as ibuprofen.
- See a lactation consultant. This professional can help you with your baby's latch and suggest treatments that promote healing. She may recommend using a nipple shield during feedings to protect your nipple, help with the latch, and encourage a flat nipple to protrude. She may suggest using special nipple creams or a hydrogel dressing (a gel-like pad that may increase comfort and speed healing). If infection or allergy may be the cause, she may encourage you to see your caregiver, a physician specializing in breastfeeding medicine, or a dermatologist. If a tight frenulum is interfering with breastfeeding, she may refer your baby to a physician skilled in breastfeeding medicine, who may suggest clipping the frenulum (a minor procedure) to free the baby's tongue and solve the latch problem.

## Infection

Persistently sore breasts or nipples (often cracked and bleeding) are typically the result of a bacterial infection (most often *Staphylococcus aureus*), a fungal (yeast) infection, or a herpes infection.

If the infection is herpes, you *must* discontinue breastfeeding on that breast until the herpes sore heals.

To determine whether the infection is bacterial, physicians take a culture of the area. If the infection is bacterial, physicians may prescribe a topical antibiotic cream or suggest using a combination cream to treat bacterial and yeast infections and reduce inflammation. They occasionally recommend oral antibiotics.

Yeast infections cause soreness less often than other infections. If you have a yeast infection, your nipples may look dark pink, shiny, and irritated, or they may look normal. Small blisters may appear. Antibiotic therapy often precedes yeast infections, and a vaginal yeast infection can lead to a yeast infection of the nipples. Yeast infections also occur when a baby has a yeast diaper rash or has a yeast infection of the mouth (thrush).

For a yeast infection, both you and your baby need treatment. Consult with your caregiver or a lactation with consultant for suggestions. Eating yogurt is one home remedy you may try, either by itself or in combination with other treatments. Be sure the yogurt contains live cultures, particularly acidophilus and bifidus, to restore the delicate balance of microorganisms in your body. Stress or antibiotic use can upset this balance and cause an overgrowth of yeast. Experts haven't determined just how much yogurt you should eat to see improvement or a cure, but it doesn't harm you to eat a comfortable amount.[51] If you don't care for yogurt, consider taking acidophilus pills or probiotics.

Your caregiver also may prescribe an oral medication for you and may suggest using a topical over-the-counter anti-fungal cream to treat your nipples and your baby's diaper rash. Your baby's caregiver may prescribe a liquid medication, such as nystatin suspension, to apply to your baby's mouth. If these treatments don't work, your lactation consultant can suggest other treatment options.

## BREAST PAIN CAUSED BY LET-DOWN

At the beginning of a feeding, some women experience a sharp, deep pain behind the areola that subsides when the milk begins to flow. This pain doesn't indicate a problem and usually disappears over time without treatment. Oxytocin is probably the cause; the release of this hormone shortens and widens the ducts, thereby increasing pressure as milk flows through them. If you had breast surgery, let-down may stretch scar tissue and cause pain. Slow breathing may help relieve pain (see page 224).

## LEAKING

During the first few weeks or months of breastfeeding, your breasts may leak milk. As your breasts "learn" how much milk to make and when to let down, the leaking usually subsides. Leaking typically occurs when your breasts are very full, when you hear your baby cry, or when you're sexually aroused. Here are some suggestions for preventing or minimizing leaking:

- When you start to feel your milk let down, discreetly press your hands or forearms firmly against your breasts to slow the milk flow.
- Compress your nipple between your thumb and index finger to stop the flow.
- To prevent soaking your clothes, wear washable cotton or wool nursing pads or disposable pads and change them when they become damp. Avoid using nursing pads with plastic liners; they retain moisture, which contributes to nipple soreness. Some mothers like using silicone pads that exert gentle pressure over the areolae to stop leaking. (Lilypadz is a popular brand.)

## PLUGGED DUCTS

If your breast gradually develops a tender, swollen lump or a sore area (but you don't have a fever), you probably have a plugged duct. The area near the plugged duct may be reddened. These suggestions help relieve discomfort:

- Apply a warm, moist washcloth to the sore area before and during feedings.
- Feed from the sore breast first.
- Press from behind the sore area toward the nipple during feedings. (See page 421.)
- Nurse your baby in a different position so his mouth puts pressure on different places on the breast.
- While showering, massage your breast, pressing from the plugged duct toward the nipple.
- Avoid wearing poorly fitting bras; they may obstruct milk ducts. Also, check the fit of your baby carrier. Some carriers' straps press on your breasts and affect milk flow.
- Pay attention when using a breast pump. Pressing the flange unevenly on your breast can reduce milk flow in one area.

It may take a few days to clear a plugged duct, but have your caregiver evaluate any lump that doesn't disappear within a week or two.

## MASTITIS

*Mastitis* is an infection of the breast that appears suddenly and can occur any time while you're nursing. Besides a tender, reddened breast, symptoms include fever, chills, fatigue, headache, and sometimes nausea and vomiting. Health care providers consider these flu-like symptoms in a breastfeeding woman to be mastitis until proven otherwise. If you have these symptoms, call your caregiver. He or she may prescribe antibiotics and advise you to do the following:

- Continue to nurse from both breasts. The milk isn't infected and doesn't harm your baby.
- Take all the prescribed antibiotics. If you stop taking the antibiotics when you start to feel better, the infection will return.
- Rest in bed until you feel better. Drink plenty of fluids.
- Apply a warm, wet washcloth on the painful area to help increase blood circulation to the breast.
- Take ibuprofen or acetaminophen to reduce fever, pain, and inflammation.
- Avoid wearing constricting bras and clothing so milk can flow easily. During feedings, massage or gently rub your breasts if pressure around the sore area feels good.

If you don't feel better within twenty-four hours after starting antibiotic treatment, call your caregiver. You may need a different antibiotic.

# Expressing and Storing Breast Milk

When your baby isn't available or able to nurse, you need to *express* your milk to relieve fullness and maintain your milk supply. Although expressing your milk by hand or by pump may seem daunting, both become easier with practice. For either method, all you need are clean hands, clean equipment, and clean containers for storing your milk.

## HAND EXPRESSION

This method is effective, inexpensive, and always available. (See page 420.) When you first learn to express by hand, you may get only drops of milk. You soon express a steady spray of milk after a little practice. Collect your milk in a measuring cup or special milk-collecting device.

## WHEN PUMPING IS HELPFUL OR NECESSARY

In the following situations, using a pump to express your milk is more efficient and desirable than hand-expressing:

- You must leave your baby because of travel or work outside your home.
- Your baby is in the neonatal intensive care unit (NICU) or special care nursery and can't breast-feed or can't yet feed frequently or vigorously.
- You're trying to build or rebuild your milk supply.
- Your baby can't get enough milk by breastfeeding alone and must have supplemental breast milk.
- You're having a medical procedure that requires you to take a medication that's unsafe for your baby. You may need to temporarily stop breastfeeding, but you can still maintain your milk supply by pumping until breastfeeding is safe to resume. In this case, you *don't* save the pumped milk for your baby to drink later.

# FINDING AND USING A BREAST PUMP

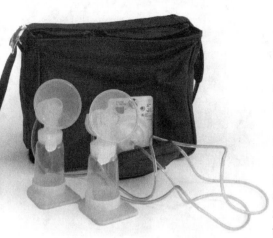

A lactation consultant, La Leche League Leader, or your caregiver can help you select a pump. (You may also visit http://www.kellymom.com for a discussion on pump selection.) If your baby needs only an occasional bottle, hand expression or a manual pump is sufficient to collect the milk. If you need to pump several bottles a day or if you're building or maintaining your milk supply, you may need an electric pump. Commercial-grade electric double breast pumps are the most efficient and effective; they're available to rent. Or you can purchase a personal-use model, which is almost as effective. Be sure to follow the directions for use.

When using a pump, always center your nipple in the pump cup (flange). When the nipple isn't centered, friction on the areola causes soreness. Use only enough suction to make milk flow well. Too much suction stretches the areola and pulls it too deeply into the pump cup, possibly injuring the tissue and causing nipple soreness. Many pumps come with different-size pump cups to fit different breasts. Some have a soft silicone insert to increase comfort. If your pump's cup seems too large or too small, check with the pump manufacturer to find the right size for you.

If you want to multitask while pumping, you can buy a device to hold an electric pump's cups in place so you can use your hands for other tasks. To make your own "handsfree" device, buy an inexpensive sports bra and cut slits in the center of each bra cup that are wide enough to hold the pump cups snugly against your breasts.

The following suggestions may help increase milk flow when pumping:
- Find a private, warm environment that's free of interruptions and distractions.
- Before pumping, cup your breasts and gently but firmly stroke them from your chest toward your areola. You can also jiggle or gently shake your breasts, or stroke them lightly with your fingertips to simulate the sensations of let-down.
- Develop a pumping ritual such as having a cup of tea or listening to relaxing music.
- Imagine you're nursing your baby or look at photos of your baby and visualize your milk flowing.

## STORING BREAST MILK

You can store expressed breast milk in clean glass bottles or jars, plastic bottles, or feeding bags designed for breast milk storage. Experts debate whether glass or plastic is the safest container for breast milk; see page 436 for further information.

## USING STORED BREAST MILK

Use stored breast milk in the following order:
1. Freshly expressed milk
2. Newly refrigerated milk, then all other refrigerated milk
3. Frozen milk (use oldest container first, to keep your entire supply as fresh as possible)

## How to Store Breast Milk

The following guidelines explain where and how long to store breast milk for healthy, full-term babies. (Mothers whose babies are ill or premature may need to follow other storage guidelines.) When storing milk for longer than a day, label the container with the collection date.

- For ten hours in a room whose temperature ranges from 66°F to 72°F (19°C to 22°C)
- For eight days in a refrigerator set at 32°F to 39°F (0°C to 3.8°C)
- For three to six months in a standard freezer set to the coldest setting (Place the milk at the back, where the temperature remains coldest. Also, before freezing breast milk, leave room at the top of the container for expansion. Don't refreeze thawed milk.)
- For six months in a deep freezer set to 0°F (-18°C) or colder. (Frozen milk is an excellent source of nutrition for up to six months.[52,53])

To warm refrigerated breast milk or thaw frozen milk, never use a microwave or a stove. Using either appliance to heat the milk can destroy many important anti-infective properties and may heat the milk unevenly, increasing the risk of hot spots that can burn your baby. Instead, place the milk container in a bowl of warm water. As the water cools, replace it with more warm water. Your baby can drink breast milk that's at room temperature or slightly warmer. When the breast milk is warmed, before giving the bottle to your baby swirl it gently to mix the fat (which rises to the top during storage) back into the milk. You can safely store thawed breast milk in the refrigerator for up to twenty-four hours, but don't refreeze it.[54]

Breast milk does lose some (but not all) of its anti-infective and nutritional properties over time and with freezing and heating. Regardless, it's still far more nutritious than formula.

# Feeding Your Baby Expressed Breast Milk or Supplemental Formula

Whenever a breastfed baby can't nurse or needs extra milk, providing expressed breast milk is best. When that's not possible, an appropriate formula is acceptable.

How you feed your baby expressed breast milk or formula depends on many factors, including your baby's age and maturity, how long you're apart from her, and whether the supplementation is permanent or temporary. In complicated situations, a lactation consultant can help you figure out how best to feed your baby. The following are ways to give a supplemental feed to your baby:

**Tubes**

For this method, you use paper tape to attach tubes next to your nipple. Depending on the device used, you either pin the milk container (syringe, bottle, or bag) to your shirt or hang it from a cord around your neck. As your baby nurses, she draws milk from the container through the tubes. A tube device may be for temporary use, but if you persistently can't produce

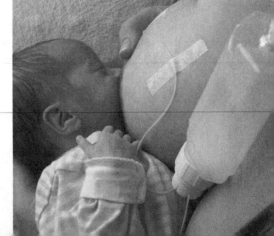

enough milk during a feeding, you can use the device for as long as necessary. A lactation consultant can show you how to use it.

**Droppers, spoons, and small cups**

You can use these items to feed your baby small amounts of supplemental milk. They provide a temporary solution for supplementation and prevent an early introduction to bottle nipples, which may cause nipple confusion.

**Bottles**

If your baby needs help feeding or gaining weight, you can use bottles to provide supplemental breast milk or formula. If you're gone for an extended time (such as when you return to work), your baby can feed from bottles.

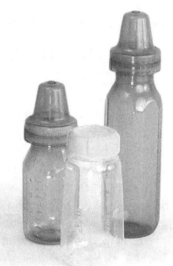

If possible, wait to introduce a bottle until you're certain your baby is nursing well and gaining weight steadily (usually four weeks or so after you've begun breastfeeding). Begin introducing a bottle about two weeks before your baby will need to feed from it while you're away. The first bottle-feeding may be challenging for you or your partner, friend, or child-care provider. Some babies learn quickly; others suck only once then stop. It may take a while for your baby to learn to bottle-feed or accept a bottle. See page 436 for more information on bottle-feeding.

## When Your Breastfed Baby Refuses a Bottle

If your baby is reluctant to take a bottle, consider these suggestions:

- Let your baby learn to suck from a bottle when he's calm.
- Choose a bottle and nipple brand that seems durable and easy to clean, then stick with it until your baby becomes familiar with it.
- Introduce a bottle before expecting your baby to take his entire feeding from it. At first, offer ½ to 1 ounce of milk after a breastfeeding session.
- Warm the bottle and nipple with running warm water.
- Your baby may accept a bottle if you hold him as you do for breastfeeding. Or he may better accept it if you distract him by talking, singing, or doing something else you *don't* do while breastfeeding.
- If your baby absolutely refuses the bottle, don't force him to take it. Use a dropper, cup, or spoon to feed him enough milk to take the edge off his hunger, then try again later with the bottle. Until he accepts this method of feeding, engage the help of someone experienced with bottle-feeding.
- If you want to continue breastfeeding, make sure your baby has more opportunities to breastfeed than bottle-feed.

# Situations That May Make Breastfeeding Challenging

Sometimes circumstances leave breastfeeding mothers and their babies needing more support and persistence than usual to establish or continue breastfeeding. Ask your caregiver, a childbirth educator, or your baby's caregiver to refer you to a lactation consultant who can help in challenging situations such as the following.

## CESAREAN BIRTH OR DIFFICULT LABOR AND BIRTH

Recovering from a cesarean can be challenging (see Chapter 14) as can recovering from a long and difficult labor and birth. In either case, you may be exhausted and require more medical and nursing care. Repairing your incision, episiotomy, or lacerations or resolving any medical emergency (such as hemorrhaging) may delay your first breastfeeding, which in turn may delay when your milk comes in.[55] If you had a cesarean, the smaller and less frequent releases of oxytocin and minimal rise in prolactin levels may also delay your milk.[56]

Despite the challenges, studies show that women who had cesareans or difficult labors and births—and who have a solid commitment to breastfeeding—tend to breastfeed for as long as women who had uncomplicated vaginal births.[57]

To help establish breastfeeding after a cesarean or difficult labor and birth, ask to see, hold, and nurse your baby as soon as possible. Breastfeeding before the epidural or spinal anesthetic wears off helps reduce any pain you may feel. Nurse your baby frequently while lying on your side and take advantage of any help offered.

After you and your baby are home, concentrate on rest, comfort, and feeding your baby. Arrange for help with household chores. You may find it most comfortable to breastfeed while lying down or sitting upright with your back supported and a pillow on your lap.

Continue to take your pain relief medication, which appears in breast milk in only trace amounts. Unrelieved pain can make breastfeeding and baby care more difficult.[58]

## PREMATURE, ILL, OR HOSPITALIZED BABIES

If your baby is premature, ill, or hospitalized, you may feel sad and worried about her well-being. Breastfeeding lets you care for your baby in an important way by giving her the closeness and comfort she needs, and your breast milk helps bolster her immune system and protect against infections.

When compared to mothers of full-term babies, mothers of premature babies produce milk that's higher in protein, nitrogen, sodium, calcium, fat, and calories. Because hospitalized premature babies are at risk for infection, breast milk's protective components are especially important. Breastfed premature babies have lower rates of infection and serious bowel problems than do formula-fed premature babies.[59] Also, when compared to formula-fed premature babies, breastfed premature babies have higher IQ scores at age eight.[60]

If your baby can't nurse or can't yet suckle well, express your colostrum or milk with a pump. As soon as your baby can take nourishment by mouth, feed her the expressed colostrum and milk by tube or dropper until she can nurse. Spend time in the hospital nursery with your baby to expose yourself to some of the organisms that can cause infection in her. Your mature immune system can make antibodies to protect you from these organisms. The antibodies appear in your breast milk and protect your baby from infection when she consumes it. Your ability to make antibodies increases when you hold your baby skin-to-skin. (See page 293.)

To establish and maintain your milk supply and to overcome obstacles you may encounter, secure the continuing support of your partner, the nursing staff, or a lactation consultant. Other parents of premature or hospitalized infants can help immensely by giving advice on breastfeeding and on other practical matters.

## NURSING WHILE PREGNANT

If you become pregnant while nursing another child, you need to decide whether to continue breastfeeding or to wean your child. Breastfeeding doesn't harm a pregnancy; at birth, babies whose mothers nursed through a pregnancy are of similar size to babies whose mothers weaned before becoming pregnant.[61]

You may find that early pregnancy symptoms, especially sore nipples and fatigue, interfere with breastfeeding. In addition, as the hormones produced during pregnancy decrease the volume of your milk and cause its flavor to change, your child may become less interested in nursing. But generally, if you're healthy and well nourished, you may have no difficulty nursing through your pregnancy.

If you choose to wean your child, see page 433.

## TANDEM NURSING

A mother who breastfeeds a newborn and older child at the same time is *tandem nursing*. Sometimes, the older child's desire to nurse is temporary as she adjusts to the new baby; sometimes, she just wants to nurse occasionally. In these situations, tandem nursing provides an opportunity for the mother, older child, and baby to bond together.

When you tandem nurse, feed your newborn first to satisfy his needs for colostrum and breast milk. Encourage the older child to wait until the baby has finished feeding. Once your mature milk is in and you're breastfeeding your newborn without problems, you can nurse both children at the same time.

Tandem nursing is challenging when the older child nurses very frequently and can't wait to feed. In this case, get support from La Leche League, a lactation consultant, or a childbirth or parent educator to help and reassure you.

## BREASTFEEDING MULTIPLES

Breastfeeding multiples is more complex than breastfeeding one baby, especially if the babies were born prematurely. However, nursing twins or triplets is very possible; even exclusive breastfeeding is feasible.

As soon as you discover you're pregnant with multiples, begin seeking the help you'll need after the babies are born. Contact a lactation consultant to learn about the special challenges of feeding multiples and about useful equipment that makes

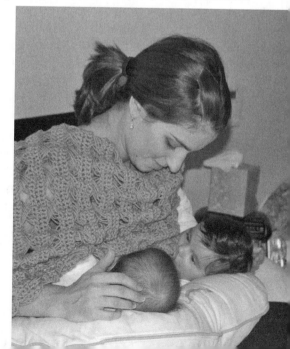

feeding easier (such as breastfeeding pillows). A lactation consultant also can help you arrange for support in the early days and weeks after the birth. Postpartum doulas are especially helpful to mothers of multiples (see page 27) as are support groups for parents of multiples.

In the beginning, it may be easier to feed one baby at a time. As you become comfortable with breastfeeding, nursing two babies at once (if they're willing) saves you time.

Make sure to eat well and eat enough; your caloric needs are greater than those of mothers feeding one baby. (See page 417.)

## BREASTFEEDING WHEN YOU'RE ILL OR HOSPITALIZED

Depending on your condition and the treatments you're receiving while hospitalized, you may have several options for baby care and feeding. Speak with the hospital's lactation consultant for guidance. If your baby can stay with you, you can breastfeed her or pump your milk and have a chance to cuddle her. Many hospitals let your partner stay in your room and care for your baby. If separated from your baby, you may be able to pump your milk so your baby can have it at home.

## TAKING MEDICATIONS AND DRUGS DURING LACTATION

With few exceptions, any medication or drug you take is present to some degree in your breast milk. Some medications do affect your baby, but most don't. For example, pain relief medications used after birth are generally safe for breastfeeding, and it's important to take them for your comfort. Likewise, stool softeners and hemorrhoid medications don't significantly affect breast milk.

Before taking any prescription or over-the-counter medications or any herbal remedies, always consult with your and your baby's caregivers or a lactation consultant about the safety of taking the medication or drug while breastfeeding. You should always avoid taking street drugs (cocaine, heroin, methamphetamines, and so on), because the effects of these drugs pose serious health risks for you and your breastfeeding baby.

Health care experts consider most vaccinations safe for breastfeeding mothers. One exception, however, is the smallpox vaccination. Breastfeeding mothers should avoid this vaccination because it causes a sore to develop at the vaccination site. If a baby is exposed to the sore, it may cause sores to develop on his skin. If you want a flu shot or a vaccination against mumps, measles, and rubella (MMR), both are safe to have if breastfeeding.[62]

If you take oral contraceptives, avoid those containing estrogen. These birth control pills can decrease your milk supply. Progestin-only contraceptives, including the mini-pill and Depo-Provera, don't interfere with milk production.

Smoking affects babies in two ways: by ingesting breast milk containing nicotine and other chemicals in tobacco and by breathing in smoke. Even though smoking can create problems for a baby (such as increased fussiness[63]), a mother who smokes should still breastfeed her baby. Breast milk produced by a smoker better protects a baby's health than formula does. Formula-fed babies of smoking mothers are seven times more likely to develop respiratory illnesses than are breastfed babies of smokers.[64]

If you smoke, try to quit or at least cut down the number of cigarettes you smoke each day. When you do smoke, avoid doing so around your baby. Secondhand smoke increases a baby's risk of sudden infant death syndrome (SIDS) and incidences of respiratory infections and ear infections.

# Questions about Medications and Breastfeeding

Before taking any medication or herbal remedy, ask your caregiver or lactation consultant the following questions:

- Do I absolutely need this medication now? Can I delay taking it until my baby is more mature and can better handle its effects?
- Is there a safer alternative to the medication?
- Can I take the medication topically (rubbed on the skin) instead of orally? (When compared to oral medications, topical medications usually pass into your bloodstream and breast milk in lower levels.)
- Can we schedule the timing of the medication or the feedings so the smallest amount of the drug is in my breast milk when feeding? (Time-release medications and some drugs take a long time to leave the body.)
- When I take medications that are unsafe for breastfeeding, should I temporarily stop nursing? (If the answer is yes, you can pump and discard your milk until the treatment is complete and the medication is out of your system.)
- What symptoms and possible side effects from medication should I watch for in my baby?
- Do you have access to the most accurate information about medication use during breastfeeding? (For example, *Medications and Mothers' Milk* by Thomas W. Hale is a regularly revised book on the subject that's well respected in the medical community.)

## WORKING OUTSIDE THE HOME

When you work outside your home, breastfeeding your baby is possible with planning and support. The extra effort to nurse your baby during the workday, or to express and store your milk, pays off in the following ways:

- By keeping up your milk supply
- By providing your baby with nourishment that can protect him from acquiring infections while in day care
- By maintaining the closeness with your baby that comes with breastfeeding

In general, a lengthy maternity leave and a flexible job make it easier to combine breastfeeding and work. Continuing breastfeeding while working is less difficult when a maternity leave lasts at least until the baby nurses less frequently and on a more predictable schedule (for example, when he starts eating table foods).

Most industrialized countries provide mothers with maternity leaves that last a year or more, allowing time for babies to naturally reduce their need to nurse and better adjust to long breaks between feedings. In the United States, however, maternity leaves are often very short (usually no longer than twelve weeks).

Political action groups such as MomsRising (http://www.momsrising.com) are working to increase the length of parental leave, but until that change occurs, breastfeeding parents in the

United States must make the most of whatever leave they're granted and plan how they'll continuing breastfeeding when the leave is over. Before returning to work, research your workplace's policy and attitudes (as well as your legal rights) about breastfeeding.

When planning a return to the workplace, you have several options for continuing breastfeeding. For example, consider switching to part-time employment or discuss with your employer the possibility of telecommuting part- or full-time. Either option will make you available to nurse your baby regularly during the workday. To further persuade your employer of the importance of breastfeeding, you may also want to let him or her know that women who breastfeed take less time off, because their breastfed children get sick less often.

If your workplace is close to where your baby is during the workday, arrange to work longer hours so you can take one to two long feeding breaks during the day. Either your baby can come to you (if your workplace supports that option) or you can go to your baby. If your baby is in day care, choose one that supports breastfeeding and won't mind if you stop by to nurse your baby.

If feeding your baby during the workday isn't an option, speak with your employer to arrange for time and privacy to express or pump milk at work. Mother-friendly workplaces often provide a room other than a restroom for working mothers to pump. Follow the guidelines on page 426 to store your milk. Mothers who can't pump at work can still breastfeed by feeding frequently when at home. Many babies of these mothers go on a "reverse feeding" schedule; that is, they nurse infrequently during the day and feed mostly in the evenings and at night.

Some working mothers decide to breastfeed while at home and supplement with formula while away. As long as you continue to nurse frequently when you're with your baby, you should produce enough milk. If your milk supply begins to dwindle, increase the number of feedings to stimulate your milk production.

For more information on breastfeeding while working, contact La Leche League or check if a local hospital, clinic, or health department offers a class on breastfeeding and returning to work. Talk with women who have returned to work and breastfed successfully.

# RELACTATION

If breastfeeding has been interrupted long enough to stop your milk production, it's possible to restart it—but it requires persistence, commitment, and a baby interested in nursing.

Frequent, around-the-clock nursing is the most effective method to reestablish lactation. You may use a tube-feeding device to encourage your baby to suckle at an empty or near-empty breast while receiving supplemental formula. (See page 426.) The suckling stimulates milk production while the device provides your baby with nutrition. Using an electric breast pump after a feeding may also increase your milk supply, as may taking herbal medications and prescribed medications (see page 416). If you decide to reestablish breastfeeding, contact a lactation consultant for support and advice.

Mothers of adopted babies can use these same methods to try to produce milk, even if they've never been pregnant or nursed a baby. Although these mothers usually don't produce a full supply, they may produce some milk. Feeding a baby even a small amount of breast milk reduces her likelihood of having problems that are common with formula-fed babies (such as constipation). If a mother can't produce milk to feed her adopted baby, she can still experience breastfeeding to a large degree by using a tube-feeding device to feed her formula.

# BREASTFEEDING AND FERTILITY

For as long as you exclusively breastfeed your baby, you greatly reduce your chance of becoming pregnant. You have less than a 2 percent chance of becoming pregnant if:

- Your baby is less than six months old.
- You don't menstruate until after fifty-six days postpartum.
- You're nursing frequently (at least every four hours during the day and every six hours at night).
- You rarely supplement your baby's feedings and give him tastes of foods or fluids only occasionally.[65]

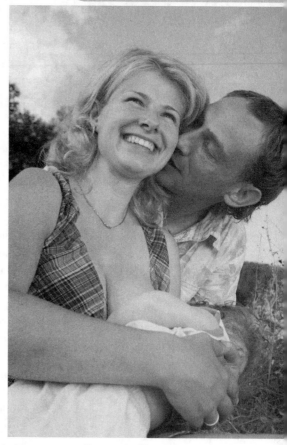

After your baby has begun eating table foods, you can extend some of breastfeeding's contraceptive benefits by nursing before offering table foods and by continuing to breastfeed throughout the day and night.

After giving birth, you may ovulate before you have your first menstrual period. If preventing pregnancy is essential or desirable, talk to your caregiver about contraception. Barrier methods (condoms and diaphragms), intrauterine devices (IUDs), and progestin-only pills and injections (mini-pill and Depo-Provera) don't interfere with breastfeeding. Birth control pills containing estrogen, however, can reduce your milk supply.[66]

Identifying your body's fertility signs is trickier when you're nursing because of the fluctuating hormone levels required for breastfeeding, but it can be done. If you're interested in learning about fertility awareness techniques, the excellent book *Taking Charge of Your Fertility: The Definitive Guide to Natural Birth Control, Pregnancy Achievement, and Reproductive Health* by Toni Weschler may give you the information you need.[67]

# WEANING

You may have heard that it's okay to wean your baby when she's six months old (or has teeth) because breast milk is most beneficial up to that time—but this information is incorrect. Breast milk benefits your baby for as long as you decide to breastfeed. In fact, the American Academy of Pediatrics (AAP) recommends breastfeeding babies for the first year or longer.

Making the decision to wean is complex; don't make your decision based on other's opinions or suggestions. You may decide to wean because you want to become pregnant and can't while breastfeeding. Or you may decide that demands at work make it difficult to continue nursing. Sometimes, the decision to wean isn't the mother's: Perhaps the child is no longer interested in nursing. Or, in very sad cases, the child has died.

## Fact or Fiction?

*You should continue to breast-feed your baby after he has begun to eat other foods.*

**Fact.** The American Academy of Pediatrics recommends that mothers exclusively breastfeed their babies for the first six months. When their babies are around six months old, parents can gradually begin introducing table foods, including foods rich in iron. However, breast milk or formula is still the most important food in a baby's diet for the rest of the first year. After the first year, mothers and babies can continue breastfeeding for as long as they desire. If babies are weaned before their first birth-days, they should consume an iron-fortified cow milk formula.

When you decide to wean your child, here are some practical tips to make the transition easier:

- Wean slowly. This way, if you change your mind and want to resume breastfeeding, you can rebuild your milk supply.
- First cut out the feeding you and your baby enjoy least. After your baby and you have adjusted to that change, continue to slowly cut out feedings one at a time, leaving the best-loved feeding (such as the first feeding of the day or the one that's part of the bedtime ritual) for last.
- When preparing bottles, gradually replace breast milk with formula or whole cow or goat milk, depending on your baby's age.
- Use the comfort measures discussed on pages 419 to treat swollen breasts.
- If you're thinking of weaning your child in the winter, wait until the spring to give her the best chance of staying healthy during the cold and flu season.
- Think of the ways you cuddled with your baby as you breastfed her. For example, you may have read a book together in a rocking chair, bathed together, or napped together. You can still do these special things while weaning your baby.
- Honor the time you nursed. Write your baby a letter about what nursing her meant to you.
- As you wean, your hormone levels change, bringing about the return of your menstrual cycle. Expect your emotions to fluctuate as your body adjusts.
- After weaning, some milk remains in your breasts. It gradually disappears over the following weeks to months.

### When You Need to Wean

Sometimes, mothers must wean after the occurrence or development of an unexpected event, such as the death of a baby or a serious medical condition in the mother. In these cases, there is sadness, grief, and uncertainty.

If a mother must wean because of a medical reason or to begin infertility treatments, it's possible to wean gradually over several days. If a baby has died, a mother doesn't need to immediately suppress milk production. After a baby's death, a mother may experience a "second grieving" for the baby who's no longer there to nurse. Some women find comfort in donating their expressed milk to a milk bank in remembrance of their babies. (For more on infant death, see page 303.)

To comfortably suppress milk production, wear a snug-fitting supportive bra (such as a sports bra) to provide comfort as your breasts swell. Apply ice packs to your breasts over your bra or light clothing and take ibuprofen to reduce inflammation. Sore breasts may last for a day or two, but you may leak milk for a week or longer. For more on lactation suppression, see page 334.

# Formula Feeding and Bottle-feeding

When breastfeeding isn't possible or desired, parents typically bottle-feed their baby formula (when breast milk isn't available) or expressed breast milk.

## TYPES OF FORMULAS AND FORMULA PREPARATION

For families who feed their babies formula, the American Academy of Pediatrics (AAP) recommends using formulas that are iron-fortified and commercially prepared to feed babies younger than one year.[68] Evaporated milk mixtures don't suit a baby's nutritional needs. Whole, 2 percent, 1 percent, or fat-free cow milk or goat milk lack many important and necessary nutrients, and are difficult to digest for babies younger than one year. Because commercially prepared formulas are fortified with vitamins and minerals, babies who consume them don't require a vitamin and mineral supplement.

Your baby's caregiver can give you guidelines on how much to feed your baby. A rule of thumb is that in a 24-hour period, a baby needs 2 to 2½ ounces for every pound he weighs.

## TYPES OF FORMULAS

Most infant formulas are made of cow milk or soybeans, and many are fortified with iron to reduce a baby's risk of becoming anemic (having low iron). Contrary to myth, consuming iron-fortified formula doesn't increase the incidence of colic, constipation, diarrhea, fussiness, or vomiting. In fact, research suggests that babies who consumed low-iron formula have lower cognitive test scores at age five than do their peers who didn't consume low-iron formula.[69] Except when a baby has a rare medical condition, the best formula for a baby's overall health is one fortified with iron and preferably made of cow milk.

Some parents switch brands of formula after noticing one brand seems to make their baby gassy or fussy. Switching formulas, however, does *not* decrease gas or reduce fussiness. All babies—breastfed and formula-fed—are gassy and fussy at times, and parents should stick with the brand of formula that their baby tolerates.

Sometimes, formulas truly don't agree with babies. For example, if your baby seems allergic to iron-fortified, cow milk formula, his caregiver may suggest hypoallergenic formulas, which are more expensive than other formulas.

If your baby can't digest lactose (galactosemia) or if your family eats a vegan diet (doesn't include animal protein), your caregiver may recommend an iron-fortified soymilk formula. Because up to 25 percent of babies with a milk allergy are also allergic to soy,[70] health care providers recommend using soy formulas in only these cases.

To learn more about formula, visit http://www.infantformula.org/.

## PREPARING FORMULA

Formulas are available in ready-to-feed bottles or cans, canned liquid concentrates, and powdered forms. When prepared as directed, all three forms have equal nutritive value. Powdered formula is least expensive and ready-to-feed formula is most expensive, with concentrated formula slightly less so.

When preparing formula, carefully follow the package directions. Make sure your hands and all equipment are clean. Always use the correct amount of water to mix powdered or concentrated formula. If you use too little water, you can cause diarrhea, dehydration, and other problems for your baby. If you use too much water, you dilute the formula and your baby doesn't receive enough calories and nutrients to thrive. Formula-fed babies don't need extra water until they begin eating table foods.

If your water supply is fluoridated, mix formula with distilled, purified water that's free of minerals and ions, or water that's been filtered by reverse osmosis. The American Academy of Pediatric Dentistry reports that using fluoridated water to prepare formula can permanently discolor teeth when babies consume fluoride in greater than optimal amounts.[71]

## BOTTLES AND NIPPLES

Although bottles come in many shapes and styles, most are made of either glass or plastic. Because plastic bottles are lightweight and don't crack or break easily, they seem the more practical choice. But the current debate on the toxicity of clear plastic bottles made of polycarbonate (which contains the chemical bisphenol A, or BPA) may persuade some parents to choose glass bottles or BPA-free plastic bottles.

Experts are split on the dangers of BPA. On one side, the National Institutes of Health reports that BPA may affect the neurology and behavior of babies and children, and the Environment California Research & Policy Center recommends that parents avoid giving their children plastic bottles or cups made of polycarbonate.[72] On the other side, the U.S. Food and Drug Administration (FDA) finds the use of BPA in plastic bottles and cups of no concern.

If you want to limit your baby's exposure to BPA, consider using glass bottles, which are stain-proof and easy to clean but are heavy and can break. If plastic bottles are more practical for you, avoid using those that have the recycling symbol 7; they contain BPA. Instead, choose bottles with the recycling symbols 1, 2, or 5; they're made of polyethylene or polypropylene.

Some parents use a feeding-bag system to avoid using bottles, even though it's harder to prepare formula this way. Some feeding units consist of a disposable plastic bag (for the formula) inside a plastic container, and it's not as easy to mix formula in a bag as it is in a bottle. If you choose this system, check the manufacturer's information to determine if the bag and container are BPA free. For other feeding supplies that don't contain BPA, visit http://www.thesoftlanding.com.

Like bottles, nipples also come in various shapes and sizes. Select one your baby likes and then stay with that type of nipple. Before feeding your baby a bottle, check that the breast milk or formula drips adequately from the nipple. If it flows in a stream, the nipple hole is too big and your baby may consume too much too fast and she may spit up. If the milk drips very slowly or not at all, your baby may tire of sucking and not consume enough (or any) milk. If the nipple hole is too large, discard the nipple. If it's too small, remove any dried breast milk or formula that may be clogging the hole or enlarge the hole with a clean needle, then check the drip again.

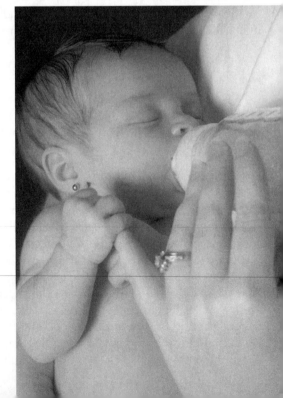

If your water supply is safe for drinking, you don't need to sterilize bottles and nipples. You can wash bottles by hand or in the dishwasher. Clean nipples with a nipple brush and hot soapy water; rinse them with hot water and dry.

Heat bottles in warm water; don't use a microwave or stove. These appliances may produce hot spots that can burn your baby. Plus, if using plastic bottles, the high heating is more likely to release chemicals into the breast milk or formula.

## TIPS FOR BOTTLE-FEEDING

Giving your baby a bottle can be an enjoyable experience. Cuddle your baby during feedings or even hold him skin-to-skin to give him the closeness he needs, promote bonding, and provide you with wonderful memories.

You can make your baby's feedings consistently successful and happy by doing the following:

- Hold your baby so he's semi-reclined. This position is more comfortable for him than lying on his back and prevents him from swallowing too much air.
- To promote normal development of your baby's eye muscles and symmetrical development of his neck muscles, hold him sometimes in your right arm and sometimes in your left.
- Burp your baby about halfway through a feeding. Babies that gulp air need to burp more often. As he grows, he'll begin to burp on his own and won't need your help. See pages 410–411 for tips on burping your baby and preventing spitting up.
- Trust that your baby knows how much he needs to eat. For the first few days after the birth, full-term babies feed eight to twelve times in twenty-four hours. As they grow, they consume more at each feeding and eat less often. Your baby might not want to consume the same amount at each feeding. If he doesn't finish a bottle, don't coax him to do so if he seems satisfied. When your baby rapidly and consistently finishes a bottle at each feeding, add more breast milk or formula (typically 1 ounce) to the bottle for the next feeding. Your baby's caregiver can give you guidelines on how much to feed your baby at each feeding.
- Offering your baby warmed (but not hot) breast milk or formula can make the feeding more comfortable. As he grows, he may begin to prefer a bottle that's cool or at room temperature.
- Never prop a bottle to feed your baby. Interacting with you and others during feedings helps him thrive emotionally and develop trust.
- Never mix cooked or raw honey into your baby's bottle (or dip his pacifiers in honey). Infant botulism can occur in babies younger than one year.

# Key Points to Remember

- Feeding your baby has far greater significance than simply providing for her physical growth. Consistently responding to her feeding cues develops her sense of trust, security, and well-being. Cuddling your baby during feedings, while smiling and talking to her, promotes emotional development and stimulates her senses.
- Feeding your baby also provides many opportunities for her to coo, grin, pat, and otherwise express affection toward you, fostering bonding and strengthening family ties.
- Under most circumstances, breastfeeding is the best way to feed babies. With more than two hundred nutrients, breast milk is easily digestible, promotes your baby's overall health, and helps prevent some illnesses and diseases. Breastfeeding also offers unique health benefits to you.
- Breastfeed your baby whenever she shows feeding cues (typically eight to twelve times a day for a newborn). Let her feed for as long as she wants on the first breast (ten to thirty minutes), then offer the second breast. Count the number of wet and poopy diapers and monitor her weight gain to know she's getting plenty of milk.
- Many breastfeeding challenges have several effective remedies. Lactation consultants, physicians specializing in breastfeeding medicine, and your caregiver can help you remedy most breastfeeding problems.
- In most cases when using formula, you should feed your baby an iron-fortified cow milk formula.
- When bottle-feeding your baby, feed her whenever she shows feeding cues and always hold her to provide the emotional interaction and love she needs.

# CHAPTER 19

# When You're Pregnant Again

When you find out that you're expecting another child, you may feel just as you did after confirming your first pregnancy, or you may have a completely different reaction. You may be happy with the news or surprised by it. You may feel confident that you can handle pregnancy and birth again, or you may wonder how this pregnancy and birth will differ from your previous experience. You may have many questions and concerns about caring for another child. You may be unsure how your older child will adjust to a baby brother or sister. This chapter describes what you can expect emotionally and physically from another pregnancy, and it offers suggestions for preparing your child for your growing family.

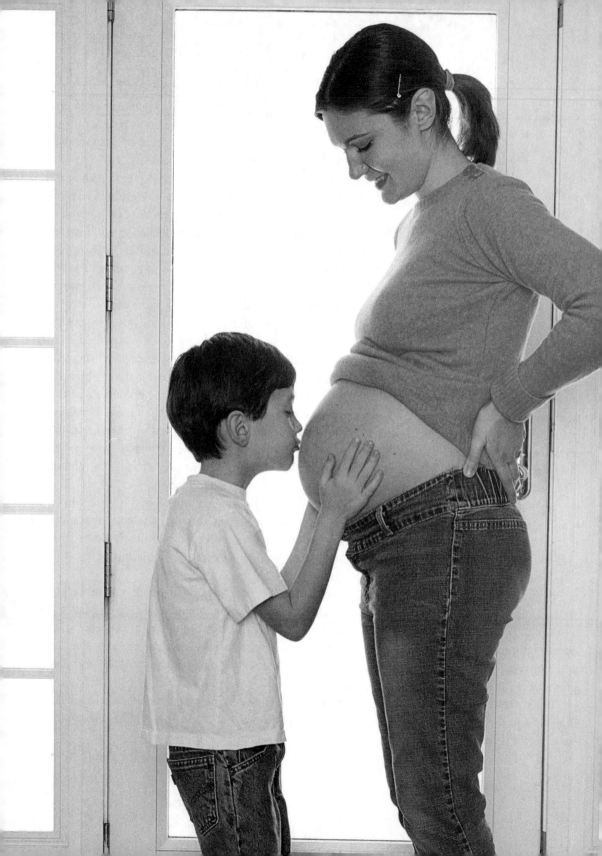

# What to Expect with This Pregnancy and Birth

After you've been pregnant once, you may think that you'll know exactly what to expect when you're pregnant again. But every pregnancy is unique; a second pregnancy won't be exactly like your first.

Subsequent pregnancies, however, do share some predictable characteristics that make them different from a first pregnancy. Physical changes may occur sooner, but you might or might not notice them. For example, you may feel the baby's movements about a month earlier, because you recognize the sensation sooner. Or you may miss the early flutters because you're not as preoccupied with this pregnancy. Your abdominal muscles relax more easily, so your belly enlarges sooner and your pregnancy becomes noticeable earlier. Your pelvic ligaments may soften sooner, and you may feel that you're carrying the baby lower. Braxton-Hicks contractions may be more noticeable and numerous, especially toward the end of pregnancy, which can make it difficult to know when they indicate the start of labor.

On average, subsequent pregnancies are a few days shorter than a first pregnancy. Labor is typically faster, and pushing is much faster. Most women report that the first stage of labor is less painful than they experienced the first time (possibly because they're less anxious), but that second-stage pushing is as painful or more so (possibly because it's faster). Despite these general observations, it's impossible to predict how labor will go in subsequent pregnancies. Each labor may be virtually identical to a previous one, or it may be completely different.

If your previous birth was a positive experience, you'll of course hope that this birth will be, too. But if your previous birth was difficult or disappointing, you naturally may worry that problems will arise again. It's common to feel anxious about labor, regardless of how many times you've given birth. Talking about your concerns with your partner, caregiver, or childbirth educator can raise your confidence and help make this birth a positive experience.

Even if you had excellent childbirth preparation classes for your first birth, it may be helpful to take another series. These "refresher" classes will not only review coping techniques for labor, but they'll also prepare you for how this labor may differ from your first. In addition, classes provide updated information about maternity care, offer ideas for preparing your older child for the birth and managing your growing household, provide opportunities to talk to other parents, and give you time to bond to your new baby before the birth.

If you choose not to attend classes, refresh your memory by reading Chapters 9 through 14. If a previous birth ended in a cesarean section, see pages 323–327 to learn about having another baby after a cesarean.

# Your Emotional Reactions to Having Another Baby

Compared to your first pregnancy, you may find that this pregnancy isn't as emotionally exhilarating. Pregnancy discomforts may seem more annoying, or you may be too busy to notice them. You may think less about being pregnant, partly because your older child requires your attention. Instead of thinking about your developing baby, you may think ahead to her as a newborn, because you already have a clear picture of yourself as a new mother. Your partner may be less attentive to you, possibly because he or she has greater confidence in your well-being this time around.

Like many mothers expecting a second child, you may worry that you won't have enough love for your new baby. Or you may wonder if your love for your older child will lessen with the new arrival. It's helpful to know that you can never run out of love. Think of all the people you care for. Your love expanded to include each of them, and it will continue to do so to include all your children.

You also may worry that there isn't enough time in the day to care for another child. It's true that your growing family will keep you busy, but you'll be surprised to discover that caring for a baby while parenting an older child isn't as hard as you may have imagined. With your first child, it took a while to learn about baby care and time management. With your second child, these skills will come quickly, allowing you to adapt to parenting two children more easily.

# Including Your Child in Your Pregnancy

When you're pregnant again, it's best to prepare your child for the pregnancy, birth, and new baby in a realistic and age-appropriate manner. The following sections offer ways to get your child ready for your family's new addition. Use the suggestions that best match your personal preferences and your child's maturity level.

One main question you may have is: *When's the best time to tell my child that I'm pregnant?* Some parents choose to announce a pregnancy after the first trimester, when the likelihood of miscarriage is reduced. They also delay the announcement to shorten the wait for a young child who doesn't understand the length of time until the birth. Other parents choose to announce the pregnancy earlier in the first

## Two Views on Being Pregnant Again

With my first pregnancy, we took all the classes, read all the books, and prepared the nursery—everything! With this pregnancy, I've barely had any time to think about it at all. I worry that this baby is getting shortchanged.

—*Mary*

I'd heard that it's easier to care for a new baby and a toddler than it is to take care of a toddler while pregnant. I agree. I'm not so tired and sore now that the baby is here, and taking care of a newborn isn't nearly as stressful as I remembered.

—*Heidi*

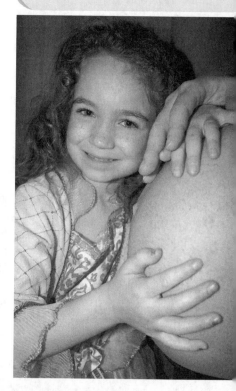

## Books for Children about Pregnancy and Birth

*Waiting for Baby* by Annie Kubler (2000). Designed for preschoolers and younger children, this board book uses only pictures to tell the story of a child who's waiting for the birth of a sibling.

*How Was I Born?* by Lennart Nilsson and Lena Katarina Swanberg (1996). This book is about fetal development (including photos), birth, and the baby's homecoming.

*Hello Baby* (formerly *Welcome with Love*) by Jenni Overend and Julie Vivas (2004). Beautifully illustrated, this story tells of a child's experience attending a home birth.

*Mommy Has to Stay in Bed* by Annette Rivlin-Gutman (2006). This story helps children understand the reasons for bed rest during pregnancy.

*Hello Baby!* by Lizzy Rockwell (2000). For ages two to five, pictures and simple explanations help children learn about pregnancy, hospital visits, and what to expect when the baby comes home.

*Runa's Birth: The Day My Sister Was Born* by Uwe Spillmann and Inga Kamieth (2006). This wonderfully illustrated story of birth is told from a child's point of view.

*Waiting for Baby* by Harriet Ziefert (1998). For ages three to seven, this story is about a boy who has trouble awaiting his baby sister's birth.

trimester, especially if there's frequent vomiting, in order to reassure the child that his mother isn't ill. If you choose to delay announcing the news to your child, be careful not to wait *too* long, as he may hear about the pregnancy from someone else.

Another question you may have is *What's the best way to tell my child about the pregnancy?* Once you decide to tell your child that you're pregnant, first talk to him about families, babies, and big brothers and sisters. When you see a family with two children, point them out to your child. Discuss families he knows who have a new baby. For example, you may say, "Did you see Cole's new sister, Maya, when his mommy picked him up at preschool?" or "Pretty soon, Aunt Heidi will have a new baby, and Amelia will be a big sister." Comments like these will help your child realize that it's normal for families to have more than one child.

To help make the wait for the birth more understandable to your child, try linking your due date to a special event or season. For example, you may say, "The baby will arrive sometime when there's snow on the ground." Also consider making a calendar so you can count down the days together.

Use the time until the birth to include your child in the pregnancy by helping him develop positive feelings and realistic expectations about the baby. Here are some suggestions:

- Talk to your child about pregnancy and birth. Depending on his age, find out what he already knows, correct any misconceptions, fill in gaps in his understanding, and answer his questions. Use appropriate terms, such as by saying that the baby is in your uterus or "a special place," not in your stomach. At the same time, avoid overwhelming your child with too much information.
- Attend a sibling preparation class, if available in your community. This class typically gives a demonstration of a birth using a doll, which can help your child understand the process.

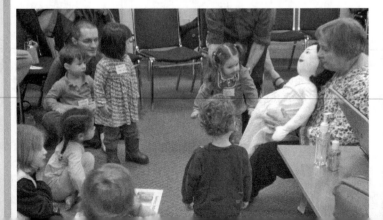

- Read together children's books about pregnancy and birth, about families having another baby, and about becoming a big brother or sister. (See pages 442 and 446.)
- Show your child where you'll give birth. If appropriate, talk about the possibility of his visiting you there after the baby is born.
- Let your child feel the baby move. Point out when the baby has the hiccups. Talk about how the baby can suck his thumb, wiggle, kick, and hear voices. Encourage your child to rest his cheek on your belly and talk or sing to the baby. Bring your child to a prenatal visit to hear the baby's heartbeat.
- Show your child photos or DVDs of himself as a baby—especially ones showing you caring for him as a newborn. Help him make a picture book about families with two or more children.
- Talk about the care a newborn needs. Have your child interact with a friend's baby to see how small a baby is and what a baby can and can't do.

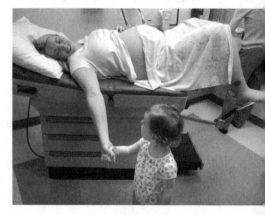

- If the baby's arrival will change where your child sleeps, move him to his new room or make new sleeping arrangements months before the birth to prevent your child from feeling suddenly displaced. Also, because accidents can happen with your child when you're busy with the baby, safety-proof your home if you haven't already done so.

## IF YOUR CHILD IS YOUNGER THAN TWO

If your child is younger than two, she can't easily tell you how she's feeling—but she probably understands more than you think. Use simple terms to talk about babies and to explain to her about becoming a big sister. You also may try the suggestions on page 442 and above, or simplify them.

A younger child's adjustment to a new baby usually occurs more rapidly than an older child's adjustment. In fact, a younger child may have trouble remembering her life without the baby. However, when the baby is older and begins playing with her sibling's toys, you may notice a period of adjustment, especially if your older child is still younger than three and has trouble sharing toys.

Although caring for multiple young children can be challenging and exhausting, the upside is that the overall duration of the babyhood phase will be shorter for your family than for families with siblings who are many years apart in age.

# Including Your Child at the Birth

Many parents feel that a birth is a family event. They believe that including their older child at the birth will help him bond to his new sibling and encourage positive, healthy attitudes about birth.

Other parents feel that birth is a process that's too complicated or too disturbing for their child to witness. They worry how their child would react to seeing his mother's discomfort in labor or the blood from the birth. They wonder about the logistics of his care during the event. What if he became bored? What if he needed a nap? What if he began to disturb the staff? Who would care for him?

Most home birth providers and birth centers welcome the inclusion of children at births, as do some hospitals. They support the idea that having a child spend time with his mother and sibling soon after the birth will reduce separation anxiety and help him adjust to the change in the family structure.

Even if your caregiver is fine with including your child at the birth, only you and your partner (and your child, if he's old enough to have a say) can decide whether your child *should* attend. To help you make your decision, assess your child's physical health, emotional readiness, personality, and maturity. Whether you choose to include your child at the birth or decide that he shouldn't attend, the following sections offer suggestions for preparing your child for the event.

# IF YOU PLAN TO HAVE YOUR CHILD ATTEND THE BIRTH

If you decide to include your child at the birth, following these guidelines can help ensure a positive experience for everyone.

- Take childbirth preparation classes or review what you learned in previous classes. To make your child feel comfortable at the birth, you'll need to be confident in your ability to cope with labor.
- Choose a birth setting that easily allows for your child's inclusion. An ideal setting is one that provides ample space and flexibility to come and go if your child becomes bored or uncomfortable. To reduce stress, set clear guidelines for your child's participation and familiarize your child with the birth setting, your caregivers, and any equipment that may be used at the birth. Make sure to bring your child's favorite toys and comfort items, such as a special blanket, to the birth.
- Arrange for someone to look after your child during the birth and help explain what's going on to her. This person should not be your partner or another labor-support person, whose sole job is to tend to your needs.
- Let your child know what to expect at the birth. Tell her what labor and birth are like (long and boring, yet exciting at times). Prepare her for the sights and sounds (such as the presence of blood and your groans, grunts, and cries). Suggest things that she can do during labor, such as bring you juice or a cool cloth, walk with you, play music, take photos with a disposable camera, be quiet when asked, and so on. Prepare her for the baby's appearance and behavior immediately after the birth (see Chapter 17). If you plan to breastfeed the baby, explain the process to your child in terms she can understand. If your child is also breastfeeding, see page 429 for information on tandem nursing.

  Children's books or DVDs on birth also can help prepare your child for the event. During the birth, your child's support person can refer to them to help explain what's happening. For example, he or she may say, "Your mommy's working hard to push the baby out. She's making noises just like those we heard on the DVD!"
- Avoid making promises about the birth that you might not be able to keep. For example, don't say, "You will be there to see your new brother being born." Instead, say, "We hope you can be with us when our baby is born."
- Let your child know what will happen if circumstances prevent her from attending the birth (for example, she's at school, asleep, or ill), if she changes her mind about attending, or if complications develop in your pregnancy or during labor or birth. See page 445 for more information.
- Expect that your child will behave as usual during your labor. Don't expect the experience to change her character or suddenly make her more mature. She'll still fuss at times, need to be taken to the restroom, say no to requests, and want you to cuddle her.

# IF YOUR CHILD WON'T BE AT THE BIRTH

The following guidelines will help you plan for your child's care while you're away and prepare him to meet his new sibling.

- During the last weeks of your pregnancy, let your child know you'll be leaving when it's time to have the baby. Unless you're having a scheduled induction or cesarean, explain that the exact time will be a surprise—it may happen during the night or day. Tell your child whether he'll be at home or stay at another person's home while you're away. Let him know who'll care for him. Your child will be less anxious if he knows and trusts this person.

- If your child will be staying at someone's home, help him pack a bag with his favorite clothes, toys, and comfort items. If you like, have him help you pack your suitcase or the baby's bag to involve him in the birth preparations.

- When labor begins, tell your child when you'll be leaving and where you'll be going. Let him know that you may leave while he's asleep so he'll be prepared for your absence when he awakens.

- Prepare for the possibility of separation anxiety if you'll be giving birth in a hospital. A one- or two-day stay after a vaginal birth is typical, as is a three- or four-day stay following a cesarean birth. During that time, your child's ability to tolerate the separation will depend on his age, how often he's been separated from you before, how long this separation will last, how comfortable he is with the person caring for him, how comfortable he is with the place of care (if not cared for at home), and how well he understands what's happening. Separation anxiety may lead to fretting, crying, sadness, clinging, irritability, sleeping difficulties, and tantrums. Let the person who'll care for your child know about these normal reactions.

- Plan to have your child visit you and the new baby. Birth centers and most hospitals allow children to visit after the birth.

- Have realistic expectations when your child visits. Seeing you and the baby will probably reassure him and let him respond in a positive way. But it's possible that he may ignore you and the baby, cling excessively, or cry uncontrollably when it's time to leave. If he responds in this manner, you may feel that it'd have been easier to avoid the visit entirely. However, it's healthier for your child to see you briefly than to be separated from you for a longer period.

- Consider having a gift for your child to open when he visits you or when you phone him to announce the baby's arrival. Tell him the gift is from the baby.

- If your hospital stay lasts longer than expected or if your child can't visit, try to talk to him by phone. You also may want to connect with him by providing photos of you and the new baby.

## Books for Children about Babies and Siblings

*I'm a Big Brother* and *I'm a Big Sister* by Joanna Cole and Maxie Chambliss (1997). For ages two to six, these books talk about the importance of a family. Except for the sex of the main character, the stories are identical.

*My New Baby* by Annie Kubler (2000). This board book uses only pictures to tell the story of a family in which the mother breastfeeds and the father helps with housework and baby care. It's for preschoolers and younger children.

*The New Baby* by Mercer Mayer (2001). For ages one to five, this story uses simple language to explain what it's like to have a new baby and ways a sibling can play with the baby.

*The New Baby* by Fred Rogers (1996). This book talks about a new baby joining the family.

# Helping Your Child Adjust to the New Baby

After the arrival of a new sibling, your child may have mixed feelings. Sometimes she may show fondness for the baby. Other times, she may express jealousy and resentment toward this tiny person who requires almost constant care, especially if your child had your undivided attention for several years.

If your child is angry and distressed by the baby's arrival, she may react by having tantrums, seeking attention, becoming excessively preoccupied with the baby, withdrawing, showing aggression toward you or the baby (hitting, biting, throwing things, and so on), changing her eating and sleeping patterns, or reverting to outgrown behavior such as thumb sucking, wanting a pacifier, feeding from bottle or breast, or wetting herself. This behavior will typically be new for your child and may catch you by surprise.

How and when your child expresses this negative behavior (if she does) depends on her age. A child younger than three tends not to fully resent a new arrival's presence until the baby begins crawling and interfering in her play. A child who's at least three years old often immediately recognizes the impact a new baby has on her relationship with her parents, and she typically has little difficulty showing her displeasure. Even preteens can feel resentment toward a new sibling, although they usually feel guilty about it and may successfully hide their feelings from their parents.

What can you do if your child isn't adjusting well to her new position in your family? Because it's difficult to avoid your child's feelings of displacement, focus instead on helping her deal with the stress. Try to accept her behavior as a normal reaction to the changes in her life. The following are tips to ease your child's adjustment:

- Give your child a doll so she has a "baby" to care for, too.
- Have a party to celebrate both the birth of the baby and the "birth" of a big sister or brother. Provide a cake or treats and give a gift to your child. Encourage her to make a gift for the baby or choose one to buy. When visitors bring gifts for the baby, let your child open them for the baby, or delay opening the gifts until she's not around.
- Before the birth, have your partner provide more of your child's daily care, such as giving her a bath or reading her a bedtime story, to help establish a routine that won't be disrupted by the baby's arrival.
- Schedule time to be alone with your child and let her decide what you'll be doing together.
- Respond to your child's requests, comments, and actions. Ignoring her when you're busy may upset her at this vulnerable time. If you can't respond right away, try not to blame the baby. Don't say, "We can't go to the park now because the baby is eating." Instead, say, "We'll go to the park later, because I think it will be sunnier then."

- Correct negative behavior as you always have. Familiar rules and routines reassure young children. If you suddenly become permissive, the change may confuse your child.
- Help your child express her feelings by saying what you think she's feeling. For example, you may say, "New babies make a lot of noise" or "Sometimes it's hard to have a tiny baby around." Reading books about new siblings with your child may help her find words to describe her emotions. (See page 446.)
- If your child wants to avoid the baby, let her. If she wants to help with baby care, include her in age-appropriate tasks. If she's older, she can hold the baby and help with diapering, dressing, or burping. Children of all ages can entertain the baby by smiling, singing, talking, and making funny faces. Teach your child how to recognize engagement cues that show the baby wants to play and disengagement cues that show the baby is overwhelmed. (See pages 377–378.)
- Use the time when you're feeding the baby to read, talk, or share a snack with your child. Consider providing special toys, books, or snacks that are just for feeding times.
- Think of stimulating activities that you and your child will enjoy doing together, such as planting seeds, blowing bubbles, or making cookies. Working together on useful tasks (even small ones) may help remind her that she's still important to you.
- While your older child is listening, talk about her to the baby. For example, say, "Lily, today we're going to the zoo with your big sister, and she's going to show you all her favorite animals." Also, praise your child within her hearing. You may say something such as, "Grandma, did you see how Adelyn smiles when Kate talks to her? Kate is such a big help when she plays with her baby sister."

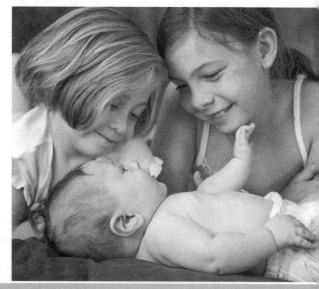

Although adjusting to a new baby may be difficult for your child, it's an opportunity for her to learn healthy ways of handling stress. With time and guidance, your child will adapt to the new family structure and eventually develop a lasting bond with her sibling.

## *Key Points to Remember*

- Physical changes occur earlier when your body has gone through pregnancy before.
- After you've told your child that you're pregnant, use the time until the birth to help him develop realistic expectations about the baby and to include him in the preparations.
- The decision to include your child at the birth is one that's best made by you, your partner, and your child.
- Whether your child attends the birth or stays with someone else, preparing him for the event will help him understand and accept the new addition to your family.
- The arrival of a baby will forever change your child's life. Help him adjust by accepting any negative reactions to the change and helping him find new, positive coping skills.

# Appendixes

# Common Medications Used for Pain Relief during Labor[1]

Effects and side effects vary for all medications, depending on the drug, total dosage, timing, your baby's condition, and your reaction to the medication. For more information on any of these medications, see Chapter 10 and visit our web site, http://www.PCNGuide.com.

## Systemic Medications

### IV Narcotics or Narcotic-like Analgesics

| How and When They're Given | Drugs Used | Benefits | Possible Risks | Additional Precautions and Interventions |
|---|---|---|---|---|
| • Given intravenously by direct injection or injection into an IV line. Sometimes, a patient-controlled analgesia (PCA) device is used. Can also be given by intramuscular (IM) injection.<br>• Given in early to active labor, when it's believed that the birth is at least 2 hours away. Also given after a cesarean birth. | • Morphine<br>• Fentanyl (Sublimaze)<br>• Meperidine (Demerol)<br>• Butorphanol (Stadol)<br>• Nalbuphine (Nubain)<br><br>(Stadol and Nubain are combination drugs—a narcotic plus a narcotic antagonist, which reduces some of the narcotic's side effects.) | • During active labor, the drugs reduce your awareness of pain and promote relaxation between contractions.<br>• Large doses of narcotics (especially morphine) may be used in a prolonged prelabor in hopes of slowing or stopping contractions and allowing you to rest. | **To you**<br>• May cause itching, nausea, vomiting, drowsiness, hallucinations, dizziness, or a feeling of being "high."<br>• May lower your heart rate, respiratory rate, and blood pressure.<br>• May affect your ability to use self-help comfort techniques.<br>• May temporarily slow labor progress.<br>**To your baby before birth**<br>• May make his heart rate readings appear abnormal.<br><br>**To your baby after birth**<br>• May slow his breathing and alter his behavioral responses (for example, poor suckling) for several days. | **For you**<br>• Possible restriction to bed and IV fluids<br>• Frequent monitoring of your blood pressure and your baby's heart rate<br>• Frequent reminders for you to breathe deeply, and help to keep you oriented<br>• Narcotic antagonists, if needed to reduce side effects<br><br>• Changes in your position or administration of oxygen to improve your baby's heart rate pattern<br><br>• Discontinuation of medications at least 2 hours before birth to reduce their effects on your baby<br>• Oxygen and resuscitation equipment on hand if your baby is born within 4 hours after narcotics are given<br>• Narcotic antagonists, if needed to reverse side effects |

### Additional Systemic Medications That Are Less Commonly Used in Labor

- Sedatives and barbiturates such as Nembutal or Phenobarbital, which are given by pill or injection. Used for anxiety or, in larger doses, to help you sleep during a slow, painful prelabor. May be used before 4 cm cervical dilation, but should be discontinued before active labor, to reduce effects on your baby. Rarely used in the United States and Canada.
- Tranquilizers such as Phenergan, Versed, or Valium, which are given by pill or injection. Used for anxiety in early labor or following a cesarean section. Not used in active labor because of their effects on newborns.
- Inhalation analgesia (nitrous oxide), which is inhaled through a mask. Doesn't eliminate pain, but the effects on your mental state mean you're less troubled by the pain. Drug is rapidly metabolized, which means few or no side effects on your baby. Rarely used in the United States, but common in Canada.
- Narcotic antagonists, such as Narcan, which are given by injection in labor if a narcotic medication is causing adverse side effects, or by injection to a newborn with breathing problems caused by narcotics given shortly before birth.
- General anesthesia, in which an induction agent is given intravenously, then an inhalation agent is inhaled through a mask. Causes unconsciousness as well as complete numbness. Used in less than 10 percent of cesarean births.

## Local Anesthetics

### Local Perineal Block

| How and When It's Given | Drug Used | Benefits | Possible Risks | Additional Precautions and Interventions |
|---|---|---|---|---|
| • Given by injection around the vaginal opening.<br>• In the second stage, given before an episiotomy; in the third stage, given for repair of the episiotomy or tear. | • Lidocaine (most often) | • Numbness in perineum<br>• Relief of pain during crowning, episiotomy, or stitching after the birth | **To you**<br>• Injections may sting.<br>• If given during the second stage, the drugs may increase swelling in your perineum and increase the likelihood of vaginal tears.<br>**To your baby**<br>• Minimal to none | • Postpone use until after the birth and use only if stitches are necessary. |

### Additional Local Anesthetics That Are Less Commonly Used

• Pudendal block, which is given by injection deep into the vagina. Numbs vagina and perineum during the birth. Rarely used, except with a forceps delivery.
• Paracervical block, which is given by injection into the cervix. Numbs cervical pain and pressure in your lower uterus. Given between 5 and 9 cm cervical dilation. Rarely used, because of the effects on the baby.

# Neuraxial Medications (Epidural or Spinal)

### Epidural Analgesia with Combination of Narcotics and Anesthetics

| How and When It's Given | Drugs Used | Benefits | Possible Risks[2] | Additional Precautions and Interventions |
|---|---|---|---|---|
| • Given by epidural catheter. See page 198 for information on placement and procedures. <br>• Typically given in active labor until birth. | • A combination of a narcotic and a "-caine" anesthetic (To learn more about the effects of narcotics and analgesics, see pages 197 and 448.) | • Decreased pain and numbness (or reduced sensation) in your abdomen, back, and perineum <br>• Increased ability to relax and sleep <br>• Mental clarity | **To you** <br>• Reduced mobility <br>• Drop in blood pressure <br>• Fever <br>• Discomforts such as itching, nausea, and vomiting (caused by narcotics) <br>• Slowed labor progress <br>• Decreased urge to push, which may lead to a forceps delivery or vacuum extraction <br>• Spinal headache caused by an epidural needle that has been inserted too far (2 percent chance) <br>• Secondary side effects from precautions and additional safety interventions (see next column) <br>**To your baby** <br>• *Same as for IV narcotics and narcotic-like analgesics (although effects are milder), plus:* <br>• Worrisome changes to her heart rate pattern <br>• Fever | **Routine** <br>• Restriction of food and drink <br>• IV fluids <br>• Bladder catheter <br>• Restriction to bed <br>• Various devices to closely monitor you and your baby <br>**Used as needed** <br>• Oxygen by mask <br>• Pitocin to speed labor <br>• Episiotomy, vacuum extraction, forceps delivery, cesarean section <br>• Blood patch for spinal headache (a small amount of your blood is injected in the epidural space near the dural puncture) <br>• Additional medications to control itching and nausea <br>**If your baby is showing effects of narcotics** <br>• *Same as for IV narcotics and narcotic-like analgesics* <br>**If your baby is born with a fever** <br>• Admittance to special care nursery for 48 hours for observation and antibiotics <br>• Septic workup to check for infection (blood test and spinal tap) |

## Spinal (Intrathecal) Narcotic Analgesia

| How and When It's Given | Drugs Used | Benefits | Possible Risks[3] | Additional Precautions and Interventions |
|---|---|---|---|---|
| • Given by spinal injection.<br>• Given in early to active labor. | • Narcotic only | • Decreases your perception of pain.<br>• Allows for the ability to move freely in bed. You may be able to stand with assistance (if policy allows).<br>• You still feel sensations other than pain (touch, pressure, temperature).<br>• When compared to IV narcotics, you receive more pain relief with less medication.<br>• Effects last up to 2 hours. | **To you**<br>• Itching, nausea, and vomiting<br>• Weakness in legs or loss of balance while walking<br>• Possible altered mental state, but less so than with IV narcotics and narcotic-like analgesics<br>• Spinal headache (less than 1 percent chance)<br>**To your baby**<br>• *Same as for IV narcotics and narcotic-like analgesics (although effects are milder)* | **If you have a spinal headache**<br>• Blood patch (see page 452)<br>• Lying flat for hours or days<br>**If your baby is showing effects of narcotics**<br>• *Same as for IV narcotics and narcotic-like analgesics* |

## Combined Spinal-Epidural (CSE)

| How and When It's Given | Drugs Used | Benefits | Possible Risks[4] | Additional Precautions and Interventions |
|---|---|---|---|---|
| • See details of placement on page 198.<br>• Given by spinal as injection as early 2 cm cervical dilation, with addition of anesthetic at 5 to 8 cm. | • Spinal narcotics are given first; epidural analgesia is given when needed. | • *Same as for spinal narcotics and epidural analgesia* | • *Same as for spinal narcotics and epidural analgesia* | • *Same as for spinal narcotics and epidural analgesia* |

## Spinal Block

| How and When It's Given | Drugs Used | Benefits | Possible Risks[5] | Additional Precautions and Interventions |
|---|---|---|---|---|
| • Given by spinal injection.<br>• Used for a planned cesarean section. | • "-caine" drugs | • Total numbness from your chest to toes, although you may still feel some pressure or pulling during the delivery of your baby.<br>• Provides excellent pain relief without impairing your mental awareness.<br>• Can be administered quickly and takes effect almost immediately.<br>• Effects last a few hours. | **To you**<br>• Drop in blood pressure<br>• Occasional feeling of being unable to breathe (because your chest becomes anesthetized)<br>• Spinal headache (1 percent chance)<br>**To your baby**<br>• Fetal distress<br>• Subtle neurobehavioral effects for days | • *Same as for spinal narcotics and epidural analgesia, plus:*<br>• Assisted ventilation if breathing difficulties arise |

## Additional Neuraxial Anesthetics That Are Less Commonly Used

• Epidurals that use an anesthetic only (more commonly used for a cesarean section than for labor)
• Epidurals that use narcotics only

# Summary of Normal Labor without Pain Medications

*Note:* If you're planning to have an epidural, use this chart until you receive the anesthesia. Then see Chapter 10, which explains how medications will affect the remainder of your labor.

## Prelabor

| What physical changes and events occur | How you may feel and how you may respond | What you can do to cope | What your partner or doula can do to help you |
|---|---|---|---|
| • Your cervix begins to ripen, efface, and move forward.<br>• You have nonprogressing contractions and may have restless back pain, soft bowel movements, and menstrual-like cramps.<br>• May last for days. | • You feel tired, discouraged, anxious. You may be unable to sleep through contractions.<br>• May overestimate labor progress, start rituals, and go to birthplace (or call home birth midwife) too early.<br>• May focus more than necessary on the contractions. | • Engage in distracting activities and projects.<br>• Alternate distracting activities with restful ones such as taking a bath, listening to music, lying down, having a massage, and so on.<br>• Use labor-stimulating measures (only if you feel pressured to get into labor).<br>• Eat if you're hungry (mostly carbohydrates).<br>• Drink to quench your thirst. | • Review the route to the birthplace.<br>• Encourage you to eat and drink.<br>• Pack the vehicle; be sure there's enough fuel in it.<br>• Time your contractions (five or six at a time) every few hours or when your labor seems to have changed.<br>• Ensure that you aren't left alone. Help make this time pleasant for you.<br>• Alert your doula to be ready to come when you need her, if she's not already with you.<br>• Enhance emotional security and reduce stress by creating a soothing, safe, private, and loving atmosphere. |

## First Stage of Labor: Early Labor

| What physical changes and events occur | How you may feel and how you may respond | What you can do to cope | What your partner or doula can do to help you |
|---|---|---|---|
| • Denotes the time from the onset of labor until your cervix is dilated to about 4 to 5 cm.<br>• Contractions are progressing, usually mild at first, then becoming longer, stronger, closer together.<br>• Your cervix continues ripening, effacing, and begins to dilate.<br>• May have bloody show.<br>• Your membranes may rupture (10 percent chance), but this usually happens later in labor.<br>• May have back pain with contractions. | • *Same as in prelabor, plus:*<br>• Have mixed feelings—excitement, confidence, and optimism; or anxiety and distress—often all at the same time.<br>• As contractions intensify, you can no longer be distracted during them. | • Begin using planned rituals (relax, breathe, and focus through each contraction) when the intensity of contractions stops you from doing distracting activities.<br>• Use slow breathing, releasing tension with each exhalation.<br>• Ask your doula for help.<br>• Contact your caregiver or birthplace as instructed, typically when your contractions have reached the 5-1-1 or 4-1-1, pattern (see page 244).<br>• Use comfort measures to relieve back pain. | • Continue timing your contractions periodically. Call caregiver or birthplace when your contractions reach designated intensity, frequency, and length, or if your membranes rupture.<br>• Focus on you during contractions as soon as you begin doing a planned ritual.<br>• Give you constructive feedback, not false praise.<br>• Help you release tension in a selected area of your body with each exhalation.<br>• Remind you of positions and comfort techniques (see Chapter 11). |

## First Stage of Labor: Getting into Active Labor

| What physical changes and events occur | How you may feel and how you may respond | What you can do to cope | What your partner or doula can do to help you |
|---|---|---|---|
| • Your cervix is dilated 4 to 5 cm.<br>• Your contractions intensify and occur every 3 to 4 minutes, lasting 1 minute or longer.<br>• Your labor progress should begin to speed up when your cervix is 5 cm dilated. | • You probably head for your birthplace or call your home birth midwife.<br>• May struggle to remain "in control" and worry that labor is too hard and long.<br>• May become serious, withdrawn, and focused on your labor.<br>• You may recognize that labor isn't within your control, leaving you feeling trapped. You may weep.<br>• You can no longer be distracted during contractions; you need your partner's or doula's undivided attention during them.<br>• Find unnecessary conversation annoying.<br>• May want pain medications.<br>• Can release control and accept your labor if you can move freely, feel safe and uninhibited, and have good support. | • Try to release your need to be in control; let labor happen as you discover what helps you cope (finding your spontaneous ritual).<br>• Maintain a rhythm with your breathing and movements, letting your partner or doula help as necessary.<br>• Try to continue slow breathing if you find it restful.<br>• Remember that labor progress should speed up soon.<br>• If you planned for an early epidural, you can probably receive it during this phase. | • Drive to the birthplace carefully!<br>• Use massage (hand or foot), double hip squeeze, counter-pressure, slow dancing, and so on to help you cope (see Chapter 11).<br>• Rhythmically murmur soothing, encouraging words to you.<br>• Guide you with visualizations, imagery, rhythmic talk, or breath-counting—whatever helps you respond well.<br>• Help you keep a rhythm in your breathing, moaning, swaying, tapping, or whatever action you choose.<br>• Refrain from asking questions during contractions, and ask only simple yes-or-no questions between contractions.<br>• Help with your ritual (for example, stroking you, holding you, or talking to you through contractions) or simply stay by you if that's all you require.<br>• Help you follow your preferences on pain medications (see page 187). |

## First Stage of Labor: Active Labor

| What physical changes and events occur | How you may feel and how you may respond | What you can do to cope | What your partner or doula can do to help you |
|---|---|---|---|
| • Your cervix dilates from 5 to 8 cm.<br>• Lasts on average 3 to 5 hours.<br>• If your baby is occiput posterior or her head is tilted to one side, dilation of your cervix may pause as your baby corrects her position.<br>• May have back pain (30 percent chance). | • You become calmer than before, now that you've discovered how to get through contractions.<br>• May enter the "birth zone" and become aware of little other than your labor. | • *Same as for early labor and getting into active labor, plus:*<br>• Take a bath for relaxation and pain relief.<br>• Stay hydrated by taking frequent sips of water or juice. | • *Same as for getting into active labor, plus:*<br>• Stay by your side.<br>• Offer you liquids.<br>• Remind you to empty your bladder. |

## First Stage of Labor: Transition

| What physical changes and events occur | How you may feel and how you may respond | What you can do to cope | What your partner or doula can do to help you |
|---|---|---|---|
| • Your cervix dilates from 8 to 10 cm.<br>• Your baby begins to descend toward your vaginal opening.<br>• Contractions are long and very close together.<br>• Pain and intensity of labor is probably at its maximum.<br>• Likely lasts less than 2 hours if this is your first birth, or less than 1 hour if you've given birth before.<br>• As your cervix completes dilation, you may have a "lip" that remains. | • May feel scared or lost in labor; may be angry or frustrated.<br>• May want more help from others.<br>• May feel that you've reached your limit.<br>• May lose your rhythm and ritual.<br>• May cry out, tense, weep, or protest.<br>• May feel hot, then cold; may tremble.<br>• May feel nauseated; may vomit. | • Keep a rhythm.<br>• Follow your partner's or doula's lead with Take Charge Routine (see page 256).<br>• Hang in there! Remember that you're almost ready to push and will feel better soon. If you can keep a rhythm and follow a ritual now, you're better able to continue laboring without medications (if that's your wish and if your labor progress remains normal).<br>• If you want an epidural, you can get it at this time as long as your labor isn't moving too fast. | • Maintain a confident, calm, optimistic manner; keep eye contact with you.<br>• Use the Take Charge Routine (see page 256) if you're panicky or if your eyes are clenched shut and your expression is anguished, or if you can't maintain a rhythm.<br>• Remind you that transition means you're almost ready to push out your baby.<br>• Hold you tightly (but not rub your body), if that's what you want.<br>• Keep encouraging you and never give up.<br>• Let you weep, if you must, while acknowledging your pain. |

## Second Stage of Labor: Resting Phase

| What physical changes and events occur | How you may feel and how you may respond | What you can do to cope | What your partner or doula can do to help you |
|---|---|---|---|
| • Denotes the time from complete dilation to when you begin to push.<br>• For up to 20 minutes, you may have few noticeable contractions (if any) or have no urge to push.<br>• After your baby's head has slipped through your cervix, your uterus may need time to tighten around the rest of your baby's body before you can begin to push. | • Feel relief, optimism, confidence, and pain-free.<br>• Have renewed energy, enthusiasm, hope, even if you don't experience a pause in contractions.<br>• No longer in the "birth zone"—you're clearheaded, talkative, and more aware of your surroundings. | • Rest or doze, if you can.<br>• If you want to push spontaneously when you have the urge, remind your nurse or caregiver of this preference.<br>• Review positions; review how to push and how to relax your pelvic floor muscles.<br>• If the resting phase lasts more than 20 minutes, change to upright positions to encourage an urge to push. | • Should match your enthusiasm (but not overly so).<br>• Use this lull to renew energy (drink a beverage, close eyes and rest for a moment, use the restroom, and so on). If leaving the room, return promptly.<br>• Help you change positions, if necessary or desired. |

## Second Stage of Labor: Descent Phase

| What physical changes and events occur | How you may feel and how you may respond | What you can do to cope | What your partner or doula can do to help you |
|---|---|---|---|
| • Your baby rotates and descends into your birth canal.<br>• Oxytocin surges cause an urge to push, which may be mild at first, but becomes compelling and irresistible. You begin to push reflexively with contractions.<br>• Contractions aren't as close together as they were in transition, and they may be shorter.<br>• May last for a few minutes or up to 2 hours.<br>• At first, your baby's head can't be seen, then it appears at your vaginal opening when you push and retreats between pushes.<br>• Your caregiver supports your perineum, applies warm compresses, and may direct your pushing. | • May feel inadequate in pushing until you get the hang of it.<br>• May find this phase rewarding, but you may find it painful and tedious. Either way, you're working hard.<br>• May find the pressure in your vagina alarming and fear it will worsen, making you "hold back" from pushing (see page 262).<br>• May feel less pain as your baby's head repositions. | • Hold your breath and strain when the contraction makes you feel that you can't avoid pushing. You may bellow or cry out with the effort.<br>• Try to bulge your pelvic floor (see page 96).<br>• Consider touching your baby's head or watching her progress in a mirror.<br>• If you're holding back, or if pushing is painful, try to push into the pain and through it. Doing so will feel better than stopping when it hurts.<br>• Change your position every 30 minutes for comfort or to speed up labor progress.<br>• Consider directed or pro-longed pushing if your labor isn't adequately progressing with spontaneous bearing down.<br>• If using directed pushing, follow the directions for when and how long to hold your breath and strain. | • Encourage and praise your efforts. (Should *not* yell, "Push!").<br>• Apply cool, damp cloths to your forehead, cheeks, neck, and chest.<br>• Report on your progress (as soon as your baby's head is visible).<br>• Remind you to release tension in your perineum.<br>• Remind your caregiver of your feelings about episiotomy, if appropriate.<br>• Support your position and help you change positions.<br>• If pushing is ineffective, remind you to open your eyes and look toward where your baby is emerging (may use a mirror). |

## Second Stage of Labor: Crowning and Birth

| What physical changes and events occur | How you may feel and how you may respond | What you can do to cope | What your partner or doula can do to help you |
|---|---|---|---|
| • Your baby's head emerges; it no longer retracts into your vaginal opening between contractions.<br>• Your perineum and area around your urethra are most vulnerable to tearing in this phase.<br>• Your caregiver either supports your perineum (often with warm compresses) or does an episiotomy (unlikely). | • Feel excited because your baby's birth will be very soon.<br>• May feel a burning sensation from vaginal stretching.<br>• May have mixed feelings: You may be tempted to push hard to get the birth over with, despite the burning. Or you may fear the burning feeling and become reluctant to push. | • Recognize the burning as a sign that labor is almost over.<br>• Use your partner's help with positions.<br>• To slow the birth of your baby's head and protect your perineum, stop pushing and pant or blow when your caregiver tells you to do so.<br>• Rejoice in your baby's birth! | • Support you as you change positions.<br>• Refrain from rushing you; help you keep from pushing as needed.<br>• Say little or nothing when your caregiver is directing you to slow the birth of your baby's head.<br>• Rejoice in your baby's birth! |

## Third Stage of Labor

| What physical changes and events occur | How you may feel and how you may respond | What you can do to cope | What your partner or doula can do to help you |
|---|---|---|---|
| • Lasts up to 30 minutes. | • Feel relief that labor is over. | • Move away clothing so your baby can lie skin-to-skin with you. | • Help you get your baby onto your bare abdomen. |
| • Your baby's umbilical cord is clamped and cut. | • Become engrossed with your baby. | • Don't rush breastfeeding. Your baby needs time to acclimate before she's ready to feed. Let her show you she's ready to start suckling (see page 410). | • Help you breathe and focus through any painful procedures. |
| • Your baby's condition is evaluated using the Apgar score. | • Feel concern over trembling. | | • Get you a warm blanket if you're trembling. |
| • If your baby is fine and hospital policy allows, your baby is placed on your bare abdomen or chest. | • Feel alarm if contractions are still painful. | | • Open shirt and snuggle skin-to-skin with your baby, if you can't hold her right away. |
| • Your uterus contracts and shrinks, the placenta separates from your uterine wall. You expel the placenta with a few pushes. | • Feel surprise at the discomfort when your caregiver examines your birth canal or massages your uterus after the placenta is expelled. | • Ask for a warm blanket to stop trembling. | • Request that routine newborn procedures (such as weighing your baby or giving her a bath) be delayed for at least an hour so you can bond with your baby. |
| • You may briefly tremble uncontrollably. (This is a normal reaction to giving birth.) | | • Use light breathing and focus on your partner or doula during uterine massage and the examination or stitching of your perineum. | • Enjoy this time with your new family! |
| • Your caregiver checks your uterus to confirm it's contracting, and checks your birth canal for tears. | | • Try to be patient during postpartum procedures. You'll have time to focus on your baby soon. | |

# Recommended Resources

The following is a list of the best books, web sites, and DVDs about topics discussed in this book. You can find additional resources on specific topics within the chapters. Visit our web site, http://www.PCNGuide.com, to find many more resources and more details on the resources listed here.

## GENERAL PREGNANCY AND BIRTH INFORMATION

*Ina May's Guide to Childbirth* by Ina May Gaskin (2003).

*The Official Lamaze Guide: Giving Birth with Confidence* by Judith Lothian and Charlotte DeVries (2010).

*Our Bodies, Ourselves: Pregnancy and Birth* by Boston Women's Health Book Collective and Judy Norsigian (2008).

*The Working Woman's Pregnancy Book* by Marjorie Greenfield (2008).

Childbirth Connection: http://www.childbirthconnection.org

March of Dimes: http://www.marchofdimes.com

*Healthy Birth Your Way: Six Steps to a Safer Birth* videos by Lamaze International and Injoy (2010). Visit http://www.mothersadvocate.org to watch them.

*Orgasmic Birth* DVD directed by Debra Pascali-Bonaro (2008).

*The Business of Being Born* DVD directed by Abby Epstein (2008).

Visit http://www.lamaze.org/default.aspx?tabid=53 to sign up for a weekly pregnancy e-newsletter from Lamaze International.

Visit http://text4baby.org/ to sign up for weekly texts about pregnancy and baby's first year.

## CHOOSING A BIRTHPLACE AND CAREGIVER

*Deliver This! Make the Childbirth Choice That's Right for You...No Matter What Everyone Else Thinks* by Marisa Cohen (2007).

*The Doula Book: How a Trained Labor Companion Can Help You Have a Shorter, Easier, and Healthier Birth* by Marshall H. Klaus, John H. Kennell, and Phyllis H. Klaus (2002).

Visit http://www.thebirthsurvey.com to see ratings of local caregivers and birthplaces.

Visit http://www.childbirthconnection.org to see a discussion of maternity care options.

Visit http://motherfriendly.org to see the Coalition for Improving Maternity Services' Ten Steps of Mother-Friendly Care.

See page 9 for a list of web sites that allow you to search for birthplaces and caregivers in your area.

## HEALTHY LIFESTYLE DURING AND AFTER PREGNANCY

*Essential Exercises for the Childbearing Year: A Guide to Health and Comfort Before and After Your Baby Is Born* by Elizabeth Noble (2003).

*Lose Your Mummy Tummy* by Julie Tupler and Jodie Gould (2004).

Visit http://www.mymidwife.org/pregnancy_body.cfm for information on coping with pregnancy discomforts.

Visit http://www.fitpregnancy.com for exercise and nutrition information.

Visit http://mypyramid.gov for information on nutrition recommendations based on dietary guidelines for Americans.

Visit http://www.mymidwife.org/prenatal_guide.cfm for information on prenatal testing.

United States Centers for Disease Control: 800-CDC-INFO (232-4636) or http://www.cdc.gov/ncbddd/pregnancy

United States Food and Drug Administration: 888-INFO-FDA (888-463-6332) or http://www.fda.gov

*Yoga for Pregnancy, Labor and Birth* DVD directed by Colette Crawford (2005).

## INFORMATION ON HAZARDS TO AVOID DURING PREGNANCY

**Alcohol:** Alcoholics Anonymous (AA): 212-870-3400 or http://www.aa.org

**Domestic violence:** National Domestic Violence Hotline: 800-799-SAFE (7233) or http://www.ndvh.org

**Drugs:** United States Substance Abuse and Mental Health Services Administration (SAMHSA): 800-662-HELP (800-662-4357) or http://www.samhsa.gov

**Narcotics:** Narcotics Anonymous (NA): 818-773-9999 or http://www.na.org.

**Teratogens** (medications, illnesses, and substances that can cause birth defects): http://www.otispregnancy.org/otis-fact-sheets-s13037

**Tobacco:** Smoking cessation: 800-CDC-INFO (232-4636) or http://www.smokefree.gov

**Workplace hazards:** The National Institute for Occupational Safety and Health (NIOSH): 800-CDC-INFO (232-4636) or http://www.cdc.gov/niosh/docs/99-104/

## SPECIAL CIRCUMSTANCES IN PREGNANCY AND BIRTH

**Disability:** *The Baby Challenge: A Handbook on Pregnancy for Women with a Physical Disability* by Mukti Jain Campion (1990).

**High-risk pregnancies:** http://www.sidelines.org

**Multiples:** *Twins! Pregnancy, Birth, and the First Year of Life* by Connie Agnew, Alan H. Klein, and Jill Alison Ganon (2006).

**Pregnancy after loss:** *Trying Again: A Guide to Pregnancy After Miscarriage, Stillbirth, and Infant Loss* by Ann Douglas, John R. Sussman, and Deborah Davis (2000).

**Survivors of childhood sexual abuse:** *When Survivors Give Birth: Understanding and Healing the Effects of Early Sexual Abuse on Childbearing Women* by Penny Simkin and Phyllis Klaus (2004).

**Teenage pregnancy:** *Your Pregnancy & Newborn Journey: A Guide for Pregnant Teens* by Jeanne Warren Lindsay and Jean Brunelli (2004).

**Nontraditional families:** *The Ultimate Guide to Pregnancy for Lesbians: How to Stay Sane and Care for Yourself From Pre-conception Through Birth* by Rachel Pepper (2005); also visit http://www.therainbowbabies.com.

## LABOR AND BIRTH

*Birth Day: A Pediatrician Explores the Science, the History, and the Wonder of Childbirth* by Mark Sloan (2009).

*The Labor Progress Handbook: Early Interventions to Prevent and Treat Dystocia* by Penny Simkin and Ruth Ancheta (2005).

*Listening to Mothers II: Report of the Second National U.S. Survey of Women's Childbearing Experiences* (2006) and *New Mothers Speak Out: National Survey Results Highlight Women's Postpartum Experiences* (2008) by Eugene R. DeClercq, Carol Sakala, Maureen P. Corry, and Sandra Applebaum; http://childbirthconnection.com/article.asp?ck=10068

## COPING WITH LABOR PAIN

*Birthing from Within: An Extra-Ordinary Guide to Childbirth Preparation* by Pam England and Rob Horowitz (1998).

*Comfort in Labor: How You Can Help Yourself to a Normal Satisfying Childbirth* by Penny Simkin (2007). http://childbirthconnection.com/pdf.asp?PDFDownload=comfort-in-labor-simkin

*Comfort Measures for Childbirth*, a DVD by Penny Simkin (2009). Visit http://www.pennysimkin.com to order a copy.

## MEDICAL INTERVENTIONS: EVIDENCE-BASED RESOURCES

Childbirth Connection: http://www.childbirthconnection.org

Cochrane Collaboration: http://www.cochrane.org/reviews/en/subtopics/87.html

PubMed: http://www.pubmed.gov

*Cesarean: What Every Pregnant Woman Needs to Know about Cesarean Section* by Childbirth Connection (2006). http://www.childbirthconnection.org/article.asp?ck=10164

Vaginal birth after cesarean (VBAC): *NIH Consensus Panel Statement* (2010). http://consensus.nih.gov/2010/vbac.htm

## POSTPARTUM COMPLICATIONS

**Cesarean support:** International Cesarean Awareness Network (ICAN): http://www.ican-online.org

**Postpartum mood disorders:** Postpartum Support International: 800-944-4773 or http://www.postpartum.net

**Traumatic birth:** http://solaceformothers.org/

**Loss of a baby:** *Mending Invisible Wings: Healing from the Loss of Your Baby* by Mary Burgess and Shiloh Sophia McCloud (2009).

## FATHERS AND FATHERHOOD

*The Birth Partner: A Complete Guide to Childbirth for Dads, Doulas, and All Other Labor Companions* by Penny Simkin (2008).

*The New Father: A Dad's Guide to the First Year* by Armin A. Brott (2005).

*Partnership Parenting: How Men and Women Parent Differently—Why It Helps Your Kids and Can Strengthen Your Marriage* by Kyle Pruett and Marsha Pruett (2009).

Great Dad: http://www.GreatDad.com

## NEWBORN CARE

*The Baby Book: Everything You Need to Know About Your Baby from Birth to Age Two* by William Sears and Martha Sears (2003).

*The Happiest Baby on the Block: The New Way to Calm Crying and Help Your Newborn Sleep Longer* by Harvey Karp (2008). Available in paperback or DVD.

*Mothering* magazine. http://www.mothering.com

*Your Baby and Child: From Birth to Age Five* by Penelope Leach (2010).

American Academy of Pediatrics: http://www.healthychildren.org

**Health and safety topics:** http://www.seattlechildrens.org/safety-wellness/

**Child development and learning enhancement:** http://www.parentingcounts.org/

## BREASTFEEDING

*The Nursing Mother's Companion: Revised Edition* by Kathleen Huggins (2005).

*Womanly Art of Breastfeeding* by La Leche League International (2010).

Kelly Mom: http://www.kellymom.com/

La Leche League: http://www.llli.org/

Newman Breastfeeding Clinic and Institute: http://www.drjacknewman.com

## RELATIONSHIPS AFTER THE BIRTH

*And Baby Makes Three: The Six-Step Plan for Preserving Marital Intimacy and Rekindling Romance After Baby Arrives* by John Gottman and Julie Schwartz Gottman (2008).

Bringing Baby Home workshops: Visit http://www.bbhonline.org to find a workshop near you.

# Notes

## Chapter 1: You're Having a Baby!

1. P. Simkin, "Just Another Day in a Woman's Life?" *Birth* 18 (December 1991); P. Simkin, "Just Another Day in a Woman's Life? Part II: Nature and Consistency of Women's Long Term Memories of Their First Birth Experiences," *Birth* 19 (June 1992): 64-81.

## Chapter 2: So Many Choices

1. C. Ruland and S. Bakken, "Developing, implementing, and evaluating decision support systems for shared decision-making in patient care: a conceptual model and case illustration," *Journal of Biomedical Informatics* 35(5-6) (2002): 313-21.

2. Russo et al., "Hospitalizations Related to Childbirth, 2006," Healthcare Cost and Utilization Project, Agency for Healthcare Research and Quality, http://www.hcup-us.ahrq.gov/reports/statbriefs/sb71.jsp (2009); S.R. Machlin and F. Rhode, Agency for Healthcare Research and Quality, "Health care expenses for uncomplicated pregnancies," http://www.meps.ahrq.gov/meps web/data_files/publications/rf27/rf27.pdf (2007); National Association of Childbearing Centers, *National Association of Childbearing Centers Survey Report of Birth Center Experience 2003*, National Association of Childbearing Centers (2004).

3. K. Johnson and B. Daviss, "Outcomes of planned home births with certified professional midwives: large prospective study in North America," *BMJ* 330 (2005): 1416; A. de Jonge et al., "Perinatal mortality and morbidity in a nationwide cohort of 529,688 low-risk planned home and hospital births," *BJOG* 10 (2009): 1111; Janssen et al., "Outcomes of planned home births versus planned hospital births after regulation of midwifery in British Columbia," *CMAJ* 3 (2002): 166.

4. K. Johnson and B. Daviss (see Note 3); Amelink-Verburg et al., "Evaluation of 280,000 cases in Dutch midwifery practices: a descriptive study," *BJOG* 115 (2008): 570-78.

5. Ibid.

6. Ibid.

7. Ibid.

8. E.D. Hodnett et al., "Continuous support for women during childbirth," Cochrane Database of Syst. Rev., Issue 3 (2003): CD003766.

9. K. Johnson and B. Daviss (see Note 3); A. de Jonge et al. (see Note 3); Janssen et al. (see Note 3).

10. Childbirth Connection, "The Rights of Childbearing Women," http://www.childbirthconnection.org/article.asp?ck=10084&ClickedLink=0&area=27 (2006).

11. E.D. Hodnett et al., "Continuous support for women during childbirth," Cochrane Database of Syst. Rev., Issue 3 (2003): CD003766.

## Chapter 3: Common Changes and Concerns in Pregnancy

1. K. Uvnas-Moberg, *The Oxytocin Factor*, Da Capo Press (2003).

2. B. Luke and M.B. Brown, "Elevated risks of pregnancy complications and adverse outcomes with increasing maternal age," *Human Reproduction* (8 February 2007).

3. J. Goodman, "Becoming an Involved Father of an Infant," *Journal of Obstetrical, Gynecological, and Neonatal Nursing* 34(2) (2005): 190-200.

4. S.J. Berg and K.E. Wynne-Edwards, "Changes in Testosterone, Cortisol, and Estradiol Levels in Men Becoming Fathers," *Mayo Clinic Proc.* 76(6) (June 2001): 582-92.

5. P. Simkin and P. Klaus, *When Survivors Give Birth: Understanding and Healing the Effects of Early Sexual Abuse on Childbearing Women*, Classic Day Publishing (2004).

## Chapter 4: Having a Healthy Pregnancy

1. March of Dimes, "Stress," http://www.marchofdimes.com/pnhec/159_527.asp (June 2008).

2. Talge et al., "Antenatal maternal stress and long-term effects on child neurodevelopment: how and why?" *J Child Psychol Psychiatry* 48(3-4) (2007): 245-61.

3. American College of Obstetrics and Gynecology (ACOG), "Alcohol in Pregnancy," ACOG Patient Education Pamphlet (2000).

4. M.M. Morales-Suarez-Varela et al., "Smoking habits, nicotine use, and congenital malformations," *Obstetrics and Gynecology* 107(1) (2006): 51-57.

5. E.K. Tong, L. England, S.A. Glantz, "Changing conclusions on secondhand smoke in a sudden infant death syndrome review funded by the tobacco industry," *Pediatrics* 115(3) (2005): e356-66.

6. E. Juaniaux and G.J. Burton, "Morphological and biological effects of maternal exposure to tobacco smoke on the feto-placental unit," *Early Human Development* 83 (11) (2007): 699-706.

7. International Food Information Council Foundation, "Healthy Eating During Pregnancy," http://internal.ific.org/publications/brochures/pregnancybroch.cfm (2009).

8. D.K. Li et al., "Caffeine and Risk of Miscarriage," *American Journal of Obstetrics and Gynecology* (24 January 2008); L.M. Grosso et al., "Caffeine metabolites in umbilical cord blood, cytochrome P-450 1A2 activity and intrauterine growth restriction," *American Journal of Epidemiology* 163 (2006): 1035-41; F. Sata et al., "Caffeine intake, CYP1A2 polymorphism and the risk of recurrent pregnancy loss," *Molecular Human Reproduction* 11(5) (2005): 357-60.

9. C.G. Rousseaux and H. Schachter, "Regulatory issues concerning the safety, efficacy and quality of herbal remedies," *Birth Defects Research Part B: Developmental & Reproductive Toxicology* 68(6) (2003): 505-10; C.H. Chuang et al., "Herbal medicines used during the first trimester and major congenital malformations: an analysis of data from a pregnancy cohort study," *Drug Safety* 29(6) (2006): 537-48.

10. J.G. Silverman et al., "Intimate partner violence victimization prior to and during pregnancy among women residing in 26 U.S. states: associations with maternal and neonatal health," *American Journal of Obstetrics and Gynecology* 195(1) (2006): 140-48.

11. J. McFarlane et al., "Abuse during pregnancy and femicide: urgent implications for women's health," *Obstetrics and Gynecology* 100(1) (2002): 27-36.

12. Centers for Disease Control, "The Effects of Workplace Hazards on Female Reproductive Health," CDC/NIOSH Health Bulletin (1999).

13. L.M. Frazier, "Reproductive disorders associated with pesticide exposure," *J Agromedicine* 12(1) (2007): 27-37; A.J. DeRoos et al., "Parental occupational exposures to chemicals and incidence of neuroblastoma in offspring," *Am J Epidemiology* 154(2) (2001): 106-14; G.R. Bunin et al., "Parental heat exposure and risk of childhood brain tumor: a Children's Oncology Group study," *Am J Epidemiolgy* 164(3) (2006): 222-31; W. Hanke and J. Jurewicz, "The risk of adverse reproductive and developmental disorders due to occupational pesticide exposure: an overview of current epidemiological evidence," *Int J Occup Med Eviron Health* 17(2) (2004): 223-43.

## Chapter 5: Feeling Good and Staying Fit

1. American College of Obstetrics and Gynecology, "Exercise During Pregnancy," ACOG (2003).

## Chapter 6: Eating Well

1. *Environmental Nutrition* (April 2006): 3.

2. The U.S. Department of Health and Human Services and the U.S. Department of Agriculture, "Dietary Guidelines for Americans" (2011).

3. International Food Information Council Foundation, "Carbohydrates and Sugars," http://www.ific.org/nutrition/sugars/index (2007); International Food Information Council Foundation, "Healthy Eating During Pregnancy," http://internal.ific.org/publications/brochures/pregnancybroch.cfm (2009).

4. Institute of Medicine, "Weight Gain During Pregnancy: Reexamining the Guidelines," National Academy of Sciences (2009).

5. R. Artal, C.J. Lockwood, H.L. Brown, "Weight gain recommendations in pregnancy and the obesity epidemic," *Obstetrics and Gynecology* 115(1) (2010): 152-55.

6. American Pregnancy Association, "Mercury Levels in Fish," http://www.americanpregnancy.org/pregnancyhealth/fishmercury.htm (March 2007); American Heart Association, "Fish, Levels of Mercury and Omega-3 Fatty Acids," http://www.americanheart.org/presenter.jhtml?identifier=3013797 (2010); Food and Drug Administration, "Mercury Levels in Commercial Fish and Shellfish," http://www.cfsan.fda.gov/~frf/sea-mehg.html (January 2006); D.G. Andersen, "Omega-3 Fatty Acids in Seafood," http://www.andersenchiro.com/omega3-fatty-acids-in-seafood-table.shtml (2007).

## Chapter 7: When Pregnancy Becomes Complicated

1. American College of Obstetricians and Gynecologists (ACOG), "Uterine Fibroids," ACOG Patient Education Pamphlet (March 2009).

2. A. Ohlsson and V.S. Shah, "Intrapartum Antibiotics for known Group B Streptococcal Colonization," Cochrane Database of Syst. Rev., Issue 3, Art. No.: CD007467. DOI: 10.1002/14651858.CD007467.pub2. (2009).

3. B.M. Sibai, "Diagnosis and Management of Gestational Hypertension and Preeclampsia," *Obstetrics & Gynecology* 102(1) (2003): 181-92.

4. A. Coomarasamy et al., "Aspirin for Prevention of Preeclampsia in Women with Historical Risk Factors: A Systematic Review," *Obstetrics and Gynecology* 101 (2003): 1319-32.

5. S.W. Wen et al., "Folic Acid Supplementation in Early Second Trimester and the Risk of Preeclampsia," *American Journal of Obstetrics and Gynecology*, 198(1) (2008): 45, e1-7.

## Chapter 8: Planning for Birth and Post Partum

1. K. Johnson and B. Daviss, "Outcomes of planned home births with certified professional midwives: large prospective study in North America," *BMJ* 330 (2005): 1416; Amelink-Verburg et al., "Evaluation of 280,000 cases in Dutch midwifery practices: a descriptive study," *BJOG* 115 (2008): 570-78.

2. E.D. Hodnett et al., "Continuous support for women during childbirth." Cochrane Database of Syst. Rev., Issue 3 (2003): CD003766.

3. K. Johnson and B. Daviss (see Note 1); Amelink-Verburg et al. (see Note 1); A. de Jonge et al., "Perinatal mortality and morbidity in a nationwide cohort oat 529,688 low-risk planned home and hospital births," *BJOG*10 (2009): 1111; Janssen et al., "Outcomes of planned home births versus planned hospital births after regulation of midwifery in British Columbia," *CMAJ* 166(3) (2002).

## Chapter 9: When and How Labor Begins

1. D. Briscoe et al., "Management of pregnancy beyond 40 weeks' gestation," *Am Fam Phys* 71 (2005): 1935-41.

2. P. Nathanielsz, *Life Before Birth and A Time To Be Born*, Promethean Press (1992); P. Nathanielsz, *Life in the Womb: The Origin of Health and Disease*, Promethean Press (1999).

3. E. Cluett, "Immersion in water in pregnancy, labour and birth," Cochrane Database of Syst. Rev., Issue 2, Art. No.: CD000111. DOI: 10.1002/14651858.CD000111.pub2.

## Chapter 10: Labor Pain and Options for Pain Relief

1. S. Kitzinger, "Pain in Childbirth," *Journal of Medical Ethics* 4 (1978): 119.

2. R. Melzak, "From the gate to the neuromatrix," *Pain* 6 (August 1999): S121-26.

3. N. Lowe, "The nature of labor pain," *American Journal of Obstetrics and Gynecology* 186 (2002): S16-24.

4. E. DeClercq et al., *Listening to Mothers II: Report of the Second National U.S. Survey of Women's Childbearing Experiences*, Childbirth Connection (2006).

5. B.A. Bucklin et al., "Obstetric Anesthesia Workforce Survey," *Anesthesiology* 103 (2005): 445-53.

6. E.D. Hodnett et al., "Continuous support for women during childbirth," Cochrane Database of Syst. Rev., Issue 3 (2003): CD003766.

7. A. Bolding and P. Simkin "Supporting the Laboring Woman without Injuring Oneself," *International Journal of Childbirth Education* 22(4) (2008): 17-33.

8. American Academy of Pediatrics and American College of Obstetricians and Gynecologists, *Guidelines for Perinatal Care*, 6th ed., American Academy of Pediatrics (2007).

9. M. Anim-Somuah, R. Smyth, C. Howell, "Epidural versus nonepidural or no analgesia in labour," Cochrane Database of Syst. Rev., CD000331 (2005); A. Hager, "Comparing Epidural and Parenteral Opioid Analgesia During Labor," *Journal of Family Practice* (2005); S.H. Halpern et al., "Effect of Epidural vs Parenteral Opioid Analgesia on the Progress of Labor: A Meta-analysis," *Journal of the American Medical Association* 280 (1998): 2105-10; B.L. Leighton and S.H. Halpern, "The effects of epidural analgesia on labor, maternal, and neonatal outcomes: a systematic review," *American Journal of Obstetrics and Gynecology*, 186(5) (2002): S31-68.

10. J.J. Henderson et al., "Impact of intrapartum epidural analgesia on breast-feeding duration," *Australian & New Zealand Journal of Obstetrics & Gynaecology* 43(5) (2003): 372-77; S. Torvaldsen et al., "Intrapartum epidural analgesia and breastfeeding: a prospective cohort study," *International Breastfeeding Journal* 1 (2006): 24; P. Volmanen, J. Valanne, S. Alahuhta, "Breast-feeding problems after epidural analgesia for labour: a retrospective cohort study of pain, obstetrical procedures and breast-feeding practices," *Int J Obstet Anesth*, 13(1) (2004): 25-29.

11. K. Arendt and S. Segal, "Why Epidurals Do Not Always Work," *Rev Obstet Gynecol* 1(2) (Spring 2008): 49-55.

## Chapter 11: Comfort Techniques for Pain Relief and Labor Progress

1. P. Simkin and A. Bolding, "Update on non-pharmacologic methods to relieve pain and prevent suffering during labor," *JMWH* 49 (2004): 489-504; P. Simkin and M. Klein, "Non pharmacological approaches to management of labor pain," *UpToDate* 17 (2009): 1-18.

2. W. Piper, *The Little Engine That Could*, Platt & Munk (1930).

3. M. Erikson et al., "Warm Tub Bath during Labor: A Study of 1385 Women with Prelabor Rupture of the Membranes after 34 weeks of Gestation," *Acta Obstet Gynecol Scand* 75 (1996): 642-44.

4. M. Odent, "Can water immersion stop labor?" *Journal of Nurse-Midwifery* 42 (1997): 414-16.

5. E. Cluett et al., "Randomized controlled trial of labouring in water compared with standard of augmentation of dystocia in first stage of labour," *BMJ* 328 (2004): 314-20; M. Odent (see Note 4).

6. M. Singata, J. Tranmer, G.M.L Gyte, "Restricting oral fluid and food intake during labour, Cochrane Database of Syst. Rev., Issue 1 (2010).

7. P. Simkin, "Stress, Pain and Catecholamines in Labor, Part I: A Review," *Birth* 13(4) (1986): 227-33; S. Alehagen et al., "Fear, pain and stress hormones during childbirth," *J Psychosom Obstet Gynaecol* 26(3) (September 2005): 153-65.

8. J.K. Gupta, G.J. Hofmeyr, R. Smyth, "Position in the second stage of labour for women without epidural anaesthesia," Cochrane Database of Syst. Rev., Issue 1 (2003).

9. M.M. Beckmann and A.J. Garrett, "Antenatal perineal massage for reducing perineal trauma," Cochrane Database of Syst. Rev., Issue 1 (2006).

## Chapter 12: What Childbirth Is Really Like

1. S.J. Buckley, *Gentle Birth, Gentle Mothering: The Wisdom and Science of Gentle Choices in Pregnancy, Birth, and Parenting*, One Moon Press (2005); M. Odent, *The Scientification of Love*, Free Association Books (1999); K. U. Moberg, *The Oxytocin Factor: Tapping the Hormone of Calm, Love, and Healing*, Perseus Books Group (2003); S. Taylor, *The Tending Instinct: Women, Men, and the Biology of Our Relationships*, Times Books (2002).

2. M. Odent, "Can water immersion stop labor?" *Journal of Nurse-Midwifery* 42 (1997): 414-16.

3. E.A. Friedman, "Dysfunctional Labor" *Management of Labor*, University Park Press (1993); J. Zhang et al., "Reassessing the Labor Curve in Nulliparous Women," *American Journal of Obstetrics and Gynecology* 187(4) (2002).

4. P. Simkin and M. O'Hara, "Nonpharmacological relief of pain during labor: Systematic reviews of five methods," *American Journal of Obstetrics and Gynecology* 186 (2002): S131-59; P. Simkin and M. Klein, "Nonpharmacologic approaches to management of labor pain," *UpToDate* 17 (2009): 1-18; A. Lawrence, L. Lewis, G. Hofmeyr, "Maternal mobility and positions during first stage labor," Cochrane Database of Syst. Rev., Issue 2, Art. No.: CD003934 (2009).

5. J. Mercer et al., "Evidence-based practices for the fetal to newborn transition," *JMWH*, 52(3) (2007): 262-72.

6. M. Odent, "The fetus ejection reflex," *Birth* 14 (1987): 104-05; N. Newton, "The fetus ejection reflex revisited," *Birth* 14 (1987): 106-08; S.J. Buckley (see Note 1).

7. Washington State Vital Statistics (2005).

8. J. Schaffer et al., "A randomized trial of the effects of coached vs. uncoached maternal pushing during the second stage of labor on postpartum pelvic floor structure and function," *American Journal of Obstetrics and Gynecology* 192 (2005): 1692-96.

9. C.J. Aldrich et al., "The effect of maternal pushing on fetal cerebral oxygenation and blood volume during the second stage of labour," *BJOG* 102 (1995): 448-53.

10. W. Fraser et al., "Multicenter, randomized, controlled trial of delayed pushing for nulliparous women in the second stage of labor with continuous epidural analgesia," *Obstetrics and Gynecology* 99 (2002): 409-18; S. Church and P. Stone, "A meta-analysis of passive descent versus immediate pushing in nulliparous women with epidural analgesia in the second stage of labor," *Journal of Obstetric, Gynecologic, and Neonatal Nursing* 37 (2008): 4-12.

11. J. Roberts and L. Hanson, "Best practices in second stage labor care: maternal bearing down and positioning." *JMWH* 52(3) (2007): 238-45.

12. Ibid.

13. E. DeClercq et al., *Listening to Mothers II: Report of the Second National U.S. Survey of Women's Childbearing Experiences*, Childbirth Connection (2006); B. Chalmers et al., "Use of routine interventions in vaginal labor and birth: Findings from the Canadian Maternity Experiences Survey," *Birth* 36 (2009): 13-24

14. H. Dahlen et al., "Perineal outcomes and maternal comfort related to the application of perineal warm packs in the second stage of labor: a randomized controlled trial," *Birth* 34(4) (2007): 282-90.

15. L. Albers et al., "Midwifery care measures in the second stage of labor and reduction of genital tract trauma at birth: a randomized trial," *JMWH* 50 (2005): 365-72; G. Stamp et al., "Perineal massage in labour and prevention of perineal trauma: randomised controlled trial," *BMJ* 322 (2001): 1277-80.

16. J. Mercer et al., "Evidence-based practices for the fetal to newborn transition," *JMWH*, 52(3) (2007): 262-72.

17. E. Hutton and E. Hassan, "Late vs early clamping of the umbilical cord in full-term neonates: systematic review and meta-analysis of controlled trials," *Journal of the American Medical Association* 297(11) (2007): 1241-52.

18. Ibid.

19. Ibid.

20. A.C. Yao, M. Moinian, and J. Lind, "Distribution of blood between infant and placenta after birth," *Lancet*, 294(7626) (1969): 871–73; R.J. Airey, D. Farrar, and L. Duley, "Alternative positions for the baby at birth before clamping the umbilical cord," Cochrane Database of Syst. Rev., Issue 10, Art. No.: CD007555.

21. J. Smith, F. Plaat, and N. Fisk, "The natural caesarean: a woman-centred technique," *BJOG* 115 (2008):1037–42.

22. American Academy of Pediatrics, Section on Hematology/Oncology and Section on Allergy/Immunology, "Cord blood banking for potential future transplantation," *Pediatrics* 119(1) (2007): 165-70.

## Chapter 13: When Childbirth Becomes Complicated

1. E. Mozurkewich et al., "Indications for induction of labour: a best evidence review," *BJOG* 116 (2009): 626-36; D. Sadeh-Mestechkin et al., "Suspected macrosomia? Better not tell," *Arch Gynecol Obstet* 278(3) (2008): 225-30.

2. American College of Obstetrics and Gynecology, "Practice Bulletin 22: Guidelines on Fetal Macrosomia," *Obstetrics & Gynecology* (November 2000); S. Chauhan et al., "Suspicion and treatment of the macrosomic fetus: a review." *American Journal of Obstetrics and Gynecology* 193(2) (2005): 332-46.

3. W. Grobman, "Elective induction: When? Ever?" *Clinical Obstetrics and Gynecology* 50(2) (2007): 537-46; C. Le Ray et al., "Elective induction of labor: failure to follow guidelines and risk of cesarean delivery," *Acta Obstet Gynecol Scand* 86(6) (2007): 657-65.

3a. S.L. Clark et al. "Reduction in elective delivery at <39 weeks of gestation: comparative effectiveness of 3 approaches to change and the impact on neonatal intensive care admission and still-birth," *American Journal of Obstetrics and Gynecology* 203(5) (2010):449.e1–6; American College of Obstetricians and Gynecologists (ACOG), "ACOG Issues Revision of Labor Induction Guidelines," (2009).

4. A.Vahratian et al., "Labor progression and risk of cesarean de-livery in electively induced nulliparas," *Obstet Gynecol* 105(4) (2005): 698-704.

5. J. Kavanagh, A.J. Kelly, J. Thomas, "Breast stimulation for cervical ripening and induction of labour," Cochrane Database of Syst. Rev., Issue 4, Art. No.: CD003392. DOI: 10.1002/14651858. CD003392.pub2 (2005).

6. D. Garry et al., "Use of Castor Oil in Pregnancies at Term," *Alternative Therapies* 6 (2000): 77–79.

7. L. Reveiz, H.G. Gaitan, L.G. Cuervo, "Enemas during labour," Cochrane Database of Syst. Rev., No.: CD000330. DOI: 10.1002/14651858.CD000330.pub2 (2007).

8. J.A. Duke, *The Green Pharmacy Handbook: Your Comprehensive Reference to the Best Herbs for Healing,* Rodale Press (2000).

9. T. Harper et al., "A randomized controlled trial of acupuncture for initiation of labor in nulliparous women," *J Matern Fetal Neonatal Med* 19 (2006): 465-70; M. Rabl et al., "Acupuncture for cervical ripening and induction of labor—a randomized controlled trial," *Wien Klin Wochenschr* 113 (2001): 942-46.

10. S. Gelber et al., "Mechanical methods of cervical ripening and labor induction," *Clinical Obstetrics and Gynecology* 49 (2006): 642-57.

11. M. Boulvain et al., "Membrane sweeping for induction of labour," Cochrane Database of Syst. Rev., Issue 4, Art. No.: CD000451 DOI: 10.1002/14651858. cd000451.pub2 (1997).

12. Y. Cheng et al., "Associated factors and outcomes of persistent occiput posterior position: A retrospective cohort study from 1976 to 2001," *J Matern Fetal Neonatal Med* 19(9) (2006): 563-68.

13. G.J. Hofmeyr and A.M. Gülmezogl, "Vaginal misoprostol for cervical ripening and induction of labour," Cochrane Database of Syst. Rev., Issue 1, Art. No.: CD000941. DOI: 10.1002/14651858.CD000941.2009 (2003); Z. Alfirevic and A. Weeks, "Oral misoprostol for induction of labour," Cochrane Database of Syst. Rev., Issue 2, Art. No.: CD001338. DOI: 10.1002/14651858.CD001338.pub2 (2006).

14. D.A. Wing and C.A. Gaffaney, "Vaginal misoprostol administration for cervical ripening and labor induction," *Clinical Obstetrics and Gynecology* 49(3) (2006): 627-41; Z. Alfirevic et al. (see Note 13); G.J. Hofmeyr and A.M. Gülmezogl (see Note 13).

15. M. Lin et al., "Misoprostol for labor induction in women with term premature rupture of membranes: a meta-analysis," *Obstet Gynecol* 106 (2005): 593-601; R. Levy, "Induction of labor with oral misoprostol for premature rupture of membranes at term in women with unfavorable cervix: a randomized, double-blind, placebo-controlled trial," *J Perinat Med* 35 (2007): 126-29; Z. Alfirevic et al. (see Note 13).

16. American College of Obstetricians and Gynecologists, Practice Bulletin 107, "Induction of Labor," *Obstetrics & Gynecology* (August 2009).

17. B. Shaffer et al., "Manual rotation of the fetal occiput: Predictors of success and delivery," *Obstet Gynecol*194 (2006): e7-9; C. Le Ray et al., "Manual rotation in occiput posterior or transverse positions: risk factors and consequences on the cesarean delivery rate," *Obstet Gynecol* 110(4) (2007): 873-79; O. Reichman et al., "Digital rotation from occipito-posterior to occipito-anterior decreases the need for cesarean section," *Eur J Obstet Gynecol Repro Biol* 10.1016/j.ejogrb.2006.12.025 (2007).

18. P. Simkin, "The Fetal Occiput Posterior Position: State of the Science and a New Perspective," *Birth* 37(1) (2010): 61-71; P. Simkin and R. Ancheta, *The Labor Progress Handbook,* Black-well Science (2005); Oxford. Sherer et al., (2002) *Ultrasound Obstet Gynecol* 102 (2002); Akmal et al., *Maternal Fetal Medicine* 496 (2002); Souka et al., *J Maternal Fetal Neonatal Med* 148 (2003); Kreiser et al., *Ultrasound Obstet Gynecol* 44 (2003); Akmal et al., *Ultrasound Obstet Gynecol* 64 (2003).

19. P. Simkin et al., "Selected non-pharmacologic methods of pain relief in labor: A systematic review," *American Journal of Obstetrics and Gynecology* 186 (2002): s131-59; J. Reynolds, "Intracutaneous sterile water for back pain in labor," *Can Fam Phys* 40 (1994): 1785-92; L. Mårtensson et al., "US Midwives' Knowledge and Use of Sterile Water Injections for Labor Pain,"*JMWH* 53(2) (2008): 115-22.

20. J.G.B. Russell, "The Rationale of Primitive Delivery Positions," *British Journal of Obstetrics and Gynaecology* 89 (1982): 712.

21. P. Simkin and R. Ancheta (see Note 18).

22. G. Carroli et al., "Episiotomy for vaginal birth," Cochrane Database of Syst. Rev., Issue 2, Art.No.: 000081. DOI: 10.1002/14651858. CD000081. (1997, updated 1999).

23. D. Roberts and S. Dalziel, "Antenatal corticosteroids for accel-erating fetal lung maturation for women at risk of preterm birth," Cochrane Database of Syst. Rev., Issue 3, Art. No.: CD004454. DOI: 10.1002/14651858.CD004454.pub2 (2006).

24. S. Anotayanonth et al., "Betamimetics for inhibiting preterm labour," Cochrane Database of Syst. Rev., Issue 4, Art. No.: CD004352. DOI: 10.1002/14651858.CD004352.pub2 (2004).

25. D. Papatsonis et al., "Oxytocin receptor antagonists for inhibiting preterm labour," Cochrane Database of Syst. Rev., Issue 3, Art. No.: CD004452. DOI: 10.1002/14651858.CD004452.pub2 (2005).

26. Ibid.

27. D. Grimes et al., "Magnesium sulfatetocolysis: time to quit," *Obstet Gynecol* 108 (2006): 986-89; C.A. Crowther, J.E. Hiller, L.W.Doyle, "Magnesium sulphate for preventing preterm birth in threatened preterm labour," Cochrane Database of Syst. Rev., Issue 4, Art. No.: CD001060. DOI: 10.1002/14651858.CD001060 (2002).

28. R. Lynch, "Surfactant and RDS in premature infants," *Fed Am Soc Expre Biol,* http://www.fasebj.org/cgi/content/full/18/13/1624e (2004).

29. S. Ludington-Hoe and S.K. Golant, *Kangaroo Care: The Best You Can Do to Help Your Preterm Infant,* Bantam Books (1993).

30. C. Nye, "Transitioning premature infants from gavage to breast," *Neonatal Netw,* 27(1) (2008): 7-13; A. Johnson, "The maternal experience of kangaroo holding," *Journal of Obstetric, Gynecologic and Neonatal Nursing,* 36(6) (2007): 568-73.

31. D.L. Davis and M.T. Stein, "Parent: You and Your Baby in the NICU," March of Dimes booklet (2007).

32. S. Chasen and F. Chervenak, "Delivery of twin gestations," *UpToDate* 17.3 (2009): 1-11.

33. C. Smith et al., "Knee-Chest Postural Management for Breech at Term: A Randomized Controlled Trial," *Birth* 26(2) (1999): 71–75; P. Crawford, "Case report of successful version with cold applied to fundus," *J Am Board Fam Pract* 18 (2005): 312-13.

34. M. Coyle et al., "Cephalic version by moxibustion for breech presentation," Cochrane Database of Syst. Rev. Issue 2, CD003928 (2005).

35. ICPA Staff Writer, "The Webster Technique: A technique for pregnant women," *The Chiropractic Journal* (August 2001).

36. E. Hutton and C.J. Hofmeyr, "External version for breech presentation before term," Cochrane Database of Syst. Rev., CD000084.

37. P. Crawford (see Note 33).

38. M.E. Hannah et al., "Planned cesarean section versus planned vaginal birth for breech presentation at term," *Lancet* 356 (2000): 1375-83.

39. A. Kotaska, S. Menticoglou, R. Gagnon, "SOGC clinical practice guideline on vaginal delivery of breech presentation," *JOGC* (June 2009): 557-67.

## Chapter 14: All about Cesarean Birth

1. H. Goer, M.S. Leslie, A. Romano, "Evidence basis for the ten steps of mother-friendly care. Step 6: does not routinely employ practices, procedures unsupported by scientific evidence," *Journal of Perinatal Education* 16(1s) (2007): 32-64.

2. Villar et al., "Maternal and neonatal individual risks and benefits associated with caesarean delivery: multicentre prospective study," *BMJ* 335: 1025; Maternity Center Association, "What Every Pregnant Woman Needs to Know about Cesarean Section" (2004); National Institutes of Health, "Final Statement from NIH State-of-the-Science Conference on Cesarean Delivery on Maternal Request" (2006); National Institute for Clinical Excellence, "Cesarean Section: Clinical Guidelines. Royal College of Obstetricians and Gynaecologists" (2004); MacDorman et al., "Infant and neonatal mortality for primary cesarean and vaginal births to women with 'no indicated risk,'" *Birth* 33(3) (2006): 175-82; Villar et al., "Caesarean delivery rates and pregnancy outcomes: the 2005 WHO global survey on maternal and perinatal health in Latin America,"*Lancet* 367 (2006): 1819-29; S. Liu et al., "Maternal mortality and severe morbidity associated with low-risk planned cesarean delivery versus planned vaginal delivery at term," *CMAJ* 176(4) (2007): 455-60.

3. P. Lumbiganon et al., "Method of delivery and pregnancy outcomes in Asia: the WHO global survey on maternal and perinatal health 2007–08," *Lancet* DOI:10.1016/S0140-6736(09) 61870-5 (January 2010).

4. MacDorman et al. (see Note 2)

5. National Institute for Clinical Excellence (see Note 2).

6. Public Health Service Task Force, "Recommendations for Use of Antiretroviral Drugs in Pregnant HIV-Infected Women for Maternal Health and Interventions to Reduce Perinatal HIV Transmission in the United States" (2006).

7. S. Liu et al. (see Note 2).

8. National Institutes of Health (see Note 2).

9. Villar et al. (see Note 2).

10. Ibid.

11. M. Siddiqui et al., "Complications of Exteriorized Compared With In Situ Uterine Repair at Cesarean Delivery Under Spinal Anesthesia," *Obstetrics & Gynecology* 110 (2007): 570-75.

12. D.J. Lyell et al., "Peritoneal Closure at Primary Cesarean Delivery and Adhesions," *Obstetrics & Gynecology* 106 (2005): 275-80; K. Hamel, Incidence of adhesions at repeat cesarean delivery," *American Journal of Obstetrics and Gynecology* 196(5) (May 2007): e31-32.

13. D. Patolia et al., "Early feeding after cesarean: randomized trial," *Obstet Gynecol* 98 (2001): 113-16; W. Teoh, M. Shah, C. Mah,

"A randomized controlled trial on beneficial effects of early feeding post-cesarean delivery under regional anesthesia," *Singapore Med J* 48 (2007): 152-57.

14. J. Riordan, *Breastfeeding and Human Lactation*, 3rd ed., Jones and Bartlett Publishers, Inc. (2005): 204; Leung et al. (2002); DiMatteo et al. (1996); Dewey et al. (2003); Perez-Escamilla et al. (1996); Verstermark (1991); Wiederpass et al. (1998); Evser-Hadani et al. (1994).

15. National Institutes of Health, Consensus Development Statement, "NIH Consensus Development Conference: Vaginal Birth After Cesarean: New Insights," http://consensus.nih.gov/2010/ images/vbac/vbac_statement.pdf (2010).

15a. American College of Obstetricians and Gynecologists (ACOG), "Practice Bulletin No. 115: Vaginal Birth after Previous Cesarean Delivery." *Obstetrics and Gynecology*, August 2010, 116:2: 450–63.

16. A. Smith et al., "The natural caesarean: a woman-centred technique," *BJOG* 115(8) (2008): 1037-42.

17. Childbirth Connection, "Tips and Tools: VBAC or Repeat C-Section," http://childbirthconnection.org/article.asp?ck= 10214 and ck=10214 (2006).

18. National Institutes of Health (see Note 15).

19. Ibid.

20. Ibid.

21. Ibid.

22. International Cesarean Awareness Network, "Your Right to Refuse: What to Do If Your Hospital Has 'Banned' VBAC," http://www.ican-online.net/resources/white_papers/wp_ vbacbanqa.pdf.

23. Childbirth Connection (see Note 17).

24. Agency for Healthcare Research and Quality, "Vaginal Birth After Cesarean (VBAC). Summary, Evidence Report/Technology Assessment: Number 71," AHRQ Publication Number 03-E017 (March 2003); National Institutes of Health (see Note 15).

25. American College of Obstetricians and Gynecologists (ACOG), "Clinical management guidelines for obstetrician-gynecologists: Vaginal birth after previous cesarean delivery," ACOG Practice Bulletin 5 (July 1999).

26. R. Roberts et al., "Changing Policies on Vaginal Birth After Cesarean: Impact on Access," *Birth* 34(4) (2007): 316-22; National Institutes of Health (see Note 15).

27. E. DeClercq et al., *Listening to Mothers II: Report of the Second National U.S. Survey of Women's Childbearing Experiences*, Childbirth Connection (2006).

28. A. Tita et al., "Timing of Elective Repeat Cesarean Delivery at Term and Neonatal Outcomes," *New England Journal of Medicine* 360(2) (2009): 112-20.

## Chapter 15: What Life Is Like for a New Mother

1. E. Noble, *Essential Exercises for the Childbearing Year*, New Life Images (1995).

2. J. Tupler, *Maternal Fitness: Preparing for a Healthy Pregnancy, an Easier Labor, and a Quick Recovery*, Fireside (1996); J. Tupler and J. Gould, *Lose Your Mummy Tummy*, Da Capo Press (2005).

3. E. Noble (see Note 1).

## Chapter 16: When Post Partum Becomes Complicated

1. C.M. Glazener et al., "Conservative management of persistent postnatal urinary and faecal incontinence: randomized controlled trial," *BMJ* 323 (15 September 2001): 593-96.

2. Ibid.; S. Morkved and B. Kari, "Prevalence and treatment of postpartum urinary incontinence," *Norsk Epidemiologi* 7(1) (1997): 123-27.

3. C. MacArthur et al., "Faecal incontinence after childbirth," *British Journal of Obstetrics and Gynaecology* 104 (1997): 46-50.

4. C.M. Glazener et al. (see Note 1).

5. E.J. Corwin, L.E. Murray-Kolb, J.L. Beard, "Low hemoglobin level is a risk factor for postpartum depression," *J. Nutr* 133 (2003): 4139-42.

6. L.A. Matthys, K.H. Coppage, M.D. Lambers et al., "Delayed postpartum preeclampsia: an experience of 151 cases," *American Journal of Obstetrics and Gynecology* 190(5) (2004): 1464-66.

7. L. Magee and S. Sadeghi, "Prevention and treatment of postpartum hypertension," Cochrane Database of Syst. Rev., Issue 1 (2005).

8. R. Gentry, "Psychiatric complications in pregnancy and postpartum," presentation at REACHE conference (November 2002).

9. E.J. Corwin, L.E. Murray-Kolb, J.L. Beard (see Note 5).

10. K. Kendall-Tackett, "A new paradigm for depression in new mothers: the central role of inflammation and how breastfeeding and anti-inflammatory treatments protect maternal mental health," *International Breastfeeding Journal* 2(6) (2007): 1-14.

11. J.M. Twenge, W.K. Campbell, C.A. Foster, "Parenthood and marital satisfaction: a meta-analysis," *Journal of Marriage and Family* 65 (2003): 574-83; P. Cowan and C. Cowan, *Normative Family Transitions, Normal Family Process, and Healthy Child Development in Normal Family Processes*, 3rd ed., Guilford Publications (2003).

12. P. Cowan and C. Cowan, *When Partners Become Parents* Routledge (2000); P. Cowan and C. Cowan (see Note 11).

13. P. Cowan and C. Cowan, "Interventions to ease the transition to parenthood: why they are needed and what they can do," *Family Relations* 44 (1995): 412-14; P. Cowan and C. Cowan, (see Note 12); M. Cox, M. Owen, M. Lewis et al., "Marriage, adult adjustment and early parenting," *Child Development* 60 (1999): 1015-24.

14. National Coalition Against Domestic Violence, http://www.ncadv.org/learn/TheProblem_100.html.

15. A. Gielen, P. O'Campo, R. Faden et al., "Interpersonal conflict and physical violence during the childbearing year," *Soc SciMed* 39 (1994): 781-87.

16. J. O. Johnson and B. Downs, Maternity leave and employment patterns: 1961-2000," Current Population Report, U.S. Census Bureau (2003): 70-203.

## Chapter 17: Caring for Your Baby

1. American Academy of Pediatrics, Committee on Fetus and Newborn, "Controversies Concerning Vitamin K and the Newborn," *Pediatrics* 112 (2003): 191-92.

2. American Academy of Pediatrics and American College of Obstetricians and Gynecologists, *Guidelines for Perinatal Care*, 4th ed., American Academy of Pediatrics (1997).

3. American Academy of Pediatrics (see Note 1).

4. American Academy of Pediatrics and American College of Obstetricians and Gynecologists (see Note 2).

5. American Academy of Pediatrics, "Breastfeeding and the use of human milk," *Pediatrics* 115 (2005): 496-506.

6. American Academy of Pediatrics and American College of Obstetricians and Gynecologists (see Note 2).

7. National Newborn Screening and Genetics Resource Center, http://genes-r-us.uthscsa.edu/.

8. J. H. Dussault, "Screening for Congenital Hypothyroidism," *Clinical Obstetrics and Gynecology* 40(1) (March 1997): 117-23.

9. American Academy of Pediatrics, Committee on Genetics, "Newborn Screening Fact Sheet," *Pediatrics* 118 (2006): 934-63.

10. American Academy of Pediatrics, Task Force on Circumcision, "Circumcision Policy Statement," *Pediatrics* 103(3) (1999): 686-93.

11. American Academy of Pediatrics, Committee on the Fetus and Newborn and Section on Surgery and Canadian Pediatric Society and Fetus and Newborn Committee, "Policy statement: prevention and management of pain in the neonate: an update," *Pediatrics* 118(5) (2006): 2231-41.

12. A. Taddio et al., "Efficacy and Safety of Lidocaine-Prilocaine Cream for Pain during Circumcision," *New England Journal of Medicine* 336 (1997): 1197-1201.

13. American Academy of Pediatrics, (see Note 10).

14. L. Pisacane et al., "Breast-feeding and Urinary Tract Infection," *Journal of Pediatrics* 120 (1992): 87-89.

15. Centers for Disease Control (CDC), "Male circumcision and risk for HIV transmission: implications for the United States," CDC Fact Sheet (March 2007).

16. http://www.nytimes.com/2010/08/17/health/research/17circ.html?_r=2. (Accessed October 2011).

17. T. Penny-MacGillivray, "A Newborn's First Bath," *Journal of Obstetric, Gynecologic and Neonatal Nursing* 25 (1996): 481-87; S. G. Cole et al., "Tub Baths or Sponge Baths for Newborn Infants?" *Mother Baby Journal* 4(3) (1999): 39-43.

18. S. Dore et al., "Alcohol versus Natural Drying for Newborn Cord Care," *Journal of Obstetric, Gynecologic, and Neonatal Nursing* 27 (1998): 621-27.

19. H. Karp, *The Happiest Baby on the Block: The New Way to Calm Crying and Help Your Baby Sleep Longer*, Bantam (2002).

20. P. Franco et al., "Influence of swaddling on sleep and arousal characteristics of healthy infants," *Pediatrics* 115(5) (2005): 311-18.

21. Wessel et al., "Paroxysmal fussing in infancy, sometimes called 'colic,'" *Pediatrics* 14(5) (1954): 421-35.

22. T.B. Brazelton, *Touchpoints Birth to 3*, Perseus Books Group (2002).

23. Ibid.

24. T. J. Metcalf et al., "Simethicone and the Treatment of Infant Colic: A Randomized, Placebo-Controlled, Multicenter Trial," *Pediatrics* 94 (1994): 29-34.

25. L. van Vlimmeren et al., "Risk factors for deformational plagiocephaly at birth and at 7 weeks of age: a prospective cohort study," *Pediatrics* 119(2) (2007): e408-18.

26. M. Klaus and P. Klaus, *Your Amazing Newborn*, Perseus Books Group (1998).

27. J. G. Cole, "What Can Babies See at Birth?" *Mother Baby Journal*, 2(4) (1997): 45-47.

28. Centers for Disease Control (CDC), "Mercury and Vaccines (Thimerosal)," CDC Fact Sheet (October 2007).

29. D.S. Greenes and G.R. Fleisher, "Accuracy of a noninvasive temporal artery thermometer for use in infants," *Arch Pediatr Adolesc Med* 155(3) (2001): 376-81; G.K. Siberry et al., "Comparison of temple temperatures with rectal temperatures in children under two years of age," *Clin Pediatr* 41(6) (2002): 405-14.

30. American Academy of Pediatrics, Task Force on Sudden Infant Death Syndrome, "The changing concept of sudden infant death syndrome: diagnostic coding shifts, controversies regarding the sleeping environment, and new variable to consider in reducing risk," *Pediatrics* 116(5) (2005): 1245-55.

31. Ibid.

32. Ibid.

33. Academy of Breastfeeding Medicine, "Protocol #6: Guideline on co-sleeping and breastfeeding," http://www.bfmed.org/ace-files/protocol/cosleeping.pdf (2003).

34. American Academy of Pediatrics, Task Force on Sudden Infant Death Syndrome (see Note 30).

35. B. D. Gessner and T.J. Porter, "Bed sharing with unimpaired parents is not an important risk for sudden infant death syndrome," *Pediatrics* 117(3) (2006): 990-91; J.J. McKenna and T. McDade, "Why babies should never sleep alone: a review of the co-sleeping controversy in relation to SIDS, bed sharing and breast feeding," *Paediatr Respir Rev* 6 (2005): 134-52.

## Chapter 18: Feeding Your Baby

1. American Academy of Pediatrics, Policy Statement, "Breastfeeding and the use of human milk," *Pediatrics* 115 (2005): 496-506.

2. G. Bauer et al., "Breastfeeding and Cognitive Development of Three-Year-Old Children," *Psychological Reports* 68 (1991): 1281; R. A. Lawrence, "Can We Expect Greater Intelligence from Human Milk Feedings?" *Birth* 19(2) (1992): 105-06; A. Lucas et al., "Randomized Trial of Early Diet in Preterm Babies and Later Intelligence Quotient, *British Medical Journal* 28 (1998): 1481-87; M. C. Tenbury et al., "Influence of Breastfeeding on the Infant's Intellectual Development," *J Pediatr Gastroenterol Nutr* 18 (1994): 32-36.

3. E.L. Mortenson et al., "The association between breastfeeding and adult intelligence," *Journal of the American Medical Association* 287 (2002): 2365-71.

4. U. M. Saarinen and M. Kajosaari, "Breastfeeding as Prophylaxis against Atopic Disease: Prospective Follow-Up Study until 17 Years Old," *Lancet* 346 (1995): 1065-69.

5. F.R. Greer, S.H. Sicherer, A.W. Burks and the Committee on Nutrition and Section on Allergy and Immunology, "Effects of early nutritional interventions on the development of atopic disease in infants and children: the role of maternal dietary restriction, breastfeeding, timing of introduction of complementary foods, and hydrolyzed formulas," *Pediatrics* 121 (2008): 183-91.

6. American Academy of Pediatrics (see Note 1).

7. A. Chen and W.J. Rogan, "Breastfeeding and the risk of postneonatal death in the United States," *Pediatrics* 113(5) (2004): e435-39.

8. American Academy of Pediatrics (see Note 1).

9. E. A. Mitchell et al., "Results from the First Year of the New Zealand Cot Death Study," *New Zealand Medical Journal* 104 (1991): 71-75; M. Vennemann et al., "Does Breastfeeding Reduce the Risk of Sudden Infant Death Syndrome?" *Pediatrics* 123(3) (2009).

10. American Academy of Pediatrics (see Note 1).

11. P. A. Newcomb et al., "Lactation and a Reduced Risk of Premenopausal Breast Cancer," *New England Journal of Medicine* 330 (1994): 81-87; National Institutes of Health Consensus Conference, "Ovarian Cancer: Screening, Treatment, and Follow-Up," *Journal of the American Medical Association* 273(6) (1995): 491-97; H. Jernstrom et al., "Breast-feeding and the risk of breast cancer in BRAC1 and BRAC2 mutation carriers," *J Natl Cancer Inst* 96 (2004): 1094-98.

12. R. G. Cumming and R. J. Klineberg, "Breastfeeding and Other Reproductive Factors and the Risk of Hip Fractures in Elderly Women," *International Journal of Epidemiology* 22 (1993): 684-91.

13. G. A. Weinberg, "The Dilemma of Postnatal Mother-to-Child Transmission of HIV: To Breastfeed or Not?" *Birth* 27(3) (2000): 199-205; World Health Organization Collaborative Study Team on the Role of Breastfeeding and the Prevention of Infant Mortality, "Effect of Breastfeeding on Child Mortality Due to Infectious Diseases in Less Developed Countries: A Pooled Analysis," *Lancet* 355 (2000): 450-55; American Academy of Pediatrics, Committee on Infectious Diseases, *Red Book: Report of the Committee on Infectious Disease*, 25th ed., American Academy of Pediatrics (2000).

14. J.S. Read and the American Academy of Pediatrics, Committee on Pediatric AIDS, "Human milk, breastfeeding and transmission of human immunodeficiency virus type 1 in the United States," *Pediatrics* 112: 1196-1205.

15. L. Larson, "Warnings Fail to Slow Low Iron Formula Sales," *AAP News* 11(3) (1995): 1, 14.

16. N. Mohrbacher and J. Stock, *The Breastfeeding Answer Book*, La Leche League International (2003): 16-18; P.E. Hartmanet al.,"Breast development and control of milk synthesis," *Food Nutr Bull* 17: 292-304; J. Kent, "Physiology of the expression of breast milk, part 2," presented at the Medela Innovations in Breast Pump Research Conference (July 2002).

17. N.A. Grossl, "Supernumerary breast tissue: historical perpectives and clinical features," *Southern Med J*, 93(1).

18. D.T. Ramsay et al., "Ultrasound imaging of milk ejection in the breast of lactating women," *Pediatrics* 113 (2004): 361-67.

19. C.J. Wilde, "Autocrine regulation of milk secretion by a protein in milk," *Biochem J* 305 (1995): 51.

20. J. Riordan, *Breastfeeding and Human Lactation*, 3rd ed., Jones and Bartlett Publishers, Inc. (2005): 110-11.

21. M.C. Neville, "Studies in human lactation; milk volumes in lactating women during the onset of lactation and full lactation," *American Journal of Clinical Nutrition* 48 (1988): 1375-86.

22. J. Riordan (see Note 20).

23. Ibid.

24. American Academy of Pediatrics (see Note 1).

25. A. Basile et al., "The effect of high-dose vitamin D supplementation on serum vitamin D levels and milk calcium concentration in lactating women and their infants," *Breastfeeding Medicine* 1 (2006): 1, 27-35; B.W. Hollis and C.L. Wagner, "Assessment of dietary vitamin D requirements during pregnancy and lactation," *American Journal of Clinical Nutrition* 79(5) (2004): 717-26; C.L. Wagner et al., (2006) "High-dose vitamin D3 supplementation in a cohort of breastfeeding mothers and their infants; a 6-month follow- pilot study," *Breastfeeding Medicine* 1(2) (2006): 59-70; C.L. Wagner, F.R. Greer, and the Section on Breastfeeding and Committee on Nutrition, "Prevention of Rickets and Vitamin D Deficiency in Infants, Children, and Adolescents," *Pediatrics* 122(5) (2008): 1142-52.

26. Ibid.

27. American Academy of Pediatric Dentistry, "Policy on the use of fluoride" (2007).

28. N. Mohrbacher and J. Stock, *The Breastfeeding Answer Book*, La Leche League International (2003): 470-72.

29. J. Riordan, *Breastfeeding and Human Lactation*, 3rd ed., Jones and Bartlett Publishers, Inc. (2005): 355.

30. J. Moon and S. Humenick, "Breast Engorgement: Contributing Variables and Variables Amenable to Nursing Intervention," *Journal of Obstetric, Gynecologic, and Neonatal Nursing* 18(4) (1989): 309-15.

31. Y. Yamauchi and H. Yamanouchi, "Breast-feeding Frequency during the First 24 Hours after Birth in Full-Term Neonates," *Pediatrics* 86 (1990): 171-75.

32. S. Phillips, "When Time Is of the Essence: Establishing Effective Breastfeeding before Early Discharge," *Mother Baby Journal* 1(1) (1996): 15-19.

33. J. Riordan, *Breastfeeding and Human Lactation*, 3rd ed., Jones and Bartlett Publishers, Inc. (2005): 187.

34. Ibid.

35. M. Neifert et al., "Nipple Confusion: Toward a Formal Definition," *Journal of Pediatrics* 126(6) (1995): S125-29.

36. L. Righard and M. O. Alade, "Breastfeeding and the Use of Pacifiers," *Birth* 24(2) (1997): 116-20; C.R. Howard et al., "Randomized clinical trial of pacifier use and bottle-feeding or cup feeding and their effect on breastfeeding," *Pediatrics* 111: 511-18.

37. American Academy of Pediatrics, Committee on Drugs, "The transfer of drugs and other chemicals into human milk," *Pediatrics* 108(3) (2001): 776-89.

38. V. Coiro et al., "Inhibition by Ethanol of the Oxytocin Response to Breast Stimulation in Normal Women and the Role of Endogenous Opiods," *Acta Endocrinol* 126 (1992): 213; C. Berlin, "Disposition of Dietary Caffeine in Milk, Saliva, and Plasma of Lactating Women," *Pediatrics* 73 (1984): 59-63; A. Dahlstrom, "Nicotine and Cotinine Concentrations in the Nursing Mother and Her Infant," *Acta Paediatr Scand* 79 (1990): 142-47.

39. G. Chan, *Lactation: the Breastfeeding Manual for Health Professionals*, Precept Press (1996); Institute of Medicine, "Nutrition during Lactation," National Academy of Sciences (1992): 86.

40. L.A. Basile et al. (see Note 25); B.W. Hollis and C.L. Wagner (see Note 25); C.L. Wagner et al. (see Note 25); C.L. Wagner, F.R. Greer, and the Section on Breastfeeding and Committee on Nutrition (see Note 25).

41. E. Reifsnider and S. L. Gill, "Nutrition for the Childbearing Years," *Journal of Obstetric, Gynecologic, and Neonatal Nursing* 29(1) (2000): 50-51.

42. J. Mennella and G. Beauchamp, "Maternal Diet Alters the Sensory Qualities of Human Milk and the Nursling's Behavior," *Pediatrics* 88(4) (1991): 737-44; J. Mennella and G. Beauchamp, "Early Flavor Experience: Research Update," *Nutrition Reviews* 56(7) (1998): 205-11.

43. Ibid.

44. J. Mennella and G. Beauchamp, (see Note 42); J. Mennella and G. Beauchamp, "Effects of Beer on Breast-fed Infants," *Journal of the American Medical Association* 269 (1993): 1635-36.

45. Institute of Medicine, "Nutrition during Lactation," National Academy of Sciences (1992): 73.

46. Institute of Medicine, "Nutrition during Lactation," National Academy of Sciences (1992): 86; L. B. Duskieder et al., "Is Milk Production Impaired by Dieting during Lactation?" *American Journal of Clinical Nutrition* 59 (1994): 833-40; A. Prentice et al., "Energy Requirements of Pregnant and Lactating Women," *European Journal of Clinical Nutrition* 50(1) (1996): S82-111.

47. V. Nicodem et al., "Do Cabbage Leaves Prevent Breast Engorgement? A Randomized, Controlled Study," *Birth* 20 (1993): 61-64; K. Roberts, "A Comparison of Chilled Cabbage Leaves and Chilled Gelpaks in Reducing Breast Engorgement," *Journal of Human Lactation* 11(1) (1995): 17-20; K. Roberts et al., "Effects of cabbage leaf extract on breast engorgement," *Journal of Human Lactation* 114(3) (1998): 231-36.

48. J. Riordan and K. G. Auerbach, *Breastfeeding and Human Lactation*, 2nd ed., Jones and Bartlett Publishers, Inc. (1998): 294; P. Simkin, "Intermittent Brachial Plexus Neuropathy Secondary to Breast Engorgement," *Birth* 15 (1988): 102-04; N. Mohrbacher and J. Stock, *The Breastfeeding Answer Book*, La Leche League International (2003): 492-96.

49. M. Ziemer and J. Pigeon, "Skin Changes and Pain in the Nipples during the First Week of Lactation," *Journal of Obstetric, Gynecologic, and Neonatal Nursing* 22(23) (1993): 247-56.

50. B. C. Bowles et al., "Alternate Massage in Breastfeeding," *Genesis* 9 (1988): 5-9.

51. K. Van Kessel et al., "Common complementary and alternative therapies for yeast vaginitis and bacterial vaginosis: a systemic review," *Obstet Gynecol Surv* 58(5) (2003): 351-58.

52. J. Barger and P. Bull, "A Comparison of the Bacterial Composition of Breast Milk Stored at Room Temperature and Stored in the Refrigerator," *International Journal of Childbirth Education* 2 (1987): 29-30; A. Pardou et al., "Human Milk Banking: Influence of Storage Processes and of Bacterial Contamination on Some Milk Constituents," *Biol Neonate* 65 (1994): 302-09.

53. N. Mohrbacher and J. Stock, *The Breastfeeding Answer Book*, La Leche League International (2003): 229; Academy of Breastfeeding Medicine, "Clinical Protocol Number #8: Human Milk Storage Information for Home Use for Healthy Full Term Infants" (2004).

54. Human Milk Banking Association of North America, *Recommendations for Collection, Storage, and Handling of a Mother's Milk for Her Own Infant in the Hospital Setting* (1993); Academy of Breastfeeding Medicine (see Note 53).

55. C.T. Beck and S. Watson, "Impact of birth trauma on breast-feeding: a tale of two pathways," *Nurs Res* 57(4) (2008): 228-36.

56. E. Nissen et al., "Different patterns of oxytocin, prolactin but not cortisol release during breastfeeding in women delivered by caesarean section or by the vaginal route," *Early Human Development* 45 (1996): 103-18.

57. C.G. Victora et al., "Caesarean section and duration of breast-feeding among Brazilians," *Arch Dis Child* 65 (1990): 632-43; M.H. Kearney, L.R. Cronenwett, R. Reinhardt, "Cesarean delivery and breastfeeding outcomes," *Birth* 30 (1990): 1285-90.

58. A. Karlstrom et al., "Postoperative pain after cesarean birth affects breastfeeding and infant care," *Journal of Obstetric, Gynecologic and Neonatal Nursing* 36(5) (2007): 430-40.

59. E. Buescher, "Host Defense Mechanisms of Human Milk and Their Relations to Enteric Infections and Necrotizing Enterocolitis," *Clinical Perinatology* 21(2) (1994): 247-62.

60. A. Lucas et al., "Breast Milk and Subsequent Intelligence Quotient in Children Born Preterm," *Lancet* 339 (1992): 261-64; A. Lucas et al., "Randomized Trial of Early Diet in Preterm Babies and Later Intelligence Quotient," *British Medical Journal* 317(28) (1998): 1481-87.

61. S. Moscone and J. Moore, "Breastfeeding during Pregnancy," *Journal of Human Lactation* 9(2) (1993): 83-88.

62. Centers for Disease Control, "General recommendation on immunization," *MMWR* 51: 11-36, http://www.cdc.gov/vaccines/recs/acip/downloads/preg-principles05-01-08.pdf.

63. I. Matheson and G. Rivrud, "The Effect of Smoking on Lactation and Infantile Colic," *Journal of the American Medical Association* 261 (1989): 42.

64. A. Woodward et al., "Acute Respiratory Illness in Adelaide Children: Breastfeeding Modifies the Effect of Passive Smoking," *Journal of Epidemiology and Community Health* 44 (1990): 224-30.

65. A. Perez et al., "Clinical Study of the Lactational Amenorrhoea Method for Family Planning," *Lancet* 339 (1992): 968-70.

66. P. Erwin, "To Use or Not Use Combined Hormonal Oral Contraceptives during Lactation," *Family Planning Perspectives* 26(1) (1994): 26-33.

67. T. Weschler, *Taking Charge of Your Fertility, 10th Anniversary Edition: The Definitive Guide to Natural Birth Control, Pregnancy Achievement and Reproductive Health,* HarperCollins Publishers (2002).

68. American Academy of Pediatrics, Committee on Nutrition, *Pediatric Nutrition Handbook*, 4th ed., American Academy of Pediatrics (1998).

69. American Academy of Pediatrics, Committee on Nutrition, *Pediatric Nutrition Handbook*, 4th ed., American Academy of Pediatrics (1998): 236; L. Larson, "Fail to Slow Low Iron Formula Sales," *AAP News* 11(3) (1995): 1, 14; American Academy of Pediatrics, Committee on Nutrition, *Pediatric Nutrition Handbook,* 5th ed., American Academy of Pediatrics (2004).

70. American Academy of Pediatrics, Committee on Nutrition, *Pediatric Nutrition Handbook*, 4th ed., American Academy of Pediatrics (1998): 36.

71. The American Academy of Pediatric Dentistry, Positions and Statements Guideline, "Interim guidance on fluoride intake for infants and young children" (8 November 2006).

72. The Environment California Research & Policy Center, "Toxic Baby Bottles," http://www.environmentcalifornia.org/reports/environmental-health/environmental-health-reports/toxic-baby-bottles (February 2007).

## Appendix A

1. M. Anim-Somuah, R. Smyth, C. Howell, "Epidural versus non-epidural or no analgesia in labour," Cochrane Database of Syst. Rev., CD000331 (2005); A. Hager, "Comparing Epidural and Parenteral Opioid Analgesia During Labor," *Journal of Family Practice* (2005); S.H. Halpern et al., "Effect of Epidural vs Parenteral Opioid Analgesia on the Progress of Labor: A Meta-analysis," *Journal of the American Medical Association* 280 (1998): 2105-10; B.L. Leighton and S.H. Halpern, "The effects of epidural analgesia on labor, maternal, and neonatal outcomes: a systematic review," *American Journal of Obstetrics and Gynecology*, 186(5) (2002): S31-68; E. Lieberman and C. O'Donoghue, "Unintended Effects of epidural analgesia during labor: a systematic review," *American Journal of Obstetrics and Gynecology*, 186(5) (2002): S31-68; E. Liu and A. Sia, "Rates of caesarean section and instrumental vaginal delivery in nulliparous women after low concentration epidural infusions or opioid analgesia: systematic review" *BMJ* 328: 1410 (2004); L.J. Mayberry, D. Clemmens, A. De, "Epidural analgesia side effects, co-interventions, and care of women during childbirth: a systematic review," *American Journal of Obstetrics and Gynecology* 186 (2002): S81-93.

2. Ibid.

3. Ibid.

4. Ibid.

5. Ibid.

# Glossary

The following are terms that are used to describe pregnancy, childbirth, and newborn care. For further discussion of these terms and their definitions, see the pages noted within the parentheses.

**4-1-1 or 5-1-1 rule**
This rule means that your labor contractions are intense enough to require you to focus and breathe rhythmically through them, and are *four or five* minutes apart with each lasting at least *one minute* for a period of *one hour*. This pattern signals to you that your labor may be progressing and it's time to call your caregiver or birthplace. (244)

**active labor**
The second phase of the first stage of labor. When your cervix is dilated to 4 to 5 centimeters, your contractions usually reach the 4-1-1 or 5-1-1 pattern. During this phase, dilation usually speeds up, contractions typically become painful (but manageable), and labor progresses with each contraction. (248)

**acupuncture**
An ancient Chinese medicine technique that uses needles placed at strategic points along meridians, or energy flow lines, in your body to guide it toward wellness and balance. (279)

**advanced practice nurse practitioner**
A maternity caregiver who provides prenatal and postpartum care, but doesn't attend women during labor. (17)

**afterpains**
As your uterus contracts after birth to its nonpregnant size (a process called involution), you may experience periods of discomfort or pain. Although this pain is common and isn't nearly as intense as labor contractions, you may need to use slow breathing to help manage it in the first few days. (269, 334)

**alveoli**
Glands in the breast that produce and store milk. (401)

**amniocentesis**
A medical procedure in which a needle is used to withdraw a small amount of amniotic fluid from your uterus. A laboratory analyzes the surfactant levels in the fluid to determine whether your baby's lungs are mature enough to function outside your womb. (292)

**amnioinfusion**
A procedure in which fluids are infused into your uterus to dilute any meconium that was expelled in the amniotic fluid , or to remove pressure on the cord caused by your baby's head or trunk. (288)

**amniotic fluid**
The fluid that surrounds your baby in the amniotic sac. It protects your baby by absorbing bumps from the outside, maintaining an even temperature, providing a medium for easy movement, and allowing your baby to develop her lungs by "breathing" the fluid. (39)

**amniotic sac**
Made up of the membranes (amnion and chorion) that create the sac that surrounds your baby. Also called "bag of waters." (39)

**amniotomy**
See *artificial rupture of membranes (AROM)*. (280)

**analgesia**
Any effect that reduces your perception of pain. In this book, this term is used to refer specifically to medications that act on the brain so you don't recognize pain stimuli or don't interpret them as pain. (193)

**androgens**
Male hormones that signal the development of a baby boy's scrotum and penis. (39)

**anemia**
A condition in which the number of red blood cells is lower than normal, reducing the blood's capacity to carry oxygen. (353)

**anesthesia**
Indicates a loss of sensation, including pain sensation. Anesthetic medications block nerve endings from sending pain impulses to your brain. (193)

**antibodies**
Proteins that protect your body from bacteria and toxins. During pregnancy and breastfeeding, your baby receives antibodies from you, which will protect him against diseases to which you're resistant or immune. (164)

**Apgar score**
Within one minute after your baby's birth and again at five minutes, your caregiver will evaluate your baby's well-being by conducting this routine newborn assessment, which assesses how well she's adapting to life outside your womb. (266)

**areola**
The darker skin surrounding each nipple. (36, 401)

**arrest of labor**
A condition in which labor stops progressing, as measured by cervical dilation. (276)

**artificial rupture of membranes (AROM)**
A procedure in which your caregiver breaks your bag of waters with an amnihook (a long plastic device that resembles a crochet needle) in the attempt to speed up the labor process. Also called *amniotomy*. (280)

**asymmetrical**
One side of your body is doing something different from the other side. For example, the lunge, side-lying, and semi-prone positions are asymmetrical positions. (230)

**asynclitic**
A position in which your baby's head is tilted and the top of it isn't centered on the cervix. Can lead to a prolonged labor. (286)

**augmentation**
Speeding up a slow labor by using self-help methods or interventions such as artificial rupture of membranes (AROM) or Pitocin. (281)

**auscultation**
Listening to sounds inside your womb, such as your baby's heartbeat. In labor, intermittent auscultation describes how your nurse or caregiver listens to your baby's heartbeat during and between contractions with a Doppler ultrasound stethoscope. At the same time, he or she may place a hand on your abdomen to feel your contractions, then count your baby's heartbeats, noting whether they speed up or slow down and recording the findings. (252)

**baby blues**
Emotional changes or mood swings that are common in new parents during the first few weeks after the birth of a baby. For example, going from elation to sadness in a matter of minutes isn't uncommon for new parents. (348)

**benefit-risk analysis**
A process by which your caregiver considers whether treatment will achieve the desired results or create problems, then weighs the treatment's benefits against its risks before forming his or her recommendation for treatment. (8)

**beta-endorphins**
Your body's natural painkillers, these hormones are secreted when you experience pain, stress, and physical exertion. Also called "endorphins." (242)

**birth ball**
A large inflatable plastic physical therapy or fitness ball that provides a soft yet firm place to sit comfortably. Used as a comfort tool in labor to enhance mobility and labor progress. (212)

**birth doula**
Someone (typically a woman) who's trained and experienced in supporting women and their partners during labor and birth. (23)

**birth plan**
A one- to two-page letter to your caregiver and staff that describes your fears and concerns as well as your wishes and priorities for the treatment of you and your baby. Also called a "birth preference list," "wish list," or "goal sheet." (148)

**blastocyst**
After conception, the fertilized egg quickly divides from one cell into two, then four, eight, sixteen, and so on until it becomes a multicellular structure called a blastocyst, which begins to implant in your uterus about five to nine days later. Once it's fully implanted, a blastocyst is called an *embryo*. (38)

**Body Mass Index (BMI)**
A measurement of the relative amounts of fat and muscle in your body. It's calculated by using a ratio of your height to your prepregnancy weight. (117)

**Braxton-Hicks contractions**
Contractions of the uterine muscle that become more frequent and intense in the third trimester, and that make your uterus hard for about a minute but aren't painful. Unlike labor contractions, Braxton-Hicks contractions don't cause changes in your cervix. (42)

**breech presentation**
When your baby is positioned with his buttocks, legs, or feet over your cervix, instead of head down (vertex). (295)

**castor oil**
A strong laxative that causes powerful bowel cramps and contractions, which may initiate uterine contractions to induce labor. (278)

**catecholamines**
Stress hormones, including epinephrine (adrenaline), norepinephrine, and dopamine. High levels of stress hormones can slow labor progress. (215, 242)

**cephalo-pelvic disproportion (CPD)**
A condition in which your baby's head is believed to be too large to fit through your pelvis. This diagnosis may be made by your caregiver based on observations during pregnancy, or may be used as a retrospective diagnosis after a prolonged labor that resulted in the birth of a large baby. (313)

**certified nurse-midwife (CNM)**
A maternity caregiver who has graduated from nursing school, passed an exam to become a registered nurse, and completed one or more years of additional training in midwifery. (16)

**certified professional midwife (CPM)**
A maternity caregiver who has received training from a variety of sources, including apprenticeship, school, and self-study, and has been the primary attendant at twenty or more births. A CPM practices outside hospitals and provides care similar to that of a licensed midwife. (17)

**cervical ripening balloon**
A silicone catheter that's placed within the cervix, then inflated with saline solution. Used to induce labor by accelerating cervical dilation. (279)

**cervix**
The lower part of the uterus, which protrudes into the vagina. (34)

**cesarean birth**
The experience of giving birth by a surgical procedure in which your baby is delivered through incisions in your abdomen and uterus. The procedure is also called a "cesarean section," "C-section," "cesarean delivery," or simply "cesarean." (306)

**circumcision**
The surgical removal of the foreskin covering the glans (tip) of the penis. (372)

**code word**
A word that you choose in advance and share with your caregivers. By saying the word during labor, you communicate that, despite your original plan to birth without pain medications, you now want help getting medicated pain relief. (189)

**colic**
Prolonged crying in a young baby. Typically defined as three or more crying episodes each week for three or more weeks, with each episode lasting three hours or longer. (379)

**colostrum**
The first breast milk: a highly nutritious yellowish fluid that's low in volume, but high in antibodies and the nutrients your baby will need for the first few days of life before your milk supply increases in volume. (43, 164, 401)

**combined spinal-epidural (CSE)**
A method for delivering pain medication. CSE uses a spinal narcotic in early labor (which may allow for more mobility), then an epidural anesthetic later in labor, when you need more pain relief. (197)

**complicated labor**
A labor that is longer, more painful, or more difficult than a normal labor, and may require medical help to ensure the well-being of you and your baby. (274)

**conception**
Occurs when a sperm fertilizes an egg. The beginning of pregnancy. (35)

**contraction**
Tightening of the uterine muscle. During labor, these muscle contractions help open your ripe, effaced cervix and help your baby descend. Contractions become more frequent and more intense as labor progresses. (241)

**corticosteroids**
Medications that may be given to speed up the maturation of your baby's lungs if a preterm birth can't be prevented. (292)

**corticotropin-releasing hormone (CRH)**
Comes from your baby, the placenta, and tissues within your uterus. Increased levels of CRH in late pregnancy may help initiate labor. (37)

**crowning**
The third phase of the second stage of labor. It begins when the widest part of your baby's head is visible at the vaginal opening and no longer retreats between pushes, and it ends with her birth. (263)

**delayed pushing**
An option for the second stage of labor, in which a woman who doesn't have an urge to push (such as after receiving an epidural) may wait an hour or two, or until her baby's head crowns, before pushing actively. Also called *passive descent*. (259)

**descent**
The downward movement of your baby into your pelvis. (168)

**diagnostic test**
Term used to describe a test that is more specific and more reliable than a screening test in identifying a woman with a pregnancy complication or a baby with a problem. (65)

**dilation**
The opening of the cervix, which allows your baby to pass through for birth. (169)

**directed pushing**
An option for the second stage of labor, in which your caregiver tells you how long and how hard to push. This method is used if you can't feel your contractions and delayed pushing isn't an option or if spontaneous pushing isn't effective. (259)

**Doppler ultrasound**
A device that uses sound waves to monitor your baby's heart rate. Typically used at prenatal visits as well as during labor and birth. (68)

**due date**
An estimate of when your baby will be born. The majority of babies are born in the period from two weeks before their due dates to two weeks after their due dates. (36)

**early labor**
Usually the longest phase of the first stage of labor, often because contractions are further apart, shorter, and less intense than they'll be later in labor. Contractions are generally more than five minutes apart, and you can walk and talk during them. Also called the *latent phase*. (242)

**ectopic**
An ectopic pregnancy occurs when the fertilized egg implants itself outside the uterus, usually in the wall of a fallopian tube (called a tubal pregnancy) but sometimes in the cervix, ovary, or abdomen. Most ectopic pregnancies can't develop into a live birth and typically require medical intervention to manage. (127)

**effacement**
The thinning and shortening of the cervix in preparation for birth. (169)

**elective induction**
An induction done without a medical reason, either because a woman requested induction or because her caregiver recommended it. Also called a "social induction." (276)

**electronic fetal monitoring (EFM)**
Used to monitor your baby's heart rate and your contractions, to assess how your baby is responding to labor. There are two types of EFM. External EFM uses belts to hold two sensors on your abdomen, and the less commonly used internal EFM uses two sensors placed inside your uterus. (252)

**embryo**
By two weeks after conception, your baby is called an embryo. (38)

**engagement**
About two weeks before the birth, your baby descends deeper into your pelvis. You may feel less pressure on your diaphragm and find breathing and eating easier. Also called *lightening* or "dropping." (46, 168)

**engorgement**
Painful swelling of the breasts. (405, 419)

**epidural catheter**
A tube inserted into the epidural space near the spinal nerves and used to deliver pain medication. (196)

**episiotomy**
A surgical incision of the perineum that enlarges the vaginal outlet. Once common practice, now the majority of caregivers use it only when medically necessary to deliver the baby quickly. (289)

**estrogen**
A hormone that promotes the growth of the uterine muscles and their blood supply, encourages production of vaginal mucus, and stimulates the development of the ductal system and blood supply in the breasts. In late pregnancy, rising estrogen levels increase the uterus's sensitivity to oxytocin and help start labor. (37, 170)

**evert**
To draw out your nipple to allow your baby to latch on well for nursing. Typically occurs when your baby suckles. (405)

**expression**
Removing milk from the breast by hand or by using a pump. May be used to relieve fullness, maintain milk supply, or store milk for your baby's consumption. (424)

**expulsion breathing**
A way to breathe during spontaneous bearing down. During the pushing stage, use relaxed breathing when you don't have the urge to push. When you have an urge to push, you may briefly hold your breath and bear down, or you may exhale with an open throat while pushing. (232)

**external version**
A procedure used to attempt to manually turn a baby from a breech or transverse position to a head-down position (vertex). (297)

**failure to progress**
Term used either to describe a labor that's taking longer than expected for the cervix to dilate to 10 centimeters, or to describe a pushing stage that's taking longer than expected. May be treated with augmentation or cesarean delivery; however, if your baby is handling labor well, you may also ask whether self-help measures can effectively help with labor progress. (312)

**fallopian tubes**
Provide the path for an egg to travel from your ovaries to your uterus. (34)

**false positives**
Describes situations in which test results for a condition are positive, but the condition isn't present (for example, the fetal heart rate pattern indicates distress, but your baby turns out to be fine). (314)

**family physician**
A physician who has graduated from medical school or a school of osteopathic medicine and has completed two or more years of additional training in family medicine, including maternity and pediatric care. (16)

**feeding cues**
How your baby shows he's hungry. Include rooting, mouthing, tongue thrusts, sucking, and increased activity levels. Crying is a late feeding cue, used when the other cues have gone unnoticed. (410)

**fetal intolerance of labor**
See *nonreassuring fetal heart rate*. Also called "fetal distress." (287, 313)

**first stage of labor**
The period that begins when contractions are becoming longer, stronger, and closer together (progressing) and ends when your cervix is completely dilated. (240)

**forceps**
A tool (steel tongs) that's used to assist with a vaginal birth. (290)

**foremilk**
Breast milk produced early in the feeding. Foremilk is lower in fat and higher in sugar than hindmilk. (403)

**fourth stage of labor**
Begins after the placenta is delivered and ends one to several hours later, when your and your baby's conditions have stabilized. (240)

**freestanding birth center**
A birth center unaffiliated with a hospital. (14)

**fundus**
The top of your uterus. (42)

**general anesthesia**
A systemic medication that causes a total loss of sensation and consciousness. (194)

**gestation**
Another term for pregnancy, which lasts an average of 280 days or forty weeks after the first day of your last menstrual period. (36)

**gestational age**
The age of your baby from the first day of your last menstrual period. Note that conception occurs within twelve to twenty-four hours after ovulation, which typically occurs fourteen days after the beginning of your last period. So, two weeks after conception your baby's gestational age is four weeks. (38)

**gestational hypertension**
High blood pressure that develops during pregnancy, defined as at least two consecutive readings that are over 140/90. This condition affects 10 percent of pregnant women in the United States. Also called *pregnancy-induced hypertension (PIH)*. (140)

**glycemic index**
An index that ranks foods according to how quickly and significantly they elevate your blood sugar. (115)

**Group B streptococcus (GBS)**
A type of bacteria. If you test positive for GBS in pregnancy, you may be given antibiotics during labor. (131)

**hemorrhoids**
Swollen varicose veins in the rectal area that may be as small as a pea or as large as a grape. (335)

**Heparin Lock**
Involves inserting an intravenous (IV) catheter, but doesn't require hooking it to an IV bag and pole until IV fluids are needed. Also called "Hep-Lock." (250)

**hindmilk**
Breast milk produced later in a feeding session, released with the let-down reflex. This milk provides most of the calories and contains more fat and protein than foremilk. (403)

**homeopathy**
A complementary medicine technique that uses diluted derivatives of natural substances to stimulate your body to respond in a way that heals or corrects a specific problem, such as a labor that won't start. (279)

**human chorionic gonadotropin (hCG)**
A hormone produced only during pregnancy. It ensures that your ovaries produce estrogen and progesterone for the first two to three months of your pregnancy, until your placenta matures and produces the appropriate amount. (37)

**hyperventilation**
Overbreathing. If you find yourself feeling lightheaded or dizzy while using a breathing technique, try either slowing down your breathing, focusing on the exhalation rather than the inhalation, or breathing into your cupped hands. (224)

**immunization**
See *vaccination*. (386)

**incompetent cervix**
A cervix that shortens and opens in midpregnancy without preterm labor contractions. (138)

**incontinence**
A condition that causes you to leak urine when you have a full bladder, exercise, cough, or sneeze (urinary incontinence) or uncontrollably pass gas or leak stool (fecal incontinence). (352–353)

**induction**
An intervention used to start labor. (275)

**infant cues**
Your baby's nonverbal communication. For example, when she's overstimulated, she may close his eyes, yawn, get glassy-eyed, turn away, or stiffen. If you miss these cues and continue to stimulate her, she may begin a prolonged bout of crying. (377)

**informed choice**
See *informed decision*. (8)

**informed consent**
After becoming informed about an option or treatment, you agree to it. (8)

**informed decision**
The decision you make to refuse or consent to a health care option or medical treatment, after becoming informed about it through research and consultation with your caregiver and other knowledgeable medical professionals, as well as with supportive friends and family. Also called *informed choice*. (8)

**informed refusal**
After becoming informed about an option or treatment, you refuse it. (8)

**inhalation medication**
A gas you breathe to receive pain medication. (192)

**intervention**
A medical procedure used to intervene in the natural labor process, such as induction, augmentation, episiotomy, or cesarean surgery. (274)

**intramuscular (IM) medication**
A shot given into a muscle to deliver medication. (192)

**intrathecal space**
The space inside the dura (the membrane that surrounds your spinal cord) that's filled with cerebrospinal fluid. It's where spinal medications are injected. (198)

**intravenous (IV) catheter**
A tube that's inserted into a vein through a needle, allowing fluids and medications to be given directly into your circulatory system. (250)

**intravenous (IV) medication**
An injection into a vein, often through an IV catheter, to deliver medication. (192)

**involution**
After the birth, your uterus begins the six-week process of contracting to its nonpregnant size. (269, 333)

**jaundice**
An excess of bilirubin that causes your baby's skin or the whites of his eyes to become yellow by the third or fourth day after the birth. (389)

**Kegel**
An exercise used to maintain the tone of your pelvic floor muscles, improve blood circulation in that area, decrease the incidence and severity of hemorrhoids and incontinence, and support your uterus and other pelvic organs. (95)

**lactation consultant**
A breastfeeding expert. (400)

**lanugo**
Fine, downy hair that develops on your baby's arms, legs, and back while in the womb. (42)

**latch**
Your baby's connection with the breast to feed. A good latch permits your baby to nurse effectively. (409)

**latent phase**
See *early labor*. (242)

**lay midwife**
A maternity caregiver who might or might not be legally registered with the state or province, and whose qualifications and standards of care might or might not meet state or provincial standards. Also called "empirical midwife." (17)

**Leopold's maneuvers**
The technique your caregiver uses to determine the baby's position by feeling your abdomen. (45)

**let-down reflex**
When your baby nurses, the suckling stimulates your pituitary gland to release oxytocin, which makes your milk-producing cells contract and release (let down) milk for your baby to drink. (402)

**leukorrhea**
A thin, liquid mucus discharge from the vagina. (173)

**licensed midwife (LM)**
A maternity caregiver who has completed up to three years of formal midwifery training according to state requirements. (17)

**lightening**
See *engagement*. (46, 168)

**local anesthetic**
Injection or application of pain medication that affects a specific, relatively small part of your body. (193)

**lochia**
The heavy red discharge that flows from your vagina in the six weeks after the birth. It's made of the extra blood and fluid that supported your pregnancy and the uterine lining that sustained your baby. (269, 334)

**malposition**
When your baby is in an unfavorable position in the womb, which may lead to a prolonged labor. Can often be corrected by changing positions frequently. (285)

**mastitis**
An infection of the breast. (424)

**meconium**
Your baby's first bowel movements, a collection of digestive enzymes and residue from swallowed amniotic fluid. Appears as a sticky, greenish-black substance. (42, 287, 369)

**membranes**
The amnion and chorion membranes create the amniotic sac that surrounds your baby in your uterus. (39)

**miscarriage**
The unexpected death and delivery of a baby before the twentieth week of pregnancy. Also called "spontaneous abortion." (127)

**misoprostol (Cytotec)**
A medication used to induce labor. (281)

**Montgomery glands**
Small bumps on your areolae that secrete a lubricating substance that keeps the nipple supple and prevents infection. (40, 401)

**morning sickness**
Nausea and vomiting in the early months of pregnancy. Despite its name, morning sickness can occur at any time of day. (40)

**moxibustion**
A version of acupuncture that doesn't use needles but instead uses burning herbs placed close to the acupuncture points. (279)

**mucous plug**
Mucus that fills the cervical opening during pregnancy to provide a barrier to help protect your baby. (39)

**multipara**
A woman who has given birth more than once. (167)

**multiples**
Two or more babies gestating in the same womb. (53)

**narcotics and narcotic-like drugs**
Medications that reduce the transmission of pain messages to the pain receptors in your brain. (194)

**naturopathic doctor (ND)**
A health care provider who has completed three to four years of postgraduate training in natural medicine. May also have taken an additional year of midwifery training to be able to provide prenatal care and attend births. (17)

**neonatal intensive care unit (NICU)**
A hospital unit where medically challenged newborns stay for monitoring and treatment until they can breathe on their own, stay warm at room temperature, and breastfeed or take a bottle. (293)

**neuraxial medications**
Drugs that are injected into the space surrounding the spinal cord (neuraxis), such as epidurals and spinal blocks. (192, 196)

**nipple confusion**
A condition experienced by some babies who have difficulty adapting to different sucking patterns and flows of liquid, when they're fed alternately by a bottle and at the breast. (412)

**nonreassuring fetal heart rate**
Term used when your baby's heart rate isn't responding to contractions in a reassuring way. Doesn't necessarily indicate that something is wrong with your baby (there's a high rate of "false positives"); however, it does indicate the need for closer monitoring and a possible need for intervention in labor. (287, 313)

**nullipara**
A woman who has never given birth. (167)

**obstetrician/gynecologist (OB-GYN)**
A physician who has graduated from medical school or a school of osteopathic medicine and has had three or more years of additional training in obstetrics and gynecology. (16)

**occiput anterior**
The back of baby's head (occiput) is toward the front of your body. (167)

**occiput posterior**
The back of baby's head (occiput) is toward your back. (167)

**oral medication**
A pill or liquid you swallow to receive a medication. (192)

**ovaries**
Female sex glands where eggs are produced. (34)

**ovulation**
When a ripened egg is released into your fallopian tubes. On average, this happens fourteen days after the first day of your last menstrual period. If you have intercourse between four days before and one day after ovulation, there's a chance of conception. (34)

**ovum**
An egg produced by a woman. When an egg is fertilized by a sperm, conception occurs. (34)

**oxytocin**
A hormone produced in your pituitary gland, which stimulates uterine contractions to help trigger the onset of labor and promote labor progress. Also present during orgasm and during breastfeeding, it's often called "the love hormone." (37, 170, 242)

**pain modifiers**
External stimuli that affect your awareness and perception of pain. (179)

**parity**
Describes the condition of having given birth. (167)

**passive descent**
See *delayed pushing*. (259)

**patient-controlled epidural analgesia (PCEA)**
A device that allows you to increase your epidural dosage when you need more pain relief. (198)

**pediatric and family nurse practitioner**
A registered nurse who has additional training in pediatrics or family health. Provides well-child care and treats common illnesses. (25)

**pediatrician**
A physician who specializes in children's health care. (24)

**pelvic floor muscles**
Muscles attached to the pelvis that support your abdominal and pelvic organs. These muscles form a figure-eight around your urethra, vagina, and anus. (34, 95)

**perinatologist**
An obstetrician/gynecologist (OB-GYN) who has received further training and certification in managing very high-risk pregnancies and births. (16)

**perineal massage**
A massage that stretches the inner tissue of your lower vagina. Can be used during pregnancy or the second stage of labor to relax the tissue so it will stretch around your baby's head. (235)

**perineum**
The external genitals (labia, urethra, clitoris, vaginal opening) and anus. (34)

**phototherapy**
A medical procedure used to treat jaundice that shines a special type of cool light on your baby's skin, causing the bilirubin level to drop. (389)

**Pitocin**
Commonly referred to as "Pit," this is a synthetic version of oxytocin. (281)

**placenta**
An organ that develops in pregnancy, the placenta produces hormones and exchanges oxygen, nutrients, and waste products for your developing baby. It's released and delivered shortly after your baby's birth. (39)

**position**
Refers to where the back of your baby's head (occiput) is in relation to your body. (167)

**positive signs of labor**
Include contractions that become longer, stronger, and more frequent (progressing) and the rupture of membranes in a gush of amniotic fluid. These are the only reliable signs that labor has begun and your cervix is dilating. (171)

**possible signs of labor**
Occur in late pregnancy and may indicate that the hormonal changes described on page 170 are underway but cervical changes aren't yet occurring. These signs occur intermittently for days or weeks, but they don't indicate labor. (171)

**post-date pregnancy**
A pregnancy that has lasted to at least forty-two weeks. Although the average length of pregnancy is forty weeks, many pregnancies last longer. Caregivers may misuse the term "post-date" as early as forty weeks. (49, 275)

**postmaturity**
A condition in which the placenta stops functioning well, the baby's growth slows or stops, and the risk of stillbirth increases. True postmaturity is rare even in babies born two weeks after their due dates. "Postmature babies" at birth have an absence of lanugo, scant vernix caseosa; long fingernails and toenails; and dry, peeling, or cracked skin. (49, 275)

**postpartum depression**
A condition that generally presents itself between two weeks to one year after the birth. Symptoms vary in severity among women. (357)

**postpartum doula**
Someone (typically a woman) who's trained and experienced with helping a woman and her family adjust to postpartum life by teaching them about newborns' needs and abilities, and about infant feeding, sleep, and cues, while providing assistance with household tasks. (26)

**postpartum hemorrhage**
The excessive loss of blood (more than 500 milliliters or 2 cups) during the first twenty-four hours after the birth. (299)

**postpartum mood disorders (PPMD)**
Emotional conditions that can develop in the first year after birth, such as anxiety and panic disorder, obsessive-compulsive disorder, postpartum depression, bipolar disorder, and post-traumatic stress disorder. (357)

**postpartum psychosis**
A rare condition that occurs in women after the birth and requires immediate care and psychiatric treatment. Symptoms include severe agitation, mood swings, depression, and delusions. (361)

**precipitate birth**
A birth that results from a very fast labor. For a first-time mother, may be defined as an entire labor that lasts six hours or less, but it's more often applied to a labor that is three hours or less. For a woman who has previously given birth, it's one hour or less. (257)

**preeclampsia**
High blood pressure and protein in the urine. A multi-organ condition with mild to severe symptoms that affects 5 to 8 percent of pregnancies. Previously called "toxemia." (140)

**pregnancy-induced hypertension (PIH)**
See *gestational hypertension*. (140)

**prelabor signs of labor**
Indicate that your cervix is probably moving forward, ripening, or effacing. These signs may progress into positive labor signs the same day they begin, or they may simply alert you that labor will begin in a few days or weeks. (171)

**prelabor**
A period of hours or days in which you experience contractions, but your cervix isn't actively dilating. It's likely that these contractions are getting your cervix ready to dilate by moving it forward and helping it ripen and efface. Prelabor contractions may range from as little as thirty seconds long and twenty minutes apart, to as much as one or two minutes long and five to eight minutes apart. However, the contractions change very little in length, frequency, and intensity over time (nonprogressing). (171)

**premature**
A baby that's born before the thirty-seventh week of pregnancy. (392)

**presentation**
Describes the part of your baby that's lying over your cervix and will emerge from your body first. Also called *presenting part*. (167)

**presenting part**
See *presentation*. (167)

**preterm labor**
A labor that begins before the thirty-seventh week of pregnancy. (136)

**primigravida**
A woman who is pregnant for the first time. (167)

**primipara**
A woman who has given birth once. (167)

**progesterone**
A hormone that relaxes your uterus during pregnancy, keeping it from contracting too much. It also relaxes the walls of blood vessels (helping you maintain a healthy blood pressure) and the walls of your stomach and bowels (allowing for greater absorption of nutrients). (37, 170)

**progressing contractions**
Contractions that become longer, stronger, and more frequent over time. (172)

**prolactin**
A hormone that's produced after the birth and stimulates the production of breast milk. (242, 401)

**prolapsed cord**
A rare condition that occurs when the water breaks and the umbilical cord slips below the baby so it's either in the vagina or lying between the baby and the cervix. Requires a call to 911 and transport to the hospital for an immediate cesarean. (302)

**prolonged labor**
A labor that progresses more slowly than expected. Diagnosis is somewhat subjective. (245)

**prolonged prelabor**
Prelabor that lasts longer than a day. (171)

**prostaglandin**
A hormone produced in your amniotic membrane. Increased levels in late pregnancy ripen your cervix in preparation for labor and stimulate muscles in your uterus and bowels to begin labor. (37, 170)

**quickening**
Describes the moment when you feel your baby's movements for the first time, during the second trimester. (42)

**regional anesthetic**
Pain medication that affects a large area of your body. (193)

**relaxin**
A hormone from your ovaries that relaxes and softens your ligaments, cartilage, and cervix, making these tissues more stretchable during pregnancy and letting your pelvic joints spread during birth. (37)

**respiratory distress syndrome (RDS)**
A condition in which a newborn infant has difficulty breathing and is unable to get sufficient oxygen due to immature lungs. The most common complication of premature birth, it requires immediate medical treatment. (292)

**rhythm**
Women who cope well in labor rely on rhythm in various forms. Rhythmic activity calms the mind and lets a woman work well with her body. (206)

**ripening**
The softening of the cervix. (169)

**ritual**
The repetition of a meaningful rhythmic activity during contractions to increase your ability to cope. (206)

**routine**
Procedures or treatment that's offered to all pregnant women and their newborns, regardless of medical status. (8)

**rupture of membranes**
Breaking of the bag of waters that may manifest itself either as the leaking of a small amount of amniotic fluid from the vagina, or as a gush of fluids. Rupture may happen before labor or may signal the onset of labor, or it can happen at any point during labor and birth. (172)

**screening test**
A medical test that can rule out a particular condition or may indicate an increased chance that the condition is present. In the latter case, a diagnostic test confirms the condition. (65)

**second stage of labor**
The birth of your baby. This stage begins when your cervix is fully dilated and ends when your baby is born. (240)

**serial induction**
Medication to induce labor is given during the day, but is discontinued at night to allow you to eat and sleep. (281)

**shared decision-making**
A collaborative approach to making an informed decision, in which you and your caregiver discuss the medical risks and benefits of treatment and any possible alternatives. (8)

**special care nursery**
A hospital unit for newborns who need extra medical monitoring or support, but don't need the intensive care of a NICU. (293)

**spinal block**
An injection of anesthetic near the spinal nerves that takes effect quickly and lasts for an hour or two. (196)

**spit up**
When a baby expels a dribble or more of milk (up to 2 to 3 tablespoons is common) after a feeding. (411)

**spontaneous bearing down**
An option for the second stage of labor, in which you naturally bear down or strain for five to six seconds at a time and take several breaths between efforts. This type of pushing makes more oxygen available to your baby than if you hold your breath and bear down for as long as possible. (259)

**spontaneous rituals**
Methods of coping invented by you over the course of your labor and reinforced by your support team. May include positions, movement, repeated words or sounds, specific kinds of touch, and so on. (207, 248)

**station**
Refers to the location of the top of your baby's head (or other presenting part) within your pelvis. Descent is measured by station. (168)

**sterile water block**
An alternative option for relief of back pain during labor. A caregiver or nurse injects tiny amounts of sterile water into four places on your lower back. The injections cause severe stinging for a minute or more, but then provide pain relief by rapidly increasing endorphin production. (286)

**sudden infant death syndrome (SIDS)**
The sudden death of a baby younger than one year that remains unexplained after a thorough investigation. There are steps that can be taken to further reduce the rare chance of SIDS; however, for about 1 in 2,000 babies, it appears to be impossible to predict or prevent. (391)

**supine hypotension**
When lying on your back makes your uterus press on the abdominal vein that carries blood from your legs to your heart (inferior vena cava), causing a drop in blood pressure. (89)

**surfactant**
A substance that allows your baby's lungs to expand during an inhalation and remain partially inflated during an exhalation. (293)

**synthetic prostaglandins**
Medications that mimic the hormone prostaglandin. (281)

**systemic**
Describes a medication that affects your entire body. (193)

**tandem nursing**
Breastfeeding two children at the same time (such as twins or your baby and toddler). (429)

**telemetry monitoring**
Wireless electronic fetal monitoring, which allows you to walk and use the shower or bath. (283)

**tension spots**
Body areas that you habitually tense when stressed. For example, your shoulders, forehead, mouth, jaw, or fists. (216, 243)

**third stage of labor**
Begins with the birth of your baby and ends with the delivery of the placenta. (240)

**Three Rs: relaxation, rhythm, and ritual**
A theory about how women cope with labor when given support and freedom to explore coping options. You stay as relaxed as possible throughout labor, until you discover your coping rhythm. Your partner's role is to reinforce this ritual for as long as it continues to help you. (206, 245)

**tocolytic medication**
A drug used to slow or stop contractions; for example, during preterm labor. (288)

**transition**
Final phase of the first stage of labor, which serves as the transition to the second stage of labor. Your cervix is reaching complete dilation, and your baby is beginning to descend into your birth canal. Contractions are ninety seconds to two minutes long and two to three minutes apart. (254)

**transverse incision**
The most common incision (cut) for a cesarean birth. Horizontal incision on the lower abdomen (at the "bikini line") through the bottom of the uterus. (316)

**transverse lie**
When your baby is positioned sideways in the uterus, with his back or shoulder closest to the cervix. Only occurs in 1 in 2,500 births. Your caregiver will attempt an external version to turn your baby, and if unsuccessful, your baby will be delivered by cesarean. (167, 295)

**triage**
Observation area in the hospital, where an admitting nurse assesses your condition, your pattern of contractions, your dilation (with a vaginal exam), and your baby's well-being, in order to determine whether you're ready to be admitted to the hospital, or whether you should return home with instructions on when to return. (249)

**trial of labor after cesarean (TOLAC)**
When a woman with a prior cesarean chooses to let labor begin and progress, with the hope of having a vaginal birth after cesarean (VBAC). (323)

**trimesters**
Pregnancy is divided into three trimesters, each one lasting about three months. (38)

**ultrasound**
See *Doppler ultrasound* and *ultrasound scan*. (68)

**ultrasound scan**
Equipment that uses intermittent transmission of sound waves to help your caregiver "see" inside the uterus. Can be used as a screening test or a diagnostic test for evaluating your baby's development. (68)

**umbilical cord**
Links the placenta to your baby's navel, and together the umbilical cord and placenta pass oxygen and nutrients from you to your baby. While the placenta provides a barrier against most (but not all) bacteria in your bloodstream, most viruses and drugs cross to your baby. The placenta also exchanges waste products from your baby, which your blood then carries to your kidneys and lungs for excretion. (39)

**urge to push**
The most significant sign of the second stage of labor. You may find yourself holding your breath and straining or grunting during each contraction. (258)

**uterine atony**
Poor uterine muscle tone. The most frequent cause of postpartum hemorrhage. (300)

**uterine rupture**
The separation of a uterine incision from a previous cesarean or uterine surgery. (323)

**uterus**
A hollow, muscular organ the size and shape of a pear in which a baby develops. (34)

**vaccination**
An administration of a vaccine to prevent illness. Also called *immunization*. (386)

**vacuum extractor**
A tool (silicone suction cup) that's used to assist with a vaginal delivery. (290)

**vaginal birth after cesarean (VBAC)**
A vaginal birth after a previous cesarean, as a result of a successful trial of labor after cesarean (TOLAC). (323)

**vernix caseosa**
A white, creamy substance that protected your baby's skin in your womb. (264, 366)

**vertex**
Presentation in which the top of your baby's head is down over your cervix. (167)

# Index

# Also from
# Meadowbrook Press

***100,000+ Baby Names*** is the #1 baby name book and is the most complete guide for helping you name your baby. It contains more than 100,000 popular and unusual names from around the world, complete with origins, meanings, variations, and famous namesakes. It also includes the most recently available top 100 names for girls and boys, as well as over 300 helpful lists of names to consider and avoid.

***The Official Lamaze® Guide: Giving Birth with Confidence*** Finally, a book that tells you what to expect, not what to fear, during pregnancy and birth! In it, leading childbirth educators Lothian and DeVries show pregnant women how to have confidence in their ability to give birth naturally. It provides expectant couples with detailed information on how to handle whatever issues arise.

***Baby Play & Learn*** Child-development expert Penny Warner offers 160 ideas for games and activities that provide hours of developmental learning opportunities. It includes bulleted lists of skills baby learns through play, step-by-step instructions for each game and activity, and illustrations that demonstrate how to play many of the games.

***Feed Me! I'm Yours*** is an easy-to-use, economical guide to making baby food at home. More than 200 recipes cover everything a parent needs to know about teething foods, nutritious snacks, and quick, pleasing lunches. Now recently revised.

***First-Year Baby Care*** is one of the leading baby-care books to guide you through your baby's first year. It contains complete information on the basics of baby care, including bathing, diapering, medical facts, and feeding your baby. Now recently revised.

***Baby & Child Emergency First Aid*** edited by Mitchell J. Einzig, MD. This user-friendly book is the next best thing to 911, with a quick-reference index, large illustrations, and easy-to-read instructions on handling the most common childhood emergencies.

**We offer many more titles written to delight, inform, and entertain.
To order books or browse our full selection of titles, visit our web site at:**
# www.meadowbrookpress.com
**For quantity discounts, please call: 1-800-338-2232**

Meadowbrook Press